Dr S.V. Smirnov
Department of Phar...
St Thomas's Hospi...
ext 156...

Pharmacology of Vascular Smooth Muscle

Pharmacology of Vascular Smooth Muscle

Edited by
C. J. Garland
Department of Pharmacology
University of Bristol

and

J. A. Angus
Department of Pharmacology
University of Melbourne
Victoria, Australia

Oxford   New York   Tokyo
OXFORD UNIVERSITY PRESS
1996

Oxford University Press, Walton Street, Oxford OX2 6DP
Oxford   New York
Athens   Auckland   Bangkok   Bombay
Calcutta   Cape Town   Dar es Salaam   Delhi
Florence   Hong Kong   Istanbul   Karachi
Kuala Lumpur   Madras   Madrid   Melbourne
Mexico City   Nairobi   Paris   Singapore
Taipei   Tokyo   Toronto
and associated companies in
Berlin   Ibadan

Oxford is a trade mark of Oxford University Press

Published in the United States
by Oxford University Press Inc., New York

© The editors and contributors, 1996

All rights reserved. No part of this publication may be
reproduced, stored in a retrieval system, or transmitted, in any
form or by any means, without the prior permission in writing of Oxford
University Press. Within the UK, exceptions are allowed in respect of any
fair dealing for the purpose of research or private study, or criticism or
review, as permitted under the Copyright, Designs and Patents Act, 1988, or
in the case of reprographic reproduction in accordance with the terms of
licences issued by the Copyright Licensing Agency. Enquiries concerning
reproduction outside those terms and in other countries should be sent to
the Rights Department, Oxford University Press, at the address above.

This book is sold subject to the condition that it shall not,
by way of trade or otherwise, be lent, re-sold, hired out, or otherwise
circulated without the publisher's prior consent in any form of binding
or cover other than that in which it is published and without a similar
condition including this condition being imposed
on the subsequent purchaser.

A catalogue record for this book is available from the British Library

Library of Congress Cataloging in Publication Data

The pharmacology of vascular smooth muscle/edited by C. J. Garland
and J. A. Angus. — 1st ed.
Includes bibliographical references.
1. Vascular smooth muscle — Effect of drugs on.   2. Cardiovascular
agents — Mechanism of action.   I. Garland, C. J.   II. Angus, J. A.
[DNLM: 1. Muscle, Smooth, Vascular — drug effects.   2. Endothelium,
Vascular — drug effects.   3. Vascular Diseases — drug therapy.   WE
500 P5365 1996]   RM345.P49 1996   615'.773 — dc20   DNLM/DLC
for Library of Congress   95-36657   CIP

ISBN 0 19 262387 7

Typeset by Colset Pte Ltd, Singapore

Printed in Great Britain by Bookcraft Ltd., Midsomer Norton, Avon

Preface

Pharmacology is an integrated science that draws on the knowledge and advances in physiology, biochemistry, anatomy, and chemistry. It is concerned with the actions of drugs on cells. In this book we are concerned specifically with the pharmacology of vascular smooth muscle cells; timely we believe, because of the revolution in our thinking of the way that the reactivity of smooth muscle cells in the blood vessel wall is modulated. This revolution started with Dr Robert Furchgott and his colleagues, when they showed that acetylcholine relaxed a segment of rabbit isolated aorta only if endothelial cells were present. This now classic organ bath observation has excited molecular biologists, neuroanatomists, and enzyme biochemists as they unravel the role of nitric oxide (NO) and nitric oxide synthase, touching every major area of biology including neurotransmission in the CNS and the enteric nervous system. The expansion of the knowledge base and the potential physiological and pathological roles for NO and control of NO synthase in the vasculature has been spectacular.

In defining the goal and structure of this book we have broadly covered four themes: (1) the **principles** and **techniques** of analytical pharmacology; isolated tissue techniques, single cell and electrophysiological techniques and *in vivo* techniques in animals and man specifically concerned with vascular pharmacology; (2) the **mechanisms of receptor–effector response** including receptor characterization, membrane ion channels, and second messengers, plus two chapters on neurotransmitter release and post-synaptic specialization, and the topical area of co-transmission and NANC transmission; (3) **specialized pharmacology** of selected **major vascular beds** including the general role of the endothelium and the cerebral, coronary, and renal vasculature; (4) **vascular pharmacology in disease**, including atherosclerosis, cerebral ischaemia, endotoxic shock, myocardial infarction, hypertension, and pulmonary hypertension. These latter chapters, in a sense, draw the book together and, in the context of the earlier chapters, highlight how information on vascular drug mechanisms gained from isolated cells, membranes, or tissue provide the foundation for the understanding of drug action in the clinical setting.

With constraints on space we have had to be selective in the topics presented. We trust that much of the material on techniques and the analytical approach to vascular pharmacology will remain relevant for some time to come. The book should appeal to pharmacologists and to physicians interested in learning more about the approach to mechanisms which underlie drug action in the vasculature and the methods employed to study them.

We thank the editorial staff at Oxford University Press especially Stuart McRobbie, and all the authors who have allowed the idea behind this book to become a reality. We hope you enjoy the intellectual stimulation that their work provides.

Bristol   C. J. G.
Melbourne   J. A. A.
May 1995

Contents

List of contributors   ix

1. Pharmacological principles for analysing responses of vascular smooth muscle   1
   Graeme R. Martin and Heather Giles

2. Isolated tissue techniques   25
   Michael J. Lew and Grant A. McPherson

3. Single cell techniques   42
   Alison M. Gurney

4. In vivo techniques and analysis   70
   J. A. Angus, C. E. Wright, K. Sudhir, and G. J. Jennings

5. Initiation of smooth muscle response   103
   A. M. Shaw and J. C. McGrath

6. Membrane ion channels in vascular smooth muscle excitation–contraction coupling   136
   Philip I. Aaronson and Sergey V. Smirnov

7. Cell signalling pathways involved in the regulation of vascular smooth muscle contraction and relaxation   160
   Kevin Malarkey, Dorothy Aidulis, Christopher M. Belham, Anne Graham, Angela McLees, Andrew Paul, and Robin Plevin

8. Neuroeffector transmission in arteries, arterioles, and veins   184
   Susan E. Luff, G. D. S. Hirst, and T. C. Cunnane

9. Cotransmission   210
   G. Burnstock and V. Ralevic

10. Endothelium-dependent vasodilator mechanisms   233
    T. M. Cocks

11. Pharmacology of the cerebral circulation   252
    P. A. T. Kelly and C. J. Garland

12. **Pharmacology of human isolated large and small coronary arteries** — 276
    J. A. Angus and T. M. Cocks

13. **Pharmacology of the renal circulation** — 306
    David P. Brooks and Richard M. Edwards

14. **Atherosclerosis** — 328
    Xiao-Jun Du and Anthony M. Dart

15. **Vessel wall injury and growth: pharmacological considerations in atherosclerosis and collateral artery function** — 341
    Norman K. Hollenberg

16. **The cerebral microvascular endothelium in ischaemia** — 357
    A. Lorris Betz and Fausto Iannotti

17. **Regulation of vascular smooth muscle tone in sepsis** — 369
    Richard G. Bogle and Patrick Vallance

18. **Hypertension** — 387
    Jaye P. F. Chin and Anthony M. Dart

19. **Pulmonary hypertension** — 402
    George Cremona and Tim Higenbottam

Index — 431

Contributors

Philip I. Aaronson
Department of Pharmacology, St Thomas's Hospital Medical School, Lambeth Palace Road, London SE1 7EH, UK.

Dorothy Aidulis
Department of Physiology and Pharmacology, University of Strathclyde, 204 George Street, Glasgow G1 1XW, UK.

J. A. Angus
Department of Pharmacology, University of Melbourne, Parkville, Victoria 3052, Australia.

Christopher M. Belham
Department of Physiology and Pharmacology, University of Strathclyde, 204 George Street, Glasgow G1 1XW, UK.

A. Lorris Betz
Crosby Neurosurgical Laboratories, The University of Michigan, Ann Arbor, MI 48109-0532, USA,

Richard G. Bogle
Department of Clinical Pharmacology, St George's Hospital Medical School, London SW17 ORE, UK.

David P. Brooks
Department of Renal Pharmacology, SmithKline Beecham, PO Box 1539, King of Prussia, PA 19406, USA.

G. Burnstock
Department of Anatomy and Developmental Biology, University College London, Gower Street, London WC1E 6BT, UK.

Jaye P. F. Chin
Baker Medical Research Institute, PO Box 348, Prahran, Victoria 3181, Australia.

T. M. Cocks
Department of Pharmacology, University of Melbourne, Parkville, Victoria 3052, Australia.

Contributors

George Cremona
Regional Pulmonary Physiology Laboratory, Papworth Hospital, Papworth Everard, Cambridge CB3 8RE, UK.

T. C. Cunnane
Department of Pharmacology, University of Oxford, Mansfield Road, Oxford OX1 3QT, UK.

Anthony M. Dart
Baker Medical Research Institute, PO Box 348, Prahran, Victoria 3181, Australia.

Xiao-Jun Du
Baker Medical Research Institute, PO Box 348, Prahran, Victoria 3181, Australia.

Richard M. Edwards
Department of Renal Pharmacology, SmithKline Beecham, PO Box 1539, King of Prussia, PA 19406, USA.

C. J. Garland
Department of Pharmacology, University of Bristol, School of Medical Sciences, University Walk, Bristol BS8 ITD, UK.

Heather Giles
Receptor Pharmacology Group, Glaxo-Wellcome, Gunnels Wood Rd. Stevenage, Herts, SG1 2NY.

Anne Graham
Department of Physiology and Pharmacology, University of Strathclyde, 204 George Street, Glasgow G1 1XW, UK.

Alison M. Gurney
Department of Physiology and Pharmacology, University of Strathclyde, 204 George Street, Glasgow G1 1XW, UK.

Tim Higenbottam
Regional Pulmonary Physiology Laboratory, Papworth Hospital, Papworth Everard, Cambridge CB3 8RE, UK.

G. D. S. Hirst
Department of Zoology, University of Melbourne, Victoria 3052, Australia.

Norman K. Hollenberg
Brigham & Women's Hospital, 75 Francis St, Boston, MA 02115, USA.

Contributors

Fausto Iannotti
Clinical Neurological Sciences, Wessex Neurological Centre, Southampton General Hospital, Tremona Road, Southampton, UK.

G. J. Jennings
Baker Medical Research Institute, PO Box 348, Prahran, Victoria 3181, Australia.

P. A. T. Kelly
Department of Clinical Neurosciences, University of Edinburgh, Western General Hospital, Crewe Road, Edinburgh EH4 2XU, UK.

Michael J. Lew
Department of Pharmacology, University of Melbourne, Parkville, Victoria 3052, Australia.

Susan E. Luff
Baker Medical Research Institute, PO Box 348, Prahran, Victoria 3181, Australia.

J. C. McGrath
Institute of Physiology, University of Glasgow, Glasgow G12 8QQ, UK.

Angela McLees
Department of Physiology and Pharmacology, University of Strathclyde, 204 George Street, Glasgow G1 1XW, UK.

Grant A. McPherson
Department of Pharmacology, Monash University, Clayton, Victoria 3168, Australia.

Kevin Malarkey
Department of Physiology and Pharmacology, University of Strathclyde, 204 George Street, Glasgow G1 1XW, UK

Graeme R. Martin
Receptor Pharmacology Group, Biology Division, The Wellcome Research Laboratories, Langley Court, Beckenham, Kent BR3 3BS, UK.

Andrew Paul
Department of Physiology and Pharmacology, University of Strathclyde, 204 George Street, Glasgow G1 1XW, UK.

Robin Plevin
Department of Physiology and Pharmacology, University of Strathclyde, 204 George Street, Glasgow G1 1XW, UK.

Contributors

V. Ralevic
Department of Anatomy and Developmental Biology, University College London, Gower Street, London WC1E 6BT, UK.

A. M. Shaw
Department of Biological Sciences, Glasgow Caledonian University, Cowcaddens Road, Glasgow G4 0BA, UK.

Sergey V. Smirnov
Department of Pharmacology, St Thomas's Hospital Medical School, Lambeth Palace Road, London SE1 7EH, UK.

K. Sudhir
Baker Medical Research Institute, PO Box 348, Prahran, Victoria 3181, Australia.

Patrick Vallance
Department of Clinical Pharmacology, St George's Hospital Medical School, London SW17 0RE, UK.

C. E. Wright
Department of Pharmacology, University of Melbourne, Parkville, Victoria 3052, Australia.

1. Pharmacological principles for analysing responses of vascular smooth muscle

Graeme R. Martin and Heather Giles

INTRODUCTION

Numerous methods exist which enable the vascular effects of drugs to be studied *in vivo* as well as *in vitro*. However, the quantitative study of drug-receptor interactions in blood vessels requires precise control over the experimental conditions and this is best achieved using isolated, intact vascular tissues physiologically maintained in an organ-bath. Fortunately, carefully prepared blood vessel segments retain much of their functional integrity making it possible to assess, in a meaningful way, the effects of vasoactive drugs in the target tissue. This chapter outlines the pharmacological principles underlying the quantitative study of agonist and antagonist drug effects on vascular smooth muscle and looks at specific practical conditions which must be observed to ensure that the information obtained is robust and reliable.

DRUG-RECEPTOR THEORY

Principles of agonist- and antagonist-receptor interactions

In terms of traditional occupancy theory, the ability of an agonist drug to elicit an effect in a tissue or cell involves two distinct steps; *binding* to a cell surface receptor followed by *transduction*, the process by which receptor occupancy is translated into a cellular response through propagation of an intracellular biochemical cascade.

Drugs which bind to the receptor, but are incapable of initiating the transduction step, are antagonists. It is now widely accepted that the binding of agonist and antagonist drugs to receptors is a saturable phenomenon which follows the Law of Mass Action (Clark 1937):

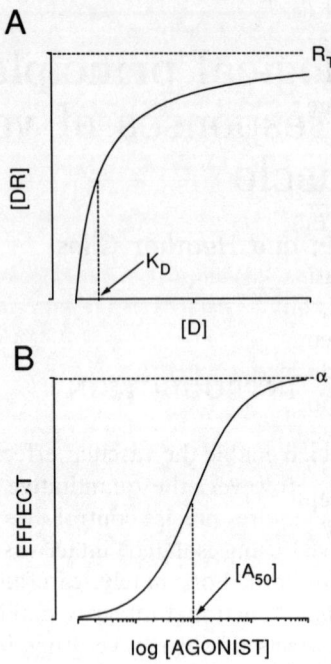

Fig. 1.1 (A) The $[DR]/[D]$ relation. Assuming a simple bimolecular interaction between drug and receptor, the relation is rectangular hyperbolic with a midpoint defined by K_D and an asymptote defined by R_T. (B) The $E/[A]$ relation. In linear space concentration–effect curves also generally conform to a hyperbola but, as here, are typically converted to a logistic form by plotting in semi-logarithmic space. $[A_{50}]$ defines the agonist curve midpoint and α the upper asymptote.

$$\frac{[DR]}{[R_T]} = \frac{[D]}{K_D + [D]} \tag{1.1}$$

$[D]$ = concentration of drug available for binding
$[DR]$ = concentration of receptors occupied by D
$[R_T]$ = total concentration of receptors
K_D = equilibrium dissociation constant for DR.

Fig. 1.1A plots eqn (1.1) and illustrates that the concentration of drug-occupied receptors, $[DR]$, is a rectangular hyperbolic function of drug concentration, $[D]$, with the asymptote defined by $[R_T]$ and the midpoint corresponding to K_D, i.e. the value of $[D]$ producing 50% occupancy of the receptors. Two important assumptions are made:

- $[D] \gg [R]$ i.e. binding to the receptors does not significantly diminish $[D]$
- equilibrium conditions pertain

In general, agonist–effect ($E/[A]$) curves plotted in arithmetic space also conform to a hyperbola, but are typically presented in logistic (sigmoid) form by plotting in semi-logarithmic space (Fig. 1.1B). This observation lead to the early belief (Clark 1937) that tissue response must be a simple, linear function of receptor occupancy such that:

$$\frac{E}{E_M} = \frac{[AR]}{[R_T]} = \frac{[A]}{K_A + [A]} \qquad (1.2)$$

where $[A]$, the concentration of agonist, simply takes the place of $[D]$ in eqn (1.1), E denotes effect, and E_M is the maximum possible effect achievable through that receptor system.

This simple relation predicts that when $[A] \gg K_A$, E/E_M approaches unity, implying that all agonists should be capable of eliciting the same maximum effect (i.e. E_M) through a given receptor system. The realization that this is not always the case prompted Ariëns (1954) to propose that agonist response must therefore be related to fractional receptor occupancy by a proportionality constant which he termed **intrinsic activity** (α):

$$\frac{E}{E_M} = \alpha \frac{[AR]}{[R_T]} = \frac{\alpha[A]}{K_A + [A]}. \qquad (1.3)$$

By definition, when $\alpha = 1$ the agonist can elicit the maximum possible effect and is a **full agonist**; when $\alpha < 1$ the agonist elicits less than the maximum possible effect and behaves as a **partial agonist**. When $\alpha = 0$ the drug is an **antagonist**.

This concept of intrinsic activity accounts for the ability of different agonists to achieve different maximum effects in a tissue, but it also implies that the maximum response to an agonist requires all available receptors to be occupied and that the concentration of agonist required to produce a half of its own maximum effect ($[A_{50}]$) will always equal the K_A. However, in many tissues inactivation of a fraction of the receptor population (e.g. by use of an irreversible receptor antagonist) simply decreases agonist potency without reducing the maximum effect (Furchgott 1954; Nickerson 1956). In these cases it is clear that only a small proportion of the receptors need to be activated to elicit a maximum response, consequently $[A_{50}]$ can be a much smaller value than K_A (see Fig. 1.2). Tissues in which this situation pertains are said to contain 'spare' receptors, more often referred to as a **receptor reserve**.

To accommodate this feature of agonist behaviour, Stephenson (1956) introduced the concept of stimulus (S) which he related to fractional receptor occupancy by the proportionality constant, e, (**efficacy**). The resulting tissue response was assumed to be related to S by some undefined, saturable function, f, such that:

$$S = e\frac{[A]}{K_A + [A]} \quad \text{and hence:} \quad \frac{E}{E_M} = f(S) = f\left(e\frac{[AR]}{[R_T]}\right). \qquad (1.4)$$

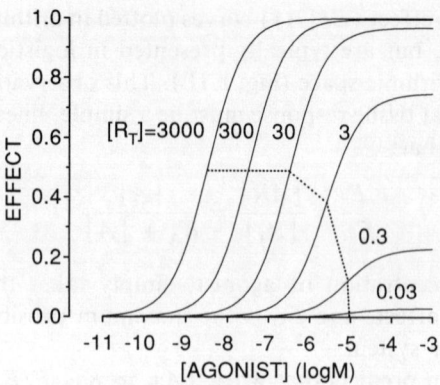

Fig. 1.2 Computer simulations illustrating the effect of changing tissue receptor density ($[R_T]$) on the shape and location of agonist $E/[A]$ curves. The lines depicting the $E/[A]$ curves at each value of $[R_T]$ were obtained using eqn (1.8) in which E_M, n, and K_E were set at unity, K_A was set at 10^{-5} M. The dotted line connects $E/[A]$ curve $[A_{50}]$ values and shows that as $[R_T]$ is progressively reduced, $[A_{50}]$ approaches and eventually coincides with K_A.

It is clear from this that equivalent responses can be elicited by two agonists which exhibit different fractional receptor occupancies provided they produce equal stimuli. Recognizing that both tissue and drug factors contribute to Stephenson's definition of efficacy, Furchgott (1966) later separated e into **intrinsic efficacy** (ϵ), the specific and *constant* property of the drug, and **receptor concentration** $[R_T]$, the specific, but *variable* property of the tissue (i.e. $e = \epsilon[R_T]$). Therefore:

$$\frac{E}{E_M} = f(S) = f\left(\epsilon[R_T]\frac{[AR]}{[R_T]}\right). \tag{1.5}$$

Expressed in this way, it is evident that the response of a given tissue to an agonist drug is dependent upon two drug factors, ϵ and K_A, and two tissue factors, f and R_T. The importance of the former two parameters to drug–receptor classification is obvious, because, in theory, they are unique for a particular agonist–receptor pair and are independent of species, the tissue type under study, and the response being measured.

Although the nature of the function f linking stimulus to effect was not originally described explicitly there is a wealth of evidence to suggest that it is hyperbolic in form (e.g. Kenakin and Beek 1980):

$$\frac{E}{E_M} = \frac{S}{\beta + S} \tag{1.6}$$

where β describes the efficiency with which a given tissue translates stimulus into effect. Substituting for S as defined in eqn (1.5) yields:

$$\frac{E}{E_M} = \frac{[AR]}{(\beta/\epsilon) + [AR]}.\qquad(1.7)$$

Here, β/ϵ defines the midpoint of the $E/[AR]$ relation and therefore determines the sensitivity with which receptor occupancy is translated into effect. This equation is essentially the same as the 'operational model of agonism' deduced by Black and Leff (1983) where β/ϵ is replaced by a single constant K_E, which is clearly agonist and tissue-dependent. Making this substitution and defining $[AR]$ in terms of $[A]$ (see eqn 1.1) yields the familiar form of the operational model:

$$\frac{E}{E_M} = \frac{\tau^n [A]^n}{(K_A + [A])^n + \tau^n [A]^n}\qquad(1.8)$$

where $\tau = [R_T]/K_E$. Tau (τ) provides an overall definition of efficacy and n, the slope parameter of the $E/[AR]$ relation, is introduced to account for $E/[A]$ curves that are steeper or flatter than a rectangular hyperbola (when $n = 1$). All the parameters in the expression can be estimated experimentally therefore the operational model provides an explicit, theoretical framework for analysing and quantifying agonist–receptor interactions.

Analysis of agonist effects: estimation of potency and maximum effect

$E/[A]$ curves plotted in semi-logarithmic space are generally symmetrical and conform to a sigmoid (see Fig. 1.1B). They can therefore be described by a logistic equation, which normally takes the following form:

$$E = \frac{\alpha [A]^m}{[A]^m + [A_{50}]^m}.\qquad(1.9)$$

Here, agonist *potency* is defined by $[A_{50}]$, the value of $[A]$ required to produce 50% of α, the *maximum effect* achieved by A. The slope parameter m is related to the slope at the midpoint of the $E/\log[A]$ curve. The maximum possible effect that can be produced through a particular receptor system is defined as E_M. When expressed as a fraction of E_M (defined by the effect of a full agonist), α is equivalent to Ariëns' intrinsic activity. However, it should be recognized that the value of α/E_M for a given agonist will be tissue-dependent, since its value will depend upon the receptor density and the efficiency of receptor–effector coupling. This is illustrated in Fig. 1.3A which shows that in ring preparations of rabbit jugular vein, the selective prostaglandin DP receptor agonist 572C85 can behave as a full agonist, i.e. $\alpha/E_M \simeq 1$ in some vessel segments, yet is unable to elicit any measurable effect ($\alpha/E_M \simeq 0$) in others (although it still binds to the receptor and would behave as a competitive antagonist: Giles unpublished). Between these extremes intermediate values of α/E_M are obtained and the compound behaves as a partial agonist. This presumably reflects vessel segment differences in DP receptor density and/or efficiency of occupancy–effect coupling.

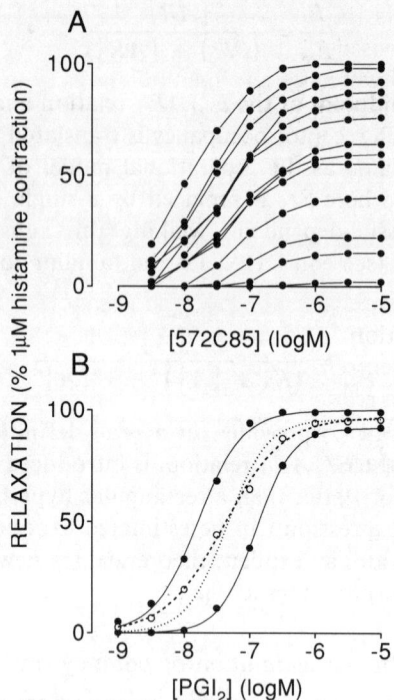

Fig. 1.3 Between-preparation variation in efficacy. (A) $E/[A]$ curves to the prostaglandin DP receptor agonist 572C85 obtained in ring preparations of rabbit jugular vein. In some vessel segments 572C85 behaves as a full agonist, in others it is a partial agonist, and in yet others it fails to elicit a response, presumably because of tissue–tissue variability in DP receptor density and/or coupling efficiency. (B) $E/[A]$ curves to PGI_2 (●) obtained in two different rings of rabbit jugular vein. The solid lines were produced by fitting eqn (1.9) to each data set; average parameter estimates for the two curves were then used to produce the dotted line which depicts the correct shape and location of the mean data set. The dashed line was produced by fitting eqn (1.9) to the mean data for the two curves (○). The slope of this line is clearly flatter than either individual curve.

On an important practical point, when replicate $E/[A]$ curve data are fitted to eqn (1.9) to provide estimates of $[A_{50}]$, α, and m, it is important to fit each $E/[A]$ curve separately and then average the resulting parameter estimates. If the mean data are fitted to a single logistic function, underestimation of the slope parameter may result, especially if there is a large between-tissue variation in potency (Fig. 1.3B).

Analysis of agonist effects: estimation of affinity and efficacy

Graphical methods Analysis of agonist $E/[A]$ curves in the manner described above provides valuable information about the agonist and tissue in question, but $[A_{50}]$ estimates provide little information about agonist affinity or efficacy because **potency** reflects the combined effect of these two properties. Various methods have been devised to estimate K_A and efficacy for full agonists (see Kenakin 1984), most of which involve manipulations to make the agonist behave as a partial agonist. When the agonist already behaves as a partial agonist, the parameters can also be estimated by comparison with a full agonist using either 'comparative' (Barlow et al. 1967) or 'interactive' (Stephenson 1956) methods. In each case, the purpose is to enable equi-effective concentrations of agonist(s) to be compared before and after a manipulation that simply changes agonist efficacy.

The simplest and most reliable approach is Furchgott's (1966) method of receptor fractional inactivation. The use of an irreversible receptor antagonist to reduce the functional receptor concentration results in right-shift of the agonist curve and, eventually, a reduction in the maximum response (see Fig. 1.2). Equi-effective concentrations of agonist before ($[A]$) and after ($[A']$) this treatment can then be compared according to the following relation:

$$\frac{1}{[A]} = \frac{1}{[A']} \cdot \frac{1}{q} + \frac{1}{[K_A]} \cdot \frac{1-q}{q} \qquad (1.10)$$

where q is the fraction of functional receptors remaining after receptor inactivation. A plot of $1[A]$ against $1[A']$ yields a straight line from which $K_A =$ (slope $-$ 1)/intercept.

An estimate of agonist efficacy (e or $\epsilon . R_T$) can also be obtained using this method, but because this parameter is tissue- as well as ligand-dependent, it is not particularly useful for receptor classification purposes. However, the ligand-dependent property of agonism, *intrinsic efficacy* (ϵ), can be measured relative to a standard agonist in the same tissue because under these circumstances the tissue-dependent factors are the same for each agonist. For this procedure K_A estimates for each agonist must be available. In the case of two agonists, A_1 and A_2, $E/[A]$ curves to both agonists are generated, ideally in the same tissue. The respective fractional receptor occupancies ($[AR]/[R_T]$) required to give equal responses can then be calculated using eqn (1.2). Since equal responses are produced by equal stimuli, then $S_{A1} = S_{A2}$. Given that $S = \epsilon . R_T . \rho$ (eqn 1.5, where $\rho =$ fractional receptor occupancy), then at equal effect $\epsilon_{A1} . R_T . \rho_{A1} = \epsilon_{A2} . R_T . \rho_{A2}$ from which $\rho_{A1}/\rho_{A2} = \epsilon_{A2}/\epsilon_{A1}$. A plot of response against log ρ for each agonist enables relative efficacy to be measured from the horizontal displacement of the curves (Furchgott and Bursztyn 1967).

Direct model-fitting methods Fitting the 'operational model of agonism' (eqn 1.8) directly to agonist response curve data provides a powerful alternative approach to the aforementioned graphical methods for agonist affinity and efficacy estimation (Black and Leff 1983; Leff 1987; Leff et al. 1990). To date model-fitting has been shown to yield results comparable to those obtained using null methods in a variety of experimental situations. In principle, model-fitting also offers several advantages; first all of the agonist curve data are used (not just that on the linear portion of the curve), enabling quantitative analysis of agonists with low intrinsic activity. Secondly, only experimentally determined data are used (not interpolated data points). Thirdly, untransformed experimental data are analysed, avoiding problems associated with the double-reciprocal ($1/[A]$ versus $1/[A']$) plot — a linear transformation of the data which heavily weights the most unreliable data at the start of an $E/[A]$ curve. Finally, the procedure is much less laborious than traditional methods since the affinity and efficacy for several agonists can be estimated simultaneously.

Analysis of antagonist effects: estimation of antagonist affinity

Graphical methods The pA scale, introduced by Schild in 1949, was the first independent scale for antagonist potency estimation, from which the most widely used parameter has been pA_2, the negative logarithm of the concentration of antagonist ($[B]$) required to produce a twofold shift to the right of the control $E/[A]$ curve. However, pA_2 is an empirical measure of antagonist potency which provides no information on the nature of the antagonism. This limits its use in receptor classification studies. By contrast, an estimate of K_B, the antagonist–receptor dissociation equilibrium constant, can be made for antagonists which compete with agonist for unoccupied receptors in a simple, reversible manner. In this case, agonist occupancy of the receptor is modified by the factor $1 + [B]^n/K_B$ (Gaddum 1937), where n is generally taken to be unity, based on the reasonable assumption that the antagonist–receptor interaction is a simple bimolecular one. Hence:

$$\frac{[AR]}{[R_T]} = \frac{[A]}{[A] + K_A\left(1 + \frac{[B]^n}{K_B}\right)} . \qquad (1.11)$$

Clearly, in the presence of antagonist, the concentration of agonist has to be raised in order to achieve the same fractional receptor occupancy and this manifests as a parallel rightward displacement of the agonist $E/[A]$ curve with no change in its asymptote (see Fig. 1.6A). Arunlakshana and Schild (1959) subsequently showed that the relation between the magnitude of agonist curve rightshift and antagonist concentration could be described by:

$$\log(r - 1) = n \cdot \log[B] + pK_B \qquad (1.12)$$

where r (concentration ratio) $= [A']/[A] =$ the concentration of agonist required to elicit an equal effect in the presence ($[A']$) and absence ($[A]$) of the antagonist and pK_B is the negative logarithm of K_B. This equation describes a linear relation between $\log(r - 1)$ and $\log[B]$ so that graphical presentation as a Schild plot yields a straight line with a slope of unity (i.e. $n = 1$) and an intercept on the abscissa of pK_B. Since the zero value on the ordinate is obtained when $r = 2$, the pK_B corresponds to pA_2. It bears emphasis that when the Schild plot slope is *not* unity, but is insignificantly different from this value, the slope of the Schild regression should be constrained to unity in order to provide an estimate of pK_B. When this is constraint is not applied, or the slope is significantly different from one, the value of the intercept still provides an estimate of pA_2, but it is no longer valid to estimate pK_B.

Direct model-fitting methods Estimates of K_B can be obtained by fitting a rearranged form of eqn (1.15) directly to agonist $[A_{50}]$ values obtained in the absence ($[A_{50}]^C$) or presence ($[A_{50}]^T$) of a competitive antagonist:

$$\log[A_{50}]^T = \log[A_{50}]^C + \log(1 + [B^n]/K_B). \qquad (1.13)$$

In circumstances where only a single $E/[A]$ curve can be obtained in each tissue preparation so that several dose-ratios must be calculated by reference to one control $E/[A]$ curve, this method avoids overweighting the control curve $[A_{50}]$ value.

EXPERIMENTAL CONSIDERATIONS

It should be clear from the foregoing that reliable estimates of affinity and efficacy can be obtained provided the effects of the drugs are reproducible and measured under equilibrium conditions. Factors which need to be considered include the method of tissue preparation as well as the experimental design and conditions used (see Furchgott 1968; Kenakin 1984). This section deals with experimental considerations that are especially pertinent to the study of isolated blood vessels.

Tissue preparation

Blood vessel geometry

Experiments with isolated blood vessels are most often performed using transverse ring segments or helical strips. Since the smooth muscle layers of a vessel are in different orientations, the angle at which helical strips are cut can have a profound influence on the magnitude of the tissue response to agonists. The importance of the angle of cut is illustrated in Fig. 1.4 which shows that, at an extreme, paradoxical relaxation can be obtained in a vessel expected to develop contraction. This emphasizes the impact that the method of tissue preparation can have on the precision of experimental data.

The endothelium

The endothelium profoundly influences both the resting tonic state and pharmacological reactivity of blood vessels, so much so that the passive or stimulated release of nitric oxide, cyclo-oxygenase products, or autacoids previously sequestered from the circulation can obscure the true behaviour of drugs acting at vascular smooth muscle receptors. For example, low efficacy partial agonists may elicit little or not detectable response in vessels with an intact endothelium,

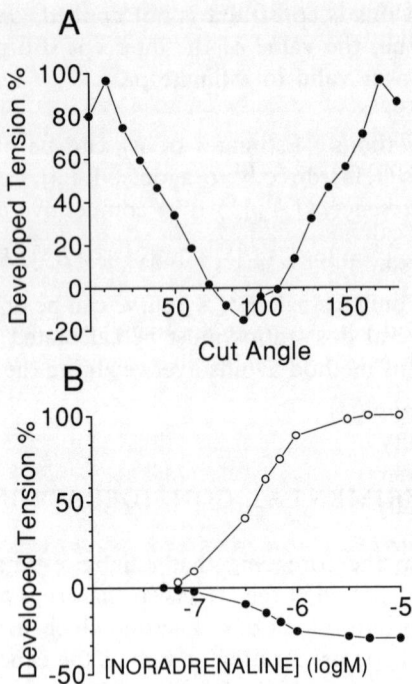

Fig. 1.4 (A) Influence of the angle of cut on contractile responses of dog femoral artery to noradrenaline (100 μM, in the presence of β-adrenoceptor blockade). (B) Concentration–effect curves to noradrenaline obtained in either circumferential (open circles) or longitudinal strips (closed circles). Adapted from Ohashi and Azuma (1980), with permission.

but produce an effect in endothelium-denuded tissues (Martin *et al.* 1986). The potential for confounding receptor classification when rank orders of potency include partial agonists is obvious. It is therefore in the interests of consistency and quantitative rigour to either retain or remove the endothelium at the outset of an experiment. In cases where an intact endothelium is required, criteria that define its functional integrity need to be established.

Practical conditions

The viability of blood vessels *in vitro* is dependent upon the provision and maintenance of a stable 'physiological' environment. In addition to elementary requirements concerning pH, temperature, and oxygen tension, the following need specific consideration.

Drug disposition mechanisms

A primary assumption of receptor theory is that the concentration of drug added to an organ-bath is the concentration of drug available for receptor interaction. A number of drug- and tissue-related properties need to be controlled to ensure this assumption remains valid.

Drug related   Some drugs, e.g. catecholamines and indolalkylamines, undergo spontaneous degradation in the organ-bath. Oxidation promoted by divalent cations can be slowed or prevented by inclusion of cation chelators (e.g. disodium EDTA) or anti-oxidants (e.g. ascorbic acid). Other drugs such as lysergic acid diethyl amide and the calcium channel blocker nifedipine are susceptible to photolysis, hence their stability is dependent upon the exclusion of light.

Tissue related   In blood vessels the receptor biophase concentration of drugs can be affected by both extra- and intracellular metabolic degradation.

   1. *Extracellular metabolism.* This is an important disposition route for acetylcholine and a variety of peptide transmitters, e.g. angiotensin, bradykinin, substance P, but, in general, is easily circumvented by use of selective enzyme inhibitors or metabolically stable hormone mimetics.

   2. *Intracellular sequestration or metabolism.* Sequestration (e.g. in the dense granules of sympathetic neurones) and/or metabolism (e.g. by monoamine oxidase (MAO) or catechol-*O*-methyltransferase (COMT)), follow the active transport of catecholamines and indolamines into sympathetic nerve terminals (via Uptake1), smooth muscle cells (via Uptake2) or endothelial cells. These uptake processes are saturable, consequently failure to block them can lead to $E/[A]$ curve distortion as well as significant underestimation of agonist and antagonist affinities. Even in the absence of an active uptake process, less polar drugs may access intracellular enzymes by lipophilic penetration of cell membranes. For example, at the 5-HT$_2$ receptor mediating contraction of the rabbit aorta, tryptamine agonist potencies decrease in the order (p$[A_{50}]$): 5-HT (6.8) $\gg$ 5-carboxamidotryptamine (5.6) > tryptamine (5.4) > *N*-methyltryptamine (5.3), but when intracellular metabolism by MAO is irreversibly blocked using pargyline, the order changes to: 5-HT (6.8) $\gg$ tryptamine (6.0) > *N*-methyltryptamine (5.8) > 5-carboxamidotryptamine (5.7) (our unpublished data).

This emphasizes the importance of routinely inhibiting uptake processes and metabolic pathways, even in circumstances where metabolism appears to play no role in the disposition of the natural receptor agonist.

Indirect actions of ligands

It is assumed that the measured effect of a drug is due to a direct interaction with a specific receptor. However, some drugs elicit responses indirectly, e.g. tyramine produces vascular contraction by displacing noradrenaline from perivascular sympathetic neurones. Fig. 1.5 shows that 5-HT also has this property. Inhibition of Uptake1 with cocaine blocks the tyramine-like effect of 5-HT, but reveals that at high concentrations, the amine produces a second phase of contraction by activating α_1-adrenoceptors directly. Treatment of the tissue with

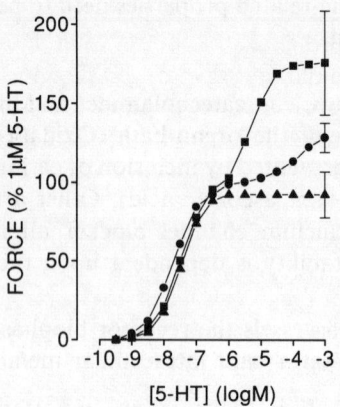

Fig. 1.5 Contractile effects of 5-HT in ring preparations of rabbit saphenous vein. In untreated tissues (■) the $E/[A]$ curve is clearly flat, extending over four orders of magnitude. Following inhibition of neuronal uptake with cocaine (30 μM: ●), the 5-HT $E/[A]$ curve becomes biphasic with a clear inflection at ~1 μM. The second phase of contraction is blocked by prazosin (30 μM) consistent with a direct action of 5-HT at α_1-adrenoceptors (not shown). Treatment of tissues with phenoxybenzamine (0.1 μM, 30 min ▲) inactivates both the uptake carrier and α_1-adrenoceptors, unmasking the action of 5-HT at 5-HT$_1$-like receptors mediating vasocontraction.

phenoxybenzamine irreversibly blocks both indirect actions of the agonist, enabling 5-HT$_1$-like receptor interactions to be studied in an unconfounded way.

Multiple receptors

It is a safe assumption that no ligand, endogenous or synthetic, displays absolute selectivity for a particular receptor type. Multiple receptor subtypes subserve the effects of most known transmitters, and receptor types apparently unrelated to the transmitter being studied can also be activated. The ability of 5-HT to activate α-adrenoceptors is one such example. PGF$_{2\alpha}$-induced vascular contraction via TP receptors is another, as is the overlap of actions at α-/β-adrenergic and dopaminergic receptors demonstrated by noradrenaline, adrenaline, and dopamine. Precautions therefore need to be taken to ensure that agonist effects measured over the entire range of concentrations used reflect an action at the target receptor only. Use of a suitably selective receptor antagonist provides confidence that this situation pertains.

Stability of tissue response

It is mandatory that tissue responses remain stable and reproducible during the time course of the experiment. In isolated blood vessels, smooth muscle responses tend to be well sustained allowing agonist concentration–effect relationships to be determined by cumulative drug additions. Endothelium-dependent responses, in contrast, appear to be susceptible to rapid desensitization, effects 'fading' rapidly in the continued presence of agonist. Cumulative agonist additions may therefore give rise to cumulative error due to desensitization and in such cases consideration should be given to constructing curves by separate additions of each agonist concentration (see below). A time-related change in tissue sensitivity may also be evident. Providing this occurs in a predictable fashion, satisfactory correction can usually be made.

Experimental design

Careful consideration must be given to the information required from a study and the experimental design should ensure the best chance of obtaining, reproducible quantitative data. Factors which can influence reproducibility of tissue responses, in addition to those already described, include age and weight of the animal, the portion of blood vessel used — receptor density may change along the length of a vessel — and the dimensions of the vessel ring or strip. A useful way of normalizing responses between tissues involves addition of a maximally effective concentration of a full agonist to define E_M for the receptor system under study in each vessel segment (see p. 3). All subsequent responses can be expressed as a per cent of this challenge. However, when E_M cannot be defined, it may be more appropriate to normalize agonist effects to a response which is independent of the receptor system under study (e.g. KCl contraction). Subsequent experimental design is generally in one of three forms:

(a) **Single exposure drug additions**. Responses to single concentrations of the drug are measured at different concentrations until a full $E/[A]$ curve is defined. Where practicable, the order of additions should be randomized. This design is commonly used when the drug effect is poorly maintained, but nevertheless requires that responses are reproducible and rapidly reversible following washout.

(b) **Cumulative drug additions: single curve**. A single, cumulative concentration-effect curve is constructed in each preparation. This design is useful in tissues where agonist effects are not easily reversed, or where responses to repeated administration of agonist are not reproducible. It is only appropriate in vessels which do not display large between-tissue variation in agonist potency.

(c) **Cumulative drug additions: paired curves**. A control curve is constructed by cumulative addition of agonist. After washout of drug a second curve is generated, usually following a pharmacological intervention. This design is particularly useful in vessels with large between-tissue differences in receptor density, but relies upon first and second curves being stable and reproducible.

CLASSIFICATION OF RECEPTORS

The use of drugs which selectively mimic or block the actions of endogenous hormones offers a simple and direct way to gain further understanding of physiological and pathophysiological processes. It was this approach that led Alquist (1948) to propose the existence of α- and β-adrenoceptors and this, in turn, led to the evolution of operational (functional pharmacological) criteria for classifying hormone receptors and the drugs which act upon them. Whilst it is now recognized that a definitive classification and nomenclature scheme also requires structural (molecular) and second messenger (biochemical) information about the receptors to be available, this in no way diminishes the importance of operational information obtained with agonist and antagonist drugs (see for example Humphrey *et al.* 1993). This section deals with the *analytical criteria* that help to provide confidence that the practical conditions outlined above have been fulfilled and that estimates of affinity and efficacy are therefore reliable.

Classification using antagonists

The dissociation equilibrium constant (K_B) is a chemical term derived from the rates of onset and offset of antagonist binding to the receptor. In principle, it is independent of receptor function and location, therefore estimation of K_B offers an unambiguous way of positively identifying a particular receptor type.

Analytical criteria

Confidence in the quality of K_B estimates is obtained from three well-defined criteria that should be regarded as necessary, though not sufficient evidence for simple, competitive antagonist behaviour (Schild 1968; Black *et al.* 1983). These criteria are illustrated by the interaction between 5-HT and the antagonist trazodone at the 5-HT$_2$ receptor in rabbit aorta (Fig. 1.6):

(a) Increasing concentrations of antagonist should produce successive, parallel rightward displacements of the agonist concentration–effect curve with no depression of the maximum, i.e. the fractional increase in agonist concentration required to overcome the effects of the antagonist should be independent of agonist concentration (Fig. 1.6A).

(b) The antagonist affinity should be independent of concentration, so that presentation of the data in the form of a Schild plot (Arunlakshana and Schild 1959) yields a straight line of unit slope (Fig. 1.6B). The antagonist concentration range should be as wide as possible,- ideally 1000-fold.

(c) The antagonist affinity should be independent of the agonist used, because the agonist simply titrates receptor sites unoccupied by the antagonist (Fig. 1.6B).

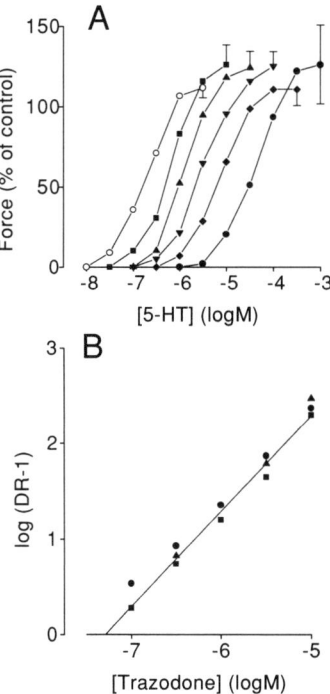

Fig. 1.6 Antagonism by trazodone of 5-HT$_2$ receptors in rabbit aorta. (A) Simple, competitive antagonism of 5-HT $E/[A]$ curves by increasing concentrations of antagonist (control ○, 0.1 ■, 0.3 ▲, 1.0 ▼, 3.0 ♦ and 10.0 μM ●). (B) Schild plot transformation of these data demonstrating that antagonism is independent of the agonist used (■ 5-HT, ● 5-methoxytryptamine, ▲ α-methyl-5-HT).

Detection of anomalous behaviour

The Schild regression offers a powerful means of identifying and diagnosing erroneous antagonist behaviour. In general, anomalies are identified by changes in the slope or asymptote of the $E/[A]$ curve in the presence of antagonist and/or by a deviation of the Schild plot regression line from a slope of unity indicating that equilibrium conditions do not pertain or that drug interactions involve more than a single receptor type. Careful attention to the nature of these Schild slope deviations enables diagnosis of the likely source of the problem (Kenakin 1982). This is exemplified in Fig. 1.7 which illustrates antagonism of isoprenaline relaxations of rabbit jugular vein by the β_2-selective antagonist ICI 118 551. In this example the Schild plot line obtained appears to be curvilinear, concave down (slope ≪ 1), a result that is typical of an interaction at two receptors (see Fig. 1.7 legend). However, in certain circumstances the Schild slope line may be unity, but the resulting estimate of K_B wrong. Outcomes that are often

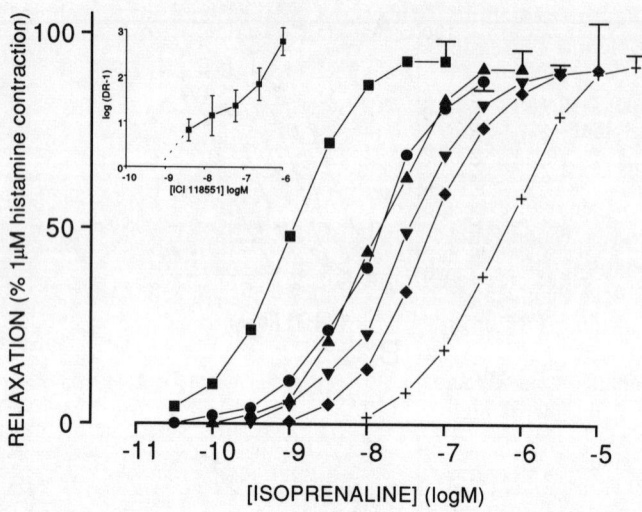

Fig. 1.7 Antagonism of isoprenaline relaxations by ICI 118 551 (control ■, 0.004 ●, 0.015 ▲, 0.06 ▼, 0.25 ♦, and 1.0 + μM) in rings of rabbit jugular vein. A low concentration (0.004 μM) of antagonist produces an impressive right-shift of the isoprenaline $E/[A]$ curve, but increasing concentrations (0.015–0.25 μM) produce little further curve displacement until, at the highest antagonist concentration tested (1.0 μM), curve displacement is once again observed. The profile results from an action of isoprenaline at both β_1- and β_2-adrenoceptors in this tissue, the agonist displaying marginal selectivity for β_2-adrenoceptors. At a low concentration of the selective antagonist ICI 118 551, β_2-adrenoceptor effects of isoprenaline are blocked shifting the response curve to higher concentrations which activate β_1-adrenoceptors. No further right-shift of the agonist curve is obtained until ICI 118 551 is raised to a concentration that is also capable of blocking β_1-adrenoceptors.

encountered, and their possible causes, are summarized in Table 1.1 (see Kenakin 1993 for more detail).

Complexities and exceptions

The utility of antagonists in receptor classification lies in the stability of their affinity estimates. However, consistent behaviour is not always observed. Important complexities and exceptions include the following.

1. *Variable pharmacodynamics at the same receptor type.* Some antagonists exhibit simple competitive antagonism in one tissue, but insurmountable antagonism (i.e. a decrease in the $E/[A]$ curve asymptote) in another. Unfortunately, a variety of mechanisms can be, and have been, proposed to explain unsurmountable antagonism: allosteric receptor modulation (e.g. Kaumann 1989), 'hemi-equilibrium' in the absence of receptor reserve (Paton and Rang 1966), and antagonist-induced changes in the receptor–effector coupling inverse agonism: Schutz and Freissmuth 1992) are just three examples. In only a few cases

Table 1.1 Factors which may confound pK_B estimation, and their effect on the slope of the Schild regression

Slope of Schild regression	Cause of slope anomaly	Possible reasons for anomalous plot
Steep	Smaller than expected concentration ratio (r) at low $[B]$	(i) Slowly associating antagonist, not at equilibrium at low $[B]$ (ii) Saturable antagonist loss, e.g. uptake
	Larger than expected r at high $[B]$ or at all $[B]$	(i) Additional, non-competitive antagonist properties of antagonist or agonist
Flat	Smaller than expected r at middle or high $[B]$	(i) Saturable agonist uptake or loss (ii) Agonist action at two receptors, antagonist of low affinity or without affinity for less potent site of agonism (iii) Additional properties of agonist or antagonist
Unity		(i) Irreversible antagonism or pseudo-irreversible antagonism, particularly when agonist has high efficacy (ii) Functional antagonism (iii) Under-equilibration of antagonist when diffusion is rate limiting (iv) Presence of another drug, e.g. uptake blocker (citalopram) — which is also a competitive antagonist

(e.g. verapamil, Leff and Morse 1987) can this behaviour be attributed to additional pharmacological properties of the antagonist and in the absence of such mechanistic understanding, unsurmountable antagonism cannot usefully contribute to receptor classification. Indeed, the use of the empirical term pD'_2 ($-\log$ of the antagonist concentration required to produce 50% depression of the agonist curve maximum) has resulted previously in misclassification because values obtained are tissue dependent.

2. *Variable affinities.* Even when the practical and analytical criteria for simple competitive antagonism are fulfilled, antagonists may exhibit significantly different affinities at the same receptor type in different tissues. This has been illustrated for a variety of 5-HT_2 receptor antagonists in rat and rabbit vascular preparations, where affinity estimates differed between species by more than tenfold (Leff and Martin 1986). There is increasing evidence from molecular biological studies to suggest that this variability is species-related, resulting from phylogenetic variations in the primary structure of the receptor protein (Adham et al. 1992).

Classification using agonists

1. *Agonist relative potencies.* Agonist rank orders of potency have long been used in receptor characterization (e.g. Alquist 1948), but do not provide a reliable basis for differential classification. For example, tryptamine agonist potencies follow the order 5-CT > 5-HT $\gg$ α-Me-5-HT at three distinct vascular 5-HT receptors (Craig and Martin 1993; Martin 1994). Agonist potency-ratios, on the other hand, might be expected to distinguish between the three receptors because, in principle, potency-ratios are constant for a given receptor type. This holds true only if each of the agonists is a full agonist in the system. If, as is often the case, receptor–effector coupling efficiency varies between tissues so that one or more of the agonists behaves as a partial agonist in some instances, potency-ratios will also vary. This is because a given decrease in the efficiency of receptor–effector coupling produces a uniform right-shift of full agonist curves, but simply depresses the maximum of curves to partial agonists without substantially changing their position on the abscissa (see Fig. 1.2). The confounding effect of agonist uptake and/or metabolism on potency ratios has already been discussed.

2. *Agonist affinities and efficacies.* Estimation of agonist dissociation constants (K_As) and relative efficacies avoids the problems alluded to above and provides more robust measures for receptor classification. Hence for a small set of agonists it is possible to obtain affinity and relative efficacy 'fingerprints' which enable the differentiation and positive identification of different receptor types. This approach has been used in 5-HT receptor studies when available antagonists displayed variable behaviour precluding proper classification (Martin 1994).

Analytical criteria

Potency ratios provide reliable information for receptor classification providing:

- all agonists achieve the same maximum effect and behave as full agonists
- there is no significant difference between the slope of the $E/[A]$ curves

A variety of null methods exist for quantifying agonist affinity and efficacy (see above pp. 6–8), but, in contrast to antagonist analyses, there are no formal criteria by which to judge the quality of estimates obtained. However, model-fitting approaches do provide a means to test accordance of experimental data with theoretical expectations (see for example Black *et al*. 1985; Leff 1987; Leff *et al*. 1990). This is illustrated in Fig. 1.8, which depicts a typical experiment to determine agonist affinity using the method of partial receptor inactivation (Furchgott 1966). A number of criteria can be defined:

(a) The inactivating agent must only reduce the number of functional receptors and in no way interfere with post-receptor events. In this case the alkylating agent phenoxybenzamine produces depression and right-shift of the 5-HT concentration–effect curve. Confidence that this results solely from receptor inactivation is provided by the ability of a reversible, competitive antagonist

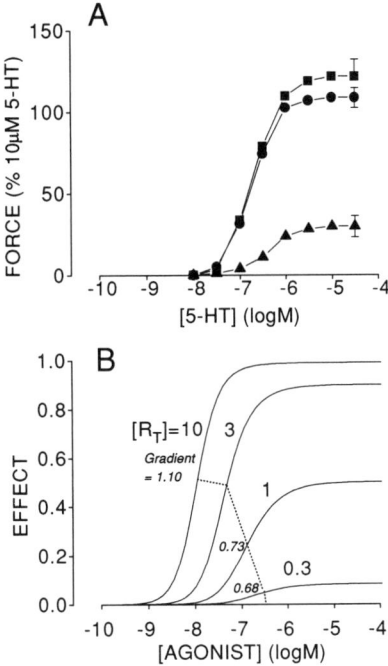

Fig. 1.8 Effect of fractional irreversible receptor inactivation on $E/[A]$ curve behaviour. (A) 5-HT contractions of rabbit aortic rings before (●) and after (▲) fractional inactivation of 5-HT$_2$ receptors with phenoxybenzamine (1 μM, 30 min). Concomitant exposure to the competitive antagonist methysergide (1 μM: ■) protects completely against the effect of the alkylating agent confirming that the latter acts exclusively to reduce receptor number. (B) Computer simulated lines depicting the effect of reducing receptor number ($[R_T]$) on $E/[A]$ curves that are inherently steep. The lines obtained at each value of $[R_T]$ were produced using eqn (1.8) with E_M and K_E set at unity, K_A set at 10^{-7} M, and $n = 2$. Progressive reduction of $[R_T]$ reduces the midpoint gradient of the $E/[A]$ curve towards that of a rectangular hyperbola (gradient = 0.576) whilst $[A_{50}]$ values, connected by the dotted line, tend to an abscissal location on the right of K_A (see Black et al. 1985).

(methysergide) to afford complete protection against the effects of phenoxybenzamine (Fig. 1.8A).

(b) Agonist curve shape changes consistent with a simple reduction of efficacy in the system should be obtained. In the example shown, 5-HT curves are inherently 'steep' but become flatter as efficacy is reduced following receptor inactivation. This accords with predictions based on the 'operational model' (see Black et al. 1985). In general, the slope parameter (m) of 'steep' curves is expected to approach that of a rectangular hyperbola (i.e. slope parameter = 1) as efficacy is progressively reduced (Fig. 1.8B). In the case of agonist curves which are rectangular hyperbolic at the outset, no change in gradient is expected.

(c) Curve behaviour should accord with a simple reduction in efficacy. With a progressive reduction in efficacy, the agonist curve midpoint ($[A_{50}]$) should approach and ultimately coincide with the value of K_A. This holds true for agonist curves that are rectangular hyperbolic at the outset (see Fig. 1.2), but when inherently 'steep' $[A_{50}]$ tends toward an abscissal intercept to the right of K_A (see Fig. 1.8B).

On a cautionary note, it should be recognized that in contrast to antagonist analyses which are truly null, any attempt to describe agonist behaviour in mathematical terms necessarily makes assumptions about the events linking receptor occupancy and effect. In the operational model (eqn 1.8) these assumptions are explicit since they are represented in the shape of the $E/[AR]$ relation. Similar assumptions are made implicitly in the traditional graphical approaches when $E/[A]$ curve data are fitted to a logistic in order to estimate equi-effective agonist concentrations. This means that any attempt to erect criteria such as those outlined above for agonist–receptor studies are only as valid as the assumptions that have been made.

Detection of anomalous behaviour

Asymmetries or irregularities in $E/[A]$ curves are often evident from visual inspection. The slope parameter m is a sensitive indicator of anomalous behaviour and its value will usually be equal to or greater than one when the agonist is acting through a single receptor type; when $m < 1$, this may be indicative of agonist actions at two distinct receptors (e.g. Fig. 1.5). Model-fitting methods also provide a basis for detecting and interpreting anomalous agonist behaviour and help to establish criteria for assessing the validity of affinity and efficacy estimates. For example, in the absence of a receptor inactivating agent, it may be feasible to attempt agonist affinity estimation using functional antagonism or receptor desensitization. To be valid, these methods must only decrease the efficacy (τ) of the receptor system under study and produce no other perturbation of the receptor–effector system, such as a change in E_M or n. If this has been achieved, then the $E/[A]$ curves should fulfil the criteria outlined above. When data does not behave in this way there are grounds to suspect that the intervention used has produced changes incompatible with valid estimation of agonist affinity.

Complexities and exceptions

In the same way that it is assumed that $[A]$ is in excess of $[AR]$, it is also assumed that, in G protein coupled systems, the concentration of $[AR]$ is vastly greater than $[G]$. If this is not the case then theoretical analysis predicts that profound errors in K_A estimates can result, sometimes in the absence of obvious deviations from the predictions of the operational model, and sometimes with a decrease in α but no change in $[A_{50}]$ in the presence of an irreversible antagonist. However, practical examples of this phenomenon have yet to be described.

In situations where antagonist affinities tend to vary at a single receptor type, the affinities of agonist hormone analogues appear to be more stable (e.g. Leff et al. 1986). However, Bevan and colleagues have shown that whilst the potency of noradrenaline at the α_1-adrenoceptor in various blood vessels from the same animal varies by more than 1000-fold, this variation could not be accounted for in terms of tissue differences in receptor–effector coupling efficiency. Rather, it appeared to result from a continual variation in ligand affinity (Bevan et al. 1989). Unfortunately these authors did not show that variable affinity was an agonist-independent feature of the α-adrenoceptor, hence it remains possible that mixed populations of receptors contributed to the phenomenon.

SUMMARY

Isolated blood vessels provide a simple and convenient way of studying the end-organ effects of vasoactive drugs and are eminently suited to quantitative analysis of drug–receptor interactions. However, it is clear that the benefits of studying drug action in functionally intact vessel segments are accompanied by potential pitfalls which can lead to misinterpretation of experimental data. Attempts to measure drug–receptor interactions under equilibrium or steady state conditions can be compromised by physiological as well as physical processes normally involved in vascular smooth muscle function (see experimental considerations, p. 9) and these must be neutralized, or taken account of, to ensure the valid quantitation of agonist and antagonist drug effects. Confidence that appropriate practical conditions have been established is provided by fulfilment of the analytical criteria outlined in the section on receptor classification, p. 14. Approached in this way, drug effects in vascular smooth muscle can be analysed in a robust and reliable way providing a secure basis for receptor classification and aiding the identification and development of new, more specific vasoactive drugs.

GLOSSARY OF TERMS

Potency	A drug property which describes the concentration range over which it has an effect — usually defined by the $p[A_{50}]$, pED_{50}, pEC_{50}, or pD_2 for agonists and pA_2, pIC_{50}, or pK_B for antagonists. Whereas agonist potency is determined by the product of efficacy and affinity, antagonist potency is usually defined simply in terms of affinity.
$p[A_{50}]$, pED_{50}, pEC_{50}, pD_2	Negative logarithm of the molar concentration of agonist required to elicit half of its own maximum effect.
pK_B, pK_A	Negative logarithm of the dissociation equilibrium constant. Defined as the molar concentration of ligand required to occupy 50% of the functional receptor pool. By convention, the subscript A is used for agonists, and B for antagonists.

Affinity	The reciprocal of the dissociation equilibrium constant.
pA_2	An empirical measure of antagonist: the molar concentration of antagonist required to cause a twofold rightward shift of an agonist $E/[A]$ curve.
E_m	A measure of the maximum possible effect that can be elicited through a given receptor system, defined by the effect of a full agonist.
Intrinsic activity (α)	A tissue-dependent, empirical term defining the maximum effect of an agonist on a scale 0–1, usually expressed relative to the maximum response of a full agonist (when $\alpha = 1$) in the receptor system under study (see Ariëns 1954).
Intrinsic efficacy	The tissue-independent, chemical property of a ligand representing its power to elicit an effect following receptor occupancy.
Efficacy	A drug and tissue-dependent property which describes the ability of a ligand to elicit an effect in a given tissue.
Partial agonist	An agonist with low intrinsic efficacy, which is unable to elicit the maximum possible effect (E_m) even when occupying all receptors; this is a drug and tissue-dependent property.

REFERENCES

Adham, N., Romanienko, P., Hartig, P., Weinshank, R. L., and Branchek, T. A. (1992). The rat 5-hydroxytryptamine$_{1B}$ receptor is the species homologue of the human 5-HT$_{1D\beta}$ receptor. *Mol. Pharmacol.*, **41**, 1–7.

Alquist, R. P. (1948). A study of the adrenotropic receptors. *Am. J. Physiol.*, **153**, 586–600.

Ariëns, E. J. (1954). Affinity and intrinsic activity in the theory of competitve inhibition. *Arch. Int. Pharmacodyn. Ther.*, **99**, 32–49.

Arunlakshana, O. and Schild, H. O. (1959). Some quantitative uses of drug antagonists. *Br. J. Pharmacol.*, **14**, 48–58.

Barlow, R. B., Scott, K. A., and Stephenson, R. P. (1967). An attempt to study the effects of chemical structure on the affinity and efficacy of compounds related to acetylcholine. *Br. J. Pharmacol.*, **21**, 509–22.

Bevan, J. A., Bevan, R. D., and Martin Shreeve, S. (1989). Variable receptor affinity hypothesis. *FASEB J.*, **3**, 1696–704.

Black, J. W. and Leff, P. (1983). Operational models of agonism. *Proc. R. Soc. London, Ser. B*, **220**, 141–62.

Black, J. W., Gerskowitch, V. P., and Leff, P. (1983). Reflections on the classification of histamine receptors. In *Pharmacology of histamine receptors* (ed. C. R. Ganellin and M. E. Parsons), pp. 1–9. John Wright, Bristol, London, Boston.

Black, J. W., Leff, P., Shankley, N. P., and Wood, J.W. (1985). An operational model of pharmacological agonism: The effect of $E/[A]$ curve shape on agonist dissociation constant estimation. *Br. J. Pharmacol.*, **84**, 561–71.

Clark, A. J. (1937). General Pharmacology. In *Handbuch der experimentelen pharmakologie*, 4. Springer, Berlin.

Craig, D. A. and Martin, G. R. (1993). 5-HT$_{1B}$ receptors mediate potent contractile responses to 5-HT in rat caudal artery. *Br. J. Pharmacol.*, **109**, 609-11.

Furchgott, R. F. (1954). Dibenamine blockade in strips of rabbit aorta and its use in differentiating receptors. *J. Pharmacol. Exp. Ther.*, **111**, 265-84.

Furchgott, R. F. (1966). The use of β-haloalkylamines in the differentiation of receptors and on the determination of dissociation constants of receptor-agonist complexes. *Adv. Drug Res.*, **3**, 21-55.

Furchgott, R. F. (1968). A critical appraisal of the use of isolated organ systems for the assessment of drug action at the receptor level. In *Importance of fundamental principles in drug evaluation* (ed. D. H. Tedeschi and R. E. Tedeschi), pp. 277-97. Raven Press, New York.

Furchgott, R. F. and Bursztyn, P. (1967). Comparison of dissociation constants and of relative efficacies of selected agonists acting on parasympathetic receptors. *Ann. N.Y. Acad. Sci.*, **144**, 882-99.

Gaddum, J. H. (1937). The quantitative effects of antagonistic drugs. *J. Physiol. (London)*, **89**, 7P-9P.

Humphrey, P. P. A., Hartig, P., and Hoyer, D. (1993). A proposed new nomenclature for 5-HT receptors. *Trends Pharmacol. Sci.*, **14**, 233-6.

Kaumann, A. J. (1989). The allosteric 5-HT$_2$ receptor system. In *The peripheral actions of 5-hydroxytryptamine* (ed. J. R. Fozard), pp. 45-71. Oxford University Press, Oxford, New York, Tokyo.

Kenakin, T. P. (1982). The Schild regression in the process of receptor classification. *Can. J. Physiol. Pharmacol.*, **60**, 249-65.

Kenakin, T. P. (1984). The classification of drugs and drug receptors in isolated tissues. *Pharmacol. Rev.*, **36**, 165-222.

Kenakin, T. (1993). In *Pharmacological analysis of drug-receptor interaction*, pp. 278-321. Raven Press, New York.

Kenakin, T. P. and Beek, D. (1980). Is prenalterol (H133/80) really a selective beta1-adrenoceptor agonist? Tissue selectivity resulting from differences in stimulus-response coupling. *J. Pharmacol. Exp. Ther.*, **213**, 406-13.

Leff, P. (1987). Can operational models of agonism provide a framework for classifying hormone receptors? In *Perspectives on receptor classification, receptor biochemistry and methodology*, 6 (ed. J. W. Black, D. H. Jenkinson, and V. P. Gerskowitch), pp. 157-67. Alan R. Liss, New York.

Leff, P. and Martin, G. R. (1986). Peripheral 5-HT$_2$-like receptors. Can they be classified with the available antagonists? *Br. J. Pharmacol.*, **88**, 585-93.

Leff, P. and Morse, J. M. (1987). Resultant pharmacological actions of verapamil: quantification of competitive 5-hydroxytryptamine antagonism in combination with calcium antagonism. *J. Pharmacol. Exp. Ther.*, **240**, 284-7.

Leff, P., Martin, G. R., and Morse, J. M. (1986). The classification of peripheral 5-HT$_2$-like receptors using tryptamine agonist and antagonist analogues. *Br. J. Pharmacol.*, **89**, 493-9.

Leff, P., Prentice, D. J., Giles, H., Martin, G. R., and Wood, J. W. (1990). Estimation of agonist affinity and efficacy by direct operational model-fitting. *J. Pharmacol. Methods*, **23**, 225-37.

Martin, G. R. (1994). Vascular receptors for 5-hydroxytryptamine. Distribution, function and classification. *Pharmacol. Ther.* **62**, 283-324.

Martin, W., Furchgott, R. F., Villani, G. M., and Jothianandan, D. (1986). Depression of contractile responses in rat aorta by spontaneously released endothelium-derived relaxing factor. *J. Pharmacol. Exp. Ther.*, **237**, 529-38.

Nickerson, M. (1956). Receptor occupancy and tissue response. *Nature (London)*, **178**, 697-8.

Ohashi, T. and Azuma, T. (1980). Paradoxical relaxation of arterial strips induced by vasoconstrictive agents. *Blood Vessels*, **17**, 16-26.

Paton, W. D. M. and Rang, H. P. (1966). The kinetic approach to drug antagonism. In *Advances in drug research* (ed. N. J. Harper and A. B. Simmonds), **3**, pp. 57-80. Academic Press, London, New York.

Schild, H. O. (1968). A pharmacological approach to drug receptors. In *Importance of fundamental principles in drug evaluation* (ed. D. H. Tedeschi and R. E. Tedeschi), pp. 257-75. Raven Press, New York.

Schutz, W. and Freissmuth, M. (1992). Reverse intrinsic activity of antagonists on G-protein-coupled receptors. *Trends Pharmacol. Sci.*, **13**, 376-80.

Stephenson, R. P. (1956). A modification of receptor theory. *Br. J. Pharmacol.*, **11**, 379-93.

2. Isolated tissue techniques

Michael J. Lew and Grant A. McPherson

INTRODUCTION

Why study blood vessels *in vitro*?

Several decades of technical innovation have given us a wide range of methods for studying the function of vascular smooth muscle with various degrees of organization ranging from intact, conscious animals down to single smooth muscle cells, and subcellular fractions. In intact animals there are many extrinsic factors that influence the behaviour of vascular smooth muscle, so in a broad way the degree of control the experimenter has is inversely related to the degree of intactness of the animal. Characterization of the intrinsic properties of arteries and arterioles can only be performed *in vitro*, but even then characterization can be made at a number of different levels of vascular integrity. For example mechanical (Harris and Warshaw 1991), electrical, and ionic (see Chapters 3 and 6) can all be assessed in isolated single smooth muscle cells as well as in isolated vascular segments, and in some cases perfused vascular beds (Bryant *et al.* 1985; Bouskela *et al.* 1991). The electrical, biochemical (second messengers), and ionic events mediating smooth muscle responses are obviously important, but ultimately it is the mechanical properties of the blood vessel that interests us most. For the purpose of this chapter we will restrict our discussion to some common *in vitro* methods involving vascular segments and perfused vascular beds. Some other methodologies used are described in other chapters of this book.

SURVEY OF METHODOLOGIES

Many methods have been developed for studying the mechanical responses of blood vessels *in vitro*. The selection of method depends on the size of the blood vessel of interest, the desired response metameter (see section on what response to measure p. 31), the desired conditions of the experiment and, in practice, the equipment available to the experimenter. For the purposes of this review, we have divided the vessels into the classes large arteries (> 1 mm diameter), small arteries (100 μm–1 mm), and arterioles (< 100 μm). These divisions are arbitrary, and are not intended to imply functional divisions.

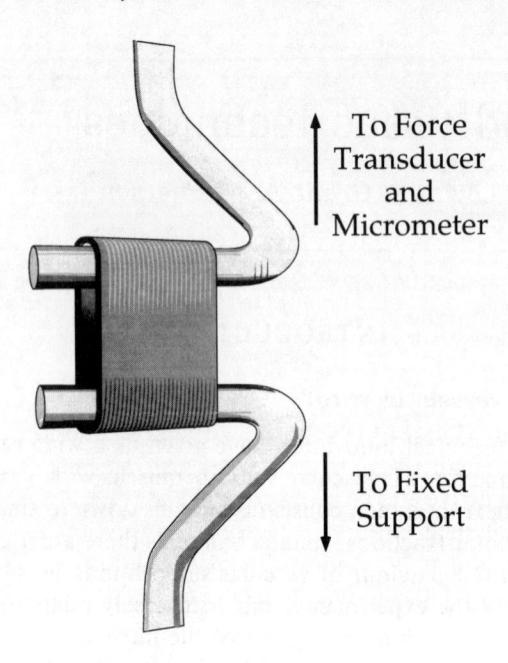

Fig. 2.1 Diagram of a large arterial ring mounted on wires. The upper wire is connected to an isometric force transducer and a micrometer for adjusting the interwire spacing.

Large arteries

For many years the most commonly used preparation of large arterial smooth muscle was the spiral-cut strip. This method was easy to use and offered the advantage that the changes in smooth muscle cell length were amplified by the mechanical arrangement of the tissue to a degree that allowed registration of these changes using isotonic kymograph recording methods. Spiral-cut strips are less commonly used now because electrical transducers and recorders are universally available, and because of recognition of the high likelihood of endothelial cell damage during the preparation of these strips (Furchgott and Zawadzki 1980). The small fractional change in diameter that most large arteries exhibit on maximal activation means that measurement of diameter and resistance of large arteries is difficult compared to smaller vessels. The most common method used for large arteries is to measure the active force developed by the smooth muscle of a short segment mounted on wires (Fig. 2.1).

Small arteries

Small arteries (frequently called 'resistance arteries') are too small to be conveniently cut into spiral strips, but can be studied by almost any other method. Myographs designed to facilitate the mounting of small arterial segments on wires have been developed by Bevan and by Mulvany and Halpern (Bevan and Osher

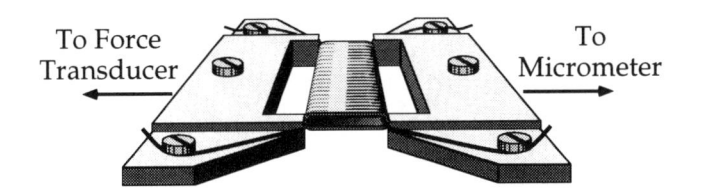

Fig. 2.2 Diagram of a small artery mounted on wires in the jaws of a small artery myograph. The left jaw is connected to a force transducer, and the right jaw is connected to a micrometer to allow graded stretch to be applied to the artery.

1972; Mulvany and Halpern 1977), and several models are commercially available. Using the small vessel myograph, vessels as small as 100 μm can be isolated and both the active and passive properties of these vessels studied *in vitro* (Fig. 2.2). The size of such small arterial segments calls for a stereomicroscope to perform the dissection and mounting. The usual approach is to insert stainless steel or tungsten wires (40 μm diameter or smaller) through the lumen of a vascular segment. One wire is attached to a stationary support driven by a hand operated or stepper-motor driven micrometer, while the other is attached to an isometric force transducer which measures force development. The incorporation of a micrometer into the design allows detailed diameter–tension curves to be constructed for different blood vessels. The use of a motor-driven micrometer allows the adaptation of the small artery myograph to isotonic or isobaric responses in addition to the normal isometric (see section on what response to measure, p. 31).

Small arteries can also be conveniently set-up as cannulated segments, either with perfusion of the lumen, or with the distal end of the artery tied off (blind-sack arrangement). With the blind-sack arrangement the only possible measurement of the mechanical behaviour of the artery is diameter, but with perfused segments either diameter or segmental perfusion resistance can be measured. Perfused arterial segments can be cannulated at both ends, or only at the upstream end. Double-cannulation offers the important advantage that the outflow tubing can be elevated to provide a basal distending pressure at the downstream end of the segment. With the outflow end uncannulated (as is the case with some preparations of rat tail artery or rabbit ear artery), the distending pressure at that end will always be zero, independent of the perfusion pressure measured upstream.

We have found that the responsiveness of small arteries can be dependent on the preparation used. Small arteries were dissected free of rat mesentery and bisected. One half was cannulated and pressurized in a blind-sack arrangement and the other half was wire-mounted in a standard small artery myograph. Concentration–response curves to methoxamine and acetylcholine were generated in both preparations. It was found that the cannulated artery segments were significantly more sensitive to methoxamine than the wire-mounted segments, but

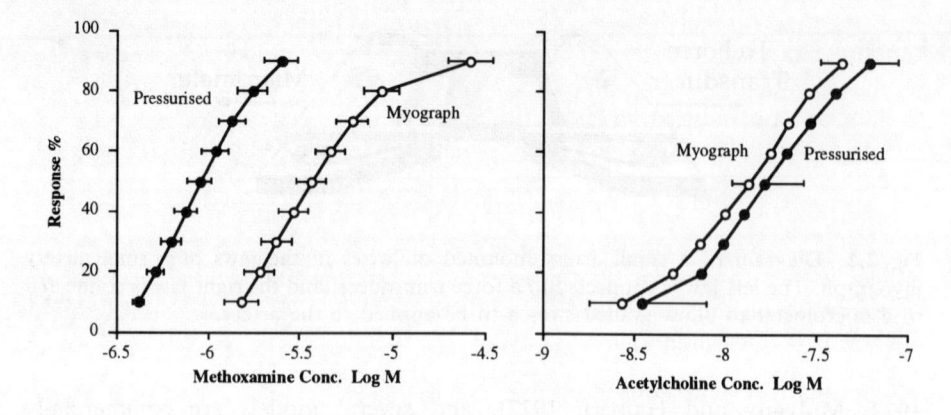

Fig. 2.3 Comparison of responses of blind-sack cannulated (pressurized) and wire-mounted (myograph) small mesenteric arteries from the rat. Arteries were bisected and one-half set-up with each method. Cannulated arteries were more sensitive to methoxamine than were wire-mounted segments (left panel), but acetylcholine was equally potent in either preparation (right panel).

the preparations were equally sensitive to acetylcholine (Fig. 2.3). Thus it is clear that the arterial responsiveness can be dependent on the way that the artery is set-up. Responsiveness can also be dependent on the way that responses are measured (see section on what to measure p. 31).

Arterioles

The size of arterioles generally precludes wire-mounting. Thus almost all of the studies of isolated arterioles have used cannulated segments, either blind-sack or perfused. While it is theoretically possible to perfuse an arteriolar segment at fixed flow and measure the perfusion pressure as an index of vasomotor tone, the very low flow rates required and the fact that many arterioles constrict to complete or near closure when maximally activated means that this method is technically difficult with arterioles. Responses of isolated arterioles are therefore usually measured as changes in diameter using a microscope and video system (Duling and Rivers 1986; Neild 1989), although other methods are possible (van Bavel *et al.* 1990). Many different schemes for cannulation of small arteries and arterioles have been used. The issues that are important are: mechanical properties such as manipulation of the vessel and the means of securing it to the cannulae; the resistance of the cannulae; the dead space in the cannulae. With respect to the mechanical manipulation of the vessel, the various concentric pipette methods (Duling and Rivers 1986) offer the advantage that the vessel can be manipulated using the pipettes alone, and thus the likelihood of damage to the tissue is reduced, and can be achieved on the stage of an inverted microscope. Tying the arteriole to a single pipette with a fine suture is possible with the aid of a powerful stereomicroscope (Osol and Halpern 1985; Kuo *et al.* 1988), and thus the need for matched specially shaped cannula pairs is obviated. The method of Sipkema *et al.* (1991) was developed to allow cannulation of small artery segments with an effective pipette resistance of zero which may be useful in elucidation of flow-induced vascular responses.

SETTING THE CONDITIONS

When setting-up vascular smooth muscle preparations *in vitro*, the experimenter must decide on the conditions under which the responses of the smooth muscle cells will be measured. The choices are:

- optimal for generation of active tension
- optimal for sensitivity to activation
- most like *in vivo* conditions
- most reproducible
- most convenient

These choices are not always addressed explicitly, but they serve as a useful framework for the discussion of *in vitro* methodology, and will be referred to below.

Wire-mounted preparations

Many studies using large wire-mounted arteries (Tallarida *et al.* 1974; Price *et al.* 1981, 1983; Herlihy and Berardo 1986) have shown that the parameters that we calculate for agonist/blood vessel interactions (e.g. agonist potency and maximum response) depend, to some extent, on the initial passive conditions under which the vessel is placed (resting tension). Therefore the quantitative outcome of an experiment can depend on the choice of initial conditions. Wire-mounted arteries are unavoidably stretched to a non-circular cross-section, and are retracted axially (Lew and Angus 1992). This altered geometry of wire-mounted arteries means that it is impossible to find conditions like those *in vivo*. None the less it is important that the conditions be chosen rationally. Experimenters commonly intend their conditions to approximate those that elicit the largest active tension (i.e. choice 1). The degree of stretch necessary for this condition can be determined directly by measuring maximal responses of each arterial segment to some stimulus (commonly potassium-induced depolarization) with several degrees of pre-stretch. The experimenter would then set the stretch to that which produced the largest response. In practice this is rarely done for each arterial segment, but is done in preliminary experiments and the average degree of stretch then used in subsequent experiments using the same type of tissue. Thus when experimenters state something like 'arteries were stretched to an initial tension of one gram which is optimal for force generation in this preparation', they are actually using choice 5 rather than their implied choice 1. It is notable that the 'optimal' stretch frequently occurs at 1, 2, or 5 g! It is also probably worth pointing out that the units of force are Newtons (one gram mass under normal gravitational conditions exerts a force of 9.8×10^{-3} N), and tension is force per unit length (i.e. Nm^{-1}).

A superior solution to the problem of setting the initial conditions was demonstrated by Mulvany and Halpern (1977) who showed that the point of maximum active tension development can be calculated empirically from the passive diameter-tension relationship. Their method for standardizing the radial stretch applied to the arteries has become ubiquitously used with small artery myographs, and is equally useful in experiments with large arteries and veins. The method involves calculation of an equivalent radial distending pressure from the measured arterial circumference and the radial force, assuming that the walls of the artery are thin and applying the Laplace relationship (tension = pressure × radius). The method is described in detail below (see section on selected methods p. 35). Calculated equivalent pressure values have the advantage over simple force or tension units that there is an inbuilt correction for the size of the vessel. Problems can occur if the calculated pressure value is taken too literally (Lew and Angus 1992), so the method does not really allow choice 3 (most like *in vivo* conditions), but this does not greatly restrict the usefulness of the method for setting the initial conditions of isolated blood vessels.

Maximum active tension development (choice 1) in the rat small mesenteric artery occurs at 0.8–0.9 times the diameter of the that the vessel would passively have at a calculated pressure of 100 mmHg. However, few studies have been performed to determine whether different vessels express maximum active tension development at the same point on the passive diameter-tension curve. Price and his colleagues (Price *et al.* 1981, 1983) have shown that in large arteries the optimal conditions for developing maximal tension and that for maximum agonist sensitivity differ (i.e. the stretch for choice 1 is different to the stretch for choice 2). A similar phenomenon has also been described for small arteries (McPherson 1992). Changes in vascular reactivity to pharmacological agents in conditions such as hypertension are of great interest particularly in arteries contributing to vascular resistance. However it is unclear at present whether the small differences in the sensitivity to vasoconstrictors of blood vessels obtained from hypertensive animals relate to intrinsic differences in the vessels or the inappropriate selection of the passive conditions under which the vessels are placed when assessing vascular reactivity. If this is the case, it may suggest that the comparison of the vascular effects of a vasoconstrictor and dilators may need to be performed under a number of different passive conditions particular when alterations in activity are small.

Cannulated arteries
For cannulated arteries the choice of initial conditions of stretch is different. The artery can simply be pressurized to a physiologically reasonable pressure. The fact that true distending pressure is measured prevents the experimenter from inadvertently setting the length of the smooth muscle cells to a value well above or below the range in which the arteries work well, but whether there is an optimum distending pressure for sensitivity to agonists is not clear. The issue of

shear stress is important to perfused artery segments. It is clear that high levels of shear can strip the endothelial cells from the artery (Fry 1968), moderate levels of shear can permeabilize the endothelium without abolishing its ability to release EDRF (Lew and Madeley 1994), and changes in shear stress in the physiological range can induce changes in the release of EDRF from the endothelial cell, and thus change the sensitivity of the artery to vasoconstrictors (Kuo *et al.* 1990). Because shear stress increases with flow velocity, it is important that the perfusion rate be kept low, but even if an artery is perfused at a fixed flow rate the shear stress can climb to damaging levels when the artery is vasoconstricted. For many experiments it is probably best to measure arterial diameter and perfuse the segment with the general method used by Kuo *et al.* (1990), (as described below) which allows independent control of the distending pressure and perfusion pressure gradient.

WHAT RESPONSE TO MEASURE

Wire-mounted arteries

In most experiments the responses of isolated arteries have been measured as active force where vessel diameter is held constant. However it is likely that the ability of a vessel to respond may depend on the conditions under which the vessel is has to operate (i.e. isobaric: constant pressure; isotonic: constant tension; isometric: constant diameter; or auxotonic: a mixture of these). In non-vascular muscles this issue was addressed as long ago as 1926 when Clark found that the concentration–response curves for acetylcholine in the frog rectus abdominus differed with isotonic and isometric recording methods (Clark 1926). In a more recent study (Michelson and Shelkovnikov 1976) it was found that the difference between isometric and isobaric concentration–response curve was large in some tissues (holothurian protractor pharynx and leach dorsal muscle) and small or absent in others (guinea-pig ileum and sea-urchin retractor dentis). Van Nueten (1980) has shown that the responses of helical strips of rat tail arteries are similar whether they are measured istonically or isometrically. This issue has now been addressed for ring segments of arteries using a motorized version of the small vessel myograph (McPherson 1992). In these experiments the manual micrometer on the small vessel myograph was replaced with a computer controlled motor. Tension in the small resistance artery was continually monitored using a computer and the equivalent transmural pressure calculated from the tension and the vessel diameter. In isobaric and isotonic mode the computer program could adjust the separation distance of the wires (and hence the vessel diameter), by the use of the inchworm motor, such that calculated pressure (isobaric) or tension (isotonic) were held constant at the desired value. In this particular series of experiments responses to methoxamine (an α_1-adrenoceptor agonist) was assessed under the three different conditions (Fig. 2.4 shows a representative trace that was obtained). The most obvious difference observed was that the potency of methoxamine was slightly greater when recorded under isometric conditions and that the maximum

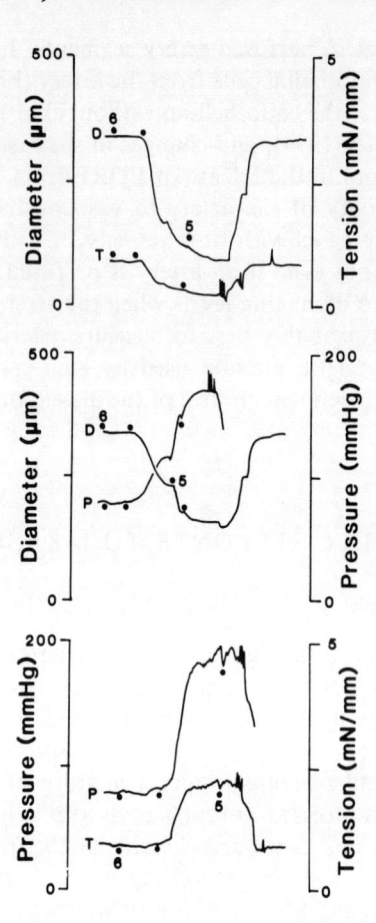

Fig. 2.4 Concentration–response curves for methoxamine in a wire-mounted rat mesenteric artery. Three separate curves were constructed with the artery held in either isotonic (*top*), isometric (*centre*), or isometric (*bottom*) conditions using a computer controlled micrometer. Under each condition the responses of the artery are expressed simultaneously as both of the other possible measurements. The concentration of methoxamine was increased cumulatively at each of the dots marked on the figure, with the concentrations indicated as −log Molar.

diameter change induced by methoxamine was greater under isobaric than under isotonic conditions. These result could be explained from the total and passive diameter–tension curves. Fig. 2.5 shows a typical set of diameter–tension curves obtained from the rat small mesenteric artery. When a vessel responds isometrically the diameter is held constant and on a plot of tension versus diameter the vessel would move from the passive tension–diameter curve to the active tension–diameter curve in a vertical direction. Under isotonic conditions, it would move horizontally along the tension–diameter curve such that tension remains constant. Under isobaric conditions, it would move down the pressure isobar such

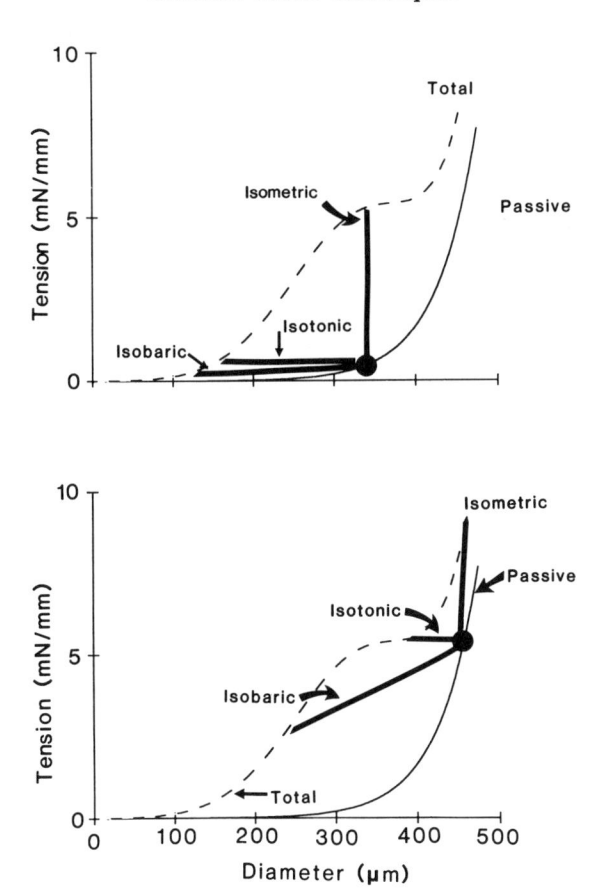

Fig. 2.5 Theoretical active and passive length–tension curves for wire-mounted arteries showing the expected changes in length and tension for arteries activated under isotonic, isometric, or isobaric conditions. See the text for a full explanation.

that pressure is held constant (Fig. 2.5). When starting at low passive tensions the two lines for isobaric and isotonic responses are almost superimposable however it is evident from Fig. 2.5 that the maximum diameter change possible under isobaric conditions will always be greater than when performed under isotonic conditions. When the passive tension is increased to relatively high value then this difference becomes more marked. In both cases this difference results from the non-linear relationship between the total and passive tension–diameter curves. From Fig. 2.5 we could predict that if pressures are increased high enough then a point is reached where responses recorded isotonically would be virtually absent while those recorded isobarically or isometrically would be maintained. While this phenomenon would only occur at relatively high passive pressures (> 140 mmHg, McPherson 1992), if the vessel is diseased or damaged then the expectation is that it may well occur closer to the blood pressure operating range of vessel.

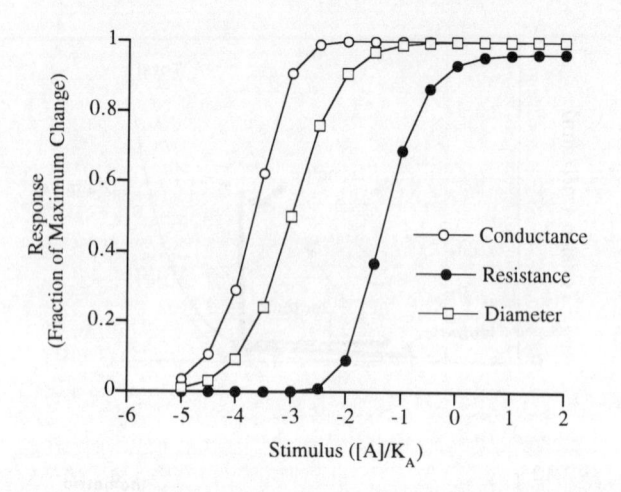

Fig. 2.6 Theoretical curves resistance–diameter and conductance–diameter curves for an artery constricted from diameter = 1 to diameter = 0.1.

Cannulated vessels

There are three sensible measurements of vascular responses can be made with perfused vessel segments: diameter, resistance, and conductance. Vessel diameter is measured directly, but resistance is usually measured as perfusion pressure with a fixed flow perfusion, and conductance would be measured as the flow rate with a fixed pressure perfusion or as a calculated reciprocal of resistance. Measurement of conductance is rarely (if ever) performed in *in vitro* experiments, although calculated vascular conductance has been very useful in some *in vivo* experiments. Although the three measurements are related by simple formula:

$$\text{conductance} = \text{resistance}^{-1} = \text{radius}^4 \times \text{constant}$$

they do not yield exactly the same information. Because of the fourth power of radius in the relationship, the conductance of a segment of artery will fall most steeply with the early diameter reductions in a vasoconstrictor concentration–response curve. Resistance will increase most steeply in the later responses (i.e. when the diameter has fallen to a low value) (Fig. 2.6). Thus for a vasoconstriction concentration–response curve when responses are scaled to a fraction of maximum, the concentration–conductance response curve will lie to the left of the concentration–resistance response curve, with the concentration–diameter curve in between (Fig. 2.7). For a vasodilator concentration–response curve, the relationship is reversed such that the resistance curve lies to the left of the conductance curve. Thus the sensitivity of the tissue to the agonist will depend on which measurement of response is used. The magnitude of the difference in sensitivity can be large, over two orders of magnitude for the example of an artery that has maximum and minimum internal diameters of 400 and 50 μm. The magnitude of the difference in sensitivity decreases as the range of diameter decreases.

Isolated tissue techniques

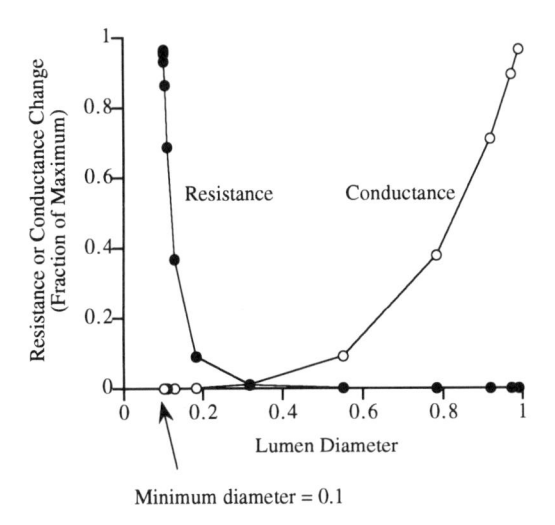

Fig. 2.7 Theoretical stimulus–response curves for an artery that contracts from diameter = 1 to diameter = 0.1. Responses were calculated as change in diameter, change in conductance, and change in resistance, and scaled as a fraction of the maximum change.

When the resistance of perfused artery segments is measured it is almost always measured indirectly as the perfusion pressure resulting from a constant perfusion flow rate. A major problem with such a system is that as the arterial lumen diameter approaches zero the perfusion pressure approaches infinity. For arteries such as rat tail and rabbit ear arteries that can constrict to spasm this means that a maximum response to a vasoconstrictor cannot be measured because the perfusion pressure builds to a level that breaks the wall of the artery. The failure appears as a sudden distension of the upstream end of the artery that gradually travels down the length of the arterial segment. An improved perfusion method that reduces this problem is described below.

METHODS

'Normalization' of initial conditions of wire-mounted arteries

If the wires have a diameter d and are separated from each others inner surface by s then the internal circumference of the vessel (L) is given by:

$$L = (\pi + 2) \cdot d + 2s. \tag{2.1}$$

From this the internal diameter of the vessel (D) can be calculated (see Fig. 2.8).

If g is the vessel length then the circumferential wall force (F) per unit length is the passive wall tension (T) which is given by:

$$T = F/2 \cdot g \tag{2.2}$$

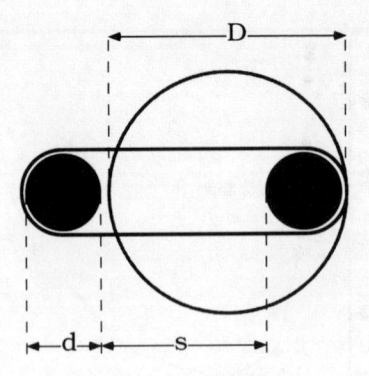

Fig. 2.8 Cross-sectional diagram of an artery mounted on wires in a myograph. Wire diameter is **d**, wire separation is **s**, and the equivalent diameter of the artery (i.e. the diameter of a circle with the same circumference as the stretched artery) is **D**.

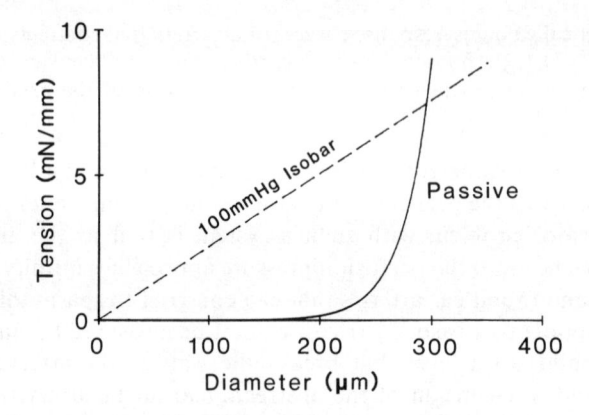

Fig. 2.9 Theoretical passive length–tension curve for a wire-mounted artery of diameter 300 μm at 100 mmHg distending pressure. The 100 mmHg isobar is indicated. The normalization routine for the arteries finds the (upper) intercept of these two lines.

For each step (i^{th}) in the normalization curve there is an estimate of the vessel diameter (D_i) and the corresponding wall tension generated (T_i). This data can be modelled to eqn (2.3):

$$T_i = A \cdot \text{Exp}\,(B \cdot D_i) \tag{2.3}$$

where A and B are the equation constants. Fig. 2.9 shows the theoretical form of this curve which is exponential. Eqn (2.3) can be solved simply by taking the logarithm of both sides of the equation, which allows linear regression to be used to calculate the values of A and B or, alternatively, non-linear curve-fitting programs (McPherson 1992), or even the iterative solving procedure of Microsoft® Excel (Solver) can be used to fit eqn (2.3) directly and thus avoids the need to transform the data.

The corresponding pressure at any point on the passive diameter–tension curve can be calculated using the Laplace equation:

$$P = T.D/2 \qquad (2.4)$$

where D is the vessel diameter, T is the passive tension, and P is the transmural pressure. Fig. 2.9 shows the form of eqn (2.4) (where P was given the value of 100 mmHg) superimposed on the diameter–tension curve. The point of intersection of the two lines gives the diameter where the vessel would experience a transmural pressure of 100 mmHg. An iterative procedure is used to calculate the point of intersection of the two lines described by eqn (2.3) and (2.4). Using other pressure isobars it was possible to calculate the equivalent transmural pressure (mmHg) for any given vessel diameter.

In practice this technique involves advancing the micrometer manually until the two mounting wires just touch, and a micrometer reading is taken. The wires are then separated using the micrometer in a stepwise fashion such that the changes in calculated transmural pressure are approximately 20 mmHg. The micrometer reading and the force (F) generated are noted at each point and the procedure repeated for approximately five steps corresponding to a total change in transmural pressure equivalent to approximately 100 mmHg. The passive diameter-tension curve is modelled and the point of intersection of the 100 mmHg pressure isobar calculated. From this the diameter at this pressure is calculated and the vessel set at 0.9 times this diameter. The use of some form of computer program greatly facilitates this normalization procedure (the authors use either a custom written stand-alone program or an Excel spreadsheet).

Constant pressure gradient perfusion

Independent control of the distending pressure and perfusion rate of small blood vessels can be conveniently achieved in doubly-cannulated preparations by attaching the upstream and downstream cannulae to elevated reservoirs of perfusate. The perfusion rate will be determined by the difference in elevation (i.e. hydrostatic head) of the two reservoirs and the total resistance of the blood vessel and the cannulae. If the resistance of both cannulae is the same then the pressure in the vessel will be the average of the hydrostatic heads of the upstream and downstream reservoirs. Thus it is simple to control the distending pressure by raising or lowering the reservoirs together, and to control the perfusion rate by raising one reservoir while lowering the other (Fig. 2.10).

Reducing effective dead space in a perfusion system

The effects of drugs on blood vessels can depend on whether they are applied to the lumen or to the abluminal surface of the vessel (de la Lande *et al.* 1967; Lew *et al.* 1989). It is therefore often of interest to apply drugs via the perfusate. With small vessels and low perfusion rates this can be made difficult by the dead space in the tubing from the pump to the artery. An arrangement that effectively

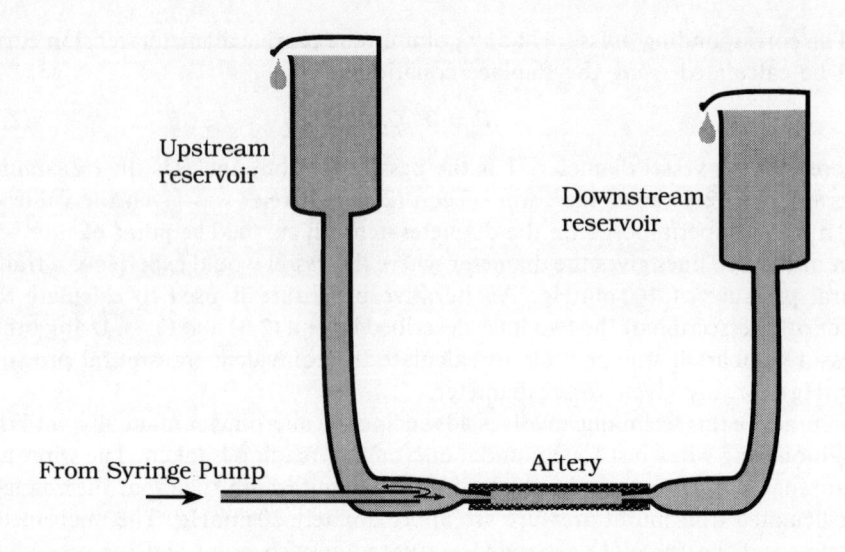

Fig. 2.10 Schematic diagram of a doubly-cannulated artery preparation where the distending pressure is determined by the average elevation of the upstream and downstream reservoirs, and the perfusion rate is a function of the difference in elevation of the two reservoirs. Also illustrated is a method of delivering perfusate to the artery with minimal effective dead space.

reduces the dead space is shown in Fig. 2.10. The tubing from the pump (which needs to be narrow compared to the lumen of the upstream cannula) is inserted into the upstream cannula such that the tube ends just short of the narrowing of the cannula. Perfusate is pumped into the upstream cannula at a high rate with most of the perfusate refluxing backwards through the upstream cannula to the upstream reservoir (where it drips to waste). A small fraction of the perfusate pumped into the system goes through the artery, and the high pump rate means that the tubing dead space doesn't lead to a long dead time. As long as the resistance of the tip of the upstream cannula is large compared to the resistance of the shank of the cannula and the tubing connecting it to the reservoir, a high pump rate can be used without significantly affecting the pressure or flow in the artery.

Improved constant flow perfusion method

Pump-perfused segments of rat tail or rabbit ear arteries are popular preparations in pharmacological experiments because they are quite sensitive to vasoconstrictor agonists, simple to set-up, and robust. However there is a major problem with such preparations: full concentration–response curves to vasoconstrictors cannot be constructed. These arteries can constrict sufficiently that the even with low perfusion rates the perfusion pressure becomes excessive with moderate activation of the arteries and can destroy the smooth muscle. To prevent this from happening,

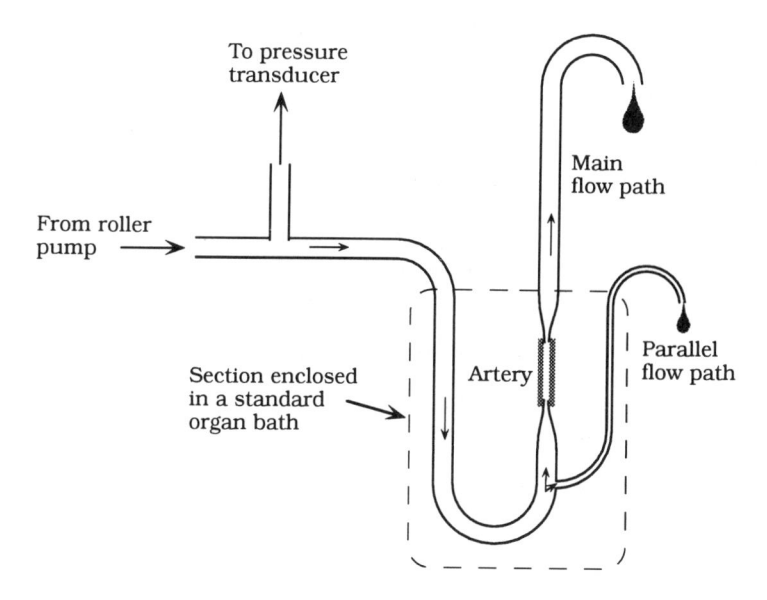

Fig. 2.11 Schematic diagram of an improved method for the perfused rat tail artery preparation. The initial pressure of the artery segment is determined by the height of the main outflow, and the perfusion pressure at maximal constriction (spasm) is determined by the resistance of the parallel outflow and the flow rate. The parallel outflow allows the tissue to be maximally activated without damage so that full concentration–response curves can be constructed.

it is normal practice with this preparation to work with only the bottom end of the concentration–response curve, and not attempt to attain a maximal constriction. This makes any changes in the maximal response of the tissue invisible, and also leads to a serious uncertainty in the position of the concentration–response curve.

This limitation can be overcome by the addition of a second flow pathway in parallel with the artery segment (Fig. 2.11). As the artery constricts flow is shunted through the parallel pathway, so the flow through the artery decreases. When the artery is totally closed, all of the flow goes through the parallel resistor, and the pressure is determined by the resistance of the parallel pathway. Thus it is possible to control the maximal pressure to which the artery is exposed by adjusting the resistance of the parallel pathway at the start of the experiment by diverting all of the flow through the parallel pathway and simply changing the length of the fine tubing until a manageable pressure (say 100 mmHg) results. This allows responses to be measured as changes in perfusion pressure without any problem of tissue damage by high pressure during maximal responses.

REFERENCES

Bevan, J. A. and Osher, J. V. (1972). A direct method for recording tension changes in the wall of small blood vessels *in vitro*. *Agents Actions*, **2**, 257–60.

Bouskela, E., Grampp, W., and Mellander, S. (1991). *In vivo* membrane potentials of smooth muscle cells in microvessels of the hamster cheek pouch. In *Resistance arteries: stucture and function*. (ed. M. J. Mulvany, C. Aalkjear, A. M. Heagerty, N. C. B. Nyborg, and S. Strandgaard). Exerpta Medica, Amsterdam.

Bryant, H. J., Harder, D. R., Pamnani, M. B., and Haddy, F. J. (1985). *In vivo* membrane potentials of smooth muscle cells in the caudal artery of the rat. *Am. J. Physiol.*, **18**, C78–83.

Clark, A. J. (1926). The reaction between acetylcholine and muscle cells. *J. Physiol. (Lond.)* **61**, 530–46.

de la Lande, I. S., Frewin, D., and Waterson, J. G. (1967). The influence of sympathetic innervation on vascular sensitivity to noradrenaline. *Br. J. Pharmacol. Chemother.*, **31**, 82–93.

Duling, B. R. and Rivers, R. J. (1986). Isolation, cannulation and perfusion of microvessels. In *Microcirculatory technology* (ed. Baker and Nastuk), pp. 265–80. Academic Press, New York.

Fry, D. L. (1968). Acute vascular endothelial changes associated with increased blood velocity gradients. *Circ. Res.*, **22**, 165–97.

Furchgott, R. F. and Zawadzki, J. V. (1980). The obligatory role of endothelial cells in the relaxation of arterial smooth muscle by acetylcholine. *Nature*, **288**, 373–6.

Harris, D. E. and Warshaw, D. M. (1991). Length versus active force relationship in single isolated smooth muscle cells. *Am. J. Physiol.*, **260**, C1104–12.

Herlihy, J. T. and Berardo, P. V. (1986). Effect of preload on rat aortic smooth muscle sensitivity to vasoactive agents. *Pharmacology*, **33**, 39–45.

Kuo, L., Davis, M. J., and Chillian, W. M. (1988). Myogenic activity in isolated subepicardial and and subendocardial coronary arteries. *Am. J. Physiol.*, **255**, H1558–62.

Kuo, L., Davis, M. J., and Chillian, W. M. (1990). Endothelium-dependent, flow-induced dilation of isolated coronary arterioles. *Am. J. Physiol.*, **259**, H1063–70.

Lew, M. J. and Angus, J. A. (1992). Wall thickness to lumen diameter ratios of arteries from SHR and WKY: comparison of pressurised and wire-mounted preparations. *J. Vasc. Res.*, **29**, 435–42.

Lew, M. J. and Madeley, L. J. (1994) The effect of high perfusion rates on the endothelial diffusion barrier in rat mesenteric arteries *in vitro*. *Clin. Exp. Pharmacol. Physiol.* **21**, 501–8.

Lew, M. J., Rivers, R. J., and Duling, B. R. (1989). Arteriolar smooth muscle responses are modulated by an intramural diffusion barrier. *Am. J. Physiol.*, **257**, H10–16.

McPherson, G. A. (1992). Optimal conditions for assessing vascular reactivity in small resistance arteries in the small vessel myograph. *Clin. Exp. Pharmacol. Physiol.*, **19**, 815–25.

Michelson, M. J. and Shelkovnikov, S. A. (1976). Isotonic and isometric responses of different agonists and antagonists. *Br. J. Pharmacol.* **56**, 457–67.

Mulvany, M. J. and Halpern, W. (1977). Contractile properties of small arterial resistance vessels in spontaneously hypertensive and normotensive rats. *Circ. Res.* **41**, 19–26.

Neild, T. O. (1989). Measurement of arteriole diameter changes by analysis of television images. *Blood Vessels*, **26**, 48–52.

Osol, G. and Halpern, W. (1985). Myogenic properties of cerebral blood vessels from normotensive and hypertensive rats. *Am. J. Physiol.*, **249**, H914–21.

Price, J. M., Davis, D. L., and Knauss, E. B. (1981). Length-dependent sensitivity in vascular smooth muscle. *Am. J. Physiol.*, **241**, H557–63.

Price, J. M., Davis, D. L., and Knauss, E. B. (1983). Length-dependent sensitivity at lengths greater than Lmax in vascular smooth muscle. *Am. J. Physiol.*, **245**, H379–84.

Sipkema, P., Hoogerwerf, N., and van der Linden, P. J. W. (1991). Perfusion of isolated small arteries: effects of flow and oxygen. In *Resistance arteries: stucture and function*. (ed. M. J. Mulvany, C. Aalkjear, A. M. Heagerty, N.C.B. Nyborg, and S. Strandgaard), pp. 347–52. Exerpta Medica, Amsterdam.

Tallarida, R. J., Sevy, R. W., Harkal, C., Bendrick, J., and Faust, R. (1974). The effect of preload on the dissociation constant of norepinephrine in isolated strips of rabbit thoracic aorta. *Arch. Int. Pharmacodyn. Ther.* **210**, 67–74.

van Bavel, Mooij, T., Giezeman, M. J. M M., and Spaan, J. A. E. (1990). Cannulation and continuous cross-sectional area measurement of small blood vessels. *J. Pharmacol. Methods*, **24**, 219–27.

Van Nueten, J. M. (1980). Comparison of isotonic and isometric measurements in isolated arterial tissues. In *Vascular neuroeffector mechanisms*. (J. A. Bevan, T. Godfraind, R. A. Maxwell, and P. M. Vanhoutte), pp. 37–9. Raven Press, New York.

3. Single cell techniques

Alison M. Gurney

INTRODUCTION

Blood vessel tone is mainly determined by the contractile activity of the smooth muscle cells of the medial layer, which are innervated by sympathetic neurones and are in close contact with endothelial cells lining the blood vessel wall. An increase in tone occurs when the smooth muscle cells contract in response to nerve stimulation, vasoconstrictor agents, such as noradrenaline, or to membrane depolarization. Vasodilators can relax vascular muscle by acting directly at the smooth muscle cells, by interfering with the release of neurotransmitter, or by causing the secretion of endothelium-derived factors on to the smooth muscle cells. Thus in intact vascular muscle preparations, studies of smooth muscle or endothelial cell function, and their responses to vasoactive substances, can be complicated by the presence of multiple cell types. By isolating single cells from the smooth muscle or endothelial layer of a blood vessel, it is possible to study signal transduction mechanisms in these cells without the need to worry about indirect effects resulting from actions on other cell types. Isolated cells also have the advantage of being more amenable to experimental techniques that can directly address questions relating to receptor mechanisms and intracellular pathways. This chapter reviews methods for isolating vascular cells and outlines techniques that are particularly well suited to single cell studies, namely voltage- and patch-clamp recording, measurement of intracellular ion concentrations, and photolysis of caged compounds. These techniques have been successfully applied to the study of endothelial and smooth muscle cell function. The aim here is to discuss the information that each technique can provide, along with their advantages and disadvantages. Technical information is kept to a minimum, because practical aspects to the application of these techniques have been covered in detail elsewhere. The reader is directed to Sakmann and Neher (1983), Ogden (1994), and Gurney (1990*a*) for detailed practical information on patch-clamp techniques. Several chapters have been published on the methodology of measuring Ca^{2+} with fluorescent probes (e.g. Gurney 1990*b*; Moreton 1991) including a book covering various aspects of Ca^{2+}-related techniques (McCormack and Cobbold 1991). Practical aspects of flash photolysis techniques are detailed in Gurney (1990*b*, 1991), while methods for the synthesis of caged compounds are given in Walker (1991).

Table 3.1 Blood vessels from which viable smooth muscle cells have been successfully dissociated — in each case relaxed cells were present at the end of the dissociation procedure

Blood vessel	Species	Reference
Aorta	Rat	Ives *et al.* 1978
Pulmonary artery	Rabbit	Okabe *et al.* 1987; Clapp and Gurney 1991
	Guinea-pig	Byrne and Large 1987
Carotid artery	Pig	Driska and Porter 1986
	Dog	Wadsworth *et al.* 1988
Coronary artery	Pig	Hirata *et al.* 1981; Katsuyama *et al.* 1991
	Cow	Van Dijk and Laird 1984
	Dog	Wilde and Lee 1989
Portal vein	Rat	Loirand *et al.* 1986
	Rabbit	Inoue *et al.* 1985; Byrne and Large 1988; Beech and Bolton 1989; Hume and Leblanc 1989
	Guinea-pig	Inoue *et al.* 1990
	Ferret	DeFeo and Morgan 1985a
	Cow	Klöckner and Isenberg 1989
Mesenteric artery	Rat	Bean *et al.* 1986; Langton *et al.* 1991
	Rabbit	Bolton *et al.* 1985; Worley *et al.* 1986; Terada *et al.* 1987; Langton *et al.* 1991
	Guinea-pig	Bolton *et al.* 1985; Benham *et al.* 1986; Ohya and Sperelakis 1989
	Human	Smirnov and Aaronson 1992
Femoral artery	Rat	Moody *et al.* 1990
Saphenous artery	Rabbit	Oike *et al.* 1992
Saphenous vein	Dog	Yatani *et al.* 1987
Ear artery	Rabbit	Benham and Bolton 1986; Droogmans *et al.* 1987
Basilar artery	Rat	Steele *et al.* 1991
	Rabbit	Worley *et al.* 1991
Pial vessels	Cow	Klöckner and Isenberg 1989

VASCULAR CELL ISOLATION

Smooth muscle cells

Smooth muscle cells have been isolated from a number of different blood vessels, some of which are listed in Table 3.1. The smooth muscle cells in a blood vessel are surrounded by extracellular connective tissue proteins such as elastin and collagen. Enzymes that break down that connective tissue are used to loosen the smooth muscle cells, so that they can be liberated by gentle trituration of the tissue. The literature contains descriptions of several methods for isolating vascular smooth muscle cells (Table 3.1), but all involve incubations for various times in enzyme solutions. Most methods use various combinations of collagenase and elastase, although some use papain, which has a broad substrate specificity, being able to hydrolyse a wide range of proteins. The usual approach is to subject small fragments of tissue to a series of incubations in enzyme solutions at 37 °C. Under these conditions the pieces of blood vessel are digested from the outside in. Thus cells from the outer regions of the tissue may become overdigested by the time the enzymes have reached deeper cells. For this reason dissociated cells need to be collected at regular intervals and the enzyme removed. The remaining tissue fragments are re-incubated for further periods in fresh enzyme solution until after the final incubation, when all of the harvested cells are washed and combined. These protocols can be quite time-consuming and the yield of viable, relaxed cells can be quite variable, as can their responsiveness to vasoactive substances. Furthermore, a cell isolation method worked out in one laboratory is often less successful when attempted in another. The reasons are not always clear, but variation in the quality of the water used to prepare solutions is often blamed. As a consequence individual laboratories have tended to develop their own procedures, and this is the main reason that so many varying methodologies exist.

In my laboratory, we have found that with relatively thin vessels, such as the rat mesenteric artery, a single 30 min incubation in a low concentration (0.25 mg/ml) of papain at 37 °C is sufficient to yield a high proportion of viable, relaxed smooth muscle cells (Fig. 3.1A), which survive storage in the refrigerator for many hours. Larger vessels, such as the rabbit pulmonary artery and aorta, yield viable cells after serial enzyme incubations, but not consistently. For this reason we set about developing a method for isolating smooth muscle cells from these arteries that would consistently yield a high proportion of relaxed, Ca^{2+}-tolerant cells. We also aimed to produce a method that would be less time-consuming than serial incubations. Our approach was to use papain (properties reviewed in Kimmel and Smith 1957), but to follow a completely different rationale, based on the fact that the proteolytic activity of papain is substantially slowed when the temperature is reduced to 5 °C. Thus by storing tissue in the presence of papain at 5 °C overnight, the enzyme might be expected to penetrate through the tissue, while causing little proteolysis. By the next morning the enzyme should be evenly distributed throughout the tissue, so that digestion should proceed quickly on warming the tissue to 37 °C. The lower enzyme concentrations and shorter 37 °C incubations required by this approach are known to result in relatively higher cell yields (Freshney 1987).

We designed the dissociation conditions to optimize the proteolytic activity of papain (Kimmel and Smith 1957) and protect the cells from damage. The dissociation medium (DM) has the following ionic composition (mM): NaCl, 110; KCl, 5; $MgCl_2$, 2; $CaCl_2$, 0.16; $NaHCO_3$, 10; KH_2PO_4, 0.5; NaH_2PO_4, 0.5; Hepes, 10; EDTA, 0.5; glucose, 10; taurine, 10. Bovine serum albumin (BSA; type V, essentially fatty acid-free, from Sigma Chemical Co., Poole, Dorset) is also added at a concentration of 0.02%. The BSA and taurine are thought to have protective effects on muscle cells during enzymatic dissociation (e.g. Isenberg and Klöckner 1982). Although cell dissociations are frequently carried

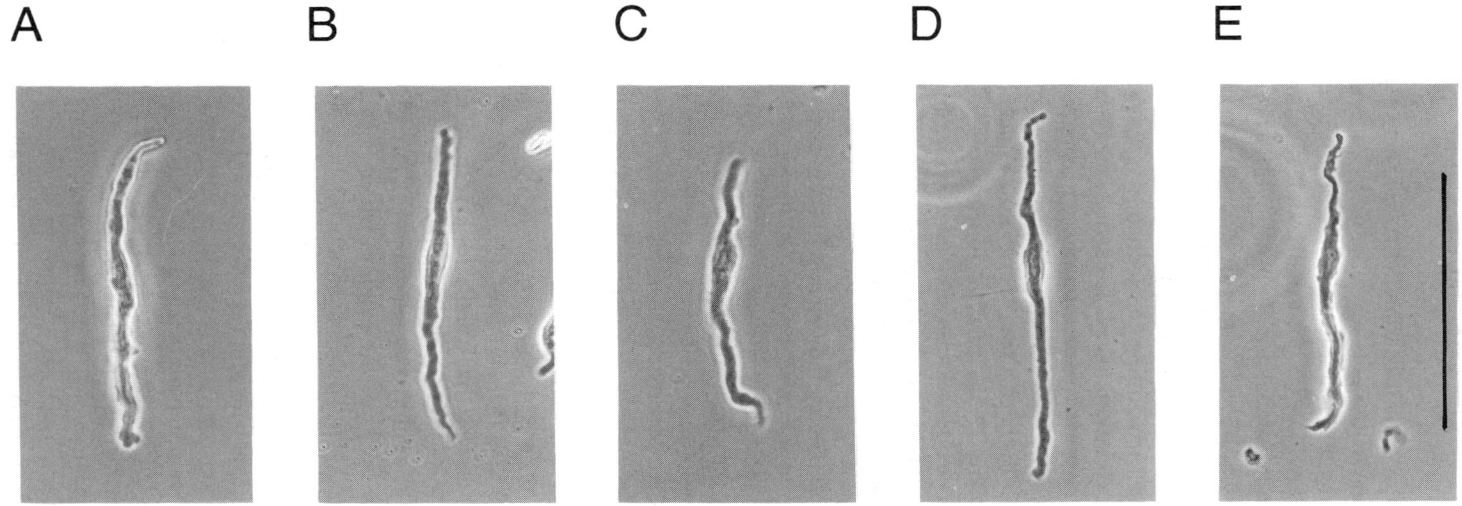

Fig. 3.1 Phase-contrast photomicrographs of smooth muscle cells isolated from rat mesenteric artery (A), rabbit mesenteric artery (B), rat aorta (C), rabbit aorta (D), and rabbit pulmonary artery (E). Cells in (A) and (B) were prepared according to the method outlined in the text, except that the overnight incubation at 5 °C was omitted and the 37 °C incubation was 30 min (A) or 40 min (B). The cells in (C), (D), and (E) were prepared as described in the text. The photographs, of freshly dissociated cells, were all taken on the same day. Calibration bar 100 μm.

out in Ca^{2+}-free media to help breakdown the connective tissues, this often results in Ca^{2+} overloading of the cells when the Ca^{2+} concentration is returned to normal at the end of the dissociation. In an attempt to prevent this, we keep the $CaCl_2$ concentration low, but do not usually omit it completely. Free sulfydryl groups on papain are essential for its proteolytic activity. Thus EDTA is added to mop up heavy metals, which bind to free sulfydryl groups and reduce enzyme activity. In addition, to maintain the sulfydryl groups in a reduced state, exposure of the papain to oxygen is minimized by pre-gassing the DM with a 95% air/5% CO_2 mixture, and then adding the reducing agent dithiothreitol (DTT) just prior to the 37 °C incubation, which is carried out at pH 7, the optimum for papain activity. We have used papain purchased from Sigma (type IV, 14.5 units/mg, Cat. No. P-4762) or Fluka Chemicals Ltd. (Glossop, Derbyshire; Cat. No. 76218, 12 units/ml). Both enzymes work at a concentration of 0.2–0.3 mg/ml, although the activity of the powder appears to gradually decline even when stored at -20 °C. The method has provided us with a high yield of isolated smooth muscle cells from rabbit and rat pulmonary arteries and aorta (Fig. 3.1). Furthermore, several (although not all) other laboratories have had success with this method.

The following procedure (Clapp and Gurney 1991) is used routinely for rabbit main pulmonary artery and aorta. The vessel is dissected from a rabbit killed by lethal injection of sodium pentobarbitone, and placed in normal physiological solution. After removing the connective tissue and adventitia, five or six strips (2–3 mm wide by ~ 10 mm long) are cut from the vessel and washed twice in DM without BSA or enzyme. The strips are then transferred into a 10 ml glass pot with an airtight lid, containing 5 ml of pre-gassed DM to which has been added 0.02% BSA and 0.25 mg/ml papain. After replacing the lid, the pot is put in the refrigerator (5 °C) and stored overnight (> 16 h). The next morning, DTT (10 μl of a 100 mM stock solution) is added directly to the pot containing the DM and tissue fragments, which is then incubated for 10 min at 37 °C. At the end of the incubation period, the muscle strips usually look rather feathery and tend to clump together. They are transferred to 2 ml fresh, gassed DM and triturated gently with a wide bore (2–3 mm) Pasteur pipette. Once a few long, relaxed, single cells can be seen in drops of the solution when viewed through a microscope, trituration is stopped. The solution containing clumps of tissue along with the isolated cells is made up to 5 ml with fresh DM, and is then stored in the refrigerator until required. Further trituration yields more cells when they are needed. Cells prepared in this way often remain viable for more than 24 hours.

This enzymatic dispersion consistently yields > 70% relaxed smooth muscle cells, with the length of rabbit pulmonary artery cells typically ranging from 60–120 μm with diameters from 5–12 μm (Clapp and Gurney 1991). A high proportion of the cells usually contract to noradrenaline (NA), adenosine 5′-triphosphate (ATP), and high K^+ concentrations. When measured in current clamp with the whole-cell patch-clamp technique, under close to normal physiological conditions, rabbit pulmonary artery smooth muscle cells have an average resting potential of -55 mV (Clapp and Gurney 1992) and an input resistance of 17 GΩ

(Clapp and Gurney 1991, 1992). These are close to the values expected from measurements made on smooth muscle cells in intact blood vessels (Casteels *et al.* 1977; Hirst and Edwards 1989). Thus the cells appear to retain their basic pharmacological, contractile, and electrophysiological properties following the dissociation procedure.

Endothelial cells

Studies of endothelial cell function have mostly employed cultured cells, which can be passaged and subcultured several times. However, freshly dissociated cells have been prepared from the endothelium of rabbit aorta (Sakai 1990; Rusko *et al.* 1992) and bovine capillaries (Bossu *et al.* 1989, 1992). The method used to isolate endothelial cells from rabbit aorta involves stripping thin sheets of endothelium from an opened vessel and incubating them in papain with DTT for 35 min at 37 °C. Cells isolated in this way retain their responsiveness to endothelium-dependent vasodilators, such as bradykinin, acetylcholine, and ATP (Sakai 1990; Rusko *et al.* 1992). The capillary endothelial cells were obtained from dispersed bovine adrenal glands by differential plating. When the dispersed adrenal cells were plated out into plastic Petri dishes, the endothelial cells adhered to the bottom surface within 3–5 h, and before other cell types, which could then be removed. The endothelial cells retained their ability to respond to K^+-induced depolarization.

ELECTROPHYSIOLOGY OF VASCULAR CELLS

Voltage-clamp

Much of our understanding of the pathways contributing to tension generation by vascular smooth muscle and the actions of vasoactive agents, has been derived from electrophysiological recordings of membrane activity in intact blood vessels. Impaling individual smooth muscle cells with a microelectrode enabled the membrane potential to be recorded, and this showed that electrical events are frequently correlated with mechanical events (reviewed in Kuriyama *et al.* 1982). To measure the membrane conductances giving rise to these activities, the membrane potential has to be controlled, since any change in current causes the membrane potential to change. This is achieved using the voltage-clamp technique, which employs a feedback amplifier to force the membrane to a chosen voltage, while recording ion flow as an electric current. Voltage-clamp separates the ionic currents flowing through the membrane from capacitive currents, which flow only when the membrane potential is changing.

In voltage-clamp experiments, the membrane voltage is usually forced to change in a step-like fashion, with the result that capacitive current flows only briefly at the onset of the step. Once the voltage is steady, there is only the ionic current, carried through membrane channels or electrogenic transport systems.

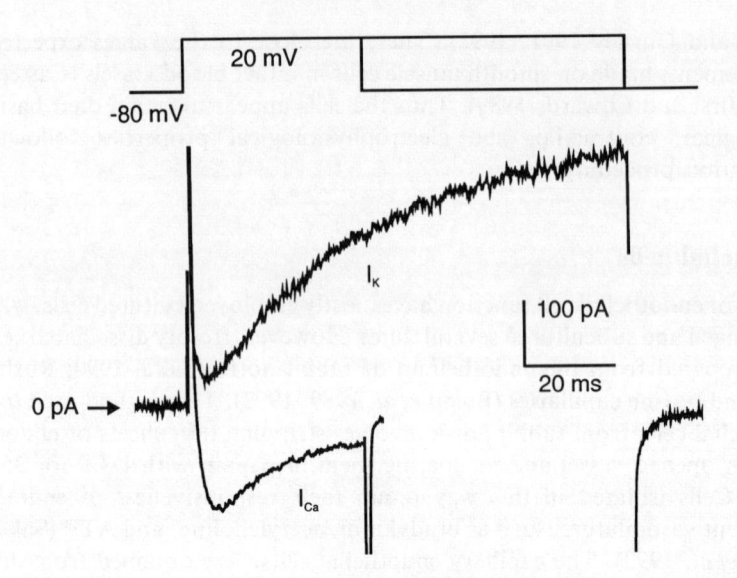

Fig. 3.2 Inward Ca^{2+} current (I_{Ca}) and outward K^+ current (I_K) recorded from isolated rabbit pulmonary arterial smooth muscle cells. Records from two separate cells, obtained using the whole-cell, patch-clamp technique have been superimposed. The extracellular Ca^{2+} concentration was 20 mM in both cases but the pipette contained Cs^+ as the main intracellular cation for I_{Ca}, while K^+ was used for I_K. The voltage protocols used are illustrated above the current traces.

Many ion channels open and close in a voltage-dependent manner, so step changes in membrane voltage result in time-dependent increases or decreases in the current flowing through these channels as the proportion of open channels relaxes to a new equilibrium. The contributions from particular ion channels can be distinguished from the kinetics and voltage dependence of the currents they give rise to, as well as from their relative permeabilities to different ions. Thus a depolarizing voltage step applied to a vascular smooth muscle cell opens voltage-gated Ca and K channels, which respectively give rise to a transient inward current and transient or delayed outward currents (Fig. 3.2).

There are clear advantages to applying voltage-clamp techniques to intact vascular preparations as opposed to isolated cells. In particular, it is only in intact preparations that excitatory junction currents (e.j.cs), arising from sympathetic nerve stimulation, can be studied. Although e.j.cs have been recorded under voltage-clamp (Finkel *et al.* 1984), there are many difficulties associated with the technique. Voltage control needs to be accurate and fast and uniform over the area of membrane containing the ion channels through which the current flows. This is difficult to achieve in intact vascular preparations, because smooth muscle cells are electrically coupled to their neighbours through gap junctions, forming a functional syncytium. Current injected into one smooth muscle cell flows through gap junctions into neighbouring cells. As the current (and the induced potential) spreads, its amplitude declines because some of the current flows out across cell membranes on the way. The length constant of vascular muscle, or the distance over which an electrotonic potential decays to about one-third of its value at the site of current injection, is around 1-1.5 mm (reviewed in Hirst and Edwards 1989). Thus, preparations as short as 1 mm would not be uniformly clamped, and current records would be distorted by channel activity in unclamped regions of the tissue. It has proved feasible to voltage-clamp short (200 μm) preparations of arterioles using a single microelectrode (Finkel *et al.* 1984; Hirst *et al.* 1986). However, due to the syncytial nature of the muscle, the capacitive currents lasted 20 ms, which is long enough to overlap with the activation of many ionic channels.

Voltage-clamp of intact vascular preparations has mostly employed sucrose gap techniques, whereby a section of muscle is electrically isolated by immersing it in isotonic sucrose. The sucrose, which has a high resistance, fills the extracellular spaces and prevents current from flowing out of the cells. This forms a conduction gap, and current originating on one side of the sucrose gap can only reach the other side by flowing through the interior of the tissue. In the double sucrose gap, a strip of tissue is placed across five chambers. The central chamber is perfused with physiological solution, with those on either side of it filled with sucrose, such that a conducting 'node' is isolated between the two sucrose pools. The solutions in the end chambers contain a high concentration of K^+ to depolarize the cut ends of the tissue and mimic intracellular solution. The membrane potential is estimated from the potential difference recorded between the node and an end chamber and the membrane in the node region is voltage-clamped by injecting current on either side of the node (at an end chamber). The current crosses the sucrose gap to the node by flowing through the interior of the tissue.

Fifteen years ago, sucrose gap was the main provider of information regarding the ionic conductances in vascular smooth muscle. Nevertheless, there was always uncertainty in the interpretation of the data, due partly to the multicellular nature of the tissue, but mainly to problems with voltage control. The width of the node is critical. Bolton (1975) found that for smooth muscle a width of less than 0.15 mm was necessary to achieve voltage uniformity during inward current flow, but with such a narrow node, non-uniformities arising in the boundary regions between the sucrose and the physiological solution contributed significantly to the signal. A further problem arises as a result of the narrow crevices that separate smooth muscle cells in intact blood vessels, which can restrict free diffusion of ions, resulting in ion accumulation particularly when currents are large. This results in a difference between the ionic composition in the extracellular spaces and the solution bathing the tissue, which can generate sufficiently large extracellular potentials to interfere with voltage control.

It was mainly the problems associated with voltage clamping intact tissue that highlighted the need to develop methods for isolating vascular smooth muscle cells. Another stimulus was the introduction of patch-clamp techniques, which required a 'clean' membrane and could be applied to small or fragile cells, such as smooth muscle or endothelial cells, that are poorly suited to impalement with microelectrodes. Only a few (e.g. Byrne and Large 1988) voltage-clamp studies have been carried out on isolated vascular cells using microelectrodes. Most have employed the patch-clamp technique.

Patch-clamp

The patch-clamp technique provides the only realistic way of voltage-clamping endothelial cells, which are extremely thin and difficult to impale with a microelectrode without causing significant damage. For similar reasons, the technique is much simpler to apply to isolated smooth muscle cells than microelectrode techniques. In addition, patch-clamp is the only technique that can resolve current flow through an individual channel, allowing the behaviour of single ion channels to be observed directly. The method was introduced by Neher and Sakmann (1976) to resolve the current passing through individual acetylcholine-activated ion channels. A small patch of membrane on an enzymatically cleaned frog muscle fibre was electrically isolated by pressing the tip of a glass micropipette against it. Current flowing through open channels in the patch of membrane flowed into the pipette and could be recorded with a low noise, high gain amplifier. It was subsequently found that if the pipette tip was first heat polished, applying suction to the interior of the pipette after it made contact with the fibre resulted in very high resistance (> 10 GΩ) seals, giving improved current resolution (Hamill et al. 1981). Further developments led to techniques for recording channel activity in excised membrane patches and for high-resolution recording of macroscopic (whole-cell) currents (Hamill et al. 1981).

The mechanical stability of the tight membrane–pipette seal means that if the pipette is withdrawn from the cell the seal remains intact, but the membrane patch containing the channel is excised with its cytoplasmic face exposed to the extracellular solution. Such a patch is referred to as 'inside out' and can be used to study the effects of cytoplasmic constituents on channel activity. Other configurations are also possible (see Fig. 3.3). After obtaining a pipette–membrane seal, the membrane under the pipette tip can be ruptured to form a low resistance pathway between the interiors of the cell and pipette. This configuration is known as 'whole-cell', because it enables current recording from channels in the entire cell membrane. Once the whole-cell configuration has been established, the pipette can be withdrawn slowly from the cell. This stretches the membrane between the pipette and the cell until it finally breaks. The membrane on the pipette then reseals to form a patch with its extracellular surface facing the bathing medium. This is known as an 'outside-out' patch, and can be used to study the effects on channels of agents that act from the extracellular surface.

Whole-cell recording

The whole-cell configuration allows electrical activity to be recorded from intact cells under voltage-clamp or current-clamp conditions. It can provide meaningful measurements of the kinetics and amplitudes of ionic currents provided the access resistance of the pipette tip is low relative to the input resistance of the cell, the

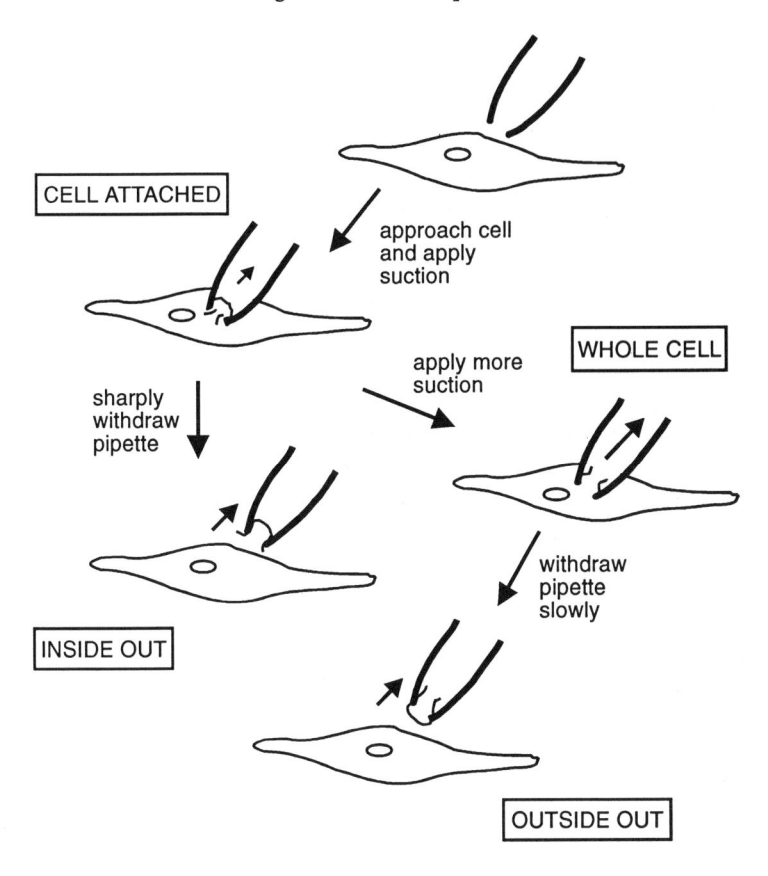

Fig. 3.3 Patch-clamp configurations and how to obtain them.

cell has a low capacitance and surface area, and the recorded currents have a small amplitude. It is possible to record from endothelial and smooth muscle cells with pipette resistances as low as 2–3 MΩ. Endothelial cells are ideally suited, since they tend to be oval or round in shape with diameters around 20 μm (Bossu *et al.* 1989; Rusko *et al.* 1992) and capacitance only 15 pF (Rusko *et al.* 1992). Most vascular muscle cells have a high input resistance, with values over 10 GΩ frequently reported. However, they are not the ideal shape for voltage-clamp. When relaxed, they are long and thin, with lengths of up to 200 μm reported for rabbit portal vein (Hume and Leblanc 1989) and human mesenteric artery (Smirnov and Aaronson 1992). Klöckner and Isenberg (1985) investigated the spatial control of voltage in bladder smooth muscle cells, which have similar dimensions and electrophysiological properties to vascular muscle cells, by measuring voltage simultaneously at both ends of a cell using two patch pipettes in the whole-cell mode. They found that membrane voltage was sufficiently homogeneous to permit inward currents as large as 1 nA to be accurately recorded. Although vascular cells have not been investigated so directly, theoretical considerations suggest that they are likely to be isopotential even during the flow of inward currents (Bolton *et al.* 1985; Toro *et al.* 1986), which rarely exceed 1 nA. Non-uniformities could however arise with larger currents. The main error in whole-cell voltage-clamp measurements results from the resistances in series with the membrane, which include the pipette resistance. In a series of recordings from rabbit pulmonary arterial smooth muscle cells using 3–7 MΩ pipettes, series resistance was found to average 13 MΩ (Clapp and Gurney 1991). This would result in a voltage error of 13 mV between the measured voltage and the actual membrane potential when recording a 1 nA current, and would be greater with larger currents. Although up to 90% of the series resistance can usually be compensated for electronically, it is a problem because it tends to fluctuate during experiments.

An advantage of the whole-cell configuration is that it allows control of the internal solution of the cell. The pipettes used for patch-clamp have a relatively large bore, so the contents of the cell and pipette are fairly readily exchanged (Pusch and Neher 1988). This property is exploited to gain more effective separation of individual ionic currents than can be achieved with other methods for recording macroscopic currents. It is common practice to fill pipettes with solutions rich in Cs^+ and free of K^+ when studying inward membrane currents; this provides a more complete block of outward K^+ currents than extracellularly applied drugs such as tetraethylammonium ions (see Klöckner and Isenberg 1985). The ready diffusion of pipette constituents into a cell is also frequently exploited to modify the intracellular concentration of putative second messengers. In this way their influence on channel function can be investigated directly. Perfusion systems have been developed that enable the exchange of solutions during an experiment, although it usually takes several minutes for complete exchange to occur (Soejima and Noma 1984). Alternatively fluorescent and/or photolabile probes can be incorporated to facilitate studies of intracellular pathways as described below.

Important constituents may also be lost from the cell during whole-cell recording, although small ions will be lost more quickly than larger molecules (Pusch and Neher 1988). The properties of some currents have been found to change as a result of washing out of cell constituents. For example Ca^{2+} (Ohya and Sperelakis 1989) and K^+ (Clapp and Gurney 1992) currents in arterial smooth muscle cells show a dependence on the intracellular ATP concentration, such that the amplitudes of these currents change with time following the washout of ATP from the cell. This can be prevented by including ATP in the solution filling the patch pipette. Receptor–channel coupling can also be disrupted. For example, when whole-cell recording is used, the noradrenaline-induced increase in membrane conductance is only seen in a few vascular smooth muscle cells, and cells usually respond only to the first noradrenaline application (Amédée *et al.* 1990*a*). This problem can be overcome using the perforated patch technique developed by Horn and Marty (1988), with which it is possible to obtain consistent responses (Amédée *et al.* 1990*b*). This method uses the anti-fungal drugs nystatin or amphotericin to puncture small holes in the membrane patch, rather than using suction to completely disrupt the patch. The perforations are large enough to enable electrical contact between the pipette and the cell (although the series resistance can be higher than with complete patch rupture), but they are small enough to prevent all but small ions from exchanging between the pipette and cell.

Single-channel recording

Single-channel recording from isolated membrane patches allows the conductance of a channel to be measured directly. It can also provide more detailed information on the permeability and kinetic behaviour of channels than can be obtained from macroscopic currents. The technique is particularly helpful in establishing the mechanisms of coupling between membrane receptors and channels. If a receptor is directly coupled to the channel, and does not require a diffusible second messenger to activate the channel, then in 'cell attached' or 'inside out' membrane patches, channel openings should be observed when the agonist is present in the patch pipette. If a diffusible second messenger is required for channel activation, then it should be possible to open channels isolated in a 'cell attached' patch when the agonist is applied in the solution bathing the rest of the cell. This kind of approach was taken to study the mechanism by which extracellularly applied ATP activates a Na^+ and Ca^{2+} permeable channel in arterial smooth muscle (Benham and Tsien 1987). ATP was found to activate channels in excised membrane patches of rabbit ear artery smooth muscle cells when it was applied to the extracellular surface of the membrane. This implies that the receptor and channel must be tightly coupled, although it does not mean that the receptor and channel are the same protein as in the case of nicotinic acetylcholine receptors. Muscarinic receptors in the heart are known to be coupled to K^+ channels through an intermediate GTP-binding protein, but acetylcholine can directly activate these channels in excised patches of cardiac cell membrane provided GTP is present at the cytoplasmic surface (Kurachi *et al.* 1986). It is not yet known if the channels coupled to ATP receptors in arterial muscle are additionally coupled to other receptors, such as α-adrenoceptors, which also gate an inward current carried by Na^+ and Ca^{2+} (Amédée *et al.* 1990*a*; Wang and Large 1991). Recent cloning studies suggest they are not (Valera *et al.* 1994).

Single-channel studies permit identification of distinct channel subtypes. For example, the smooth muscle of rabbit portal vein contains at least two Ca^{2+}-activated K channels, with similar sensitivities to cytoplasmic Ca^{2+} and voltage (Inoue *et al.* 1985). The macroscopic currents contributed by these channels would not be readily separated, but at the single-channel level they are clearly distinguishable, because one has a fivefold higher conductance than the other. There are clear advantages to studying channels in cell-free membrane patches. The solutions on both sides of the membrane can be controlled, making it easier to isolate the channel of interest. For example, the Ca^{2+} concentration in the intracellular solution can be strongly buffered to prevent opening of Ca^{2+}-activated K channels when other K channels are to be investigated. Furthermore, the solution on the side of the membrane exposed to the bath can be changed during an experiment, enabling the concentration dependence of a drug effect to be studied.

There are also drawbacks to studying channel activity in membrane patches. Channel properties may be altered in excised patches as a result of removing intracellular constituents. To resolve single Ca channel currents, a high concentration of Ba^{2+} is required. However, the sensitivity to dihydropyridine Ca antagonists and the voltage sensitivity of channel kinetics is altered under these conditions (Aaronson et al. 1988). Caution should thus be taken in relating single-channel data to the intact blood vessel. The profusion of different K channels, identified from single-channel studies as being sensitive to hyperpolarizing vasodilators like levcromakalim (reviewed in Clapp and Gurney 1993), may even have hindered our understanding of the channel responsible for the drugs' actions. In most cases, no attempt was made to determine if any of these channels could give rise to membrane hyperpolarization and tissue relaxation. Whole-cell recording in conjunction with studies on vascular muscle tension have now shown that the channel mediating hyperpolarization is sensitive to the intracellular ATP concentration (Clapp and Gurney 1992, 1993; Clapp et al. 1993; Noack et al. 1992; Silberberg and van Breemen 1992), but is not Ca^{2+} activated (Clapp and Gurney 1993; Clapp et al. 1993). Fluctuation analysis of whole-cell records has further indicated that the channel has a low conductance and is present at low density in vascular cells (Noack et al. 1992; Clapp et al. 1994). The important channel would therefore be difficult to detect with single-channel recording.

In furthering our understanding of vascular muscle pharmacology, whole-cell and single-channel recording are powerful techniques. However, neither technique can answer all the problems on its own. The most useful information can be obtained when these techniques are used in combination, and in parallel with other approaches.

MEASUREMENT OF INTRACELLULAR ION CONCENTRATIONS

A rise in the intracellular concentration of ionized Ca^{2+} is the trigger in endothelial cells for secretion and in smooth muscle cells for contraction. It is therefore important to understand how the concentration of Ca^{2+} is regulated in these cells, and how it is correlated with function. Simultaneous monitoring of the intracellular Ca^{2+} concentration ($[Ca^{2+}]_i$) and tension development in vascular muscle strips was achieved ten years ago, using the luminescent photoprotein aequorin, which was incorporated into the smooth muscle cells by reversible permeabilization (Morgan and Morgan 1982). Aequorin emits blue light when it comes into contact with Ca^{2+}, the luminescence intensity increasing as a function of the Ca^{2+} concentration. Thus when a tissue was stimulated to contract, an increase in luminescence was detected, which preceded the development of tension. These experiments revealed an unexpected relationship between $[Ca^{2+}]_i$ and tension (De Feo and Morgan 1985b), which was later confirmed using the newer $[Ca^{2+}]_i$ indicator fura-2 (see Karaki 1989). Tension is not linearly related to the smooth muscle $[Ca^{2+}]_i$, rather the relationship depends on the nature of the contractile stimulus. When the smooth muscle was depolarized by raising the extracellular K^+ concentration, a sustained elevation of both $[Ca^{2+}]_i$ and tension was observed. However, when phenylephrine was applied to activate α-adrenergic receptors, an initial increase in $[Ca^{2+}]_i$ and tension was followed by a decline in the $[Ca^{2+}]_i$ while tension was sustained. Thus for a given $[Ca^{2+}]_i$, phenylephrine generated more tension than K^+, leading to the conclusion that α-adrenergic stimulation increases the sensitivity of the contractile apparatus to Ca^{2+} (DeFeo and Morgan 1985b). These findings highlight the need to directly measure $[Ca^{2+}]_i$ to determine how it is regulated.

Monitoring $[Ca^{2+}]_i$ in intact tissues has the advantage that it permits $[Ca^{2+}]_i$ and tension to be correlated. Nevertheless, the application of $[Ca^{2+}]_i$ indicators in intact tissues is associated with a number of problems. For example, more than one cell type may contribute to the $[Ca^{2+}]_i$ signal, including cells that may have become damaged during the loading procedure, and the indicator may not be evenly distributed throughout the tissue or be restricted to cytoplasm. In addition, drugs applied to the muscle would not reach all cells simultaneously and the cells would not respond synchronously. Thus subtle patterns in the Ca^{2+} signal from the individual cells would be lost in the time averaged signal from the entire preparation. Aequorin suffers from the added disadvantage that each molecule emits light only once, so that the photoprotein may be gradually consumed during sustained tension and elevations in $[Ca^{2+}]_i$. Still, these difficulties are unlikely to account for the complex $[Ca^{2+}]_i$-force relationship observed in intact vascular muscle strips, because a non-linear Ca^{2+} sensitivity of contractile proteins has also been noted in individual gastric smooth muscle cells, from which force and $[Ca^{2+}]_i$ could be simultaneously measured (Yagi et al. 1988).

There are clear advantages to measuring $[Ca^{2+}]_i$ in isolated cells. Apart from avoiding some of the problems described above, it is the only way in which a spatial image of the subcellular distribution of Ca^{2+} can be obtained (Williams et al. 1985). Furthermore, the medium surrounding isolated cells is easily controlled. In particular, extracellular Ca^{2+} is rapidly depleted on bathing the cells with a Ca^{2+}-free solution, allowing the relative contributions of intracellular and extracellular Ca^{2+} to pharmacological responses to be determined with greater certainty. Aequorin is poorly suited to isolated vascular cells, since the signal it would generate from a single cell would be too small to be accurately detected (Cobbold and Lee 1991). The measurement of $[Ca^{2+}]_i$ in isolated vascular cells became practical with the introduction of fluorescent $[Ca^{2+}]$ indicators (Tsien et al. 1982), which have an improved signal-to-noise ratio and are easier to use than photoproteins. The fluorescent indicators can be loaded into cells in a non-disruptive way, using membrane permeant precursors (acetoxymethyl esters) that are cleaved by intracellular enzymes to release the free indicator. The probes can be loaded in this way into intact tissues and isolated cells, enabling $[Ca^{2+}]_i$ to be measured in individual, unperturbed cells. However, when incorporated in this way, the indicator can become compartmentalized into subcellular organelles (Williams et al. 1985) and fluorescence from partially hydrolysed forms of the dye (Scanlon et al. 1987) can complicate calibration of the signal. The preferred free acid form of the indicator can be microinjected, or when used in combination with patch-clamp techniques it is introduced into the cell under study by including it in the solution filling the patch recording pipette. In the whole-cell configuration, the molecule will diffuse passively into the cell, so in theory, after equilibration, the indicator concentration is known. Quin-2 (Tsien et al. 1982), the first fluorescent probe to be introduced, was soon followed by the improved indicators fura-2 and indo-1 (Grynkiewicz et al. 1985) and more recently by a variety of new indicators (Haughland 1992), including fluo-3 and rhod-2 (Minta et al. 1989). These indicators are all based on the same chemistry but with structural modifications that influence their properties. They are all well suited to measuring $[Ca^{2+}]$ in the physiological concentration range; they show high selectivity for Ca^{2+} over Mg^{2+} and are little influenced by pH.

The available probes differ mainly in their excitation and emission spectra and the effect that Ca^{2+} binding has on these spectra. For example, quin-2, fura-2, and indo-1 fluorescence display excitation maxima around 350 nm, compared with 500 nm for fluo-3 and rhod-2 (Minta et al. 1989). The latter two indicators can be used with long wavelength excitation sources, and are suitable for confocal fluorescence microscopy using visible light lasers. Excitation of the former probes requires wavelengths that are too short to be transmitted by the usual optics in epifluorescence microscopes, which often need to be upgraded for single cell measurements. In addition, autofluorescence from cells contributes more at the shorter excitation wavelengths. The effect of Ca^{2+} binding to quin-2, fluo-3, or rhod-2, is to enhance their fluorescence intensities with no clear change in their excitation or emission spectra, so $[Ca^{2+}]$ is measured from the fluorescence emitted at a single wavelength in response to excitation at a single wavelength. In contrast, Ca^{2+} binding shifts the excitation spectrum of fura-2 and the emission spectrum of indo-1 to shorter wavelengths. With these probes a measure of $[Ca^{2+}]$ can be obtained from the ratio of fluorescence at the two excitation (fura-2) or emission (indo-1) maxima. This is advantageous, because ratios provide a more sensitive indicator of $[Ca^{2+}]$ than single wavelength measurements; they amplify the fluorescence signal and are simply related to the proportion of the indicator that is bound by Ca^{2+}. Unlike single wavelength measurements, dual wavelength ratios are not sensitive to variations of the indicator concentration in the cell or the optical path length through the cell. This is important when making measurements from muscle cells, which by their nature change shape, and hence thickness, in response to variations in $[Ca^{2+}]_i$. Fura-2 is widely used as a $[Ca^{2+}]_i$ probe in vascular muscle, both in intact tissue and in isolated cells. It is currently the indicator of choice for spatial imaging of $[Ca^{2+}]_i$ in single cells (e.g. Williams et al. 1985, 1987; Papageorgiou and Morgan 1990).

Using fluorescent indicators, the resting level of Ca^{2+} in freshly isolated vascular smooth muscle cells has been estimated at around 120 nM (e.g. De Feo and Morgan 1986; Sumimoto and Kuriyama 1986; Papageorgiou and Morgan 1990; Katsuyama et al. 1991), which is close to values estimated from intact muscle strips (e.g. De Feo and Morgan 1986). The tension induced by many vasoconstrictor agents has long been known to result from a combination of Ca^{2+} influx across the plasma membrane and mobilization of intracellular stores of Ca^{2+} (Bolton 1979). In isolated cells, $[Ca^{2+}]_i$ can rise to $1\,\mu M$ in response to stimulation with noradrenaline, although the response to this and a variety of other agonists is biphasic (e.g. De Feo and Morgan 1986; Sumimoto and Kuriyama 1986; Katsuyama et al. 1991; Pacaud et al. 1992). The initial elevation of $[Ca^{2+}]_i$ is transient, and because it is little affected by removing extracellular Ca^{2+}, it is thought to originate from intracellular stores. The second phase is characterized by a sustained elevation of $[Ca^{2+}]_i$ above the resting level, which is blocked upon removal of extracellular Ca^{2+}, and is therefore due to Ca^{2+} influx. The $[Ca^{2+}]_i$ rise caused by stimulation with high K^+ is due entirely to Ca^{2+} influx and is blocked by removing extracellular Ca^{2+}. Endothelial cells show a similar biphasic $[Ca^{2+}]_i$ response to receptor stimulation, with agents that induce the release of endothelium-derived factors (reviewed in Rusko et al. 1992). Again these two phases result from a transient release of Ca^{2+} from intracellular stores, followed by sustained Ca^{2+} entry.

Single cell $[Ca^{2+}]_i$ measurements can be combined with whole-cell patch-clamp recording. The preferred indicator in this case is indo-1, because $[Ca^{2+}]$ is reported by the ratio of fluorescence emitted at two wavelengths, which can be measured simultaneously and hence with greater time resolution than fura-2. Benham (1989) used this approach to show that ATP-activated ion channels gate Ca^{2+} entry in smooth muscle cells isolated from rabbit ear artery. ATP was shown to induce an inward current, but this was only associated with a rise in $[Ca^{2+}]_i$ if the extracellular solution contained Ca^{2+}. This suggested that the action of ATP on vascular smooth muscle cells was twofold: it activates an inward current which would depolarize the cells while at the same time admitting sufficient Ca^{2+} to significantly raise the intracellular $[Ca^{2+}]$. Combined $[Ca^{2+}]_i$ and patch-clamp measurements have also been used to examine the nature of the channels giving rise to the maintained elevation of $[Ca^{2+}]_i$ induced by noradrenaline in portal vein smooth muscle cells (Pacaud et al. 1992).

Perhaps the most powerful technique for studying Ca^{2+} homeostasis and $[Ca^{2+}]_i$ responses to pharmacological agents in vascular cells is fluorescence imaging, which allows the spatial and temporal distribution of $[Ca^{2+}]$ in a cell to be resolved. Imaging can be done with an epifluorescence microscope, equipped with a sensitive video camera and computer-linked image processor to digitize and process the video images. In the processed image, variations in the $[Ca^{2+}]$ are represented as variations in brightness. The main limitation on spacial resolution ($1-2\,\mu m$) is the fluorescence in parts of the cell that are above or below the focal plane, but contribute to the fluorescence detected. In confocal microscopy (Fine et al. 1988), the excitation light is the image of a pin-hole, and the emitted fluorescence is viewed through a second pin-hole at an identical image plane. In this way, out of focus fluorescence is excluded from the detector. The confocal pin-holes scan the cell to build up a two-dimensional image point by point. This, however, limits the time resolution of the confocal microscope, in which respect the epifluorescence\microscope is presently much better. Another disadvantage of confocal microscopy is the high levels of excitation light needed. The light source is usually a visible light laser, because sufficiently powerful UV lasers are very expensive. For this reason, long wavelength fluorescent indicators, such as fluo-3, are presently the most suitable, although they cannot be used for ratio measurements. Imaging with an epifluorescence microscope and fura-2 has already provided new information on the dynamics of $[Ca^{2+}]_i$ control in vascular cells.

It is possible, in cells loaded with the fura-2 acetoxymethyl ester, to monitor Ca^{2+} levels in the nucleus and sarcoplasmic reticulum as well as cytoplasm (Williams et al. 1985; Papageorgiou and Morgan 1990), allowing interactions between these compartments to be investigated. There is evidence that $[Ca^{2+}]$ gradients exist under the plasmalemma of vascular smooth muscle cells. This comes partly from patch-clamp studies showing spontaneous activation of Ca^{2+}-activated K channels in the membrane without accompanying contraction (Benham and Bolton 1986), but also from the fact that the sarcoplasmic reticulum can fill with Ca^{2+} in the absence of muscle contraction. When imaging techniques improve, it may be possible to visualize these gradients. This may be helped by recently described derivatives of fura-2 that selectively incorporate into the cell membrane and report $[Ca^{2+}]$ in the vicinity of the membrane (Etter et al. 1994). Images of subcellular $[Ca^{2+}]_i$ signalling in cultured vascular smooth muscle (Neylon et al. 1990) and endothelial (Jacob 1990) cells obtained using fura-2, have suggested that in both cell types, agonist-induced elevations of $[Ca^{2+}]_i$ begin in a discrete region of the cell and then spread throughout the cytoplasm. However, it is not yet known if this is the case in non-cultured cells, or what physiological role it could play.

The techniques for measuring $[Ca^{2+}]_i$ with fluorescent probes can also be applied to the measurement of other intracellular ions, with indicators now available for pH as well as Mg^{2+}, Na^+, K^+, Zn^{2+}, and Cl^- (Haughland 1992). A method has also been described for fluorescence ratio imaging of cAMP in single cells (Adams et al. 1991).

FLASH PHOTOLYSIS OF CAGED COMPOUNDS

Photolabile 'caged' compounds are inert precursors of biologically active molecules, which when stimulated with near-UV light release the active species. They provide a means of bypassing diffusional delays; a cell can be pre-equilibrated with the inactive precursor and a flash of light presented to generate the active species at its site of action on demand. Available probes include caged neurotransmitters and receptor agonists. Of those, the most relevant to vascular pharmacology are caged phenylephrine, photolysis of which activates α-adrenoceptors to cause contraction (Somlyo et al. 1988), caged ATP and caged carbachol, potential probes for investigating purinergic and muscarinic receptors on smooth muscle or endothelial cells. A caged nitric oxide was also described recently, which when photolysed caused a rapid relaxation of rabbit aorta (Carter et al. 1993). Additionally, there are caged intracellular messengers, which can be loaded into cells to release the free messenger upon photolysis. Examples of these include caged nucleotides (Wootton and Trentham 1989), caged inositol trisphosphate (IP$_3$; Walker *et al.* 1987), and photolabile cation chelators that permit manipulation of the intracellular Ca^{2+} or Mg^{2+} concentration. Nitr-5 (Adams *et al.* 1988), DM-nitrophen (Kaplan and Ellis-Davies 1988) and nitrophenyl-EGTA (NP-EGTA; Ellis-Davies and Kaplan 1994) release Ca^{2+} upon photolysis, whereas diazo-2 (Adams *et al.* 1989) mops up Ca^{2+}. In each case photolysis alters the cation affinity of the molecule. Nitr-5, NP-EGTA and DM-nitrophen differ mainly in their selectivities for Ca^{2+} over Mg^{2+}, and their pre- and post-photolysis affinities for Ca^{2+}. Whereas nitr-5 and NP-EGTA are highly selective for Ca^{2+}, DM-nitrophen also binds Mg^{2+} at physiological concentrations. NP-EGTA and DM-nitrophen have a higher affinity for Ca^{2+} and show a larger loss of affinity upon photolysis than nitr-5. Thus they can produce larger Ca^{2+} 'jumps', but with DM-nitrophen a 'jump' in Mg^{2+} may also result. DM-nitrophen can, however, be used to selectively release Mg^{2+} (O'Rourke *et al.* 1992). In addition to the already available probes, new molecules and design strategies are continuously being developed (Adams and Tsien 1993).

Photolabile molecules that are inactivated by light, such as the calcium antagonist drug nifedipine, can also be exploited. The rapidity with which this drug is destroyed by photolysis allowed it to be used in cardiac cells to study its interaction with the voltage-gated Ca channel (Gurney *et al.* 1985). A similar approach has been taken to study the role of Ca^{2+} in electromechanical coupling in gastric smooth muscle (Bonev *et al.* 1988), and could be taken in vascular muscle cells, the main therapeutic target for the drug.

The power of the technique lies in the speed of the photochemical reactions and the relative ease with which the intensity, duration, and area of activating light can be varied. Millisecond time resolution is often, but not always achievable; the half-time for photolysis of caged carbachol is 0.04 msec (Milliurn *et al.* 1989) compared with 200 msec for caged phenylephrine (Walker and Trentham 1988). In theory, light could be focused on the entire cell or localized to part of the cell, allowing global or local applications. It is also possible to apply photolysis techniques to small strips of intact vascular muscle, since the cells are sufficiently transparent to permit efficient photolysis. Photolabile caged compounds have recently been reviewed (e.g. Kaplan 1990; Somlyo and Somlyo 1990; Adams and Tsien 1993; Gurney 1993). A number of caged compounds can be purchased from Molecular Probes, Oregon, USA or Calbiochem, California, USA.

Basic properties of caged compounds

The structure of most caged compounds is based on the photolabile O-nitrobenzyl moiety illustrated in Fig. 3.4. Irradiation cleaves the precursor at the benzyl carbon, freeing the active molecule along with a proton and a nitroso byproduct. Changes in pH caused by proton release can be minimized by buffering the experimental solution well. The reactivity of the nitroso product presents a potential problem, but can be avoided by adding a hydrophilic thiol, such as

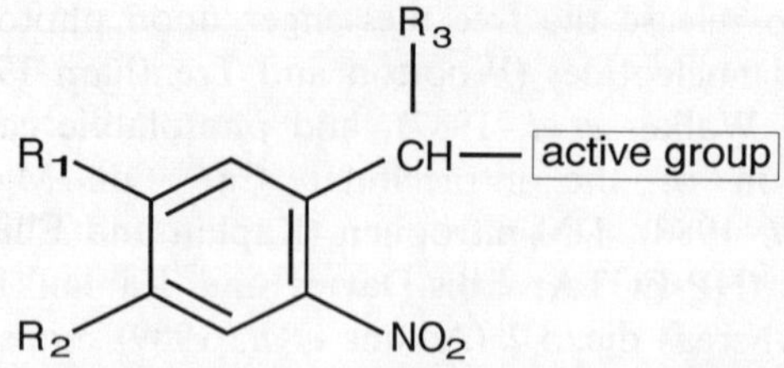

Fig. 3.4 General structure of caged compounds based on the *o*-nitrobenzyl moiety. In the nitrobenzyl (NB) derivatives $R_1 = -H$, $R_2 = -H$, and $R_3 = -H$, whereas R_3 becomes $-CH_3$ in the (nitrophenyl)ethyl (NPE) derivatives. The dimethoxy derivatives (DMNB or DMNPE) are prepared by substituting $-OCH_3$ at positions R_1 and R_2.

glutathione or DTT (Kaplan *et al.* 1978). In most experiments, only small amounts of the product are likely to be formed, because most agents work in the micromolar concentration range. Commercially available probes have a sufficiently high quantum yield to permit concentration changes in the physiological range to be produced with flash lamps or lasers. The light is usually filtered before it reaches the cell to remove wavelengths shorter than 300 nm, which can cause cell damage. Most caged compounds absorb light maximally at around 350 nm, and absorb little above 600 nm. They are therefore fairly stable under normal room lighting.

Several analogues of some molecules are available, varying in the substitutions at positions R_1, R_2, and R_3 (Fig. 3.4). For example, caged ATP can be purchased as either the O-nitrobenzyl (NB), O-nitrophenylethyl (NPE), or the dimethoxy O-nitrophenylethyl (DMNPE) ester. These modifications influence the rate and efficiency of the photochemical reaction, as well as the biological activity of the precursor and the photoproduct. For example ATP is released more rapidly from NPE ATP than from the DMNPE derivative (Wootton and Trentham 1989). However, in isolated arterial smooth muscle cells NPE ATP, but not the DMNPE analogue, acts as an inhibitor of ATP-sensitive K^+ current. Photolysis of NPE ATP produces no further block of the current, whereas in the presence of DMNPE ATP, suppression of the current is seen only after photolysis (Clapp and Gurney 1992). In contrast, NPE ATP appeared to behave simply as an inert precursor for ATP in studies of vascular muscle contraction (Somlyo *et al.* 1988). The NPE ester of cyclic GMP (cGMP) also has effects on vascular muscle that are not shared by DMNB cGMP. When applied to intact rabbit pulmonary artery, NPE cGMP induces large relaxations at low concentration, with light flashes having little further effect (Gurney 1993). Relaxation is observed in the presence of DMNB cGMP, but only after photolysis (Gurney 1993). It is not clear whether the effects of NPE cGMP are direct, or result from intracellular hydrolysis to free cGMP. Nevertheless, the DMNB ester appears to be the most appropriate for studies in vascular cells.

Most of the available probes are water soluble, so can be restricted to one side of the membrane. The exceptions are the caged cyclic nucleotides, which will permeate cells when applied to the extracellular surface. The photolabile calcium buffer, nitr-5, is available as a soluble salt and as the acetoxymethyl ester. The latter form diffuses across the cell membrane, where cytoplasmic enzymes cleave it to release the free buffer. Nitr-5 can therefore be pre-loaded using methods developed for loading fluorescent Ca indicators. With this approach, it is difficult to predict the concentration of nitr-5 achieved, and hence photolysis-induced changes in Ca^{2+} concentration. On the other hand, nitr-5 can be co-loaded with fluorescent Ca^{2+} indicators, which then report the Ca^{2+} jumps induced by flashes (Kao et al. 1989).

Application of caged compounds to vascular muscle

The delay between activation of a receptor and a cell's response can provide insight into the mechanisms coupling the receptor to the response. Using caged receptor agonists, the speed of application achieved by flash photolysis allows receptor activation to be temporally separated from receptor desensitization, and from other processes that inactivate receptor ligands. The activation of α-adrenergic receptors in vascular smooth muscle has been studied using caged phenylephrine (NPE ester), which has minimal activity before photolysis (Somlyo et al. 1988). After equilibrating intact guinea-pig portal vein with caged phenylephrine, photolysis caused the muscle strip to contract with a latency of 1.5 s, followed by a time to half peak force of 1.4 s at 20 °C. The latency was shown to be due entirely to the events linking phenylephrine binding to its receptor and the subsequent response (Somlyo et al. 1988). The contractile response is, however, quite far removed from receptor activation and it has yet to be determined if phenylephrine is released fast enough from the presently available caged precursor to permit studies of the activation of more immediate events, such as membrane conductances. These parallel studies with caged IP_3, incorporated into muscle strips by permeabilizing them with staphylococcal α-toxin, verified that IP_3 was the likely intracellular messenger mediating the response to phenylephrine (Somlyo et al. 1988; Somlyo and Somlyo 1990). Photolysis of caged IP_3 resulted in contraction that developed after a latency of only 0.5 s at 20 °C, which is significantly shorter than the latency following photolysis of caged phenylephrine. The difference in the latencies following photorelease of phenylephrine and IP_3 presumably reflects the delay between binding to α-adrenoceptors and IP_3 synthesis.

Caged IP_3 has also been used to study the kinetics of Ca^{2+} release from intracellular stores in cultured endothelial cells (Carter and Ogden 1992) and in intestinal smooth muscle cells (Komori and Bolton 1991), although it has not yet been applied to isolated vascular smooth muscle cells. In both cases, micromolar levels of IP_3 induced a Ca^{2+} response within 30 ms; elevated Ca^{2+} levels could be detected within 6 ms in the endothelial cells. Also in both cell types, the released Ca^{2+} induced an outward current, probably carried through Ca^{2+}-activated K^+ channels, which was similar to the current activated by extracellularly applied agonists. The responses to photolysis of IP_3 were consistent with a role for IP_3 in mediating the Ca^{2+} releasing action of the agonist.

A problem that we have encountered on applying photolabile probes in vascular muscle is that light frequently has effects even in the absence of the probe. In most non-vascular preparations, light at the wavelengths and intensity required for photolysis have little or no effect. However, light at those wavelengths is known to induce arterial muscle relaxation by stimulating guanylate cyclase and raising cGMP levels in the smooth muscle (Furchgott and Jothianandan 1991). The rabbit pulmonary artery frequently shows pronounced relaxation in response to 1 ms flashes of similar wavelengths and intensity to those required to photolyse caged compounds. Light also has direct effects on isolated vascular muscle cells, where it modulates membrane Ca^{2+} and K^+ currents in a similar way to nitrovasodilator drugs (Gurney 1993), which work through intracellular cGMP. This clearly complicates the application of photolabile caged compounds in vascular muscle, particularly in studies involving the cGMP cascade. However, it is possible to block these light effects with haemoglobin. It is also sometimes possible to adjust the light intensity to a level that has insignificant effects by itself, but induces sufficient photolysis. Furthermore, some responses, such as K channel inhibition by ATP (Clapp and Gurney 1992), do not appear to be influenced by light and can be studied usefully with caged compounds.

Flash photolysis is well suited to electrophysiological studies using the patch-clamp technique, either to study the activation or modulation of ion channels in isolated membrane patches or in whole cells. Caged intracellular messengers are easily incorporated into cells in the whole-cell configuration. Provided care is taken to protect the pipette from the activating light, for example by coating it with an opaque substance, the solution in the pipette provides an essentially unlimited store of unphotolysed chelator. Reproducible responses to photolysis can thus be obtained in a single cell, and it is possible to examine responses over a wide range of concentrations.

CONCLUSIONS

The techniques described all have the potential to address questions regarding the function of vascular cells and the mechanisms of action of hormones, neurotransmitters, and drugs on these cells. Although the techniques have been discussed individually, they can be applied together to study isolated cells. Thus a $[Ca^{2+}]$ indicator could be incorporated into a cell through a patch pipette, to monitor changes in $[Ca^{2+}]_i$ resulting from photolysis of a caged compound, while the associated changes in membrane conductance are monitored under voltage-clamp conditions. In this way, $[Ca^{2+}]_i$ and membrane conductance can be correlated with each other, and with activation of receptors or intracellular second messenger pathways.

ACKNOWLEDGEMENTS

I am grateful to Dr A. M. Evans for reading and criticizing an earlier draft of the chapter, and to Dr A. M. Evans and Ms F. C. Halliday for allowing me to photograph their cells for Fig. 3.1. Research in my laboratory has been funded by grants from the British Heart Foundation, the Wellcome Trust, the Royal Society, and the Medical Research Council.

REFERENCES

Aaronson, P. I., Bolton, T. B., Lang, R. J., and MacKenzie, I. (1988). Calcium currents in single isolated smooth muscle cells from the rabbit ear artery in normal-calcium and high-barium solutions. *J. Physiol.*, **405**, 57-75.

Adams, S. R. and Tsien, R. Y. (1993). Controlling cell chemistry with caged compounds. *Annu. Rev. Physiol.*, **55**, 775-84.

Adams, S. R., Kao, J. P. Y., Grynkiewicz, G., Minta, A., and Tsien, R. Y. (1988). Biologically useful chelators that release Ca^{2+} upon illumination. *J. Am. Chem. Soc*, **110**, 3212-20.

Adams, S. R., Kao, J. P. Y., and Tsien, R. Y. (1989). Biologically useful chelators that take up Ca^{2+} upon illumination. *J. Am. Chem. Soc.*, **111**, 7957-68.

Adams, S. R., Harootunian, A. T., Buechler, Y. J., Taylor, S. S., and Tsien, R. Y. (1991). Fluorescence ratio imaging of cyclic AMP in single cells. *Nature*, **349**, 694-7.

Amédée, T., Benham, C. D., Bolton, T. B., Byrne, N. G., and Large, W. A. (1990*a*). Potassium, chloride and non-selective cation conductances opened by noradrenaline in rabbit ear artery cells. *J. Physiol.*, **423**, 551-68.

Amédée, T., Large, W. A., and Wang, Q. (1990*b*). Characteristics of chloride currents activated by noradrenaline in rabbit ear artery cells. *J. Physiol.*, **428**, 501-16.

Bean, B. P., Sturek, M., Puga, A., and Hermsmeyer, K. (1986). Calcium channels in muscle cells isolated from rat mesenteric arteries: modulation by dihydropyridine drugs. *Circ. Res.*, **59**, 229-35.

Beech, D. J. and Bolton, T. B. (1989). Properties of the cromakalim-induced potassium conductance in smooth muscle cells isolated from the rabbit portal vein. *Br. J. Pharmacol.*, **98**, 851-64.

Benham, C. D. (1989). ATP-activated channels gate calcium entry in single smooth muscle cells dissociated from rabbit ear artery. *J. Physiol.*, **419**, 689-701.

Benham, C. D. and Bolton, T. B. (1986). Spontaneous transient outward currents in single visceral and vascular smooth muscle cells of the rabbit. *J. Physiol.*, **381**, 385-406.

Benham, C. D. and Tsien, R. W. (1987). Receptor operated, Ca-permeable channels activated by ATP in arterial smooth muscle. *Nature*, **328**, 275-8.

Benham, C. D., Bolton, T. B., Lang, R. J., and Takewaki, T. (1986). Calcium-activated potassium channels in single smooth muscle cells of rabbit jejunum and guinea-pig mesenteric artery. *J. Physiol.*, **371**, 45-67.

Bolton, T. B. (1975). Effects of stimulating the acetylcholine receptor on the current-voltage relationship of the smooth muscle membrane studied by voltage clamp of potential recorded by micro-electrode. *J. Physiol.*, **250**, 175-202.

Bolton, T. B. (1979). Mechanisms of action of transmitters and other substances on smooth muscle. *Physiol. Rev.*, **59**, 606-718.

Bolton, T. B., Lang, R. J., Takewaki, T., and Benham, C. D. (1985). Patch and whole-cell voltage clamp of single mammalian visceral and vascular smooth muscle cells. *Experientia*, **41**, 887-94.

Bonev, A., Boev, K., and Spassov, G. (1988). Photoinduced removal of nifedipine blockade of Ca^{2+} entry in different phases of gastric plateau action potential. *Methods Findings Exp. Clin. Pharmacol.*, **10**, 111-15.

Bossu, J.-L., Feltz, A., Rodeau, J.-L. and Tanzi, F. (1989). Voltage-dependent calcium currents in freshly dissociated capillary endothelial cells. *FEBS Lett.*, **255**, 377-80.

Bossu, J.-L., Elhamdani, A., Feltz, A., Tanzi, F., Aunis, D., and Thierse, D. (1992). Voltage-gated Ca entry in isolated bovine capillary endothelial cells: evidence of a new type of Bay K 8644-sensitive channel. *Pflügers Arch.*, **420**, 200-7.

Byrne, N. G. and Large, W. A. (1987). The actions of noradrenaline on single smooth muscle cells freshly dispersed from the guinea-pig pulmonary artery. *Br. J. Pharmacol.*, **91**, 89-94.

Byrne, N. G. and Large, W. A. (1988). Mechanism of action of α-adrenoceptor activation in single cells freshly dissociated from the rabbit portal vein. *Br. J. Pharmacol.*, **94**, 475-82.

Carter, T. D. and Ogden, D. C. (1992). Kinetics of intracellular calcium release by inositol 1,4,5-trisphosphate and extracellular ATP in porcine cultured aortic endothelial cells. *Proc. R. Soc. Lond.*, **250**, 235-41.

Carter, T.D., Bettache, N., Ogden, D., and Trentham, D.R. (1993). Photochemical release of nitric oxide from ruthenium nitrosyl trichloride: relaxation of rabbit isolated aortic rings mediated by photo-release of nitric oxide. *J. Physiol.* **467**, 165 P.

Casteels, R., Kitamura, K., Kuriyama, H., and Suzuki, H. (1977). The membrane properties of the smooth muscle cells of the rabbit main pulmonary artery. *J. Physiol.*, **271**, 41-61.

Clapp, L. H. and Gurney, A. M. (1991). A simple method for cell isolation: characterisation of the major outward currents in rabbit pulmonary artery. *Exp. Physiol.*, **76**, 677-93.

Clapp, L. H. and Gurney, A. M. (1992). ATP-sensitive potassium channels regulate the resting potential of arterial cells. *Am. J. Physiol.*, **262**, H916-20.

Clapp, L. H., Davey, R. and Gurney, A. M. (1993). ATP-sensitive K^+ channels mediate vasodilation produced by lemakalim in rabbit pulmonary artery. *Am. J. Physiol.* **264**, H1907-15.

Clapp, L. H. and Gurney, A. M. (1993) ATP-sensitive K^+ channels in the pulmonary vasculature. In *Ion flux in pulmonary vascular control* (ed. E. K. Weir). pp. 129-39 Plenum, New York.

Clapp, L. H., Gurney, A. M., Standen, N. B., and Langton, P. D. (1994). Properties of the ATP-sensitive K^+ current activated by levcromakalim in isolated rabbit pulmonary artery myocytes. *J. Memb. Biol.*, **140**, 205-13.

Cobbold, P. H. and Lee, J. A. C. (1991). Aequorin measurements of cytoplasmic free calcium. In *Cellular calcium: a practical approach* (ed. J. G. McCormack and P. H. Cobbold), pp. 55-81. IRL Press, Oxford.

DeFeo, T. T. and Morgan, K. G. (1985a). Responses of enzymatically isolated mammalian vascular smooth muscle cells to pharmacological and electrical stimuli. *Pflügers Arch.*, **404**, 100-2.

DeFeo, T. T. and Morgan, K. G. (1985b). Calcium-force relationships as detected with aequorin in two different vascular smooth muscles of the ferret. *J. Physiol.*, **369**, 269-82.

DeFeo, T. T. and Morgan, K. G. (1986). A comparison of two different indicators: quin 2 and aequorin in isolated single cells and intact strips of ferret portal vein. *Pflügers Arch.*, **406**, 427-9.

Driska, S. P. and Porter, R. (1986). Isolation of smooth muscle cells from swine carotid artery by digestion with papain. *Am. J. Physiol.*, **251**, C474-81.

Droogmans, G., Declerck, I., and Casteels, R. (1987). Effect of adrenergic agonists on Ca^{2+}-channel currents in single vascular smooth muscle cells. *Pflügers Arch.*, **409**, 7-12.

Ellis Davies, G. C. and Kaplan, J. H. (1994). Nitrophenyl-EGTA, a photolabile chelator that selectively binds Ca^{2+} with high affinity and releases it rapidly upon photolysis. *Proc. Nat. Acad. Sci. USA.*, **91**, 187-91.

Etter, E. F., Kuhn, M. A., and Fay, F. S. (1994). Detection of changes in near-membrane Ca^{2+} concentration using a novel membrane-associated Ca^{2+} indicator. *J. Biol. Chem.*, **269**, 10141-9.

Fine, A., Amos, W. B., Durbin, R. M., and McNaughton, P. A. (1988). Confocal microscopy: applications in neurobiology. *Trends Neurosci.*, **11**, 346-51.

Finkel, A. S., Hirst, G. D. S., and Van Helden, D. F. (1984). Some properties of excitatory junction currents recorded from submucosal arterioles of guinea-pig ileum. *J. Physiol.*, **351**, 87-98.

Freshney, R. I. (1987). *Culture of animal cells. A manual of basic technique.* Alan R. Liss, New York.

Furchgott, R. F. and Jothianandan, D. (1991). Endothelium-dependent and -independent vasodilation involving cyclic GMP: relaxation induced by nitric oxide, carbon monoxide and light. *Blood Vessels*, **28**, 52-61.

Grynkiewicz, G., Poenie, M., and Tsien, R. Y. (1985). A new generation of Ca^{2+} indicators with greatly improved fluorescence properties. *J. Biol. Chem.*, **260**, 3440-50.

Gurney, A. M. (1990*a*). Molecular pharmacology of ion channels using the patch-clamp. In *Receptor-effector coupling: a practical approach* (ed. E. C. Hulme), pp. 155-79. IRL Press, Oxford.

Gurney, A. M. (1990*b*). Measurement and control of intracellular calcium. In *Receptor-effecter coupling: a practical approach* (ed. E. C. Hulme), pp. 117-53. IRL Press, Oxford.

Gurney, A. M. (1991). Photolabile calcium buffers to selectively activate calcium-dependent processes. In *Cellular neurobiology: a practical approach* (ed. J. Chad and H. Wheal), pp. 153-77. IRL Press, Oxford.

Gurney, A. M. (1993). Photolabile caged compounds. In *Fluorescent probes for biological activity of living cells. A practical guide* (ed. W. T. Mason), pp. 335-48. Academic Press, London.

Gurney, A. M., Nerbonne, J. M., and Lester, H. A. (1985). Photoinduced removal of nifedipine reveals mechanisms of calcium antagonist action on single heart cells. *J. Gen. Physiol.*, **86**, 353-79.

Hamill, O. P., Marty, A., Neher, E., Sakmann, B., and Sigworth, F. J. (1981). Improved patch-clamp techniques for high resolution current recording from cells and cell-free membrane patches. *Pflügers Arch.*, **39**, 85-100.

Haughland, R. P. (1992). *Handbook of fluorescent probes and research chemicals.* Molecular Probes Inc., Eugene, Oregon, USA.

Hirata, M., Itoh, T., and Kuriyama, H. (1981). Effects of external cations on calcium efflux from single cells of the guinea-pig taenia coli and porcine coronary artery. *J. Physiol.*, **310**, 321-36.

Hirst, G. D. S. and Edwards, F. R. (1989). Sympathetic neuroeffector transmission in arteries and arterioles. *Physiol. Rev.*, **69**, 546-604.

Hirst, G. D. S., Silverberg, G. D., and Van Helden, D. F. (1986). The action potential and underlying ionic currents in proximal rat middle cerebral arterioles. *J. Physiol.*, **371**, 289-304.

Horn, R. and Marty, A. (1988). Muscarinic activation of ionic currents measured by a new whole cell recording method. *J. Gen. Physiol.*, **92**, 145-59.

Hume, J. R. and Leblanc, N. (1989). Macroscopic K^+ currents in single smooth muscle cells of the rabbit portal vein. *J. Physiol.*, **413**, 49-73.

Inoue, R., Kitamura, K., and Kuriyama, H. (1985). Two Ca-dependent K-channels classified by the application of tetraethylammonium distribute to smooth muscle membranes of the rabbit portal vein. *Pflügers Arch.*, **405**, 173-9.

Inoue, Y., Oike, M., Nakao, K., Kitamura, K., and Kuriyama, H. (1990). Endothelin augments unitary calcium channel currents on the smooth muscle cell membrane of guinea-pig portal vein. *J. Physiol.*, **423**, 171-91.

Isenberg, G. and Klöckner, U. (1982). Calcium tolerant ventricular myocytes prepared by preincubation in a 'KB' medium. *Pflügers Arch.*, **395**, 6-18.

Ives, H. E., Schultz, G. S., Galardy, R. E., and Jamieson, J. D. (1978). Preparation of functional smooth muscle cells from the rabbit aorta. *J. Exp. Med.*, **148**, 1400-13.

Jacob, R. (1990). Imaging cytoplasmic free calcium in histamine stimulated endothelial cells and in fMet-Leu-Phe stimulated neutrophils. *Cell Calcium*, **11**, 241-9.

Kao, J. P. Y., Harootunian, A. T., and Tsien, R. Y. (1989). Photochemically generated cytosolic calcium pulses and their detection by fluo-3. *J. Biol. Chem.*, **264**, 8179-84.

Kaplan, J. H. (1990). Photochemical manipulation of divalent cation levels. *Annu. Rev. Physiol.*, **52**, 897-914.

Kaplan, J. H. and Ellis-Davies, G. C. R. (1988). Photolabile chelators for the rapid photorelease of divalent cations. *Proc. Nat. Acad. Sci. USA*, **85**, 6571-5.

Kaplan, J. H., Forbush, B., and Hoffman, J. H. (1978). Rapid photolytic release of adenosine 5'-triphosphate from a protected analogue: utilization by the Na:K pump of human red blood cell ghosts. *Biochemistry*, **17**, 1929-35.

Karaki, H. (1989). Ca^{2+} localization and sensitivity in vascular smooth muscle. *Trends Pharmacol. Sci.*, **10**, 320-5.

Katsuyama, H., Ito, S., Itoh, T., and Kuriyama, H. (1991). Effects of ryanodine on acetylcholine-induced Ca^{2+} mobilization in single smooth muscle cells of the porcine coronary artery. *Pflügers Archiv.*, **419**, 460-6.

Kimmel, J. R. and Smith, E. L. (1957). The properties of papain. *Adv. Enzymol.*, **19**, 267-354.

Klöckner, U. and Isenberg, G. (1985). Action potentials and net membrane currents of isolated smooth muscle cells (Urinary bladder of the guinea-pig). *Pflügers Arch.*, **405**, 329-39.

Klöckner, U. and Isenberg, G. (1989). The dihydropyridine niguldipine modulates calcium and potassium currents in vascular smooth muscle cells. *Br. J. Pharmacol.*, **97**, 957-67.

Komori, S. and Bolton, T. B. (1991). Calcium release induced by inositol 1,4,5-trisphosphate in single rabbit intestinal smooth muscle cells. *J. Physiol.*, **433**, 495-517.

Kurachi, Y., Nakajima, T., and Sugimoto, T. (1986). On the mechanism of activation of muscarinic K^+ channels by adenosine in isolated atrial cells: involvement of GTP-binding proteins. *Pflügers Arch.*, **407**, 264-74.

Kuriyama, H., Ito, Y., Suzuki, H., Kitamura, K., and Itoh, T. (1982). Factors modifying contraction-relaxation cycle in vascular smooth muscles. *Am. J. Physiol.*, **243**, H641-62.

Langton, P. D., Nelson, M. T., Huang, Y., and Standen, N. B. (1991). Block of calcium-activated potassium channels in mammalian arterial myocytes by tetraethylammonium ions. *Am. J. Physiol.*, **260**, H927-34.

Loirand, G., Pacaud, P., Mironneau, C., and Mironneau, J. (1986). Evidence for two distinct calcium channels in rat vascular smooth muscle cells in short-term primary culture. *Pflügers Arch.*, **407**, 566-8.

McCormack, J. G. and Cobbold, P. H. (1991). *Cellular calcium: a practical approach*. IRL Press, Oxford.

Milburn, T., Matsubara, N., Billington, A. P., Udgaonkar, J. B., Walker, J. W., Carpenter, B. K., *et al.* (1989). Synthesis, photochemistry, and biological activity of a caged photolabile acetylcholine receptor ligand. *Biochemistry*, **28**, 49-55.

Minta, A., Kao, J. P. Y., and Tsien, R. Y. (1989). Fluorescent indicators for cytosolic calcium based on rhodamine and fluorescein chromophores. *J. Biol. Chem.*, **264**, 8171–8.

Moody, C. J., Dashwood, M. R., Sykes, R. M., Chester, M. Jones, S. M., Yacoub, M. H., et al. (1990). Functional and autoradiographic evidence for endothelin 1 receptors on human and rat cardiac myocytes. Comparison with single smooth muscle cells. *Circ. Res.*, **67**, 764–9.

Moreton, R. B. (1991). Optical techniques and Ca^{2+} imaging. In *Cellular neurobiology: a practical approach* (ed. J. Chad and H. Wheal), pp. 205–22. IRL Press, Oxford.

Morgan, J. P. and Morgan, K. G. (1982). Vascular smooth muscle: the first recorded Ca^{2+} transients. *Pflügers Arch.*, **395**, 75–7.

Neher, E. and Sakmann, B. (1976). Single channel currents recorded from membrane of denervated frog muscle fibres. *Nature*, **260**, 799–802.

Neylon, C. B., Hoyland, J., Mason, W. T., and Irvine, R. F. (1990). Spatial dynamics of intracellular calcium in agonist-stimulated vascular smooth muscle cells. *Am. J. Physiol.*, **259**, C675–86.

Noack, T., Edwards, G., Deitmer, P., and Weston, A. H. (1992). Potassium channel modulation in rat portal vein by ATP depletion: a comparison with the effects of levcromakalim (BRL 38227). *Br. J. Pharmacol.*, **107**, 945–55.

Ogden, D. (1994). *Microelectrode techniques. The Plymouth workshop handbook*, Company of Biologists Ltd., Cambridge.

Ohya, Y. and Sperelakis, N. (1989). ATP regulation of the slow calcium channels in vascular smooth muscle cells of guinea-pig mesenteric artery. *Circ. Res.*, **64**, 145–54.

Oike, M., Kitamura, K., and Kuriyama, H. (1992). Histamine H_3-receptor activation augments voltage-dependent Ca^{2+} current via GTP hydrolysis in rabbit saphenous artery. *J. Physiol.*, **448**, 133–52.

Okabe, K., Kitamura, K., and Kuriyama, H. (1987). Features of 4-aminopyridine sensitive outward current observed in single smooth muscle cells from the rabbit pulmonary artery. *Pflügers Arch.*, **409**, 561–8.

O'Rourke, B., Backx, P. H., and Marban, E. (1992). Phosphorylation-independent modulation of L-type calcium channels by magnesium-nucleotide complexes. *Science*, **257**, 245–8.

Pacaud, P., Loirand, G., Bolton, T. B., Mironneau, C., and Mironneau, J. (1992). Intracellular cations modulate noradrenaline-stimulated calcium entry into smooth muscle cells of rat portal vein. *J. Physiol.*, **456**, 541–56.

Papageorgiou, P. and Morgan, K. G. (1990). The nuclear–cytoplasmic $[Ca^{2+}]$ gradient in single mammalian vascular smooth muscle cells. *Proc. Soc. Exp. Biol. Med.*, **193**, 331–4.

Pusch, M. and Neher, E. (1988). Rates of diffusional exchange between small cells and a measuring patch pipette. *Pflügers Arch.*, **411**, 204–11.

Rusko, J., Tanzi, F., Van Breemen, C., and Adams, D. J. (1992). Calcium-activated potassium channels in native endothelial cells from rabbit aorta: conductance, Ca^{2+} sensitivity and block. *J. Physiol.*, **455**, 601–21.

Sakai, T. (1990). Acetylcholine induces Ca-dependent K currents in rabbit endothelial cells. *Jap. J. Pharmacol.*, **53**, 235–46.

Sakmann, B. and Neher, E. (1983). *Single-channel recording*. Plenum Press, New York.

Scanlon, M., Williams, D. A., and Fay, F. S. (1987). A Ca^{2+}-insensitive form of fura-2 associated with polymorphonuclear leukocytes. Assessment and accurate Ca^{2+} measurement. *J. Biol. Chem.*, **262**, 6308–12.

Silberberg, S. D. and Van Breemen, C. (1990). An ATP, calcium and voltage sensitive potassium channel in porcine coronary artery smooth muscle cells. *Biochem. Biophys. Res. Commun.*, **17**, 517–22.

Smirnov, S. V. and Aaronson, P. I. (1992). Ca^{2+}-activated and voltage-gated K$^+$ currents in smooth muscle cells isolated from human mesenteric arteries. *J. Physiol.*, **457**, 431–54.

Soejima, A. and Noma, A. (1984). Mode of regulation of the acetylcholine sensitive K-channel by the muscarinic receptor in rabbit atrial cells. *Pflügers Arch.*, **400**, 424–31.

Somlyo, A. P. and Somlyo, A. V. (1990). Flash photolysis studies of excitation-contraction coupling, regulation, and contraction in smooth muscle. *Annu. Rev. Physiol.*, **52**, 857–74.

Somlyo, A. P., Walker, J. W., Goldman, Y. E., Trentham, D. R., Kobayashi, S., Kitazawa, T., *et al.* (1988). Inositol trisphosphate, calcium and muscle contraction. *Phil. Trans. R. Soc. London*, **320**, 399–414.

Steele, J. A., Stockbridge, N., Maljkovic, G., and Weir, B. (1991). Free radicals mediate actions of oxyhemoglobin on cerebrovascular smooth muscle cells. *Circ. Res.*, **68**, 416–23.

Sumimoto, K. and Kuriyama, H. (1986). Mobilization of free Ca^{2+} measured during contraction-relaxation cycles in smooth muscle cells of the porcine coronary artery using quin 2. *Pflügers Arch.*, **406**, 173–80.

Terada, K., Nakao, K., Okabe, K., Kitamura, K., and Kuriyama, H. (1987). Action of the 1,4-dihydropyridine derivative, KW-3049, on the smooth muscle membrane of the rabbit mesenteric artery. *Br. J. Pharmacol.*, **92**, 615–25.

Toro, L., Gonzalez-Robles, A., and Stefani, E. (1986). Electrical properties and morphology of single vascular smooth muscle cells in culture. *Am. J. Physiol.*, **251**, C763–73.

Tsien, R. Y., Pozzan, T., and Rink, T. J. (1982). Calcium homeostasis in intact lymphocytes: cytoplasmic free calcium monitored with a new, intracellularly trapped fluorescent indicator. *J. Cell Biol.*, **94**, 325–34.

Valera, S., Hussey, N., Evans, R. J., Adami, N., North, R. A., Surprenant, A., *et al.* (1994). A new class of ligand-gated ion channel defined by P$_{2x}$ receptor for extracellular ATP. *Nature*, **371**, 516–9.

Van Dijk, A. M. and Laird, J. D. (1984). Characterisation of single isolated vascular smooth muscle cells from bovine coronary artery. *Blood Vessels*, **21**, 267–78.

Wadsworth, R. M., Crankshaw, J., Kwan, C. Y., and Daniel, E. E. (1988). Morphology and contractile properties of smooth muscle cells isolated from the dog carotid artery. *Blood Vessels*, **25**, 166–84.

Walker, J. W. (1991). Caged molecules activated by light. In *Cellular neurobiology: a practical approach* (ed. J. Chad and H. Wheal), pp. 179–203. IRL Press, Oxford.

Walker, J. W. and Trentham, D. R. (1988). Caged phenylephrine: synthesis and photochemical properties. *Biophys. J.*, **53**, 596a.

Walker, J. W., Somlyo, A. V., Goldman, Y. E., Somlyo, A. P., and Trentham, D. R. (1987). Kinetics of smooth and skeletal muscle activation by laser pulse photolysis of caged inositol 1,4,5-trisphosphate. *Nature*, **327**, 249–52.

Wang, Q. and Large, W. A. (1991). Noradrenaline-evoked cation conductance recorded with the nystatin whole-cell method in rabbit portal vein cells. *J. Physiol.*, **435**, 21–39.

Wilde, D. W. and Lee, K. S. (1989). Outward potassium currents in freshly isolated smooth muscle cell of dog coronary arteries. *Circ. Res.*, **65**, 1718–34.

Williams, D. A., Fogarty, K. E., Tsien, R. Y., and Fay, F. S. (1985). Calcium gradients in single smooth muscle cells revealed by the digital imaging microscope using Fura-2. *Nature*, **318**, 558–61.

Williams, D. A., Becker, P. L., and Fay, F. S. (1987). Regional changes in calcium underlying contraction of single smooth muscle cells. *Science*, **235**, 1644–8.

Wootton, J. F. and Trentham, D. R. (1989). 'Caged' compounds to probe the dynamics of cellular processes: synthesis and properties of some novel photosensitive P-2-nitrobenzyl esters of nucleotides. *NATO ASI series C*, **272**, 277-96.

Worley, J. F., Deitmer, J. W., and Nelson, M. T. (1986). Single nisoldipine-sensitive calcium channels in smooth muscle cells isolated from rabbit mesenteric artery. *Proc. Nat. Acad. Sci. USA*, **83**, 5746-50.

Worley, J. F., Quayle, J. M., Standen, N. B., and Nelson, M. T. (1991). Regulation of single calcium channels in cerebral arteries by voltage, serotonin, and dihydropyridines. *Am. J. Physiol.*, **261**, H1951-60.

Yagi, S., Becker, P. L., and Fay, F. S. (1988). Relationship between force and Ca^{2+} concentration in smooth muscle as revealed by measurements on single cells. *Proc. Nat. Acad. Sci. USA*, **85**, 4109-13.

Yatani, A., Seidel, C. L., Allen, J., and Brown, A. M. (1987). Whole-cell and single channel calcium currents of isolated smooth muscle cells from saphenous vein. *Circ. Res.*, **60**, 523-33.

4. In vivo techniques and analysis

J. A. Angus, C. E. Wright, K. Sudhir, and G. J. Jennings

"Life is like an onion, which one peels crying" — French proverb

INTRODUCTION

Take an onion; peel away the layers and you find perhaps, disappointingly, nothing at the centre. You are left with a pile of skins but you will have gained important knowledge of how the onion is structured and the hierarchy of each layer. Similarly, when scientists aim to understand the mechanism of action of a drug on the vascular system, they will seek the ultimate experiment in a chosen test system stripped of its layers of complex interactions to maximize analytical power and minimize external influences. With such a controlled assay design, scientists may achieve some measure of analytical certainty that their vascular drug is behaving in a direct predictable manner.

Such a bioassay system may be a smooth muscle cell membrane preparation, cell culture system, or isolated large or small artery mounted in a myograph or organ chamber (Fig. 4.1). But in the end, these scientists will, theoretically at least, have to extrapolate their findings to the more integrated (intact) system of a vascular bed and ultimately the human circulation. To reconstruct 'the onion' as a whole from the pile of skins, knowing that the information obtained in the more integrated system must 'trump' the findings in the less organized (less complex) assays, is the challenge for the *in vivo* pharmacologist. Whether the response chosen for measurement by the pharmacologist truly represents the **direct** effects of the drug or is the resultant from these direct effects plus the system's reaction to perturbation by the drug, are issues for concern in design, interpretation, and further experimentation. Here we will summarize these challenges and various approaches to measuring simply the vascular response to a drug in animals and man. Examples of different techniques, drug delivery routes, and cautionary experiences will be presented. The last part of the chapter will relate specific techniques for the *in vivo* study of vascular pharmacology in man.

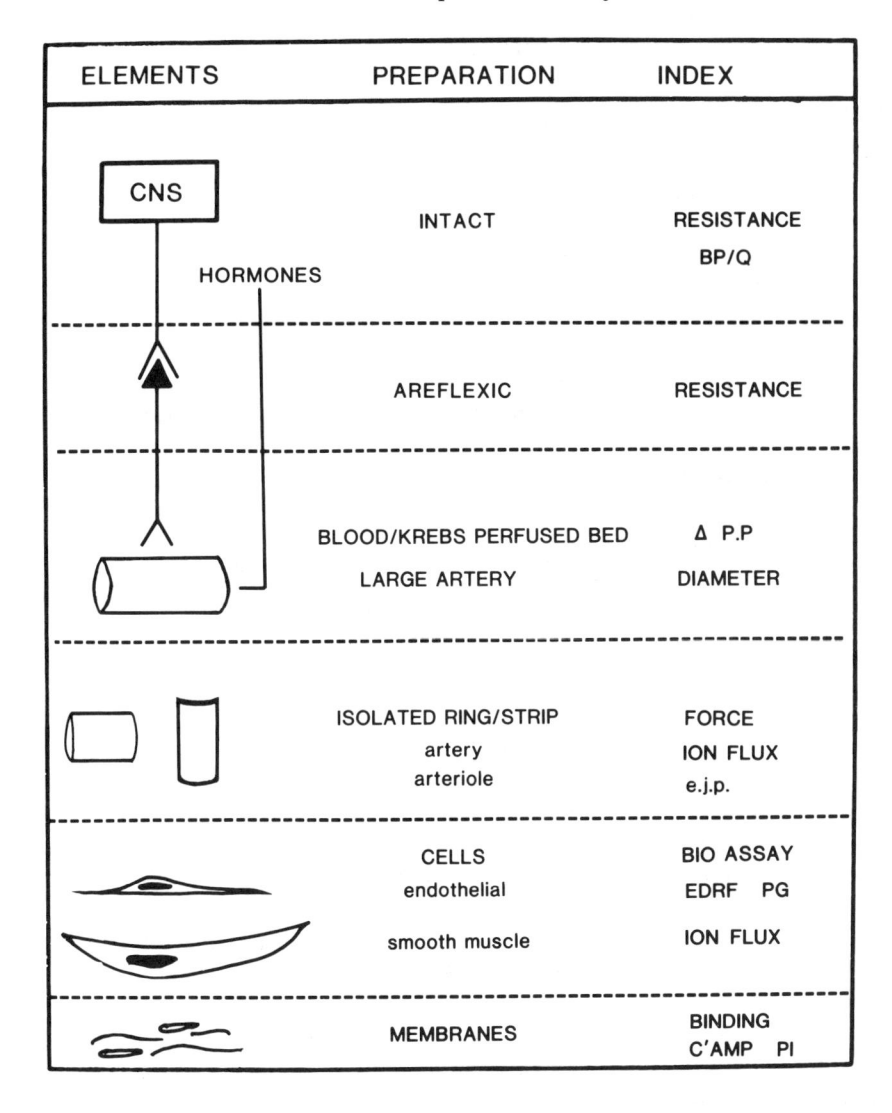

ELEMENTS	PREPARATION	INDEX
CNS / HORMONES	INTACT	RESISTANCE BP/Q
	AREFLEXIC	RESISTANCE
	BLOOD/KREBS PERFUSED BED / LARGE ARTERY	Δ P.P / DIAMETER
	ISOLATED RING/STRIP / artery / arteriole	FORCE / ION FLUX / e.j.p.
	CELLS / endothelial / smooth muscle	BIO ASSAY / EDRF PG / ION FLUX
	MEMBRANES	BINDING / C'AMP PI

Fig. 4.1 Schema illustrating the main elements, experimental preparations, and possible indices in studies of the pharmacology of the vasculature. *BP/Q* is ratio of blood pressure and flow; *ΔP.P* is change in perfusion pressure; e.j.p. is excitatory junction potential; EDRF is endothelium-derived relaxing factor; PG is prostaglandin; PI is phosphatidyl inositol (J. Angus unpublished).

DELIVERY

Intravenous route

Bolus injection and infusion. Many scientists give a vasoactive agent intravenously over a short time period of seconds to a few minutes as a bolus injection. Clearly this route offers convenience but is probably the least useful in scientific experiment. The bolus raises the concentration which wanes as the drug is diluted with the cardiac output. Plasma concentration will arguably never be at steady state with vascular receptors. Continuous infusion would theoretically have the advantage of allowing the drug to come into steady state concentration with the vascular receptors. Factors that may alter the time taken to reach steady state include recirculation, kinetics of metabolism, uptake, redistribution, or metabolism to an inactive or less active metabolite. If the drug has cardiac activity in addition to vascular actions (i.e. positive inotropy and/or chronotropy), the intravenous route would be best avoided. Confounding effects of the drug on the heart or pulmonary circulation will cloud the interpretation of vascular actions. Note that drugs may alter the coronary vasculature and indirectly alter myocardial contractility, heart rate, and cardiac output.

Intra-arterial infusion

Local infusion. This route offers many advantages over intravenous injection. It allows a steady state concentration to be achieved rapidly before significant recirculation occurs and much lower concentrations need to be used (rule of thumb: one-tenth local dose compared with intravenous dose rates). Local infusion into a specific vascular bed may include the hindquarter bed of a conscious rabbit via a chronic indwelling catheter in the lower abdominal aorta. Specific examples using this method will follow. Other specific routes are intrarenal, intracoronary, intramesenteric, or into the cerebral circulation via the vertebral artery or directly into a ventricle. In chronically instrumented rabbits we prefer to implant polyvinyl chloride catheters directly into the lower abdominal aorta via the technique of Herd and Barger (1964). This technique requires catheters to be drawn out to a very thin diameter and inserted into the lumen of 25–26 gauge needles or of 31 gauge dental needles for very small catheters. The catheter can be inserted directly through the wall of the artery, secured by a purse-string suture in the vessel wall and tied in place with a securing cuff. Catheters may remain patent for up to six weeks if heparinized saline is used to flush the catheter weekly (Wright *et al.* 1987). In conscious rabbits, we use a steady i.a. infusion via a rollerpump of 1 ml/min of ascending concentrations of agonist made up in 20 ml glass vials. Each dose step is infused for 2–3 min or until a steady state plateau has been reached. A complete concentration–response curve can be constructed in 15–20 min. It is important to state that the final concentration (C) in the artery is dependent upon the blood flow (Q) and the infused amount (A), i.e. $C \propto A/Q$ assuming perfect mixing in the artery. If the flow is measured, then the actual final concentration in the artery may be determined (see Angus and Lew 1992).

Extravascular or topical

There may be occasions where local delivery of drug is required only to a segment of artery. The drug could be applied topically by continuously applying the drug to the external surface of a large artery and measuring the external diameter by sonomicrometry. This would avoid distribution of the drug to the smaller resistance vessels (Angus *et al.* 1983). Newer techniques of delivery include pluronic gels, slow release formulation, or osmotic minipumps to release vasoactive drugs extravascularly. This latter delivery system may directly affect large vessels through their vasovasorum or may be absorbed by the microcirculation for systemic distribution. Extravascular drug delivery may be affected by a loss of drug activity due to poor distribution across the vessel wall, metabolism, or uptake by nerves especially if the receptors are located in endothelium. For example acetylcholine was 50–100-fold less potent in relaxing an artery when applied topically compared with intraluminal infusion (Angus *et al.* 1983).

DEFINING THE EXPERIMENTAL CONDITIONS

It has been argued that the *modus operandi* for *in vivo* studies is to apply a drug in the fully integrated preparation and measure the resultant amalgam response from direct, reflex, and local factors. This is, of course, a legitimate goal but it only allows a general description of the drug effect and not an interpretation of mechanism. Therefore with *in vivo* vascular preparations, one cannot escape the critical first step of asking what it is that we want to know. Defining the question is as vital in these more sophisticated preparations as in more structurally reduced isolated tissue bioassays with their added analytical power.

Therefore pharmacologists interested in vascular **reactivity** *in vivo* must decode what is:

- the DIRECT effect of the drug on the blood vessel diameter
- the influence of EXTERNAL FACTORS that may amplify or annul (say by physiological antagonism) the direct effect of the drug
- the role of LOCAL FACTORS in the environment of the blood vessel wall that may alter the DIRECT drug response

Often the roles of these factors cannot be easily determined without a perturbation of the integrated preparation, for example, by administration of a ganglion blocking drug (see below) or alternatively, by pharmacological blockade of autonomic effectors including acetylcholine, noradrenaline, angiotensin II, and vasopressin, removal of baroreceptor afferent nerves, blockade of the synthesis (or receptors) for local autacoids such as nitric oxide, prostacyclin, thromboxane A_2, and endothelin. In the following example, we sought to measure the pressor

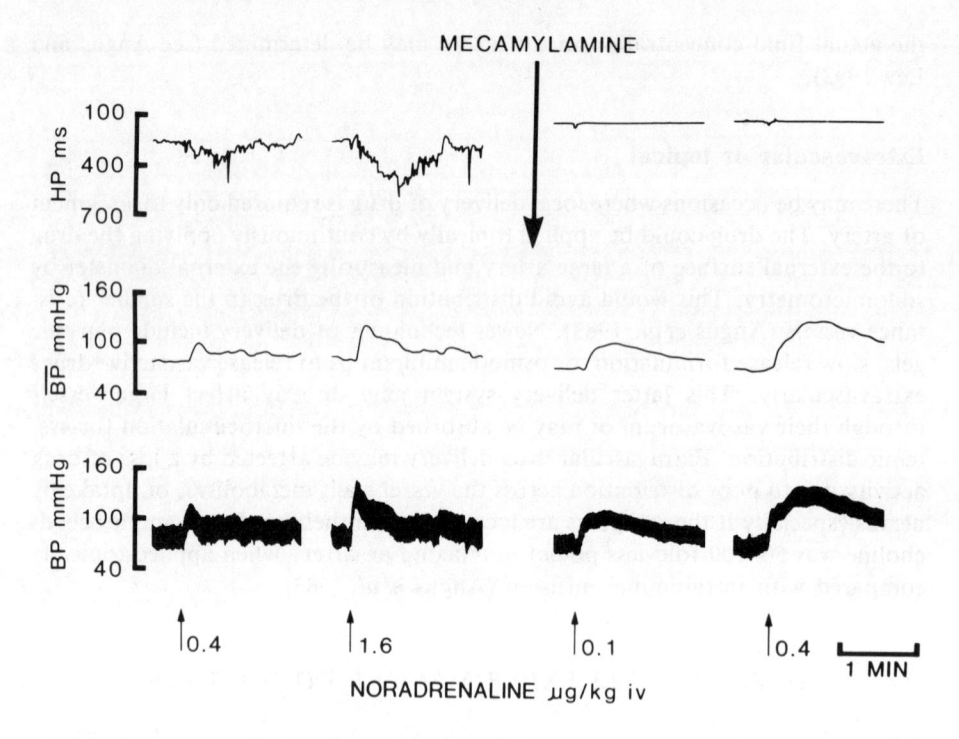

Fig. 4.2 Mecamylamine (10 mg/kg), a ganglion blocking drug, abolishes the bradycardia and increases the pressor sensitivity of conscious rabbits to noradrenaline bolus intravenous injections. *HP*, heart period msec; *BP* and $\overline{BP}$ are phasic, and mean blood pressure, mmHg. (Reproduced from Wright *et al.* 1987 with permission.)

sensitivity to noradrenaline in a conscious rabbit as part of a study of renovascular hypertension (Wright *et al.* 1987). Fig. 4.2 shows the effects of bolus intravenous injections of noradrenaline before and after the autonomic reflex loop has been opened pharmacologically by administration of the ganglion blocking drug, mecamylamine, in a conscious rabbit. Before ganglion blockade, the pressor responses to noradrenaline (0.4 and 1.6 μg/kg iv) were associated with marked bradycardia. After mecamylamine, only 25% of the dose was required to cause the same rise in blood pressure — i.e. the pressor *sensitivity* increased about four times — and there was no reflex bradycardia. This illustrates the importance of such an areflexic preparation to prevent changes in cardiac rate and force and in sympathetic vascular tone through various baroreceptor reflexes that are brought into play in the intact animal when the blood pressure changes during drug administration. Interactions between the local (direct) and reflexly-evoked effects of a drug on cardiac and vascular tone are particularly pronounced when the intravenous route of administration is employed.

EXTRAPOLATION

Importantly, pharmacologists study normal preparations and often make inferences about diseased preparations. Similarly, data from laboratory animals are extrapolated to man. These leaps of faith must be appropriately cautioned by observations that disease:

- often reduces homeostatic autonomic reflexes, e.g. hypertension attenuates the baroreceptor-heart rate reflex gain
- alters local metabolites, (such as atherosclerosis inhibiting nitric oxide)
- may change receptor populations (β_2-adrenoceptors in congestive heart failure)
- may alter the structure of vascular beds through rarefaction, collateralization, angiogenesis, or medial hypertrophy with or without lumen encroachment

Pharmacological observations — drug action — must be interpreted with the caveat that the ultimate test is in man and that there is no 'animal' model of man — rather that observations are made of specific drug interactions in a particular species. Extrapolation, while an indulgence, is fraught with error and should be treated with great caution.

ANAESTHESIA

Anaesthetics in general depress the circulation and may have direct effects on the vasculature. For example, L-type calcium channel blockade may occur with barbiturates, apart from difficulties with respiration, fluid balance, and so on. Anaesthetics may alter hormone levels, circulating catecholamines, and other homeostatic mechanisms such as baroreceptor reflexes. Nevertheless, anaesthetized preparations have a place in vascular reactivity studies especially if the preparation requires control of blood flow or if neural stimulation is desired.

MEASUREMENT

Blood pressure, blood flow, and resistance

Ultimately a blood vessel will respond to a drug by changing its internal diameter and radius (r_i) by altering the circumferential length of its medial smooth muscle. This response of the mechanical effector will alter the resistance R of that segment of blood vessel to blood flow, i.e. $R = f[1/r^4]$ (Korner and Angus 1992) according to Poiseuille's law as a first approximation. Normally segmental resistance cannot be easily measured and one extrapolates to measuring total vascular bed resistance (R_T) by determining $R_T \propto BP/Q$ where BP is systemic arterial blood pressure − venous pressure, and Q local blood flow. If cardiac output (CO) is measured, total peripheral resistance ($TPR \propto BP/CO$) can be readily determined. It is apparent that unless Q or cardiac output is constant, then resistance (and thus vascular diameter) does **not** equate with blood pressure. Experimenters who, for convenience, measure blood pressure without considering blood flow or cardiac output are at risk of poor analysis if they equate changes in blood pressure with changes in vascular diameter. Cardiac output and therefore regional flow are dependent on many factors including heart rate, myocardial contractility, pre-load, and after-load. Unless the blood flow is controlled, e.g. constant flow perfused organ (rat hindlimb preparation of Folkow *et al.* 1970) then the appropriate measure is vascular resistance or conductance (see below) requiring measurement of regional flow **and** systemic pressure.

Conductance

Conductance is the reciprocal of resistance ($C = 1/R$) and a convenient parameter to use if the blood flow (Q) approaches zero in response to a vasoconstrictor drug. By using conductance, the dose of vasoconstrictor agent that reduces the conductance by 50% (ED_{50}) can be readily determined because the range (resting baseline to zero) is known. Conversely, the response to a vasodilator drug is best described by resistance (R) since R approaches zero as blood flow increases.

In Fig. 4.3 the hindquarter resistance (lower graph) rises sharply as noradrenaline is infused into the lower abdominal aorta of a conscious normotensive rabbit and to a greater extent in the hypertensive rabbit. The same data plotted as conductance (upper graph) allow for the full range of the dose–response curve to be measured, and thus an ED_{50} determined, as flow and thus conductance approach zero.

Fig. 4.4 shows that by choosing appropriate measures of response, depending upon the nature of the vasoactive drug, estimates of the ED_{50} can be obtained because the range of dose–response curves can be defined. Moreover, in rabbits with experimental renovascular hypertension the hindquarter bed is an amplifier of resistance changes to a vasodilator but an attenuator of conductance changes to a vasoconstrictor drug (see later).

Average radius

We faced the challenge of how to combine the dose–response curve to a dilator drug with that from a vasoconstrictor drug (i.e. as in Fig. 4.3) to construct the 'FULL' stimulus–response curve from maximum dilatation to maximum vasoconstriction. In conscious animals and man most vascular beds have a resting vascular resistance to allow for active dilatation and constriction. In contrast, in crystalloid perfused rat hindquarters, the preparation is maximally dilated at the start making the analysis of the stimulus–response curve for infusion of a constrictor drug quite straightforward (see Korner and Angus 1992).

In the conscious rabbit, therefore, we have combined the data from a dilator stimulus (adenosine) with the constrictor stimulus (noradrenaline) by calculating

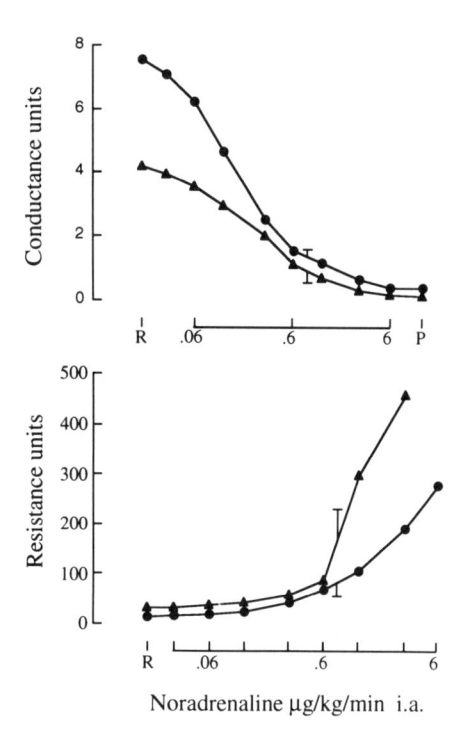

Fig. 4.3 Average resistance values from the mean arterial pressure and hindquarter blood flow in conscious, autonomically-blocked normotensive (circles) or hypertensive (diamond) rabbits during rest R and intra-abdominal aorta infusion of noradrenaline. The same data are plotted above as conductance units (P is plateau) (from Wright *et al.* 1987 with permission).

the average vascular bed radius $\bar{r}$ from the average conductance and resistance values from each separate dose–response curve,

$$\text{i.e. } \bar{r} = \sqrt[4]{C} \text{ and } \bar{r} = \frac{1}{\sqrt[4]{R}}.$$

The relationship between constrictor and dilator drug dose on the x axis and average radius, conductance, or resistance on the y axis is shown in Fig. 4.5 for a hindquarter vascular bed of a conscious rabbit (Korner and Angus 1992). Blood pressure was measured in an ear artery catheter and total hindquarter blood flow by a chronically implanted pulsed Doppler flow transducer. Drugs were infused directly into the lower abdominal aorta via an indwelling chronic catheter just proximal to the iliac bifurcation (Wright *et al.* 1987). The important features of this graphical display of a regional vascular bed reactivity are:

(a) The use of linear dose units of two arms of the dose–response curve about the resting level of $\bar{r}$, conductance, or resistance when drug = zero. One can plot the parameter of choice as the constrictor or dilator drug is infused

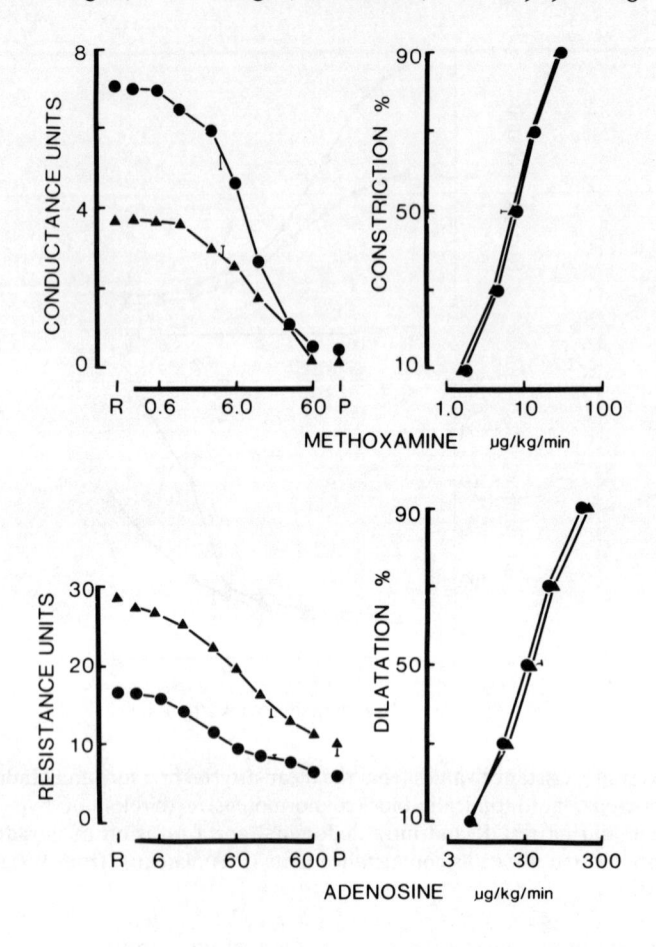

Fig. 4.4 *Top*: average values for hindquarter conductance (*Q/BP*) and *bottom*: hindquarter resistance (1/C) during intra-aortic infusion of methoxamine (*top*) and adenosine (*bottom*) in conscious normotensive (circle n = 7) or renal hypertensive rabbits (diamond n = 5) after ganglion blockade. At *right* are the corresponding sensitivity graphs (ED$_{10-90}$) computer fitted from individual curves.

intra-arterially into the lower abdominal aorta under conditions of autonomic reflex blockade with mecamylamine.

(b) Each arm of the dose–response curve can be simulated by the hyperbolic relationship $E = MA/(A + K_A)$ where E is response, M is maximum, A is dose of agonist, and K_A is dose of agonist at half maximum response

(c) The two dose–response curves will combine to provide a display of the **full** stimulation–response curve from maximum constriction to maximum dilatation in that vascular bed.

(d) The display shows that the response to a constrictor drug, for example, is

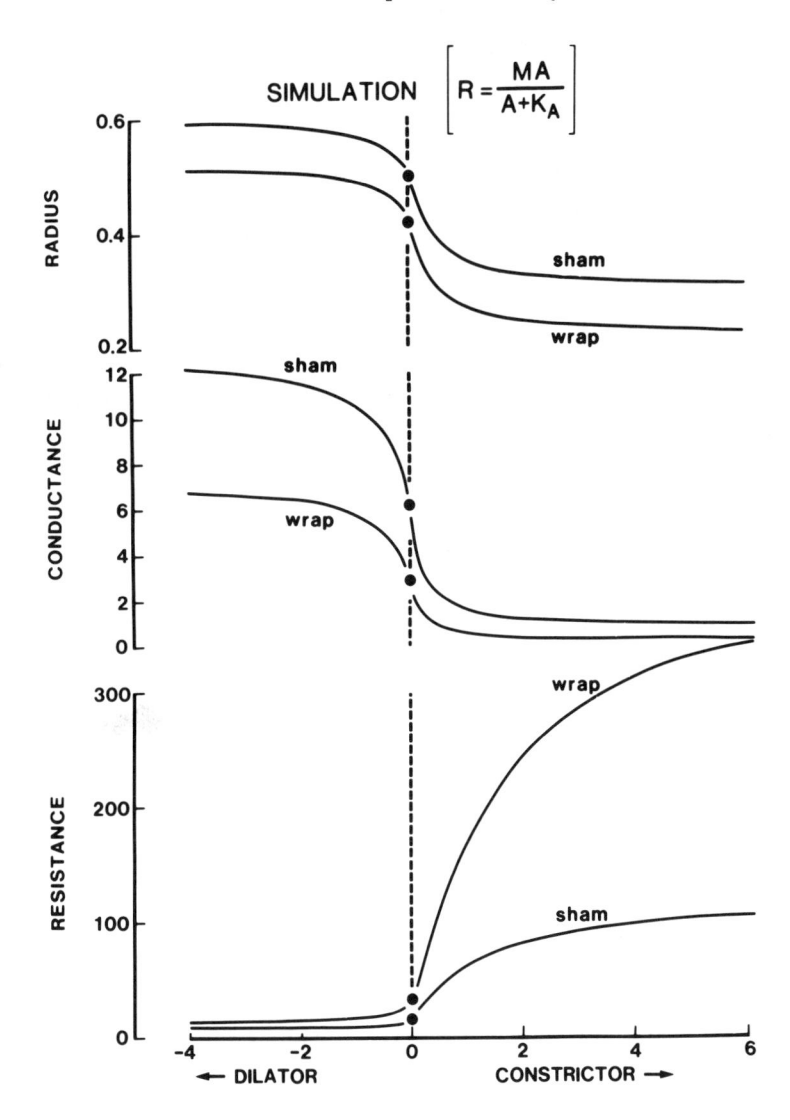

Fig. 4.5 Graphical display of the simulation of data from conscious rabbit hindquarter resistance, conductance, and average radius. From resting values (0 on x axis) linear dose units of a dilator or constrictor drug infused intra-arterially alter the three parameters as shown. Wrap are renal cellophane wrap hypertensive rabbits and sham are normotensive controls. (Reproduced from Korner *et al.* 1989.)

amplified as measured by a change in resistance in hypertensive rabbits (wrap = bilateral kidney cellophane wrap perinephritic hypertension) compared with normotensive sham rabbits but the plot of average radius values displays consistently lower internal radius throughout the stimulus–response curve compared with normotensive rabbits (Korner and Angus 1992).

The advantages of this display are that sensitivity (ED_{50}) and range of vascular reactivity to dilator and constrictor drugs can be examined recognizing the underlying importance of the vascular amplifier (or conductance attenuator) in understanding drug action. Such an approach should be feasible for all intact vascular bed studies including the human forearm. It emphasizes the **range** of response about resting tone and serves to remind the investigator of the need for stimulus-response curves rather than one or two dose-response points that may mislead interpretation.

We have used **mathematical modelling** to test various hypotheses as to how the artery wall could remodel in hypertension, i.e. medial hypertrophy with or without lumen encroachment and observe how the average $\bar{r}$, R, or C curves would be affected. These extensive analyses aid thinking and interpretation of the experimental findings (see Korner and Angus 1992).

Interpretation of regional vascular reactivity is constrained by the possible variation in response by different parts of the bed under study. In the hindquarter this might be skin versus muscle, large artery versus resistance artery, and shunts from arteriovenous anastomoses. Microspheres may go part of the way to solve this dilemma but the restriction in the number of measurements you can make (five to ten including control (baseline)) makes constructing dose-response curves almost impossible.

Large artery diameter

In animal experiments segmental large artery diameter can be continuously measured by the technique of sonomicrometry in acute or chronic preparations. Arteries of larger than 1 mm external diameter can be measured by pairs of 9 or 20 MHz quartz piezoelectric crystals (one emitter, one receiver) that are glued or stitched opposite each other to the adventitia of the artery. The time taken for the pulsed ultrasonic signal to be received is directly proportional to the distance between the inner surfaces of the two crystals (Angus *et al.* 1983).

Distending arterial pressure (transmural pressure) will directly influence the diameter of the artery. For example in Fig. 4.6 injecting a bolus of acetylcholine or sodium nitroprusside down the femoral artery of an anaesthetized dog caused a marked increase in femoral blood flow but a fall in systemic arterial pressure. However, note that the phasic and mean femoral artery diameter **falls** with both drugs because the blood pressure has fallen. If there is a large artery dilatation from nitric oxide release by acetylcholine, it is obscured because of the passive fall in diameter caused by the hypotension. In the same dog the experiment was repeated but the blood flow was now controlled by a roller pump and the pressure controlled by inserting a Starling resistor circuit in the distal femoral artery with the blood shunted to the femoral vein. Now under conditions of controlled flow and pressure acetylcholine will dilate the femoral artery without any change to side branch pressure (Fig. 4.7). Endothelial cell removal by passing an inflated intraluminal Fogarty balloon completely prevented the acetylcholine response (Fig. 4.7).

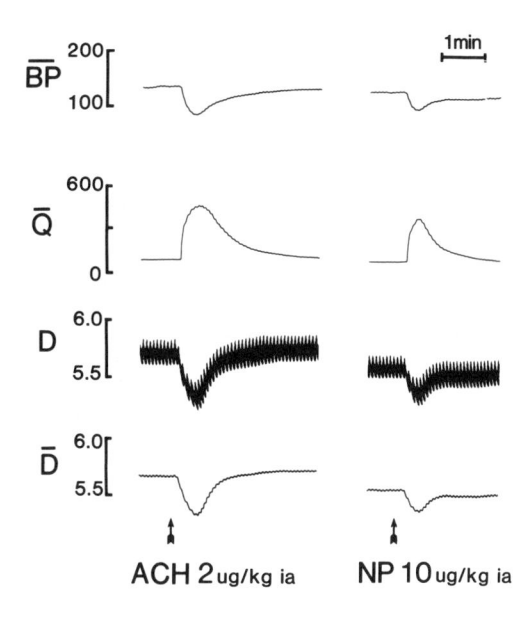

Fig. 4.6 Traces showing mean blood pressure ($\overline{BP}$ mmhg; mean femoral blood flow ($\overline{Q}$) via an electromagnetic flow meter ml/min; phasic (D) and mean external femoral artery diameter ($\overline{D}$, mm) in an anaesthetized dog. Acetylcholine (ACh) 2 μ/2g/kg and nitroprusside (NP 10 μg/kg) were given as intra-arterial bolus injections into the femoral artery. (Reproduced from Angus *et al.* 1988 with permission.)

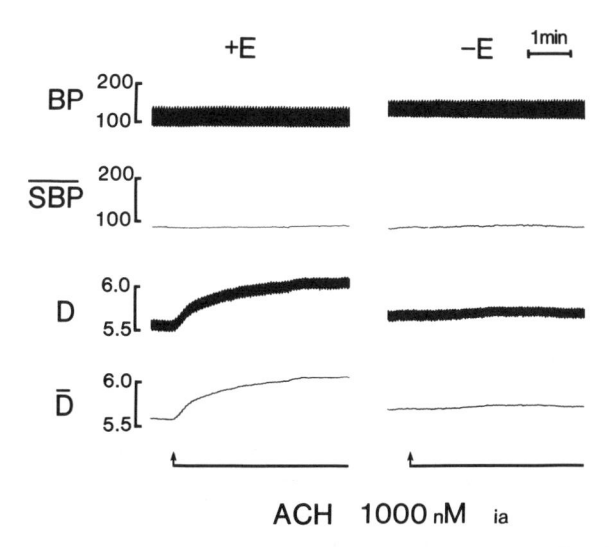

Fig. 4.7 Traces from same experiment as in Fig. 4.6 after controlling blood flow and distal resistance (see text). Traces are *BP*, systemic blood pressure mmHg; side branch femoral artery pressure $\overline{SBP}$ mmHg; and femoral artery external diameter phasic *D* and mean $\overline{D}$ mm. Acetylcholine (ACh) was infused at a final concentration of 1 μM before (+E) and after (−E) endothelial cell removal. (Reproduced from Angus *et al.* 1988 with permission.)

HEAD

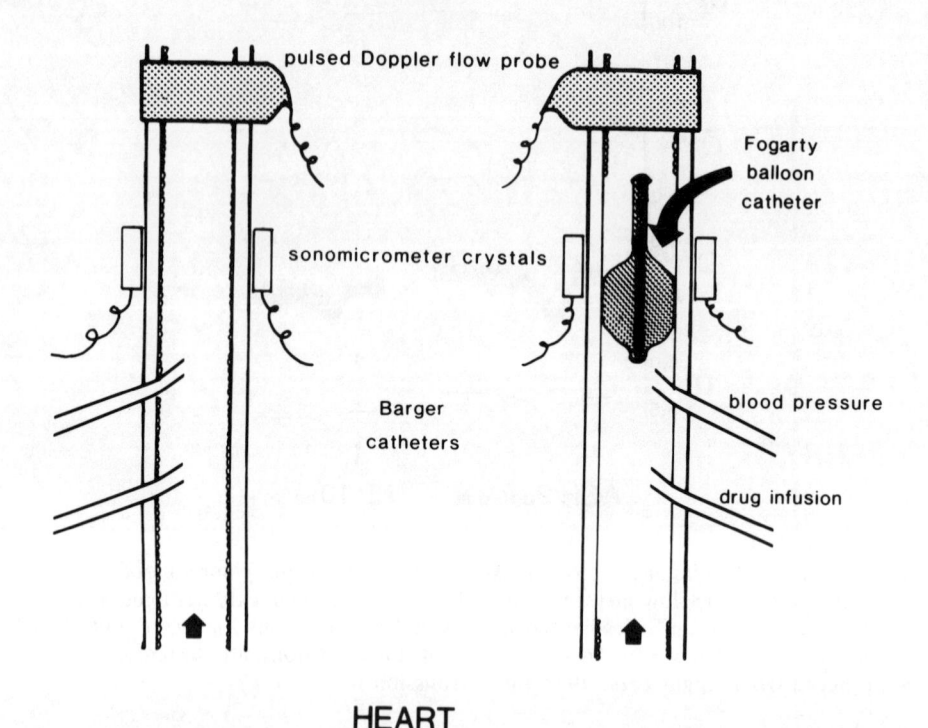

HEART

Fig. 4.8 Schematic of the bilateral instrumentation of greyhound carotid arteries with two indwelling catheters, pair of sonomicrometer crystals, and pulsed Doppler flow probe. The right carotid artery had the endothelium removed by three strokes of a Fogarty balloon catheter. Drugs were infused intra-arterially and blood pressure measured via the indwelling catheters.

Conscious dog carotid artery diameter

In the conscious dog we have explored the effects of 5-HT infusions directly into the carotid artery to establish the differential effects of 5-HT on the large artery and the resistance vessels simultaneously. Dogs were prepared with two indwelling Barger catheters sewn into the wall of both the proximal common carotid arteries and a pair of sonomicrometer crystals attached distal to these catheters (Fig. 4.8). Common carotid flow was measured by pulsed Doppler flow transducers. In addition, at surgery the right carotid artery had the endothelium removed by passing an inflated Fogarty balloon catheter three times along the length of the common carotid artery controlled via a purse-string suture. 11 days later with the dog lying quietly, 5-HT was infused into the right carotid artery. Fig. 4.9 shows how intra-arterial 5-HT caused constriction of the large carotid artery as external diameter fell with progressive doses but the carotid flow

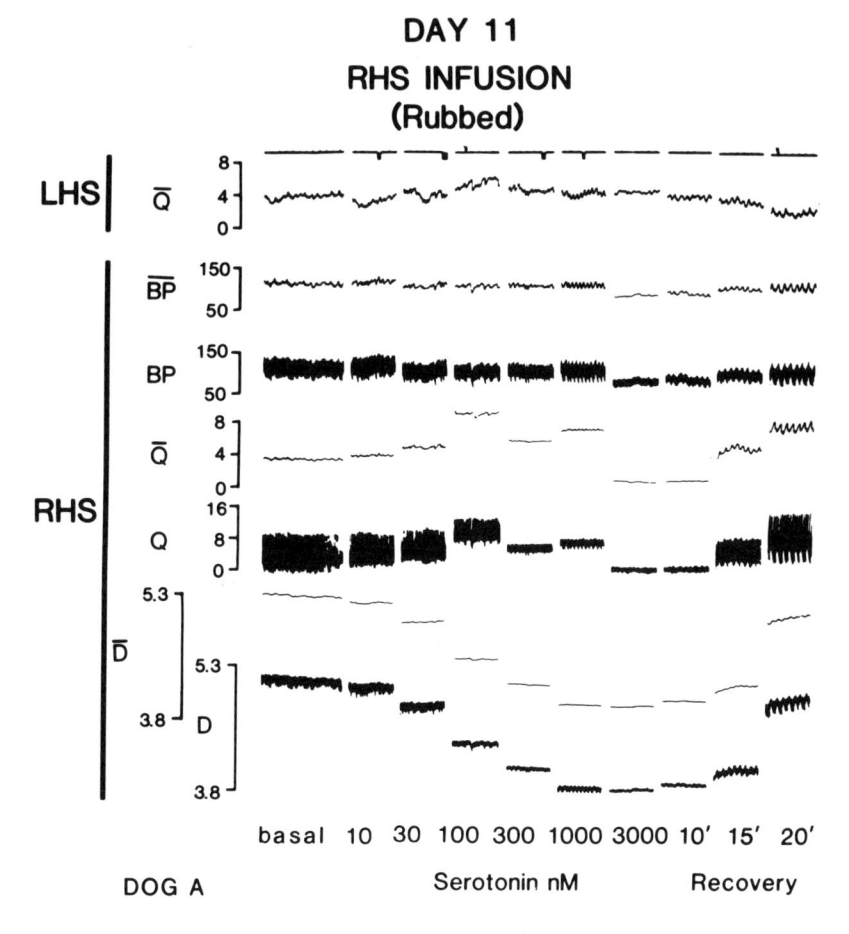

Fig. 4.9 Chart records from a conscious greyhound dog showing carotid artery haemodynamics. LHS, left-hand side mean carotid flow ($\bar{Q}$, kHz Doppler shift). RHS, right carotid mean and phasic blood pressure ($\overline{BP}$, BP, mmHg); flow ($\bar{Q}$, Q, kHz Doppler shift), and mean and phasic diameter ($\bar{D}$, D, mm). 5-HT infusion concentrations are only estimates assuming 100 ml/min flow. The RHS blood flow range was halved for 300 and 1000 nM 5-HT as the flow was >8 kHz (from J. Angus unpublished).

increased. At the highest dose (nominally 3000 nM) the flow abruptly fell to zero as the large artery constriction became flow limiting. The opposite carotid artery flow remained relatively steady.

This preparation was very useful for following the return of the endothelial response to acetylcholine (Angus *et al.* 1988) and the effect of neointimal thickening on the large artery reactivity to 5-HT in a chronic longitudinal experiment. It highlights the value of measuring large and small vessel reactivity simultaneously even though the former is a direct measure of vascular calibre while the latter is derived from changes in resistance.

REGIONAL BLOOD FLOW: METHODOLOGY

Intravenous drug administration with autonomic blockade

Changes in systemic blood pressure alone give little information about the main locus of action of a drug or, importantly, whether the drug may evoke different responses in various vascular beds. A useful technique is that of ultrasonic pulsed Doppler flow measurement. The Doppler flow cuffs can be cheaply fabricated and chronically implanted around blood vessels of interest, for instance, the lower abdominal aorta and renal, mesenteric, and carotid arteries. Changes in blood flow velocity (kHz Doppler shift) are directly related to volume blood flow after stabilization of the diameter as the wall becomes fixed to the cuff with granulation tissue (Wright *et al.* 1987). The investment in surgery, manufacture, and implantation of flow cuffs pays great dividends with longitudinal within animal experimental design. Experiments may then be performed in conscious animals without the confounding effects of an anaesthetic. Fig. 4.10 illustrates the complex haemodynamic changes elicited by bolus intravenous administration of the peptide, endothelin-1, in an anaesthetized rat and a conscious rabbit. The autonomic reflexes were obviated with mecamylamine in each animal. In both species, the responses to endothelin were biphasic — the initial effect of the peptide was a fall in blood pressure associated with *increases* in carotid (in the rat) and hindquarter vascular conductances but marked *decreases* in conductance in renal and mesenteric (in the rat) vascular beds. Fig. 4.11 illustrates the different patterns of vascular responses to intravenous steady state infusion of 5-HT in two conscious, ganglion-blocked rabbits. In both rabbits, 5-HT (30–60 μg/kg/min iv) caused vasodilatation in the hindquarter vascular bed (with little change in blood pressure), but concomitant marked falls in renal blood flow due to renal artery spasm, confirmed by angiography (Wright and Angus 1987). These examples highlight the importance of considering differences in *regional* vascular responsiveness to drugs in the absence of autonomic reflexes; information *not* reflected by changes in systemic blood pressure.

Intra-arterial drug administration with autonomic blockade

In the conscious animal, contrary to the common practice of generating dose–response relationships with only one to three points, it is possible to derive logistic agonist dose–vascular response curves where all parameters, including the range from resting value (baseline) to maximum response, ED_{50} (sensitivity) and the slope at ED_{50}, may be defined by standard pharmacological analysis (Wright *et al.* 1987). The use of local *intra-arterial* steady state infusions of drugs allows maximum dilator (or constrictor) responses to be obtained *before* decreases (or increases) in systemic blood pressure come close to life-threatening limits in the conscious or anaesthetized animal. Even with intra-arterial administration, ganglion blockade or autonomic effector blockade is still necessary, however, as the drug may have systemic effects at higher doses if it is not metabolized in the

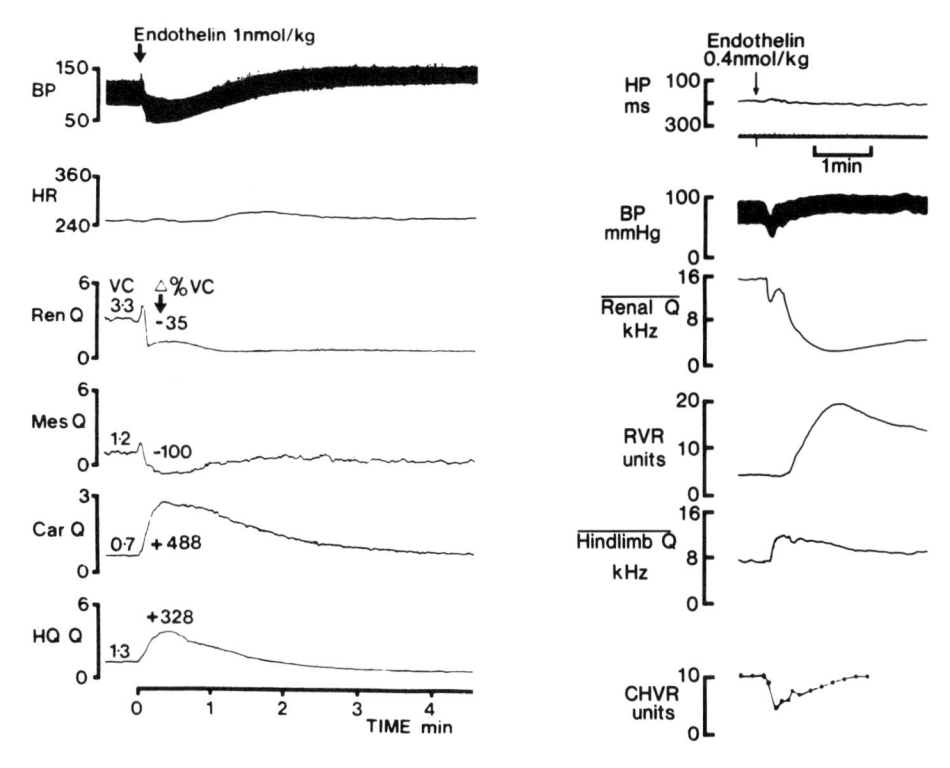

Fig. 4.10 Regional vascular responses to endothelin-1 in a ganglion-blocked, anaesthetized, spontaneously hypertensive rat (*left* panel) and ganglion-blocked conscious rabbit (*right* panel). Regional flows (kHz Doppler shift) are renal (Ren), mesenteric (Mes), carotid (Car), and hindquarter (HQ) in the rat, and the calculated vascular conductances (VC) are shown. For the rabbit, *HP* is heart period, *RVR* is analogue-computed renal vascular resistance, and *CHVR* is calculated hindlimb vascular resistance, (Reproduced from Wright and Fozard 1988 and Cocks *et al.* 1989.)

vascular bed of interest. Local intra-arterial drug infusion is possible with the chronic implantation of a catheter into the artery feeding the vascular bed of interest, for example, into the lower abdominal aorta (just above the iliac bifurcation) for the measurement of hindquarter vascular reactivity. The technique of Herd and Barger (1964) may be used to insert a fine polyvinyl chloride into the aorta (or other vessel) without any restriction to blood flow to the distal vascular bed. The catheter lead may then be tunnelled subcutaneously to the nape of the animal's neck. The catheter is filled with heparin and flushed weekly to maintain patency. On the day of the experiment, the catheter lead (and flow probe wires) may be retrieved under local anaesthetic and agonist drug infusions made directly into the vascular bed under study. Fig. 4.12 depicts ascending doses of the α_1-adrenoceptor agonist, methoxamine, by intra-arterial infusion into the hindquarter vascular bed of a conscious, ganglion-blocked hypertensive rabbit. Hindquarter vascular conductance falls to near zero with the high dose of methoxamine

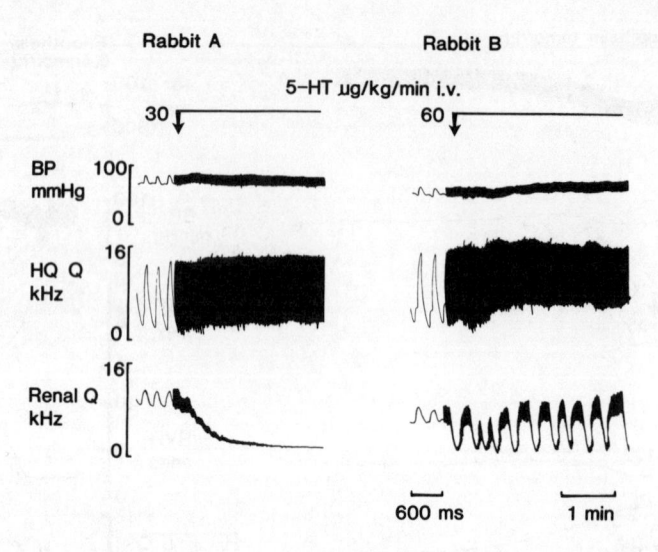

Fig. 4.11 5-HT infusion (iv) to two conscious rabbits with ganglion blockade (mecamylamine) caused renal artery spasm in rabbit A but intermittent renal artery spasm in rabbit B with increases in hindquarter flow (HQ Q). (Reproduced from Wright and Angus 1987 with permission.)

(30 μg/kg/min i.a.) *without* large increases in systemic blood pressure. Note the rapid recovery on cessation of infusion. The analysis of this experiment to determine the pharmacological parameters is shown in Fig. 4.4.

BARORECEPTOR REFLEX AND SYMPATHOLYTIC ACTIVITY

So far, examples have been given where vascular drug action has been defined in the **absence** of autonomic reflexes. However, we have recently explored the *in vivo* pharmacology of a vasodilator peptide where the dilatation was most likely due to inhibition of sympathetic constrictor tone. One convenient method to explore this sympatholytic action was the baroreceptor heart rate reflex in the conscious rabbit. Two methods of generating the control heart rate (y axis) and mean arterial pressure (x axis) curve are:

(a) By giving bolus iv injections of sodium nitroprusside (1–16 μg/kg) to lower arterial pressure and evoke reflex tachycardia and phenylephrine (1–16 μg/kg) to raise pressure and evoke reflex bradycardia (Fig. 4.13).

(b) To implant perivascular balloon cuffs on the thoracic aorta and inferior vena cava to apply steady state depressor and pressor changes to the aortic and carotid baroreceptors (Fig. 4.14) (Korner *et al.* 1972).

By alternating pressor and depressor stimuli the baroreceptor reflex curve can

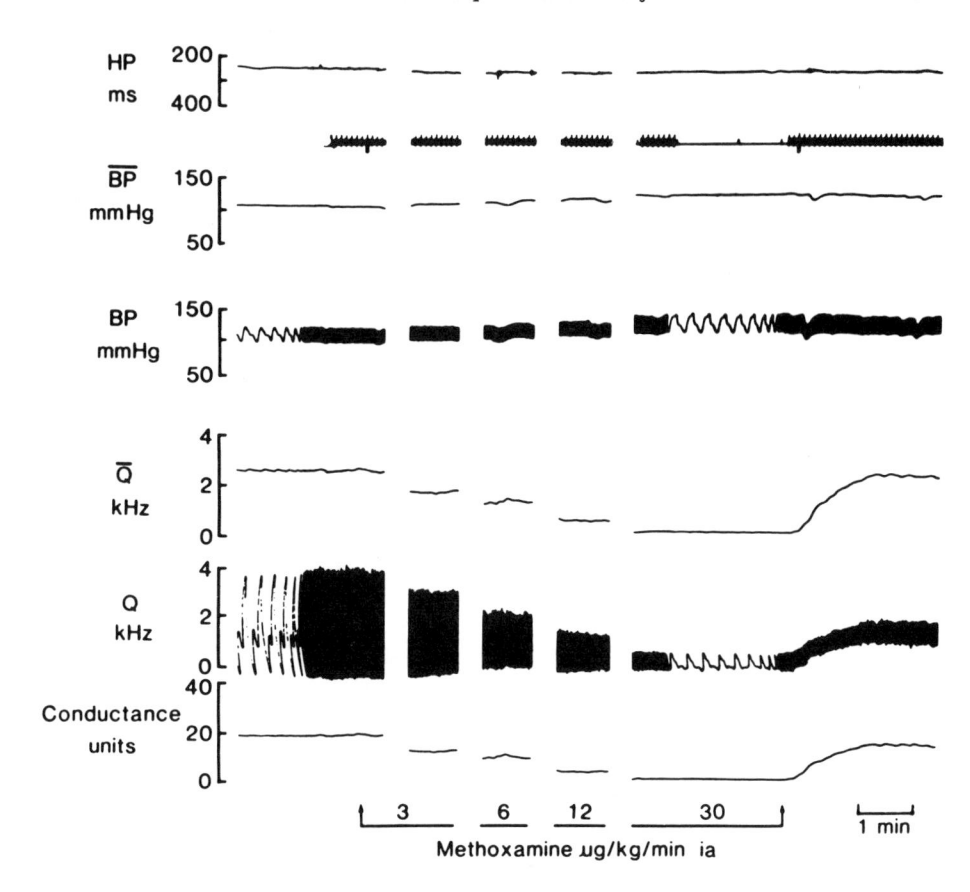

Fig. 4.12 Chart records of methoxamine infused intra-arterially (lower abdominal aorta) in a conscious ganglion-blocked hypertensive rabbit. Variables are heart period *HP*, mean and phasic blood pressure *BP*, mean and phasic hindquarter flow *Q*, kHz Doppler shift, and hindquarter conductance, $\bar{Q}/\overline{BP}$. The two portions of fast trace were recorded at 60 × the normal speed. (Reproduced from Wright *et al.* 1987 with permission.)

be easily generated and a sigmoidal logistic equation employed to characterize the heart rate range, gain, and blood pressure at half the heart rate range (Fig. 4.15) (Head and Adams 1992).

ω-Conotoxin GVIA (ω-CTX 3–10 μg/kg iv), a 27 amino acid peptide from the fish-eating cone snail *Conus geographus*, increases blood flow to the renal, mesenteric, and hindquarter vascular beds in the conscious rabbit, and attenuates the sympathetic component of the baroreceptor–heart rate reflex (Pruneau and Angus 1990*a*). The average resting blood pressure falls but the resting heart rate increases due to vagal withdrawal in spite of the sympatholytic action of the peptide (Fig. 4.15). The two methods (cuff and drug) to alter blood pressure essentially gave the same result; sympathetic component inhibited but a preserved vagal component. Higher doses of ω-CTX 10 μg/kg attenuated the sympathetic

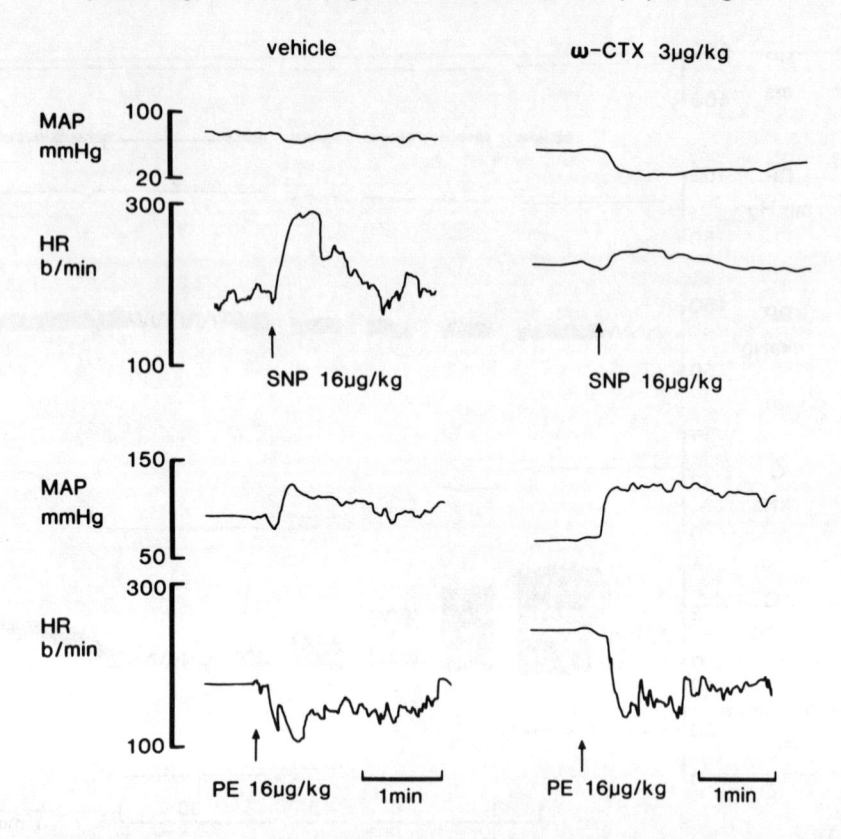

Fig. 4.13 Chart records to illustrate the drug method to raise or lower arterial blood pressure mean arterial pressure (*MAP*) in conscious rabbits causing falls or rises in heart rate (*HR*). SNP is sodium nitroprusside; PE is phenylephrine both as iv bolus injections before and after ω-conotoxin GVIA 3 μg/kg iv (Reproduced from Pruneau and Angus 1990*a* with permission.)

and vagal components (Wright and Angus 1995). This *in vivo* data and other *in vitro* data (Pruneau and Angus 1990*b*) in isolated mesenteric arteries are consistent with the view that ω-CTX blocks 'N'-type calcium channels on sympathetic varicosities to inhibit transmitter release. This example illustrates the importance of a conscious animal preparation with resting neural activity when testing sympatholytic drugs.

DRUG SELECTIVITY *IN VIVO*

Agonists selective for particular receptor subtypes are usually classified in rigorous *in vitro* bioassay systems before they are used in whole animal preparations. However, *in vivo*, other factors may come into play to alter the apparent selectivity, of the agonist. The following illustrates how an agonist, 5-carboxamidotryptamine

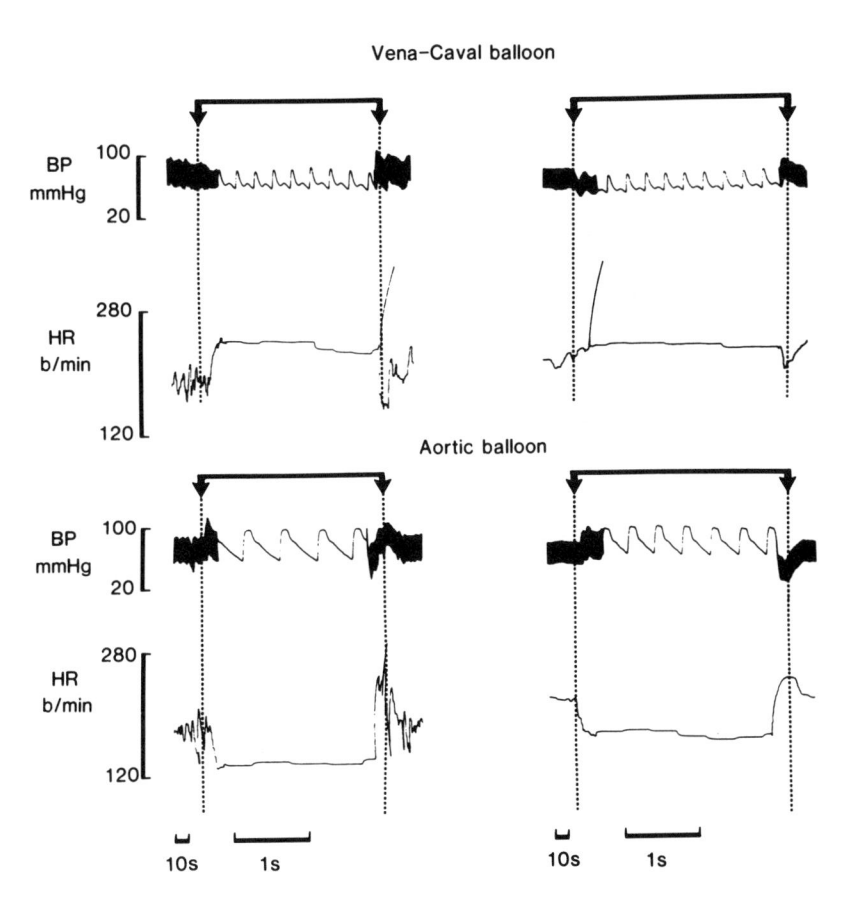

Fig. 4.14 Chart records of phasic arterial blood pressure (*BP*) and heart rate (*HR*) in a conscious rabbit during short vena caval balloon or aortic balloon inflations. ω-Conotoxin 3 μg/kg lowered the *BP* and attenuated the tachycardia to depressor (vena caval balloon) stimuli. (Reproduced from Pruneau and Angus 1990a with permission.)

(5-CT), defined at the time (1989) as a selective '5-HT$_1$-like' receptor agonist *in vitro*, becomes non-selective when administered to the conscious rabbit. Fig. 4.16 shows the effects of a steady state intravenous infusion of 5-CT to a conscious ganglion-blocked rabbit. At a dose (0.6 μg/kg/min iv) too low to elicit hindquarter vasodilatation (a '5-HT$_1$-like' receptor-mediated response in this species), 5-CT caused a dramatic fall in renal blood flow to zero, probably as a result of spasm of the renal artery (note the narrowing of the pulsatile record). This renal vascular response could be prevented by administration of the 5-HT$_2$ receptor antagonist, ketanserin (Wright and Angus 1989). Furthermore, an intravenous bolus of 5-CT (0.8 μg/kg) was able to elicit the 5-HT$_3$ receptor-mediated

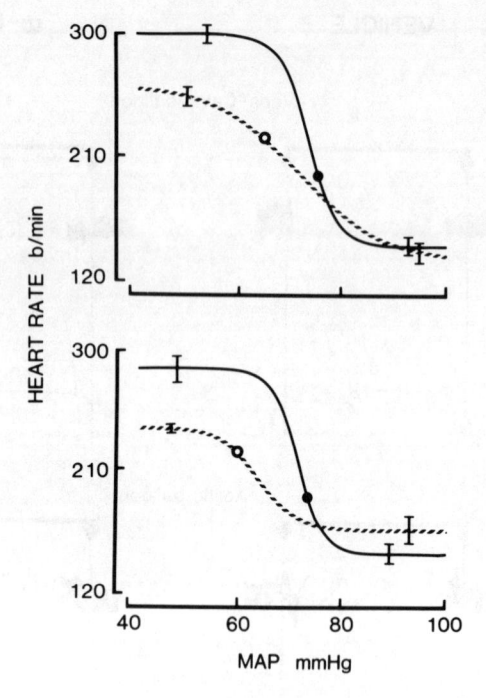

Fig. 4.15 Average baroreceptor reflex curves from conscious rabbits generated by the cuff inflation method (*bottom* panel $n = 3$) and drug method (*top* panel $n = 7$). Curves were obtained before (solid line) and after ω-conotoxin GVIA 3 µg/kg iv. Dots are at average resting heart rate and blood pressure. (Reproduced from Pruneau and Angus 1990*a* with permission.)

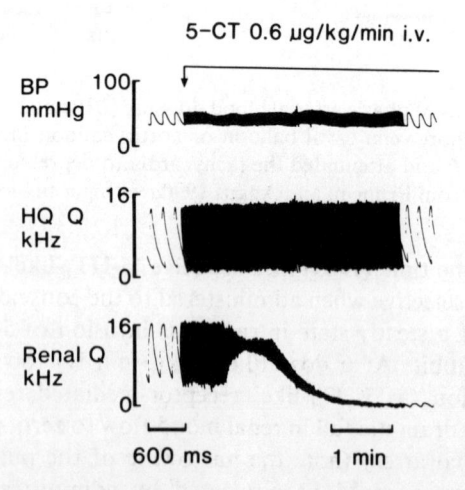

Fig. 4.16 Chart records showing renal artery spasm but no changes in the hindquarter bed (HQ Q = flow) during intravenous infusion of 5-carboxamidotryptamine (5-CT) in a conscious rabbit treated with mecamylamine. (Reproduced from Wright and Angus 1989 with permission.)

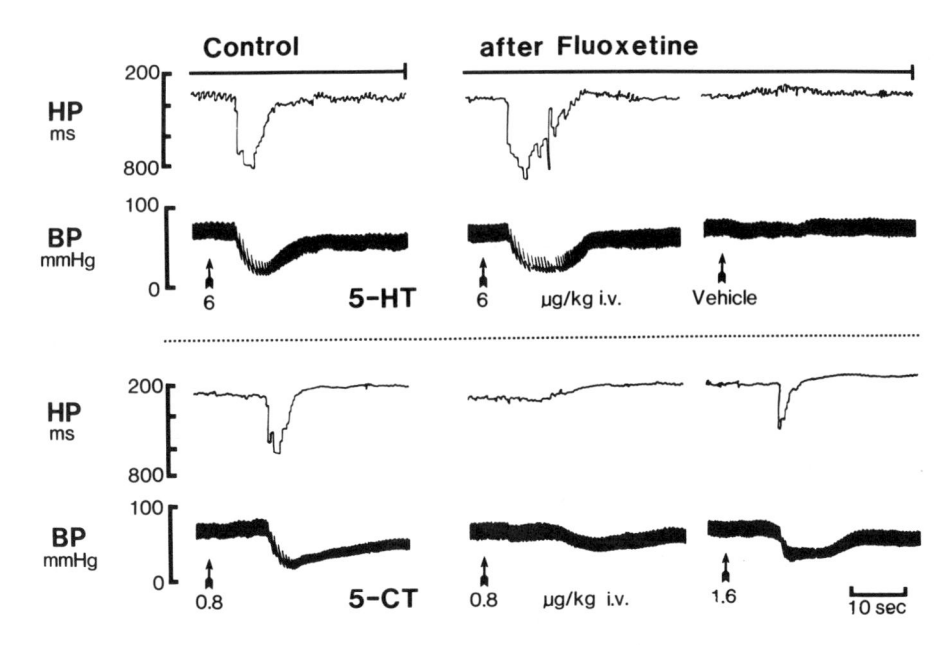

Fig. 4.17 Chart records from a conscious rabbit of heart period (*HP*) and arterial blood pressure (*BP*) during the 'Bezold–Jarisch-like' reflex evoked by 5-hydroxytryptamine (5-HT) 6 μg/kg IV bolus and by 5-carboxamidotryptamine (5-CT) 0.8–1.6 μg/kg before and 10 min after fluoxetine (1 μg/kg iv), an inhibitor of 5-HT uptake into platelets. (Reproduced from Wright and Angus 1989 with permission.)

Bezold–Jarisch-like bradycardic reflex in the conscious rabbit (Fig. 4.17). So it appeared, surprisingly, that 5-CT had 'lost' it's selectivity for '5-HT$_1$-like' receptors *in vivo*. But, these anomalous 5-HT$_2$ and 5-HT$_3$ receptor-mediated effects of 5-CT could be abolished by treatment of the rabbit with fluoxetine, a 5-HT uptake inhibitor (Fig. 4.17), or reserpine, to deplete stores of amines. These experiments suggested that 5-CT was taken up into platelets where it potently released endogenous 5-HT. Thus, 5-CT is essentially both a direct '5-HT$_1$-like' agonist and an indirectly-acting (5-HT-releasing) agonist in the rabbit. This cautionary example illustrates how apparent receptor selectivity may be lost when moving from well defined *in vitro* assays to the whole animal — an essential step in predicting the actions of novel and 'selective' therapeutic agents in man.

IN VIVO TECHNIQUES IN MAN

Studies of vascular smooth muscle pharmacology in man involve a variety of techniques directed to measurement of either vascular dimensions or blood flow. Depending on the vascular bed under study, these techniques may be non-invasive, utilizing external probes placed on the skin over the blood vessel, or invasive, requiring placement of devices in vessels of interest. In addition to assessment of dimensions and flow, techniques have been developed to measure vascular compliance, which has both structural as well as dynamic components, the latter being influenced by vascular tone.

Measurement of vessel diameter

Angiography

For many years, the gold standard for the measurement of vascular diameter has been angiography, a procedure that involves injection of a contrast agent into the blood vessel of interest to enable its radiographic visualization. Angiography has been employed, especially in the coronary vasculature, to study vascular pharmacology, by measuring changes in vascular dimensions in response to vasoactive agents. Recent advances in computer-assisted measurement techniques (quantitative angiography) have greatly increased the accuracy of this approach. For example the intracoronary injection of acetylcholine caused vasorelaxation in normal coronary arteries but impaired responses in human subjects with atherosclerosis (Ludmer *et al.* 1986). Since then we have witnessed a plethora of studies examining endothelium-dependent and independent vasomotion in the coronary circulation, that have shed new insights into our understanding of myocardial ischaemia (for review see Yeung *et al.* 1992). The major advantage of this technique is that studies can be performed as an adjunct to clinical investigation, since patients with atherosclerosis often require angiographic definition of the diseased segments of their arteries in order to plan surgical or non-surgical management.

However, angiographic estimates of *in vivo* vasomotion have several potential limitations. First, while it provides remarkably accurate estimates of vessel calibre in normal arteries and in settings of concentric disease, it is notoriously inaccurate in the more commonly encountered situation of eccentric atheroma. Multiple radiographic projections may be required to assess diameter in a region with significant narrowing. Secondly, most angiographic contrast agents induce varying degrees of vasodilatation, which may influence the assessment of vascular reactivity. Finally, the technique provides short glimpses of blood vessels over a few seconds at best and is unsuitable for continuous monitoring of vascular reactivity. Despite these limitations, angiography has yielded information over the years on vascular reactivity in response to stressors, adrenoceptor stimulation, endothelial function (Yeung *et al.* 1992), and other aspects of coronary and peripheral vascular responsiveness.

Intravascular ultrasound

Intravascular ultrasound imaging is a clinical tool that permits direct visualization of vascular pathology (Pandian *et al.* 1988; Yock *et al.* 1991). The ability of ultrasound to penetrate below the luminal surface allows imaging of the entire cross-section of an artery in real time. This technology has opened new vistas in the study of atherosclerosis and enabled direct observations of the effects of different interventions on the plaque and arterial wall. There are two basic approaches to catheter imaging, involving either solid state or mechanical designs. One solid state catheter currently available has 64 transducer elements arranged radially near the catheter tip. The mechanical catheters develop images either by directly rotating the transducer at the tip of the catheter or by rotating a reflector adjacent to the transducer. The use of high frequency (30–40 MHz) transducers in the catheter design permits high-resolution imaging and enhances the accuracy of the measurement.

Intravascular ultrasound imaging provides highly accurate estimates of vascular cross-sectional area that correlate closely with histological measurements (Tobis *et al.* 1989). This technique is therefore being increasingly used in the assessment of vascular reactivity in medium sized arteries, including the epicardial coronary circulation (Pinto *et al.* 1992). Continuous on-line imaging permits real time visualization and measurement of changes in vascular dimensions. However, its greatest advantage over angiography is that it provides information on the structure of the vascular wall, and thus has the potential to yield data on structure–function relationships that are so important in the study of pathological states like atherosclerosis and hypertension. With catheter ultrasound images of arteries, the layers of the arterial wall are distinct acoustically. In muscular arteries such as the coronaries, the media of the vessel stands out as a dark band compared to the intima and adventitia. An impressive finding in the early imaging experience of any laboratory is the amount of plaque present in a coronary artery in the so-called angiographically 'normal' reference segment. In fact, in a vessel with an angiographically 'discrete' stenosis, it is unusual to find any segment in the vessel that does not have significant plaque accumulation.

Limitations to the use of intravascular ultrasound imaging in the assessment of vascular reactivity include access to only proximal arteries because of catheter size, and the ability to visualize only one cross-sectional 'slice' of the artery. The latter problem is being addressed with the approach of three-dimensional reconstruction of arterial anatomy from a series of two-dimensional slices, thus providing information on vascular segments rather than limited cross-sections (Rosenfield *et al.* 1992).

Non-invasive high-frequency ultrasound

This technique has recently emerged as a practical non-invasive approach to the study of endothelium-dependent and endothelium-independent vasorelaxation in the brachial artery in man (Celemajer *et al.* 1992). In brief, the technique consists of interrogation of the brachial artery from the surface with a 10–12 MHz transducer, and measurement of the diameter of the vessel. Flow-mediated endothelium-dependent vasodilatation is then assessed by inflating a wrist cuff to suprasystolic pressures for a finite time period (5–10 min) and then releasing it, to allow a hyperaemic response to occur in the forearm and hand. The brachial

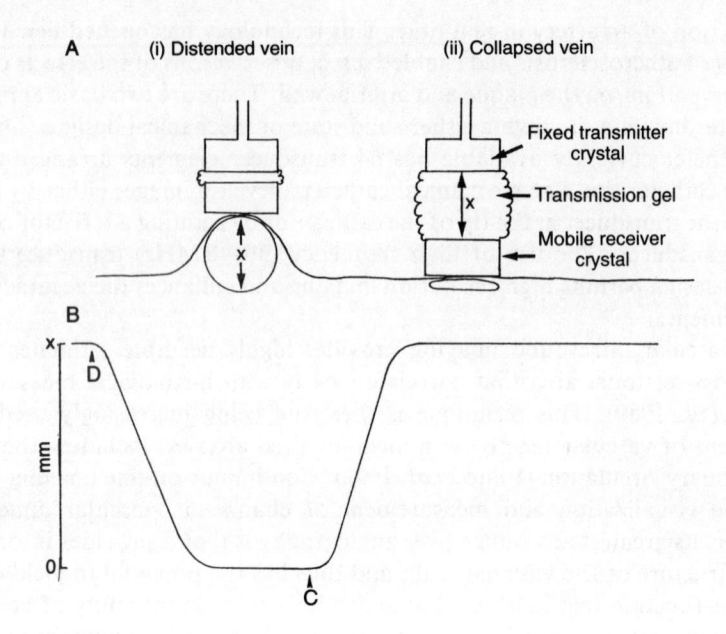

Fig. 4.18 Schematic diagram of the non-invasive measurement of hand vein diameter by sonomicrometry. Passive distention of the vein (D) by inflating an arm cuff brings the lower mobile crystal glued to the skin overlying the vein closer to the upper reference crystal. At C the cuff is released collapsing the vein and allowing the mobile crystal to move away.

artery dilates in response to this hyperaemia, and this dilatation is endothelium-dependent. Endothelium-independent vasodilatation is also assessed in the brachial artery in response to sublingual nitroglycerin. Several groups have adopted this approach for reasons of convenience and because it is non-invasive. Its limitation is that it provides information only on flow-mediated vasodilatation, which is only one aspect of endothelium-dependent vasorelaxation.

In vivo *assessment of venous reactivity*

Venous reactivity can be assessed *in vivo* by measuring changes in diameter in a venous segment maintained at constant pressure. A variety of approaches have been used, such as a microscope focused on a dot painted on the overlying skin and use of displacement transducers, including linear variable differential transducers. In our laboratory, sonomicrometer crystals placed over the vein are used to provide continuous recordings of changes in vein size in response to pharmacological agents (Hurlston and Chin 1992) (Fig. 4.18). As shown in Fig. 4.19 the vein is first partly distended passively by inflating a cuff on the upper arm to slow venous flow. When the diameter is steady, noradrenaline is infused intravenously upstream at 0.1 ml/min and continued until the contraction is steady.

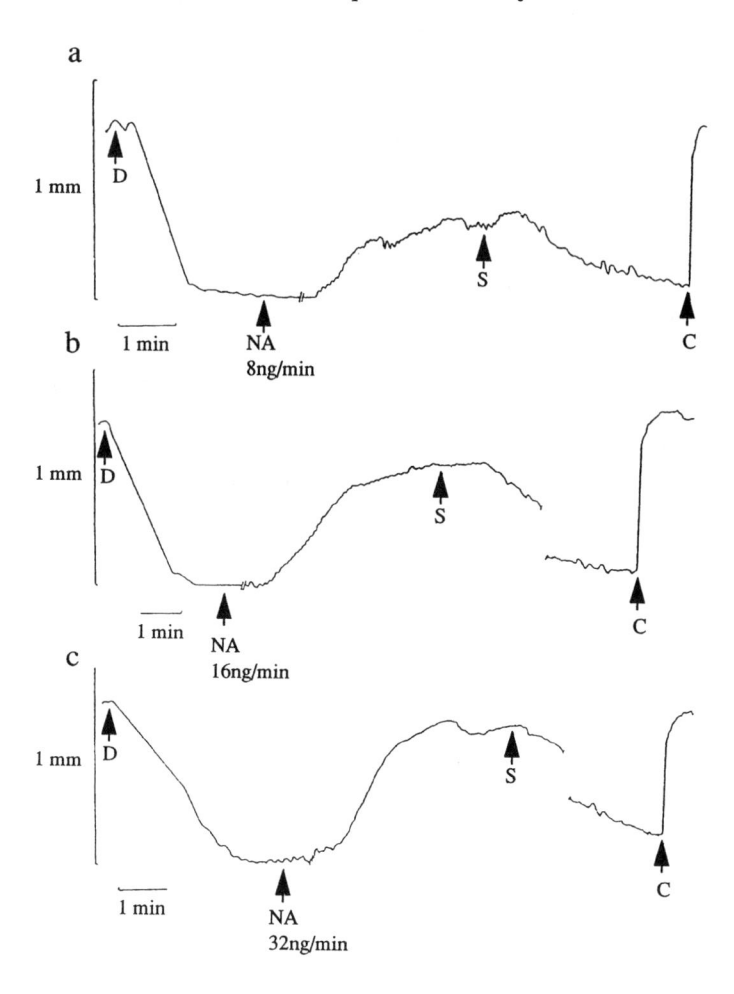

Fig. 4.19 Sonomicrometer traces of the diameter changes of a human hand vein during constriction by noradrenaline (NA) infusion 8, 16, or 32 ng/min given intravenously upstream between NA and S, Stop. At D the vein was passively distended by partly inflating an arm cuff before infusing the noradrenaline. At C the arm cuff was collapsed. Note the active contraction of the vein by progressively increasing doses of NA. (From Hurlston and Chin, Baker Medical Research Institute, unpublished.)

The cuff is then released to fully collapse the vein (Fig. 4.19). The technique measures the active constriction of the vein from the distended starting diameter. The limitation of such assays is that a suitable length of vein without branches is required. A great advantage of the approach is that the same vein or one in the vicinity can be biopsied for *in vitro* pharmacology studies providing direct *in vivo–in vitro* comparisons (Hurlston and Chin 1992).

Measurement of blood flow

The availability of a number of techniques for measurement of blood flow in man permits pharmacological studies in regional vascular beds.

Indicator dilution and thermodilution techniques

The Fick principle forms the basis for the indicator dilution method of measuring blood flow and cardiac output. A green dye (indocyanine green), a radioactive isotope, or cold saline (thermodilution, see below) is injected into one part of the circulation and measured in another. A known amount of indicator is injected and its concentration is measured downstream after the indicator has thoroughly mixed with the blood. Flow is then measured as the amount of indicator injected divided by its average concentration during its passage past the sampling site.

Thermodilution techniques utilize injection of a fluid miscible with blood and a lower temperature into the region of study at a constant rate. The resulting change in temperature is then detected a short distance downstream. The technique requires placement of specially designed catheters in regional vascular beds, such as the pulmonary circulation and the coronary sinus. The technique has the advantage of allowing measurements to be repeated at short intervals, and thus monitoring rapid changes in the circulation. However, its major disadvantage is its lack of reproducibility, limiting its use in the detection of small changes in flow.

Doppler velocimetry

More recently, a number of catheter-based approaches to the measurement of regional blood flow using Doppler velocimetry have been developed and successfully applied to pharmacological studies in regional vascular beds (Sibley *et al*. 1986; Doucette *et al*. 1992). Currently, Doppler catheters as well as guidewires are in use: these consist of piezo electric crystals mounted at the tip of catheters or extremely thin guidewires which can be positioned in the artery of interest. Flow velocity is measured from the reflection of ultrasonic waves off the erythrocytes in the vessel under study. Recent studies have shown that in combination with intravascular ultrasound imaging to measure vascular cross-sectional area, Doppler velocimetry yields highly accurate estimates of volumetric blood flow. Further, in the coronary circulation, numerous studies have shown that this combination is of great value in the study of differential drug effects on the conductance and resistance arteries (Sudhir *et al*. 1992, 1993*a,b*, 1994) (Fig. 4.20). A drug that influences epicardial cross-sectional area, but has minimal effects on blood flow must act predominantly on conductance arteries (e.g. nitroglycerin, ergonovine) (Fig. 4.21). While an agent that does not change epicardial coronary arterial dimensions but increases coronary blood flow must act predominantly on resistance arteries (e.g. adenosine) (Sudhir *et al*. 1993*a*).

A number of important considerations influence the accuracy of Doppler-derived blood flow measurements. Recent studies have shown that the method

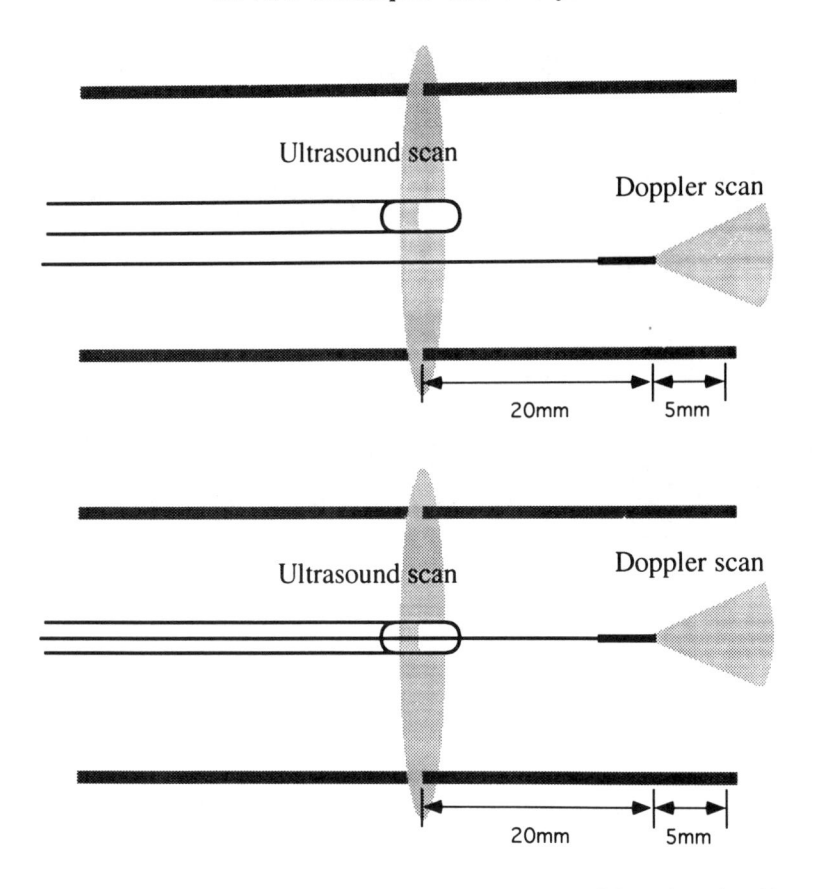

Fig. 4.20 Schema of relative positions of imaging catheter and Doppler wire. *Top*: two-dimensional imaging catheter placed alongside a 0.018 inch Doppler wire. *Bottom*: two-dimensional imaging catheter introduced over a 0.014 inch Doppler wire. (Drawn after Figure 1, Sudhir *et al.* 1993*a*.)

of analysis of the Doppler-shift signals influences the accuracy of the technique. Flow derived from fast-Fourier transformation (FFT) analysis yields highly accurate measurements, while flow derived using zero-cross detectors appear to have less accuracy (Sudhir *et al.* 1992), especially with non-uniform flow profiles. Another limitation of Doppler-derived measurements using catheter-based systems is that the catheter itself is a potential source of error, since it may interfere with flow. The disruption of blood flow would also tend to flatten the velocity profile, leading to reduced peak velocity measurements (Tadaoka *et al.* 1990). However, *in vitro* studies have shown that interference to Doppler flow velocity measurements produced by the intravascular location of a catheter are minimal at a distance of about 10 catheter diameters downstream from the catheter tip. Sample volumes in such systems are therefore usually positioned at this distance from the catheter to minimize this potential problem.

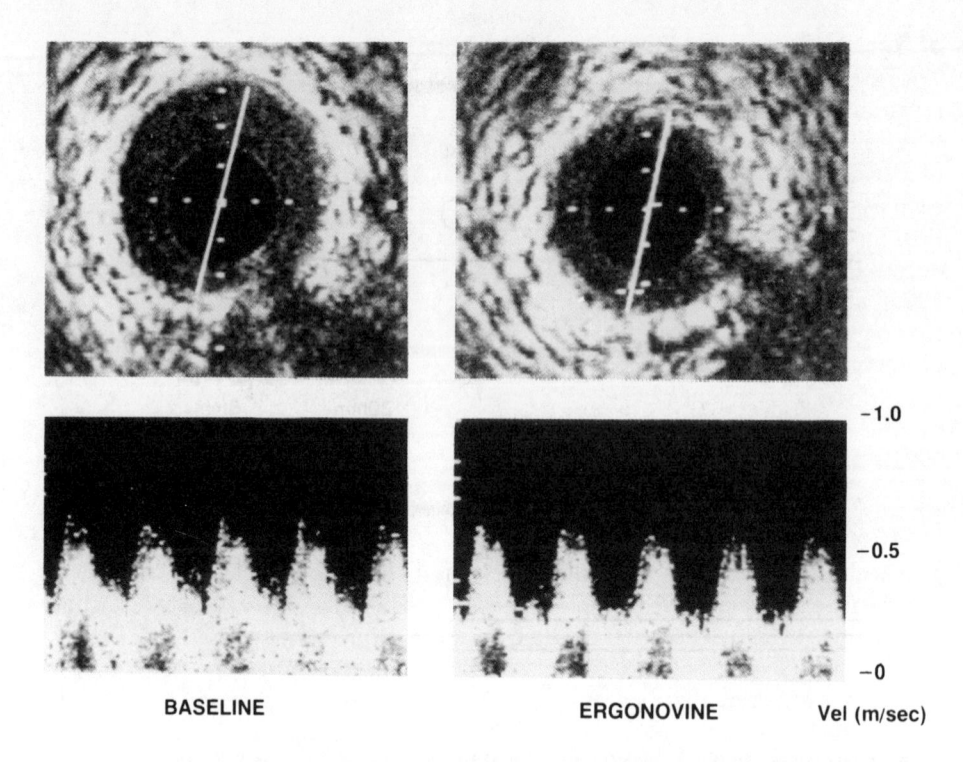

Fig. 4.21 Two-dimensional ultrasound images (*top* panels) showing cross-sections of the left circumflex coronary artery of a mongrel dog and spectral display (*bottom* panels) showing simultaneous Doppler velocimetry in the same coronary artery at baseline (*left*) and 2 min after intracoronary 200 μg of ergonovine. (Reproduced from Sudhir *et al.* 1993a with permission.)

Venous occlusion plethysmography

This is a well established technique of limb blood flow measurement that has seen a major resurgence in recent years as a method of studying responses of resistance arteries in limbs to infusion of pharmacological agents. In brief, the technique consists of blocking venous outflow from the limb using cuff occlusion, without interfering with arterial inflow. The volume changes in the limb beyond the level of occlusion are measured using a mercury-in-rubber strain gauge. The initial rate of volume increase during venous occlusion is the rate of arterial inflow. The technique can be applied to the forearm and drugs can be infused through a cannula placed in the brachial artery. Venous occlusion plethysmography has also been used to measure calf blood flow changes in response to pharmacological agents infused into the femoral artery.

The major advantage of the technique is that it is fairly easy to use. However, a number of precautions have to be taken to ensure accurate and reproducible measurement of blood flow. The measurements should be made in a quiet room to avoid variations induced by noise. Further, a small but significant component of forearm flow is skin blood flow which is influenced by ambient temperature. The use of a temperature controlled room is therefore essential to ensure reproducible results.

A fairly large body of information has been obtained on the pharmacology of peripheral resistance arteries using this technique in pathological conditions such as hypertension (Panza *et al*. 1990; Calver *et al*. 1992). The first demonstration in humans that an abnormality of endothelium-dependent vasorelaxation occurs in essential hypertension was obtained using this technique (Panza *et al*. 1990), although more recent studies with the same methodology suggest that this finding may not be universal (Cockcroft *et al*. 1994). Several studies from our group have utilized this technique to examine changes in pharmacological properties of forearm resistance arteries induced by such interventions as steroid therapy (Sudhir *et al*. 1989; Pirpiris *et al*. 1992), fish oil supplementation (Chin *et al*. 1993), and exercise.

Laser Doppler flowmetry

This technique utilizes the Doppler shift of laser light as the information carrier to measure microvascular flow in a continuous non-invasive manner. A common application of the technique is in skin pharmacology studies where skin blood flow changes following drug administration can be monitored. A major limitation of the technique is that the concentration of drug that reaches the blood vessel is unknown and might be quite different from that applied to the skin.

Determination of arterial compliance

Considerable evidence now exists that arterial compliance has both a passive component determined by the tissue content of the vascular wall, especially extracellular matrix proteins, and an active component that is a result of smooth muscle tone. With the recognition that proximal arterial compliance is significantly decreased in, and may be a determinant of, isolated systolic hypertension, there is now considerable interest in techniques that can be used to quantify arterial compliance. These vary from direct approaches to measure aortic and total body compliance using suprasternal two-dimensional echocardiographic and Doppler techniques (Dart *et al*. 1991), to more indirect techniques such as the determination of aortic and limb pulse wave velocity by **applanation tonometry**. The latter technique has the advantage of being able to detect and quantify pulse wave reflection from the periphery, which is influenced by the tone of precapillary arterioles, and is reportedly an important factor in systolic hypertension in the elderly (O'Rourke 1990). Safar and co-workers were among the first to demonstrate that mechanical properties of medium sized blood vessels can be altered by anti-hypertensive therapy (Safar *et al*. 1987). More recently, Cameron and Dart (1994) have shown that interventions such as exercise training can increase total systemic arterial compliance in humans.

ACKNOWLEDGEMENTS

The authors thank Miss Fanoula Penou for secretarial assistance and Dr Jaye Chin for preparation of some figures. The work reviewed here was supported by an Institute block grant from the National Health and Medical Research Council of Australia and Glaxo Australia Pty Ltd.

REFERENCES

Angus, J. A. and Lew, M. J. (1992). Interpretation of the acetylcholine test of endothelial cell dysfunction in hypertension. *J. Hypertens.*, **10(Suppl.7)**, S179-86.

Angus, J. A, Campbell, G. R., Cocks, T. M., and Manderson, J. A. (1983). Vasodilatation by acetylcholine is endothelium-dependent: a study by sonomicrometry in canine femoral artery *in vivo*. *J. Physiol.*, **344**, 209-22.

Angus, J. A., Cocks, T. M., Wright, C. E., Satoh, K., and Campbell, G. R. (1988). Endothelium-dependent responses in large arteries and in the microcirculation. In *Relaxing and contracting factors* (ed.) P. M. Vanhoutte, pp. 361-87. Humana Press. New Jersey.

Calver, A., Collier, J., Moncada, S., and Vallance, P. (1992). Effect of local intra-arterial NG-monomethyl-L-arginine in patients with hypertension: the nitric oxide dilator mechanism appears abnormal. *J. Hypertens.*, **10**, 1025-31.

Cameron, J. D. and Dart, A. M. (1994). Exercise training increases total systemic arterial compliance in humans. *Am. J. Physiol.*, **266**, H693-701.

Celermajer, D. S., Sorensen, K. E., Gooch, V. M., Spiegelhalter, D. J., Miller, O. I., Sullivan, I. D., *et al.* (1992). Non-invasive detection of endothelial dysfunction in children and adults at risk of atherosclerosis. *Lancet*, **340**, 1111-15.

Chin, J. P. F., Gust, A. P., Nestel, P. J., and Dart, A. M. (1993). Marine oils dose-dependently inhibit vasoconstriction of forearm resistance vessels in humans. *Hypertension*, **21**, 22-28.

Cockcroft, J. R., Chowienczyk, P. J., Benjamin, N., and Ritter, J. M. (1994). Preserved endothelium-dependent vasodilation in patients with essential hypertension. *N. Engl. J. Med.*, **330**, 1036-40.

Cocks, T. M., Broughton, A., Dib, M., Sudhir, K., and Angus, J. A. (1989). Endothelin is blood vessel selective: studies on a variety of human and dog vessels *in vitro* and regional blood flow in the conscious rabbit. *Clin. Exp. Pharmacol. Physiol.*, **16**, 243-6..

Dart, A. M., Lacombe, E., Yeoh, J. K., Cameron, J. D., Jennings, G. L., Laufer, E., *et al.* (1991). Aortic distensibility in patients with isolated hypercholesterolaemia, coronary heart disease or cardiac transplant. *Lancet*, **338**, 270-3.

Doucette, J. W., Corl, P. D., Payne, H. M., Flynn, A. E., Goto, M., Nassi, M., *et al.* (1992). Validation of a Doppler guide wire for intravascular measurement of coronary artery flow velocity. *Circulation*, **85**, 1899-911.

Folkow, B., Hallback, M., Lundgren, Y., and Weiss, L. (1970). Background of increased flow resistance and vascular reactivity in spontaneously hypertensive rats. *Acta Physiol. Scand.*, **80**, 93-106.

Head, G. A. and Adams, M. A. (1992). Time course of changes in baroreceptor heart rate reflex deficit in spontaneously hypertensive rats. *Clin. Exp. Pharmacol. Physiol.*, **19**, 587-97.

Herd, J. A. and Barger, A. C. (1964). Simplified technique for chronic catheterization of blood vessels. *J. Appl. Physiol.*, **19**, 791-2.

Hurlston, R. M. and Chin, J. P. F. (1992). Pharmacology of human hand veins: *in vivo* and *in vitro* studies (Abstract). *Clin. Exp. Pharmacol Physiol.*, **(suppl 21)**, 30.

Korner, P. I. and Angus, J. A. (1992). Structural determinants of vascular resistance properties in hypertension. Hemodynamic and model analysis. *J. Vasc. Res.*, **29**, 293–312.

Korner, P. I., Bobik, A., Angus, J. A., Adams, M., and Friberg, P. (1989). Resistance control in hypertension. *J. Hypertension* **7**, S125–34.

Korner, P. I., Shaw, J., West, M. J., and Oliver, J. R. (1972). Central nervous system control of baroreceptor reflexes in the rabbit. *Circ. Res.* **31**, 637–52.

Ludmer, P. L., Selwyn, A. P., Shook, T. L., Wayne, R. R., Mudge, G. H., Alexander, R. W., *et al.* (1986). Paradoxical vasoconstriction induced by acetylcholine in atherosclerotic coronary arteries. *N. Engl. J. Med.*, **315**, 1046–51.

O'Rourke, M. F. (1990). Arterial stiffness, systolic blood pressure and the logical treatment of arterial hypertension. *Hypertension*, **15**, 339–47.

Pandian, N. G., Kreis, A., Brockway, B., Isner, J. M., Sacharoff, A., Boleza, E., *et al.* (1988). Ultrasound angioscopy: Real-time, two-dimensional, intraluminal ultrasound imaging of blood vessels. *Am. J. Cardiol.*, **62**, 493–4.

Panza, J. A., Quyyumi, A. A., Brush, J. E. Jr, and Epstein, S. E. (1990). Abnormal endothelium-dependent vascular relaxation in patients with essential hypertension. *N. Engl. J. Med.*, **323**, 22–27.

Pinto, F. J., St. Goar, F. G., Fischell, T. A., Stadius, M. L., Valantine, H. A., Alderman, E. L., *et al.* (1992). Nitroglycerin-induced coronary vasodilation in cardiac transplant recipients: evaluation with *in vivo* intracoronary ultrasound. *Circulation*, **85**, 69–77.

Pirpiris, M., Sudhir, K., Yeung, S., Jennings, G., and Whitworth, J. A. (1992). Pressor responsiveness in corticosteroid-induced hypertension in man. *Hypertension*, **19**, 567–74.

Pruneau, D. and Angus, J. A. (1990a). ω-conotoxin GVIA, the N-type calcium channel inhibitor, is sympatholytic but not vagolytic: consequences for hemodynamics and autonomic reflexes in conscious rabbits. *J. Cardiovasc. Pharmacol.*, **16**, 675–80.

Pruneau, D. and Angus, J. A. (1990b). ω-conotoxin GVIA is a potent inhibitor of sympathetic neurogenic responses in rat small mesenteric arteries. *Br. J. Pharmacol.*, **100**, 180–4.

Rosenfield, K., Kaufman, J., Pieczek, A., Langevin, R. E., Razvi, S., and Isner, J. M. (1992). Real-time three-dimensional reconstruction of intravascular ultrasound images of iliac arteries. *Am. J. Cardiol.*, **70**, 412–15.

Safar, M. E., Toto-Moukouo, J. J., Bauthier, J. A., Asmar, R. E., Levenson, J. A., Simon, A. C., *et al.* (1987). Arterial dynamics, cardiac hypertrophy and antihypertensive treatment. *Circulation*, **75(Suppl I)**, I156–61.

Sibley, D. H., Millar, H. D., Hartley, C. J., and Whitlow, P. L. (1986). Subselective measurement of coronary blood flow velocity using a steerable Doppler catheter. *J. Am. Coll. Cardiol.*, **8**, 1332–40.

Sudhir, K., Jennings, G. L., Esler, M. D., Korner, P. I., Blombery, P., Lambert, G., *et al.* (1989). Hydrocortisone induced hypertension in man: pressor responsiveness and sympathetic function. *Hypertension*, **13**, 416–21.

Sudhir, K., Hargrave, V., Johnson, E., Aldea, G., Mori, G, Ports, T. A., *et al.* (1992). Measurement of volumetric coronary blood flow using a Doppler catheter: Validation in an animal model. *Am. Heart J.*, **124**, 870–5.

Sudhir K., MacGregor, J. S., Barbant, S. D., Foster, E., Fitzgerald, P. J., Chatterjee, K., *et al.* (1993a). Assessment of coronary conductance and resistance vessel reactivity in response to nitroglycerin, ergonovine and adenosine: *in vivo* studies with simultaneous intravascular two-dimensional and Doppler ultrasound. *J. Am. Coll. Cardiol.*, **21**, 1261–68.

Sudhir, K., MacGregor, J. S., Gupta, M., Barbant, S. D., Redberg, R., Yock, P. G., et al. (1993b). Effect of selective angiotensin II receptor antagonism and ACE inhibition on the coronary vasculature in vivo: intravascular two-dimensional and Doppler ultrasound studies. *Circulation*, **87**, 931–8.

Sudhir, K., MacGregor, J. S., DeMarco, T., Gupta, M., Yock, P. G., and Chatterjee, K. (1994). Cyclosporine impairs release of endothelium-derived relaxing factor in epicardial and resistance coronary arteries. *Circulation*. **90**, 3018–23.

Tadaoka, S., Kagiyama, M., Hiramatsu, O., et al.(1990). Accuracy of 20 MHz Doppler catheter coronary artery velocimetry for measurement of coronary blood flow velocity. *Cathet. Cardiovasc. Diagn.*, **19**, 205–13.

Tobis, J. M., Mallery, J. A., Gessert, J., Griffith, J., Mahon, D., Bessen, M. et al. (1989). Intravascular ultrasound cross-sectional imaging before and after balloon angioplasty in vivo. *Circulation.*, **80**, 873–82.

Wright, C. E. and Angus, J. A. (1987). Diverse vascular responses to serotonin in the conscious rabbit: effects of serotonin antagonists on renal artery spasm. *J. Cardiovasc. Pharmacol.*, **10**, 415–23.

Wright, C. E. and Angus, J. A. (1989). 5-carboxamidotryptamine elicits 5-HT$_2$ and 5-HT$_3$ receptor-mediated cardiovascular responses in the conscious rabbit: evidence for 5-HT release from platelets. *J. Cardiovasc. Pharmacol.*, **13**, 557–64.

Wright, C. E. and Angus, J. A. (1995). Haemodynamic and autonomic reflex effects of chronic N-type Ca^{++} channel blockade with ω-conotoxin GVIA in conscious normotensive and hypertensive rabbits. *J. Cardiovasc. Pharmacol.* **25**, 459–68.

Wright, C. E. and Fozard, J. R. (1988). Regional vasodilatation is a prominent feature of the haemodynamic response to endothelin in anaesthetized, spontaneously hypertensive rats. *Eur. J. Pharmacol.*, **155**, 201–3.

Wright, C. E, Angus, J. A., and Korner, P. I. (1987). Vascular amplifier properities in renovascular hypertension in conscious rabbits. Hindquarter responses to constrictor and dilator stimuli. *Hypertension*, **9**, 122–31.

Yeung, A. C., Raby, K. E., Ganz, P., and Selwyn, A. P. (1992). New insights into the management of myocardial ischemia. *Am. J. Cardiol.*, **70**, 8G–12G.

Yock, P. G., Fitzgerald, P. J., Linker, D. T., and Angelsen, B. A. J. (1991). Intravascular ultrasound guidance for catheter-based coronary interventions. *J. Am. Coll. Cardiol.*, **17**, 39B–45B.

5. Initiation of smooth muscle response

A. M. Shaw and J. C. McGrath

RECEPTORS AND RECEPTOR TRANSDUCTION

Regulation of vascular smooth muscle tone

The tension of vascular smooth muscle is regulated by numerous exogenous chemical agents (agonists) whose concentrations change in response to physiological and pathophysiological events in order to modulate blood flow. For experimental purposes the responses of vascular smooth muscle may be conveniently divided into stimulatory (promoting contraction) or inhibitory (promoting relaxation). *In vivo*, the degree of background tension (tone) of the smooth muscle is largely due to the interaction between those exogenous agonists promoting constriction (vasoconstrictors) and those agonists promoting relaxation (vasodilators).

The sequence of events by which most stimulatory or inhibitory agonists regulate smooth muscle activity is depicted schematically in Fig. 5.1. These events are often referred to as pharmacomechanical coupling and are defined as those mechanisms that evoke smooth muscle responses that are independent of changes in the electrical potential of the plasma membrane. Pharmacomechanical responses are achieved by agonist-induced changes in the intracellular concentration of second messenger molecules. These include cytosolic free calcium ($[Ca^+]_i$) (contraction), cyclic adenosine monophosphate (cAMP) (relaxation), cyclic guanosine monophosphate (cGMP) (relaxation), and 1,2-diacylglycerol (DG) (relaxation/contraction). Changes in $[Ca^+]_i$ may arise from the opening of Ca^+ channels in the plasma membrane allowing influx of extracellular Ca^+ or from the release of Ca^+ from intracellular organelles, such as endoplasmic reticulum. Influx of extracellular Ca^+ may be mediated through ion channels directly linked to receptors (receptor operated ion channel, ROC) or through Ca^+ channels sensitive to membrane potential (voltage operated ion channel, VOC) which open in response to membrane depolarization.

The release of intracellular Ca^+ is mediated through changes in the concentration of inositol-1,4,5-trisphosphate (Ins $(1,4,5)P_3$, IP_3) an intermediary derived from the phosphorylated inositolphospholipid phosphatidylinositol-4,5-bisphosphate (Ptd Ins $(4,5)$ P_2) by the action of phospholipase C enzymes (see Chapter 8). The hydrolysis of Ptd Ins $(4,5)$ P_2 also results in the formation of DG. DG may however arise independently of this pathway by the action of phospholipase enzymes on the membrane phospholipids phosphatidylethanolamine, phosphatidylcholine, and sphingomylin.

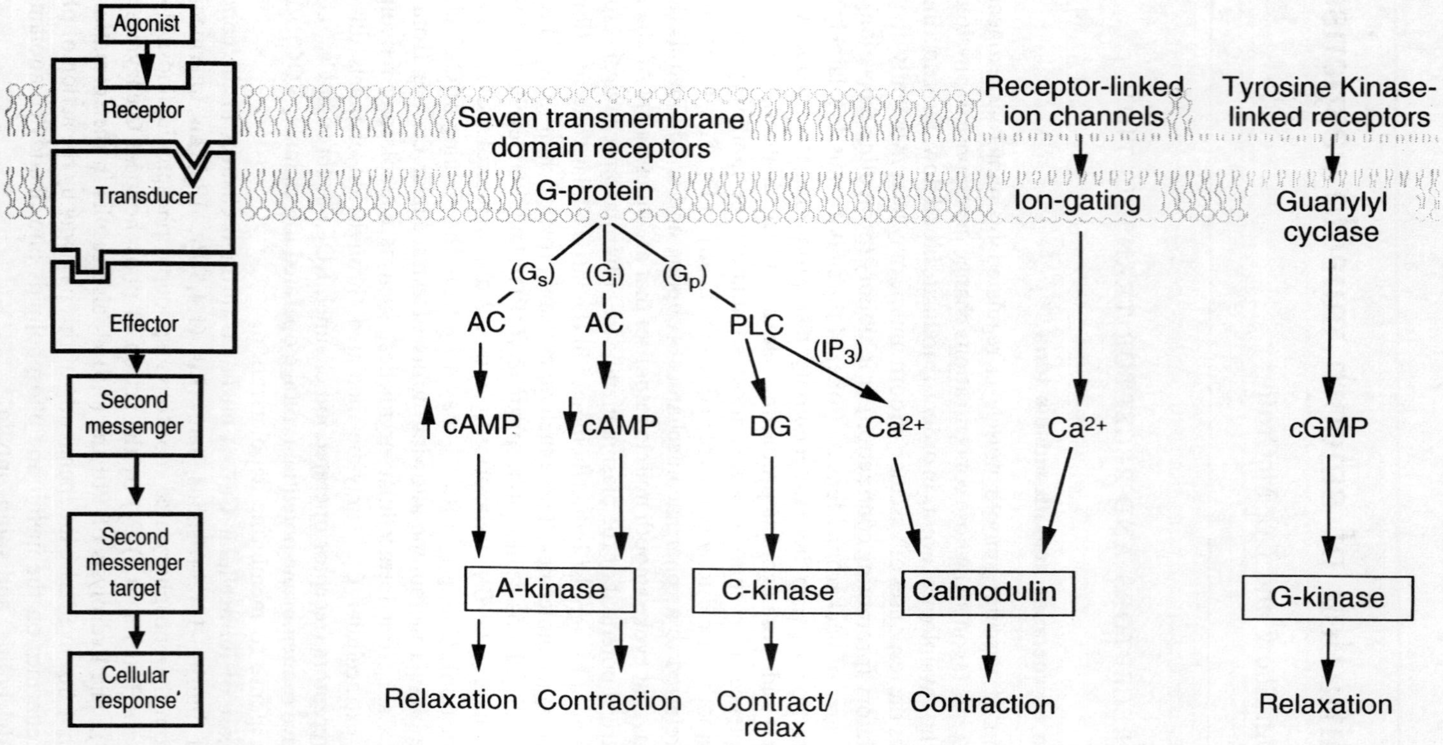

Fig. 5.1 Simplified schematic diagram showing the sequence of events underlying excitation–contraction coupling in vascular smooth muscle. AC, adenylyl cyclase; A-kinase, cyclic AMP-dependent protein kinase; C-kinase, protein kinase C-dependent kinase; G-kinase, cyclic GMP-dependent protein kinase.

These second messengers interact with specific intracellular receptors located either in the plasma membrane or on intracellular structures. The targets for second messengers are predominantly the protein kinases (and protein phosphatases) that catalyse the phosphorylation (dephosphorylation) of proteins associated with those elements of the cell, such as the contractile machinery or membrane ion channels, which mediate the functional response. Phosphorylation by protein kinases of seryl, threonyl, and to a lesser extent tyrosyl residues on these proteins results in conformational changes which initiate the functional response. Protein kinase A is the target for cAMP, protein kinase G for cGMP, protein kinase C for DG, and Ca^+-calmodulin-dependent kinase for $[Ca^+]_i$.

The initiation of this sequence of intracellular events is achieved by the interaction of external agonists with *specific membrane receptors*. Some of those agonists that are of pathophysiological importance are discussed in a later section (p. 123). They include a variety of neurotransmitters, hormones, and autacoids that are heterogeneous both in structure and in biological function. It is the primary function of membrane receptors to discriminate between the plethora of extracellular agonists to permit individual cell types to respond selectively to changes in the concentration of specific agonists.

Criteria for receptor classification

Membrane receptors can be classified using several pharmacological approaches.

(a) Rank order of agonist potency. The function of a receptor is to respond to its 'natural' agonist rather than others so this is the first line of definition. However 'natural' agonists often act at several receptors so on their own are an imprecise guide. The specificity of a receptor can often be defined by a range of structurally related agonists. For example the division of the adrenoceptors into α and β subtypes was based on the relative potency of a range of catecholamines that produce relaxation or contraction of smooth muscle. Logically, it should be possible to extend this approach to structure activity relationships. Key characteristics of the chemical composition of the ligand recognition site of the receptor can be gleaned by studying a range of related agonists with defined structural modifications. The assumption is that the agonist with the greatest efficacy (the capacity to evoke a response) is structurally more complementary with the receptor structure.

(b) High affinity antagonists: molecules devoid of intrinsic efficacy bind to the ligand recognition site and block agonist responses. This is the simplest and consequently the most widely used approach for receptor classification.

(c) Radiolabelled agonists and antagonists offer a means of quantifying the density of receptors. The labelled ligand must have a high affinity and high specificity for the receptor and must display both reversibility and saturability. The binding kinetics must be consistent with the time course of the functional response.

(d) The phenomenon of homologous desensitization also offers a convenient way to define receptor types. Almost all receptors to some extent display this phenomenon: exposure of the receptor to, usually, high concentrations of a specific agonist renders that receptor insensitive to subsequent agonist challenge. It is now clear that modification of specific domains on the receptor underlies this phenomenon (see next section p. 123).

(e) The second messenger system associated with a receptor also offers a convenient way of classifying receptors. For example, each of the receptor classes for 5-HT is coupled to a distinct transduction process (see Table 5.1). These techniques have played an important role in the classification of receptors for many agonists including acetylcholine, catecholamines, histamine, eicosanoids, etc.

(f) Classification of receptors according to their chemical structure has now been made possible through the techniques of molecular biology. The development of efficient methods for receptor isolation and purification, molecular cloning, and gene expression techniques has identified the amino acid sequence (primary structure) for many receptors. Once the primary structure of the receptor protein has been identified its tertiary structure, i.e. configuration within the membrane, can be deduced. Largely based on their tertiary configuration, receptors have been classified into three structurally distinct families. Receptors composed of seven transmembrane domains (G protein-linked receptors), receptors composed of a single transmembrane domain (tyrosine kinase-linked receptors), and receptors composed of transmembrane subunits incorporating a cation/anion channel (ion channel-linked receptors).

Seven transmembrane domain receptors (G protein-linked receptors)

Most agonists, both stimulatory and inhibitory, that regulate smooth muscle activity interact with this receptor type. Molecular cloning techniques have permitted the identification of the primary structure of many of these membrane receptors. Receptors in this class are usually glycoproteins. Their primary structure consists of a single polypeptide ranging between 359 (histamine H_2) and 560 (α_{1A}-adrenoceptor) amino acid residues. Seven hydrophobic stretches of 20–25 amino acids interspersed with hydrophilic regions are important features in defining the tertiary structure of this receptor class. The structure of the β_2-adrenoceptor is shown in Fig. 5.2. The seven hydrophobic regions pack into the membrane in α helical formation to form the transmembrane domains. Each hydrophobic domain is linked by hydrophilic loops that extend alternatively into the extracellular medium and the cytosol. A cytosolic carboxyl terminal and an extended third cytosolic loop between transmembrane domain five and six are also characteristics of this receptor class. The extracellular amino terminal on these receptors and intracellular carboxyl terminal contain several sites for glycosylation. The role of carbohydrate moieties of glycosylated receptors, which are not a feature of the rat α_{1A}-adrenoceptor, is unclear. Current evidence suggests that

Table 5.1 A summary of the principle molecular and pharmacological characteristics of the receptors/putative receptors on vascular smooth muscle

RECEPTOR	GENE	PEPTIDE ACCESSION No.	SPECIES	AMINO ACID RESIDUES	PRIMARY EFFECTOR (OTHER RESPONSE)	SELECTIVE AGONISTS	SELECTIVE ANTAGONISTS (pA2)	REFERENCES
β_1	β_1	P08588 P181090	human rat	477 466	↑ AC	Ro363	CGP20712A (9.3) Bisoprolol (8.3)	Frielle et al., (1987) Machida et al. (1990)
β_2	β_2	P07550 P10608 P18762 P04274	human rat mouse hamster	413 418 418 418	↑ AC	Procaterol	ICI118551 (9.1)	Kobilka et al., (1987) Allen et al., (1988) Chung et al., (1987) Dixon et al. (1986)
β_3	β_3-C8 β_3-C8	P13945 P25962	human mouse rat	402 388 400	↑ AC	BRL28410 BRL37344		Emorine et al. (1989) Granneman et al., (1991) Nahmias et al., (1991)
α_{1A}	$\alpha 1A$-C5	M60654	rat hamster	560	DHP-Ca^{2+} channel	Methoxamine	WB4101 (9.2)	Lomasney et al., (1991)
α_{1B}	$\alpha 1B$-C5	P15823 P18841	rat hamster	515 515	↑IP_3/DG		Prazosin CEC (irreversible)	Cotecchia et al., (1988)
α_{1C}	$\alpha 1C$-C8	P18130	bovine	466	↑ IP_3/DG		WB4101 (9.2) CEC (irreversible)	Schwinn et al., (1990)
α_{1D}	$\alpha 1A$-C20		rat	560			WB4101 (9.2)	Schwinn et al., (1992) Perez et al., (1991)
α_{2A}	$\alpha 2A$-C10	P08913 P18871	human porcine rat	450 450 450	↓ AC (↑ K^+ channel) (↓ Ca^{2+} channel)	Oxymetazoline UK14304	BRL44408 (8.8)	Kobilka et al., (1987) Fraser et al., (1989) Guyer et al., (1990)
a_{2B}	$a2B$-C2 RNG	P18825 P19328	human rat	450 453	↓ AC (↓ Ca^{2+} channel)		prazosin (7.5) ARC239 (8.0) BRL41992 (8.9)	Lomasney et al., (1990) Weinshank et al., (1990) Zeng et al., (1990)
a_{2C}	$a2C$-C4 RG-10	P19328 P18089	human rat	461 450	↓ AC		Prazosin (7.5) ARC239 (8.0)	Regan et al. (1988) Lanier et al., (1991)
a_{2D}	RG-20				↓ AC			Lanier et al. (1991)
5-HT$_{1A}$	5ht1A-G21	P08908 P19327	human rat	421 422	↓AC (↑ K^+ channel) (↑ AC)	8-OH-DPAT 5-CT	WAY100135	Kobilka et al., (1987) Fargin et al., (1988)
5-HT$_{1B}$	5ht-1B 5ht-1Bα 5ht-1Bβ	P28564 P28334	rat mouse mouse	386 386	↓ AC	CP93129 5-CT		Maroteaux et al., (1992) Voight et al., (1991) Adham et al. (1992)

Table 5.1 (Continued.)

RECEPTOR	GENE	PEPTIDE ACCESSION No.	SPECIES	AMINO ACID RESIDUES	PRIMARY EFFECTOR (OTHER RESPONSE)	SELECTIVE AGONISTS	SELECTIVE ANTAGONISTS (pA2)	REFERENCES
5-HT$_{1D}$	5ht1Dα-C1 5ht1Dβ-C6	P11614 P28222 P28565 P11614	human human rat canine	377 390 374 377	↓ AC	Sumatriptan 5-CT		Weinshank et al., (1992) Hamblin & Metcalf, (1991) Jin et al., (1992) Zgombick et al., (1991) Libert et al., (1989) Maenhault et al., (1991) Hamblin et al., (1991, 1992)
5-HT$_{1E}$	5ht1E		human	365	↓ AC			Leonhardt et al., (1989)
5-HT$_{1F}$	5ht1F		mouse human	367	↓ AC			Amlaiky et al., (1992) Adham et al., (1993)
5-HT$_{2A}$	5ht2A	P28233	human rat	471 471	↑ IP$_3$/DG	α-methyl-5-HT	Ritanserin (9.5) Ketanserin (9.3)	Pritchett et al., (1988)
5-HT$_{2B}$	5ht2B		human	479	↑ IP$_3$/DG	α-methyl-5-HT	Ly53857 (noncompetative)	Kursar et al., (1992)
5-HT$_{2C}$	5ht2C	P28335 P08909	human rat	458 460	↑IP$_3$/DG	α-methyl-5-HT	mesulergine (9.1)	Julius et al., (1988) Yagaloff & Hartig, (1985) Lubbert et al., (1987a, 1987b)
5-HT$_4$					↑ AC	5-methoxytrypt- ophan Renzapride BIMU8	GR113808 (9.5) Rs23597190 (7.8)	
m1 (M1)	m1	P11229 P12657 P08482 P04761	human mouse rat porcine	460 460 460 460	↑ IP$_3$/DG		Pipenzepine (8.0) Telenzepine (9.1)	Bonner et al., (1987) Kubo et al., (1986a) Peralta et al., (1987) Braun et al., (1987)
m2 (M2)	m2	P08172 P10980 P06199	human rat porcine	466 466 466	↓ AC (↑ K$^+$ channel)		Methoctramine (7.9) AFDX116 (7.3)	Kubo et al., (1986b) Peralta et al., (1987) Bonner et al., (1987)
m3 (M3)	m3	P20309 P08483 P11483	human rat porcine	590 589 590	↑ IP$_3$/DG		Hexahydrosiladifenidol (8.0) p-Flurohexahydrosil-adifenidol (7.8)	Bonner et al., (1987) Akiba et al., (1988)
m4	m4	P08173 P08485 P17200	human rat chick	479 478 490	↓ AC		Topicamide (7.8)	Bonner et al., (1987)

RECEPTOR	GENE	PEPTIDE ACCESSION No.	SPECIES	AMINO ACID RESIDUES	PRIMARY EFFECTOR (OTHER RESPONSE)	SELECTIVE AGONISTS	SELECTIVE ANTAGONISTS (pA2)	REFERENCES
m5	*m5*		human rat		↑ IP$_3$/DG			Bonner et al., (1988)
H$_1$	*h1*			491	↑ IP$_3$/DG		Mepyramine (9.1) Triprolidine (9.9)	Yamashita et al., (1991)
H$_2$	*h2*	P20520 P17124 P25102		359 359 358	↑ AC	Dimaprit	Ranitidine (7.2) Tiotidine (7.8)	Gantz et al., (1991) Ruat et al., (1991)
H$_3$	*h3*					α-methyl-histamine Imetit	Thioperamide (8.4) Iodophenpropit (9.6)	
AT$_1$	*at1*	P25095 P25104	human rat mouse bovine	359 359 359 359	↑ IP$_3$/DG ↓ AC		DuP753 (8.1) (losartan) SKF108566 (9.7) EXP31274 (10.0)	Murphy et al., (1991) Sasaki et al., (1991)
AT$_2$					↑ GC		CGP42112A PD123177	
V1	*v1A*		rat	394	↑ IP$_3$/DG	Felypressin	OPC21263	Morel et al., (1993)
V2	*v2*		human rat	371 371	↑ AC	Desmopressin	SKF105494 OPC31260	Barberis et al., (1993) Morel et al., (1992)
OT	*ot*		human	389	↑ IP$_3$/DG			Kimura et al., (1992)
EP$_1$					↑ IP$_3$/DG	17-phenyl-ω-trinor-PGE$_2$	SC19220 (5.6) AH6809 (6.8)	
EP$_2$					↑ AC	Butaprost AH13205		
EP$_3$	*ep3*		mouse	365	↑ IP$_3$/DG	Enprostil GR63799 MB28767		Sugimoto et al., (1992)
DP					↑ AC	PGD$_2$ BW245C ZK110841		
FP					↑ IP$_3$/DG	PGF$_{2α}$ Fluprostenol		
IP					↑ AC	PGI$_2$ Cicaprost		
TP	*tp*	P21731	human mouse	343 341	≠ IP$_3$/DG	U46619	GR32191 (8.8) SQ29548 (8.7)	Hirata et al., (1991) Namba et al., (1992)

glycosylation has no obvious influence on either ligand binding or on the ability of the receptor to activate effectors.

The functional significance of specific amino acid residues and domains in the receptor have been identified using other techniques of the molecular biologist. For example, using the technique of site-directed mutagenesis small changes are made in the DNA encoding the receptor. Expression of the modified gene produces a mutant receptor in which particular amino acid domains are deleted or substituted. Point mutations allows individual amino acids to be changed. The aim of this approach is to correlate particular structural domains with the loss or the acquisition of a distinct function. It is assumed that where loss or change of a specific function occurs, in the modified receptor, then that function may be attributed to the region or amino acid that has undergone modification. These approaches have been used to investigate the domains and amino acid residues that are important in ligand recognition, G protein interaction, and sites for modification of the receptor by protein kinases. From these investigations it is clear that the transmembrane domains contain the ligand recognition sites and that the hydrophilic loops connecting the seven hydrophobic transmembrane domains, the carboxyl terminus, and the amino terminus are not involved in ligand recognition. This explains the observation that between subtypes of the same receptor the amino acids in the transmembrane domains are highly conserved since the same agonist, e.g. 5-hydroxytryptamine or adrenaline must interact with each receptor. For example, the 5-HT_{2A} and 5-HT_{2C} receptors share 78% sequence homology; 141 out of 180 amino acids are identical (Hartig 1989). The β_2-adrenoceptor subtypes and α_2-adrenoceptor subtypes share 75% sequence homology with the α_1-adrenoceptor subtypes (Ruffolo et al. 1991). One difficulty of interpreting the results of substitution or deletion mutation experiments, particularly in the transmembrane region, is that the apparent loss of a specific function may simply be the result of changes in the tertiary structure of the receptor. One approach, which has been used to overcome this inherent problem, has been to examine chimeras constructed from structurally similar receptors. The α_2- and β_2-adreoceptors, that are both pharmacologically distinct and are linked to different transduction systems, have been used. The α_2-adrenoceptor is linked to adenylyl cyclase via an inhibitory G protein and the β_2-adrenoceptor is linked to adenylyl cyclase via a stimulatory G protein. In these experiments gene modifications allow corresponding domains to be systematically exchanged from each receptor. Because the receptors are structurally similar this exchange has minimal effect on the tertiary structure of the receptor. An assessment of the pharmacological profile of the chimera and its ability to stimulate second messenger systems can then be used to reveal the functional importance of the exchanged domains. For example, transmembrane domain VII appears to be important in antagonist recognition. Replacement of this domain in the α_2-adrenoceptor with the corresponding domain from the β_2-adrenoceptor results in a chimera which loses α_2 antagonist selectivity but acquires β_2 antagonist specificity. In contrast, replacing transmembrane domain V and VI along with the connecting loop in the α_2-adrenoceptor with the corresponding β_2 domains results in a chimera which retains α_2 ligand specificity but interacts with G_S rather than G_I (Frielle et al. 1988; Kobilka et al. 1988; Beyer, 1990; Marullo et al. 1990; Ostrowski et al. 1992).

The molecular biology of the β_2-adrenoceptors has been studied extensively (see Dohlman et al. 1991; Tota et al. 1991; Ostrowski et al. 1992 for reviews) and consequently these receptors are the best defined of the seven transmembrane domain receptors. Some of the amino acids involved in ligand recognition and G protein interaction have been identified. In these receptors four cysteine (C) residues C^{106}, located on the first extracellular loop, and $C^{184, 190, 191}$, located on the second extracellular loop, are important for both agonist and antagonist binding (Dixon et al. 1987; Raymond et al. 1990; Dohlman et al. 1991). Substitution of the aspartic acid (D) residue (D^{113}) in the third transmembrane domain dramatically decreases the affinity of the receptor for both agonists and antagonists. This acidic amino acid, which is conserved only in those receptors whose natural ligand is a biogenic amine, is thought to be the counterion that binds the cationic amine moiety of catecholamine ligands (Tota et al. 1991). Substitution of the amino acids D^{79}, serine $(S)^{204, 207, 309}$, tyrosine $(Y)^{326}$ and phenylalanine $(F)^{289, 290}$ attenuates the affinity of the receptor for agonists but not for antagonists. Substitution of $S^{204, 207}$, which are believed to form hydrogen bonds with the *meta* and *para* catechol hydroxyl moieties, respectively, on the catecholamines produces a 25-35-fold reduction in agonist binding (Tota et al. 1991). Eight amino acid residues (222-229) at the N portion and twelve (258-270) at the carboxyl portion of the third hydrophilic loop appear to be key elements of the G protein recognition site on the β_2-adrenoceptor. Deletion of these residues markedly impairs the ability of the receptor to stimulate adenylyl cyclase. Of these histidine $(H)^{269}$ and Lysine $(K)^{270}$ are reported to be of particular importance (Strader et al. 1987; Raymond et al. 1990). Substitution of C^{341} in the carboxy terminal also significantly impairs the ability of the receptor to stimulate adenylyl cyclase. The principle features of the β_2-adrenoceptor that have been deduced from these experimental approaches and a model of the proposed interaction between the β_2-receptor and adrenaline are shown in Fig. 5.2a and 5.2b.

The sensitivity of most G protein-linked receptors is subject to regulation. Numerous mechanisms contribute to the phenomenon of receptor desensitization and operate at different levels within the transduction cascade. Phosphorylation of specific residues on the receptor decreases receptor sensitivity. Two types of receptor desensitization are recognized. Heterologous desensitization is the simultaneous reduction in sensitivity to activation of more than one receptor type which share some common subsequent step. For example heterologous desensitization of the β_2-adrenoceptor is produced by any agonist that stimulates the activity of the serine kinases PKA or PKC. Residues on the third hydrophilic loop ($S^{261, 262}$) and the carboxyl terminus ($S^{345, 346}$) appear to be the targets for these enzymes (Hausdorf et al. 1990; Dohlman et al. 1991).

Homologous desensitization applies only to attenuation of responses to the desensitizing agonist and is a reduced tissue responsiveness with time despite the continuous presence of the stimulating agonist. Homologous desensitization of the β_2-adrenoceptor is mediated by a specific kinase, β-adrenergic receptor

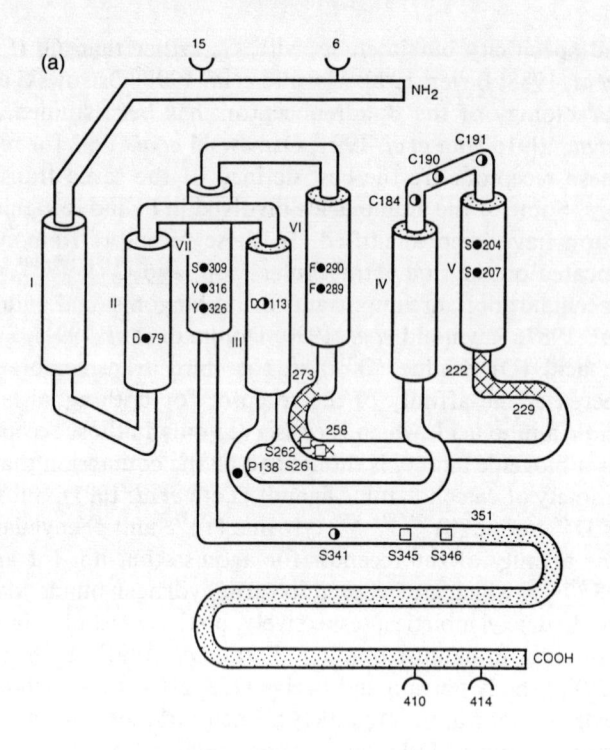

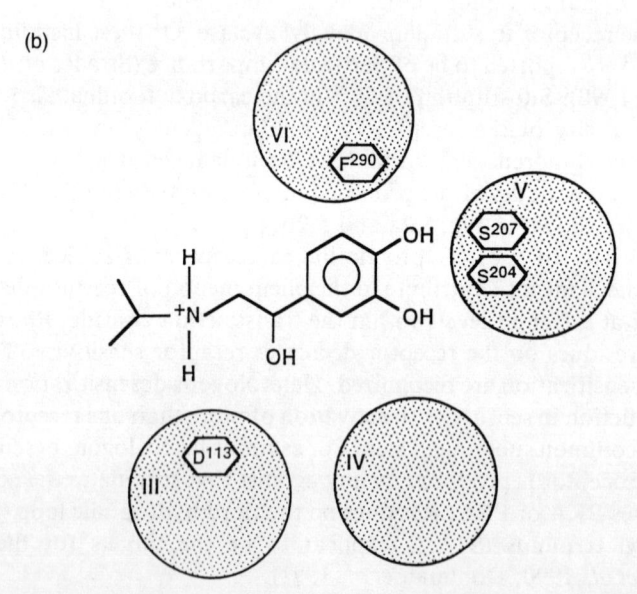

Fig. 5.2 (a) The putative structure of the β_2-adrenoceptor. The amino acid residues that are important for glycosylation (⋎), agonist (●), and antagonist (○) binding, G protein coupling (hatched regions), phosphorylation by protein kinases (□), and phosphorylation

kinase (βARK). This kinase only phosphorylates agonist-occupied receptors and appears to involve both serine and threonine residues in the carboxyl terminus. The unusually short carboxy terminus on the $β_3$-adrenoceptor may be the reason why this receptor does not exhibit homologous desensitization (Carpene et al. 1993).

Similar receptor-specific kinases appear to modulate the sensitivity of other receptors such as the acetylcholine muscarinic (AChm) receptor (Nathanson 1987) and $α_2$-adrenoceptor (Benovic et al. 1987). Interestingly the $α_2$-adrenoceptors are also substrate for βARK but lack serine and threonine residues in the carboxy terminus. However, a high density of these amino acids in the third cytoplasmic loop may suggest that this region is also important in regulating receptor sensitivity (Kobilka et al. 1988).

G proteins: properties and classification

For the seven transmembrane domain receptors the transduction of the external signal (agonist-receptor interaction) with those intracellular effectors that regulate second messenger levels is mediated exclusively through a family of guanine nucleotide binding proteins (GTP-binding proteins). Evidence for the role of GTP-binding proteins arose from investigations into the mechanisms by which the $β_2$-adrenoceptor activated adenylyl cyclase. The observation that GTP was required for $β_2$-induced stimulation of adenylyl cyclase in isolated membrane preparations (Rodbell et al. 1971) led to the isolation and purification of a protein that, in the presence of GTP, activated adenylyl cyclase. All GTP-binding proteins operate as biological switches and share the same basic principle of operation. They are activated by GTP binding and inactivated by GTP hydrolysis. The role of GTP-binding proteins in transmembrane signalling, normally abbveviated to G proteins, has been reviewed extensively (Houslay and Milligan 1990; Kaziro et al. 1991; Hepler and Gilman 1992; Clapham and Neer 1993). In addition to their role in signal transduction, GTP-binding proteins subserve many other functional roles within the cell: reviews (Bourne et al. 1991; Kaziro et al. 1991). The G proteins involved in transmembrane signalling are heterotrimers. The three subunits are designated, in order of decreasing molecular mass, $α$ (39-46 kDa), $β$ (35 kDa), and $γ$ (8 kDa). The $β$ and $γ$ subunits exist as a tightly associated complex and appear to operate as a functional unit.

$α$ Subunit   The biological activity of the G protein appears to reside predominantly within the $α$ subunit. This was originally demonstrated in reconstitution

---

by βARK (stippled regions). The large diameter segments represent the transmembrane regions. The upper and lower portion of the structure represent the extracellular and intracellular domains respectively. See text for details. Taken from Summers and McMartin (1993) with permission. (b) Cross-section through transmembrane domains III-VI showing the amino acid residues that are important for binding adrenaline. See text for details. Modified from Strader et al. (1989) with permission.

systems in which the activities of the subunits were investigated. These experiments showed that, in the presence of a non-hydrolysable GTP analogue (GTPγS), the α subunits could fully activate several effectors such as adenylyl cyclase and cGMP phosphodiesterase, whereas the $\beta\gamma$ subunit displayed little capacity to regulate effector proteins. Several experimental approaches have now uncovered many biological properties of the α subunit. The subunit contains GTPase activity and a single binding domain for guanine nucleotides. Modification of the amino terminal affects the ability of the subunit to associate with the $\beta\gamma$ whereas the carboxy terminal of the subunit contains the receptor recognition site. Currently the α subunit serves to define individual G proteins. However, the nomenclature used to identify G proteins is confusing. This has arisen because G protein α subunits were initially identified by function. For example, the receptor-linked adenylyl cyclase enzyme is regulated by two G proteins one stimulatory and one inhibitory. The G protein α subunits were therefore denoted by the subscripts 's' (stimulatory) and 'i' (inhibitory) reflecting their functional activity. G proteins that regulate K^+ channels were named G_K; those that regulate phospholipase A and C G_P. G proteins gating calcium channels were named G_Z (open) G_X (closed); the G protein coupling rhodopsin to cGMP phosphodiesterase in retinal rod and cone cells was called transducin (G_t). The introduction of cloning techniques led to the discovery of increasing numbers of subunits where knowledge of function was unknown and subsequently naming became unrelated to function. One approach used widely to classify G proteins has been the use of the bacterial toxins cholera toxin (from *Vibrio cholera*) and pertussis toxin (from *Bordetella pertussis*). These toxins possess enzymic activity that can catalyse the transfer of the ADP-ribose moiety from NAD to specific amino acid residues on certain α subunits. For example, the G protein that stimulates adenylyl cyclase is sensitive to cholera toxin whereas the G protein that inhibits adenylyl cyclase is the substrate for pertussis toxin. Cholera toxin ADP-ribosylates specific arginine (R) residues on some α subunits, an event that inactivates the GTPase activity resulting in sustained activation of the α subunit. Pertussis toxin ADP-ribosylates the cysteine residue four amino acid residues from the carboxy terminus of the $G_{i\alpha}$ subunit. Modification to this domain, the receptor recognition site, prevents the G protein from interacting with the receptor and thus inhibits the transduction of the external signal.

Sensitivity to these bacterial toxins has became an important tool for classifying G proteins. According to toxin sensitivity, G proteins α subunits can be classified into four groups, substrates sensitive to cholera toxin only, pertussis toxin only, both, or neither. Substrates sensitive to cholera toxin only include G_S and G_{olf} (similar to G_s: found in olfactory epithelium). Pertussis toxin-sensitive substrates include G_i and G_o (structurally similar to G_i: found in neuronal tissue). G_t and G_g (gusducin, similar to transducin: found in taste buds) are examples of substrates sensitive to both pertussis and cholera toxin. G proteins that are insensitive to both toxins include G_q (which activates the phospholipase $C\beta$ (PLCβ) isoenzymes), G_{12} (function unknown), and G_Z (expressed in platelets and neuronal tissue). Molecular cloning experiments have identified some 21 distinct G protein α subunits. These have now been divided into four subfamilies according to structural similarities in their amino acid sequence and are denoted by the subscripts G_s, G_i, G_q, and G_{12} (Hepler and Gilman 1992). The subscripts 's' and 'i' have been retained in this classification since the division according to toxin sensitivity is also supported by structural distinction.

$\beta\gamma$ Subunit The apparent inability of $G_{\beta\gamma}$ subunits to regulate effectors under experimental conditions and the interchangeability of $G_{\beta\gamma}$ subunits from different G proteins without loss of activity led to the belief that the $G_{\beta\gamma}$ subunit serves only as a membrane anchor stabilizing the heterotrimeric complex. Recently, however, increasing experimental evidence has indicated that $G_{\beta\gamma}$ subunits can directly regulate some effectors. These include phospholipase C (Camps et al. 1992; Katz et al. 1992), phospholipase A (Jelsema and Axelrod 1987), AChm-sensitive K^+ channels from atrial myocytes (Logothetis et al. 1987), and can regulate the various isoenzymes of adenylyl cyclase by either potentiating (type II and IV) or attenuating (type I) the stimulatory effect of $G_{s\alpha}$ (Tang and Gillman 1991) (also reviewed in Clapham and Neer 1993).

Receptors that regulate cytosolic free calcium are linked to phospholipase C (PLC) enzymes through a group of G proteins collectively referred to as G_p (p standing for phospholipid) of which G_q is a member. 16 distinct PLC enzymes have now been identified. These enzymes have been divided into three classes PLC_β, PLC_γ and PLC_δ (Rhee and Choi 1992). The $PLC_{\beta1-4}$ iosenzymes are regulated by G_q. $PLC_{\beta1-3}$ are regulated by both $G_{q\alpha}$ and also by $G_{q\beta\gamma}$ whereas $PLC_{\beta4}$ is insensitive to regulation by $G_{q\beta\gamma}$.

In addition, the identification of increasing numbers of structurally distinct G_β and G_γ subunits (Hepler and Gilman 1992) supports the view that the $\beta\gamma$ subunits may have a more direct role in signal transduction than simply acting as a membrane anchor. Currently four mammalian G_β subunits and seven G_γ subunits are known (Simon et al. 1991; von Weizsacker et al. 1992). The G_β subunits are structurally very similar sharing 80% amonio acid homology but can only form dimers with specific G_γ subunits, for example $G_{\beta1}$ can only associate with $G_{\gamma1}$ and $G_{\gamma2}$ whereas $G_{\beta2}$ can associate with $G_{\gamma2}$ but not $G_{\gamma1}$ (Schmidt et al. 1992; Pronin and Gautam 1992). The G_γ subunits are more heterogeneous than the G_β subunits. $G_{\gamma1}$ (retinal) shares only 38% sequence homology with $G_{\gamma2}$ (brain).

The G_γ subunits also differ in the degree of prenylation (Spiegel et al. 1991). This lipid modification to the G_γ subunit bestows upon the $G_{\beta\gamma}$ dimer the ability to bind to the plasma membrane, to stimulate some effectors such as adenylyl cyclase, and to interact with some G_α subunits (Inguez-Liuhi et al. 1991; Simonds et al. 1991; Muntz et al. 1992). The G_γ subunit may also determine the function of the $G_{\beta\gamma}$ dimer, for example $G_{\beta1\gamma1}$, present in retina, is functionally distinct from $G_{\beta1\gamma2}$, present in brain. Since the G_β subunits are identical it is assumed that the functional difference resides in the different G_γ subunits. One interesting observation that $G_{\beta\gamma}$ can phosphorylate the acetylcholine muscarinic receptor (AChm) by directly stimulating the activity of AChm kinase (Haga and

Haga 1992) may indicate that the $G_{\beta\gamma}$ subunit has a role in regulating receptor sensitivity. It has also been suggested that different $G_{\beta\gamma}$ subunits may specify which receptor activates a particular G_α subtype. This suggestion arose from observations that activation of both the M4 mACh and somatostatin receptors inhibit influx of Ca^{2+} through the N-type ω-conotoxin-sensitive Ca^{2+} channel. Inhibition mediated by the somatostatin receptor involves $G_{\alpha O2\beta 1\gamma 3}$ whereas the M4 mACh receptor involves $G_{\alpha O1\beta 3\gamma 4}$ (Kleuss *et al*. 1993). Inhibition of the appropriate G_α or $G_{\beta\gamma}$ subunits blocks the ability of these receptors to inhibit the Ca^{2+} channel. This prompted the suggestion that the $G_{\beta\gamma}$ subunit determines which G protein interacts with which receptor or alternatively that the N-type channel may be regulated by both subunits independently. Several observations indicate that activation of some receptors, where the transduction system is apparently well defined, results not only in the conventional signal transduction cascade mediated by the activated G_α subunit of the G protein but also results in activation of other second messenger systems. It has been suggested that the participation of the $G_{\beta\gamma}$ subunit in regulating effectors may represent a bifurcation in the signal transduction process and may be the mechanism by which some receptors can apparently activate two transduction processes (see Milligan 1993 for a comprehensive discussion).

Receptor transduction

The putative scheme of events involved in transduction of the external signals is described in brief below and depicted in Fig. 5.3. The reader should refer to Birnbaumer (1990) for more extensive reviews. The membrane receptor in Fig. 5.3 is coupled to adenylyl cyclase by a stimulatory G protein. In the quiescent state, the G protein exists in its heterotrimeric form with GDP bound to the α subunit. The receptor is unoccupied and the effector is in an inactive state (Fig. 5.3a). Agonist–receptor interaction promotes binding of the G protein to the agonist-bound receptor. This interaction stimulates the dissociation of GDP from the nucleotide binding site and in the presence of the normally high concentrations of GTP and Mg^{2+} within the cell the nucleotide binding site is occupied by GTP. The binding of GTP induces a conformational change in the α subunit ($G_{s\alpha}$). This activated state has two important consequences. First, the high affinity of the receptor for the agonist is decreased and the agonist dissociates from the low affinity receptor (Fig. 5.3b). This event only operates when the receptor is occupied by a molecule with intrinsic efficacy, i.e. an agonist. When the receptor is occupied by a molecule devoid of efficacy (i.e. pharmacological antagonists) the affinity of the receptor remains unchanged.

Secondly, the conformational change in the α subunit lowers the affinity of this subunit for the $\beta\gamma$ subunit and the subunits dissociate (Fig. 5.3c). The activated $G_{S\alpha}$ moves freely within the plane of the membrane to fulfil its primary function as a regulator of adenylyl cyclase (Fig. 5.3d). The intrinsic GTPase of $G_{S\alpha}$ is activated by the binding of GTP. The hydrolysis of the terminal phosphate of GTP to GDP and P_i reverses the conformational change

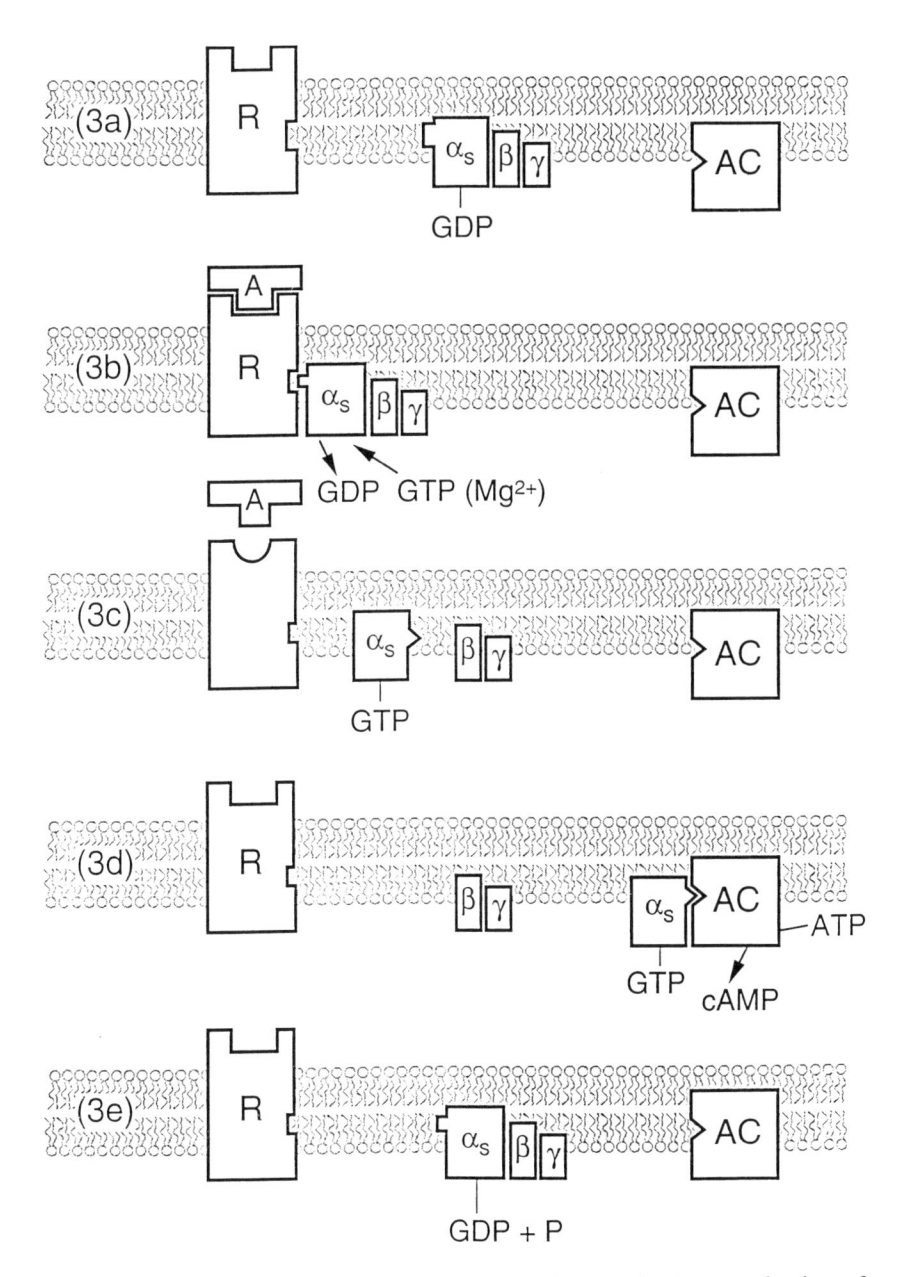

Fig. 5.3 A model showing the proposed sequence of events in the transduction of an external signal with the activation of adenylyl cyclase by the G protein G_S. See text for details.

reforming the inactive subunit and terminating the regulation of the effector. The inactive $G_{S\alpha}$ reassociates with the $\beta\gamma$ subunit (Fig. 5.3e). The duration of the active α subunit and hence the regulation of the effector protein is determined by the rate of GTP hydrolysis. The cycling between the active and inactive state, in the presence of an agonist, is largely dependent on the intrinsic activity of the GTPase enzyme of individual G proteins.

Tyrosine kinase-linked receptors (guanylyl cyclase receptors)

Whilst most external agonists that regulate smooth muscle responses do so through the G protein-linked receptor system, other receptor-linked transduction systems also operate to regulate smooth muscle responses. A second, though less well understood, transduction system is mediated through a family of tyrosine kinase-linked receptors. This receptor consists of a single polypeptide containing one hydrophobic region that forms a single transmembrane domain. The external moiety contains the agonist recognition site and the cytosolic region incorporates a tyrosine kinase enzyme. These receptors bind peptide agonists such as insulin and mitogenic growth factors such as platelet-derived growth factor (PGDF) and epidermal growth factor (EGF). A number of tyrosine kinase-linked receptors mediate their response through activation of a particulate guanylyl cyclase enzyme. Guanylyl cyclase enzymes exists in both a cytosolic and a particulate form in the cell and although the soluble guanylyl cyclase activity was first discovered some 30 years ago it is only recently that the role of particulate guanylyl cyclase enzymes has been uncovered. These enzymes were found to be activated by several peptides including bacterial enterotoxins, peptides released from sea-urchin eggs that stimulate spermatozoa motility, and a natriuretic peptide released from the atria which stimulates diuresis, naturesis, and vasodilation. Atrial natriuretic peptide (ANP) or atrial natriuretic factor (ANF) is released into the circulation in response to increased pressure in the right atrium. ANF is a potent vasodilator of large capacitance arteries but with the exception of the kidney has little effect on most vascular beds. In the kidney it contributes to diuresis by dilating the afferent arterioles and constricting the efferent arterioles of the glomeruli resulting in increased filtration pressure. The vasodilator effect of ANF is mediated through the ANF-A-R (B-ANF, ANF-R1) receptor. It is now clear that a guanylyl cyclase enzyme is an integral part of the tyrosine kinase receptor (Chinkers and Garbers 1991; Maack 1992).

The guanylyl cyclase-linked receptors consist of three distinct domains. An external moiety contains the peptide recognition site. An intracellular region contains the guanylyl cyclase catalytic domain, and located between the plasma membrane and this catalytic moiety is an amino acid sequence which is structurally similar to the tyrosine kinases enzymes. In the guanylyl cyclase-linked receptor tyrosine kinase activity has not been demonstrated and therefore the functional role of this (tyrosine kinase) domain is unclear. However, in other receptors of this class such as the insulin receptor, phosphorylation of specific tyrosyl residues on this receptor (autophosphorylation) is initiated by agonist binding and

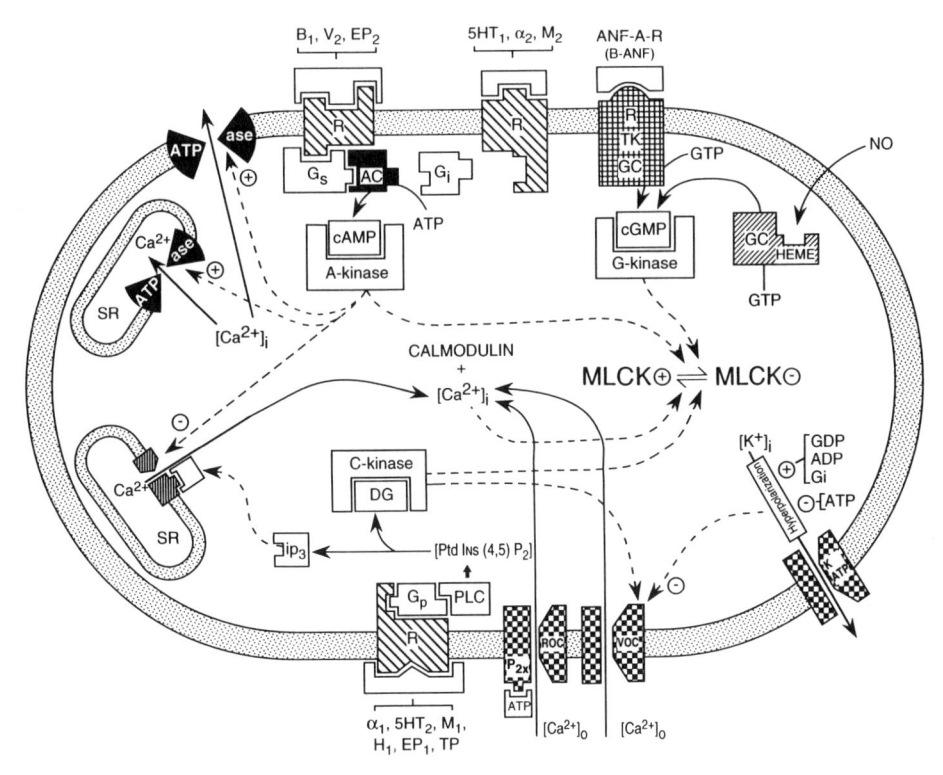

Fig. 5.4 Simplified schematic diagram summarizing some of the agonists, their associated receptors, and the various transduction mechanisms which regulate smooth muscle tone. TK, tyrosine kinase; GC, guanylyl cyclase; AC adenylyl cyclase; SR, sarcoplasmic reticulum. MLCK⊕, increased activity of myosin light chain kinase. MLCK⊖, decreased activity of myosin light chain kinase. See text for all other details.

markedly increases receptor sensitivity (Rosen 1987) suggesting that this enzyme may have a role in regulating receptor sensitivity. Activation of the guanylyl cyclase-linked receptors increases the intracellular concentration of the second messenger cyclic guanosine monophosphate (cGMP) which in smooth muscle promotes relaxation however, some agonists that act through tyrosine kinase receptors can also produce vasoconstriction. PDGF, for example, as well as inducing mitogenesis, is also a powerful vasoconstrictor. The transduction mechanisms underlying this response have not been fully elucidated but appears to involve inositol phospholipid metabolism. Both PDGF and EGF but not insulin are known to stimulate the hydrolysis of Ptd Ins (4,5) P_2 (Pandiella *et al.* 1989) which may involve the hydrolysis of a specific pool of Ptd Ins (4,5) P_2, bound to the protein profilin, by the phospholipase C enzyme $PLC_{\gamma 1}$. This enzyme is phosphorylated by tyrosine kinase enzymes, PDGF and EGF but not by insulin, and in its phosphorylated state $PLC_{\gamma 1}$ is capable of hydrolysing profilin-bound [Ptd Ins (4,5) P_2] generating IP_3 and DG (Goldschmidt-Clermont 1991). This effect on inositol phospholipid metabolism may, at least in part, underly the vasoconstrictor effect of PDGF.

Receptor-linked ion channels

Comparisons between the primary sequence of various ion channels show that they belong to a related molecular family which utilize a number of homologous transmembrane α helical domains symmetrically arranged to form a ring structure that serves as the channel pore. This protein family includes voltage operated (Na^+, K^+, and Ca^{2+}) channels, ion channels linked to 'fast' neurotransmitters, and channels that gate ion movement across intracellular organelles. The nicotinic ACh (nACh) receptor is the prototypic example of an ion channel that directly binds the external agonist. The model that has been developed for the nACh receptor suggests that it consists of four subunits $\alpha\beta\delta\gamma$ with a stoichiometry of α_2, β, δ, γ (Changeux et al. 1987). This receptor type also binds neurotransmitters such as glutamate (Hollmann et al. 1989; Moriyoshi et al. 1991), glycine (Langosch et al. 1990), GABA (Schofield et al. 1987), ACh (Galzi et al. 1991), 5-HT at 5-HT_3 receptors (Maricq et al. 1991). The interaction of an agonist with this receptor results in the opening of the transmembrane ion channel allowing the rapid movement of cations or anions down their electrochemical gradient. Since this transduction mechanism does not depend on the production and diffusion of second messengers within the cytosol the response time is very much quicker than that of biochemical transduction. In vascular smooth muscle several members of this ion channel family play an important role in regulating tone (see also Chapter 6).

Ca^{2+} channels

Vasoconstrictor agonists that are linked to PLC enzymes can regulate vascular smooth muscle tone by mobilizing intracellular Ca^{2+} through the generation of IP_3. The IP_3 receptor is a member of this ion channel family and consists of four subunits each composed of six or eight hydrophobic domains. Binding sites for IP_3 are present on all four subunits (Furuichi et al. 1992; Mikoshiba 1993).

Vasoconstrictor responses in some smooth muscles are dependent on extracellular Ca^{2+}. In general, it has been found that resistance arteries have a greater dependence on extracellular Ca^{2+} than elastic capacitance vessels (Bulbring and Tomita 1987). It is widely assumed that the initiation of contractile response in smooth muscle involves the release of intracellular Ca^{2+} (Ca^{2+} mobilization) and that maintained contractile states requires influx of extracellular Ca^{2+}. The entry of extracellular Ca^{2+} could be required to refill cytosolic stores or may enter the cytosol to directly regulate the contractile elements. Influx of extracellular Ca^{2+} may be achieved by agonist receptors that are directly linked to Ca^{2+} channels in the plasma membrane (receptor operated channels, ROC). The plasma membrane also contains Ca^{2+} channels that are sensitive to membrane potential (voltage operated Ca^{2+} channels, VOCs) that open when the membrane is depolarized. Many agonists produce a depolarization of the plasma membrane (Nelson et al. 1990a) and the subsequent influx of Ca^{2+} through VOCs is likely to contribute to the contractile event.

Receptor operated Ca^{2+} channels were originally inferred from experiments where the contractile response and inward Ca^{2+} current evoked by membrane depolarization, operating through VOCs, could be augmented by the addition of vasoconstrictor agonists. Because the additional Ca^{2+} influx and mechanical tension in response to agonists were observed in the absence of further changes in membrane polarity the increased current was assumed to be mediated through a Ca^{2+} channel directly linked to the agonist receptor (Bolton 1979). The evidence for a Ca^{2+} channel directly coupled to receptors in smooth muscle is scant and as detailed above largely indirect. However, Benham and Tsien (1987) have described an ATP-stimulated inward current carried predominantly by Ca^{2+} in smooth muscle cells from rabbit ear artery. This current was reported to be insensitive to second messengers and dihydropyridine antagonists, and was increased by membrane hyperpolarization which clearly distinguishes it from L-type VOC. P_{2X}-purinoceptors, which are believed to mediate the fast response following sympathetic nerve stimulation through the release of the cotransmitter ATP, have therefore been suggested to operate through a receptor operated Ca^{2+} channel (Benham and Tsien 1987) however, the selectivity of this channel for Ca^{2+} over Na^+ (3:1) is extremely low compared with the L-type VOC.

Voltage operated Ca^{2+} channels

Based on electrical characteristics, pharmacology, and cell distribution, four distinct voltage operated Ca^{2+} channels (L, N, T, and P) have been described (Tsien et al. 1990). Of these, the L-type channel, which is characterized by its high voltage activation and sensitivity to dihydropyridine compounds, is the most prominant Ca^{2+} channel in vascular smooth muscle (Nelson et al. 1990a). This channel consists of two high molecular weight subunits α_1 and α_2 and three β, γ, δ smaller subunits. The α_1 subunit is composed of four homologous units each containing six α helical transmembrane domains. The binding site for the dihydropyridine compounds is located on the cytosolic carboxyl terminal of this unit (Tsien et al. 1991). The ability of dihydropyridine antagonists to produce vasodilation in many arteries clearly shows the important role of this channel in maintaining vascular tone. Although the L-type VOC is regulated by membrane potential there is increasing evidence that agonists such as noradrenaline, 5-hydroxytryptamine, angiotensin II, endothelin, and acetylcholine can regulate channel activity by a mechanism unrelated to changes in the membrane potential (Tomita 1988; Nelson et al. 1990a; Worley et al. 1991; Kamishima et al. 1992). The link between activation of receptors for these agonists and activation of this channel is not yet established. Because all of these agonists are linked to a PLC enzyme it is assumed that some intermediary of the biochemical transduction pathway may regulate this Ca^{2+} channel. It is known, for example, that protein kinase C phosphorylates the α_1 and β subunits of the L-type VOC from skeletal muscle (Shearman *et al.* 1989), and although protein kinase C activators are reported to induce both vasoconstriction and vasodilation in various smooth muscle prepartions (Shearman *et al.* 1989), synthetic diglycerides (Vivaudou *et al.* 1988) and phorbol esters (Fish *et al.* 1988) have been reported to increase Ca^{2+} currents in single smooth muscle cells. Direct regulation by G protein subunits has also been reported (Hepler and Gilman 1992).

K^+ channels

The relatively recent discovery that a group of drugs (cromakalim, pinacidil, minoxidil, and diazoxide) were potent vasodilators and produced smooth muscle relaxation by increasing the membrane permeability to K^+ has led to the discovery of an important new mechanism for regulating vascular smooth muscle tone. The outward K^+ current induced by these drugs, now collectively known as K^+ channel openers (reviewed in Weston and Edwards 1992), results in hyperpolarization of the plasma membrane. Inhibition of Ca^{2+} influx through VOCs is likely to be an important part of this response but may not be the only mechanism by which membrane hyperpolarization induces smooth muscle relaxation. K^+ channels have been divided into three classes:

(a) *Delayed rectifier K^+ channels*. This K^+ channel is activated by membrane depolarization, displays time-dependent inactivation, and is sensitive to the inhibitors 4-aminopyridine and tetraethyl ammonium (TEA).

(b) K_{Ca2+} *channels* are present on most smooth muscle and are activated by increased $[Ca^{2+}]_i$, blocked by TEA and charybdotoxin, and are voltage-dependent.

(c) K^+_{ATP} *channels* were originally identified in cardiac muscle but have now been shown to be present in a number of tissues including arterial smooth muscle. Although these channels were shown to be closed down by intracellular ATP and consequently were referred to as ATP-sensitive K^+ channels (K^+_{ATP} channel) it is clear that they are regulated by a number of factors including pyridine nucleotides, cyclic AMP, nucleotide diphosphates, pH, Ca^{2+}, Mg^{2+}, and G protein subunits (Tomita 1988; Davies *et al.* 1991; Bolton and Beech 1992).

Recently K^+_{ATP} channels have been further divided into three subgroups (Beech *et al.* 1993*a*). Of these a small conductance K^+ channel which appears to be selectively inhibited by the anti-diabetic drug glibenclamide and activated by nucleotide diphosphatases such as GDP and ADP has been reported to be target for the K^+ channel opening drugs (Beech *et al.* 1993*b*). Activation of K^+_{ATP} channels by the peptide neurotransmitter, calcitonin gene-related peptide (Nelson *et al.* 1990*b*) and endothelium-derived hyperpolarizing factor (Bryden 1990 but also see Chapter 11) has been reported to be an important part of the relaxation induced by these agents.

SMOOTH MUSCLE CELL MEMBRANE RECEPTORS

The principle characteristics of smooth muscle receptors are summarized in Table 1. Figure 5.4 is a schematic representation depicting the receptors and transduction mechanisms that operate to determine smooth muscle tone.

Adrenoceptors

Ahlquist (1948) divided adrenoceptors into α and β. Four subgroups of adrenoceptors α_1, α_2, β_1, and β_2 are now universally accepted and are the subject of several comprehensive reviews (Bylund 1988; Limbird 1988; Minneman 1988; Docherty 1989; McGrath et al. 1989; Ruffolo et al. 1991; Summers and McMartin 1993). β-Adrenoceptor were divided into β_1 and β_2 subtypes on the basis of rank order of potencies of catecholamines (Lands et al. 1967) and subsequently confirmed with the development of selective agonists and antagonists. The concept of a β_3-adrenoceptor arose from observations that β-adrenoceptors on adipocytes, colon, and skeletal muscle display a low affinity for conventional β_1 and β_2 antagonists. Selective agonists have now been developed for this receptor. Three distinct human β-adrenoceptors as well as rodent homologues have been cloned.

α-*Adrenoceptors* have also been divided into α_1 and α_2. Subdivision of the α_1-receptor is based on antagonist affinity and differential requirements for extracellular calcium (McGrath 1983; Drew 1985; Flavahan and Vanhoutte 1986, Morrow and Cresse 1986; Han et al. 1987; Minneman 1988; Hanft et al. 1989).

Three α_1-receptors have been cloned from bovine, rat, and hamster genes. The hamster receptor corresponds to the α_{1B} subtype. The bovine receptor, although similar to the α_{1A} subtype is pharmacologically distinct and is not expressed in any of the rat or bovine tissue known to contain the α_{1A} receptor. This receptor is currently designated as α_{1C}. Pharmacological characterization of the receptor cloned from rat cerebral cortex indicates a novel receptor and has currently been defined as α_{1D}.

Heterogeneity within the α_2-adrenoceptor class was first suggested by Drew (1985) and subsequently supported by radioligand binding (Summer et al. 1983; Cheung et al. 1986; McKernan et al. 1986; Alabaster et al. 1986), functional (de Jonge et al. 1981; Hicks 1981; Alabaster and Peters 1984; Maura et al. 1985; Ruffolo et al. 1987; Docherty 1989), and biochemical (Fain and Garcia-Sainz, 1980; Jakobs and Schultz 1982; Lanier et al. 1988) studies, as well as differential requirement for extracellular Ca^{2+} (Han et al. 1987). Bylund (1985) proposed the division of the α_2-adrenoceptors into α_{2A}, typified by the human platelet α_2-receptor and α_{2B}-receptor, typified by the neonatal rat lung receptor. The α_2-adrenoceptor in opossum-kidney-derived cell line displayed characteristics that could not be classified as either α_{2A} or α_{2B} and was subsequently designated the α_{2C}-adrenoceptor (Blaxall et al. 1991). The α_2-adrenoceptor in the rat submaxillary gland, bovine pineal gland, and rat cortex is suggested to represent a fourth division of the α_2-adrenoceptors and has been termed the α_{2D}-subtype (Bylund et al. 1991).

The gene encoding the human platelet α_2-adrenoceptor, designated α2-C10, the postscript denoting the chromosomal location, as well as porcine and rat homologues have been cloned. Two other α_2-adrenoceptor genes reside on human chromosomes 2 and 4. The three human genes encode distinct α_2-adrenoceptors designated α2-C10, α2-C2, and α2-C4 which correlate with the pharmacologically defined α_{2A}, α_{2B}, and α_{2C} receptors respectively.

In the rat two α_{2B}-adrenoceptors exist: the α_2RNG (rat non-glycosylated) and a glycosylated receptor. The receptor expressed from the RG10 clone which is present in rat brain may correspond to the α_{2C}-adrenoceptor. The receptor, expressed from the rat RG20 gene has been classified as the α_{2D} receptor.

5-Hydroxytryptamine

These receptors were originally subdivided by Gaddum and Picarelli (1957) and later by Peroutka and Snyder (1979). Bradley and colleagues (1986) proposed the division of the 5-HT receptors into three classes 5-HT$_1$, 5-HT$_2$, and 5-HT$_3$ and based on its unique pharmacological profile Bockaert and colleagues (1992) proposed a 5-HT$_4$ receptor.

Based on pharmacological, biochemical, molecular, and electrophysiological evidence receptors for 5-HT have now been divided into four main classes 5-HT$_1$, 5-HT$_2$, 5-HT$_3$, and 5-HT$_4$ (Humphrey et al. 1993). Receptors in the 5-HT$_1$ class have been subdivided into 5-HT$_{1A}$, 5-HT$_{1B}$, 5-HT$_{1D}$, 5-HT$_{1E}$, and 5-HT$_{1F}$. In the human two genes encode structurally distinct 5-HT$_{1D}$ receptors that are pharmacologically indistinguishable even though the amino acids in the transmembrane regions of these receptors, termed 5-HT$_{1D\alpha}$ and 5-HT$_{1D\beta}$, differ by 23%. The 5-HT$_{1B}$ receptor appears to be the rodent homologue of the 5-HT$_{1D}$ receptor found in the pig, calf, and human (5-HT$_{1D\beta}$). Despite the close structural similarity between the rodent and its human homologue, these receptors display a substantially different pharmacological profile and for this reason both receptors are retained in the current nomenclature. The pharmacological difference between the two receptors may arise from a single amino acid difference threonine[355] (human)/asparagine[351] (rat) in the seventh transmembrane domain (Metcalf et al. 1992). In addition to the 5-HT$_{1B}$ receptor in the rat a 5-HT$_{1D}$ receptor has also been reported which is structurally similar to the human 5-HT$_{1D\alpha}$ receptor (Hartig et al. 1992). As yet no functional correlate exists for the cloned 5-HT$_{1E}$ and 5-HT$_{1F}$ receptors.

The 5-HT$_2$ receptors have been divided into three subtypes. These are 5-HT$_{2A}$ (formerly 5-HT$_2$), 5-HT$_{2B}$ (formerly 5-HT$_{2F}$ the receptor mediating constriction of the rat fundus), and 5-HT$_{2C}$ (formerly 5-HT$_{1C}$).

5-HT$_3$ receptor is a member of the ion channel-linked receptor family (Maricq et al. 1991). The 5-HT$_4$ receptor is the only 5-HT receptor that has not been cloned.

In addition to the current classification Matthes et al. (1993) have suggested that two receptors which they termed 5-HT$_{5A}$ and 5-HT$_{5B}$ represent a further 5-HT receptor class. Similarly, another structurally unique receptor which has been cloned (Monsma et al. 1993) and is positively linked to adenylyl cyclase has been presented as evidence for a 5-HT$_6$ receptor class.

Muscarinic receptors

Goyal and Rattan (1978) suggested that muscarinic receptors on neuronal tissue, designated M$_1$, are distinct from those present on heart and smooth muscle, designated M$_2$. Ligand binding studies support this division (Hammer et al. 1980). Doods et al. (1987) proposed the division of the muscarinic receptors into M$_1$, M$_2$, and M$_3$. Molecular cloning of porcine cerebral and atrial receptors provided structural verification that the muscarinic receptors on brain and heart were distinct. Human and rat homologues have been cloned as well as three other distinct muscarinic receptors designated m1, m2, m3, m4, and m5. Of the cloned receptors m1, m2, and m3 correlate with the pharmacologically defined and M$_1$, M$_2$, and M$_3$ receptors respectively. The muscarinic receptors on vascular smooth muscle are vasoconstrictor and appear to be similar to the M$_3$ receptor (Duckles and Garcia-Villalon 1990).

Histaminergic receptors

Ash and Schild (1966) introduced the term H$_1$ histamine receptor to describe the receptor mediating the range of responses that were sensitive to 'classical antihistamines'. The inability of these antagonists to inhibit gastric acid secretion and contraction of the rat uterus supported the belief that a distinct histamine receptor mediating these response existed. The histamine receptor insensitive to the classical antihistamines was eventually defined as H$_2$ (Black et al. 1972). The concept of a third histamine receptor H$_3$ was originally introduced to explain the atypical pharmacological profile of histamine receptors in rat cerebral cortex which regulate histamine release (Arrang et al. 1987). The H$_1$ and H$_2$ receptors have been cloned.

Angiotensin

Heterogeneity within the receptor population for AII is derived from different orders of potencies and binding affinities for the endogenous angiotensins II and III and from different susceptibilities to antagonism by peptide and non-peptide antagonists (Timmermann et al. 1991). Two distinct receptors AT$_1$ and AT$_2$ have been defined. All of the known functional roles of AII are mediated through the AT$_1$ receptor. To date no functional role has been identified for the AT$_2$ receptor. The AT$_1$ receptor has been cloned.

Vasopressin

Vasopressin (antidiuretic hormone, ADH) and oxytocin (OT) are the main peptide hormones released from the posterior pituitary. Pharmacological studies support the existence of two distinct receptors for vasopressin, V_1 and V_2 and one OT receptor. Pharmacological differences between V_1 receptors on adenohypophysial cells and those on hepatocytes led to the division of the Y_1 class into the $V_{1\alpha}$ (hepatocytes and constriction of vascular smooth muscle) and the $V_{1\beta}$ (anterior pituitary) (Jard 1988). V_2 receptors mediate the antidiuretic effect of vasopressin and relaxation of vascular smooth muscle (Liard 1990). The V_1, V_2, and OT receptors have been cloned.

Prostanoid receptors

Functional and ligand binding studies supports the existence of specific receptors for each of the natural cyclo-oxygenase products; prostaglandins (PG) PGE_2, $PGF_{2\alpha}$, PGF_2, and PGI_2 (prostacyclin), and thromboxane A_2 (TXA_2). These receptors have been defined as EP, FP, DP, and TP respectively (Coleman et al. 1990). The preceding letter denotes the prostaglandin for which the receptor is most selective. The EP receptor class into three distinct subtypes: EP_1, EP_2, and EP_3. IP, EP_2, and DP receptors produce relaxation of vascular smooth muscle whereas TP, FP, EP_1, and EP_3 receptors are vasoconstructor phospholipid turnover. At present the TP and EP_3 receptors are the only prostanoid receptors that have been cloned.

REFERENCES

Adham, N., Romanienko, P., Hartig, P. R., Weinshank, R., and Branchek, T. (1992). The rat 5-hydroxytryptamine$_{1B}$ receptor is the species homologue of the human 5-hydroxytryptamine$_{1D\beta}$ receptor. *Mol. Pharmacol.*, **41**, 1-7.

Adham, N., Kao, H.-T., Schechter, L. E., Bard, J., Olsen, M., Urquhart, D., et al. (1993). Cloning of another human serotonin receptor 5-HT$_{1F}$: A fifth 5-HT$_1$ receptor subtype coupled to inhibition of adenylyl cyclase. *Proc. Natl. Acad. Sci. USA*, **90**, 404-12.

Ahlquist, R. P. (1948). A study of the adrenergic receptor. *Am. J. Physiol.*, **153**, 586-600.

Akiba, I., Kubo, T., Maeda, A., Bujor, J., Nahai, J., Mishina, M., et al. (1988). Primary structure of porcine muscarinic acetylcholine receptor III and antagonist bindind studies. *FEBS Lett.*, **235**, 257-61.

Alabaster, V. A. and Peters, C. J. (1984). Pre- and post-junctional α_2-adrenoceptors can be differentially antagonised. *Br. J. Pharmacol.*, **81**, 163P.

Alabaster, V. A., Keir, R. F., and Peters, C. J. (1986). Comparison of the potency of α_2-adrenoceptor antagonists *in vitro*: evidence for heterogeneity of α_2-adrenoceptors. *Br. J. Pharmacol.*, **88**, 607-14.

Allan, J. M., Baetge, E. E., Abrass, I. B., and Palmiter, R. D. (1988). Iosproterenol response following transfection of the mouse β_2-adrenergic receptor gene into Y1 cells. *EMBO J.*, **7**, 33-8.

Amlaiky, N., Ramboz, S., Boschert, U., Plassat, J. L., and Hen, R. (1992). Isolation of a mouse 5-HT$_{1E}$-like serotonin receptor expressed predominantly in hippocampus. *J. Biol. Chem.*, **267**, 19761-4.

Arrang, J. M., Garbang, M., Lancelot, J. C., Lecompte, J. M., Pollard, H., Robba, M., et al. (1987). Highly potent and selective ligands for histamine H_3 receptors. *Nature*, **327**, 117-23.

Ash, A. S. F. and Schield, H. O. (1966). Receptors mediating some actions of histamine. *Br. J. Pharmacol. Chemother.*, **27**, 427-39.

Barberis, C., Seibold, A., Ishido, M., Rosenthal, W., and Birnbaumer, M. (1993). Expression cloning of the human V_2 vasopressin receptor. *Regul. Pept.*, **45**, 61-6.

Beech, D. J., Zhang, H., Nakao, K., and Bolton, T. B. (1993a). Single channel and whole-cell K-currents evoked by leycromakalim in smooth muscle cells from the rabbit portal vein. *Br. J. Pharmacol.*, **110**, 583-90.

Beech, D. J., Zhang, H., Nakao, K., and Bolton, T. B. (1993b). K Channel activation by nucleotide diphosphates and its inhibition by glibenclamide in vascular smooth muscle cells. *Br. J. Pharmacol.*, **110**, 573-82.

Benham, C. D. and Tsien, R. W. (1987). A novel receptor-operated Ca^{2+}-permeable channel activated by ATP in smooth muscle. *Nature*, **328**, 275-8.

Benovic, J. L., Regan, J. W., Matsui, H., Mayor, F., Coteccha, S., Leeblundberg, L. M. F., et al. (1987). Agonist-dependent phosphorylation of α_2 adrenergic receptor by β-adrenergic kinase. *J. Biol. Chem.*, **262**, 17252-3.

Beyer, R. M., Strosberg, A. D., and Guillet, J-G. (1990). Mutational analysis of ligand binding activity of β_2-adrenergic receptor expressed in *Escherichia coli*. *EMBO J.*, **9**, 2679-84.

Birnbaumer, L. (1990). Transduction of receptor signal into modulation of effector activity by G proteins: the first 20 years or so. *FASEB J.*, **4**, 3068-78.

Black, J. W., Duncan, W. A. M., Durant, C. J., Ganellin, C. C., and Parsons, M. E. (1972). Definition and antagonism of histamine H_2-receptors. *Nature*, **236**, 385-90.

Blaxall, H. S., Murphy, T. J., Baker, J. C., Ray, C., and Bylund, D. B. (1991). Characterization of the alpha-2C-adrenergic receptor subtype in the opossum kidney and in the OK cell line. *J. Pharmacol. Exp. Ther.*, **259**, 323-9.

Bockaert, J., Fozard, J. R., Dumuis, A., and Clarke, D. E. (1992). The 5-HT_4 receptor: a place in the sun. *Trends Pharmacol. Sci.*, **13**, 141-5.

Bolton, T. B. (1979). Mechanisms of action of transmitters and other substances on smooth muscle. *Physiol. Rev.*, **59**, 606-718.

Bolton, T. B. and Beech, D. J. (1992). Smooth muscle potassium channels: their electrophysiology and function. In *Potassium channel modulators: pharmacological, molecular and clinical aspects* (ed. A. H. Weston and T. C. Hamilton), Oxford: Blackwell Scientific Publications, Oxford. pp. 144-180.

Bonner, T. I., Buckley, N. S., Young, A., and Braun, M. R. (1987). Identification of a family of muscarinic receptor genes. *Science*, **237**, 527-32.

Bonner, T. I., Young, A. C., Braun, M., and Buckley, N. J. (1988). Cloning and expression of the human and rat m5 muscarinic acetylcholine receptor genes. *Neuron*, **1**, 403-10.

Bourne, H. R., Sanders, D. A., and McCormack, F. (1991). The GTPase superfamily: conserved structure and molecular mechanism. *Nature*, **349**, 117-27.

Bradley, P. B., Engel, G., Feniuk, W., Fozard, J. R., Humphrey, P. P. A., Midlemiss, D. N. et al. (1986). Proposals for the classification and nomenclature of functional receptors for 5-hydroxytryptamine. *Neuropharmacology*, **25**, 563-76.

Braun, T., Schofield, Shivers, B. D., Pritchett, D. B., and Seeburg, P. H. (1987). A novel muscarinic receptor identified by homology screening. *Biochem. Biophys. Res. Commun.*, **149**, 125-32.

Brayden, J. E. (1990). Membrane hyperpolarization is a mechanism of endothelium-dependent cerebral vasodilation. *Am. J. Physiol.*, **259**, H668-73.

Bulbring, E. and Tomita, T. (1987). Catecholamine action on smooth muscle. *Pharmacol. Rev.*, **39**, 50-86.

Bylund, B. D. (1985). Heterogeneity of alpha-2 adrenergic receptors. *Pharmacol. Biochem. Behav.*, **22**, 835-43.

Bylund, B. D. (1988). Subtypes of alpha 2-adrenoceptors: pharmacological and molecular evidence converge. *Trends Pharmacol. Sci.*, **9**, 356-61.

Bylund, D. B., Blaxall, H. S., Murphy, T. J., and Simmoneaux, V. (1991). Pharmacological evidence for α_{2C} and α_{2D} adrenergic subtypes. In *Adrenergic structure, mechanisms, function* (ed. E. Szabadi and C. M. Bradshaw), pp. 27-36. Birkhauser Verlag, Basel.

Camps, M., Hou, C., and Sidiropoulos, D., Stock, J. B., Jakobs, K. H., and Gierschik, P. (1992). Stimulation of phospholipase C by guanine-nucleotide binding protein $\beta\gamma$ subunits. *Eur. J. Biochem.*, **206**, 821-31.

Carpene, C., Galitzky, J., Collon, P., Esclapez, F., Dauzats, M., and Lafontan, M. (1993). Desensitization of beta-1 and beta-2, but not beta-3, adrenoceptor-mediated lipolytic responses of adipocytes after long-term noradrenaline infusion. *J. Pharmacol. Exp. Ther.*, **265**, 237-247.

Changeux, J.-P., Girauldt, J., and Dennis, M. (1987). The nicotinic acetylcholine receptor: molecular architecture of a ligand-regulated ion channel. *Trends Pharmacol. Sci.*, **8**, 459-65.

Cheung, Y.-D., Barnett, D. B., and Nahorski, S. R. (1986). Heterogeneous properties of alpha-2-adrenoceptors in particulate and soluble preperations of human platelet and rat and rabbit kidney. *Biochem. Pharmacol.*, **35**, 3767-75.

Chinkers, M. and Garbers, D. L. (1991). Signal transduction by guanylyl cyclases. *Annu. Rev. Biochem.*, **60**, 553-75.

Chung, F. Z., Lentes, K. V., Gocayne, J., Fitzgerald, M., Robinson, D., Kerlavage, A. R., *et al.* (1987). Cloning and sequence analysis of the human brain β-adrenergic receptor. Evolutionary relationship to rodent and avian β-receptors and porcine muscarinic receptors. *FEBS Lett.*, **211**, 200-6.

Clapham, D. E. and Neer, E. J. (1993). New roles for G protein $\beta\gamma$-dimers in transmembrane signaling. *Nature*, **365**, 403-6.

Coleman, R. A., Kennedy, I., Humphrey, P. P. A., Bunce, K. T., and Lumley, P. (1990). Prostanoids and their receptors. In *Comprehensive medicinal chemistry* Vol. 3, (ed. J. C. Emmett). Chapter 12.11. Pergamon Press, Oxford.

Cotecchia, S., Schwinn, D. A., Randall, R. R., Lefkowitz, R. J., Caron, M. G., and Kobilka, B. K. (1988). Molecular cloning and expression of cDNA for the hamster α_1-adrenergic receptor. *Proc. Natl. Acad. Sci. USA*, **85**, 7159-63.

Daves, N. W., Standen, N. B., and Stanfield, P. R. (1991). ATP-dependent potassium channels of muscle cells: their properties, regulation and possible functions. *J. Bioeng. Biomembr.*, **23**, 509-35.

De Jonge, A., Santing, P. N., Timmermans, P. B. M. W. M., and Van Zwieten, P. A. (1981). A comparison of peripheral pre- and post-synaptic α_2-adrenoceptors using meta-substituted imidazolines. *J. Auton. Pharmacol.*, **1**, 377-83.

Dixon, R. A. F., Kobilka, B. K., Benovic, J. L., Dohlman, H. G., Frielle, T., Bolanowski, M. A., *et al.* (1986). Cloning of the gene and cDNA from mammalian β-adrenergic receptor and homology with rhodopsin. *Nature*, **321**, 75-9.

Dixon, R. A. F., Sigal, I. S., Candelore, M. R., Register, R. B., Scattergood, W., Rands, E., *et al.* (1987). Structural features required for ligand binding to β-adrenergic receptors. *EMBO J.*, **6**, 3269-75.

Docherty, J. R. (1989). The pharmacology of α_1 and α_2 adrenoceptors: evidence for and against a further subdivision. *Pharmacol. Ther.*, **44**, 241-84.

Dohlman, H. G., Thorner, J., Caron, M. G., and Lefkowitz, R. J. (1991). Model systems for the study of seven-transmembrane segment receptors. *Annu. Rev. Biochem.*, **60**, 653-88.

Doods, H. N., Mathy, M.-J., Davidson, D., van Charldorp, K. J., de Jonge, A., and van Zwieten, P. A. (1987). Selectivity of muscarinic antagonist in radioligand and *in vivo* experiments for putative M1, M2 and M3 receptors. *J. Pharmacol. Exp. Ther.*, **242**, 257-62.

Drew, G. M. (1985). What do antagonists tell us about α-adrenoceptors. *Clin. Sci.*, **68(suppl. 10)**, 15S–19S.

Duckles, S. P. and Garcia-Villalon, A. L. (1990). Characterization of vascular muscarinic receptors: Rabbit ear artery and bovine coronary artery. *J. Pharmacol. Exp. Ther.*, **252**, 608–13.

Emorine, L. J., Marullo, S., Briend-Sutren, M. M., Patey, G., Tate, K., Delavier-Klutchko, C., *et al.* (1989). Molecular characterization of the β₃-adrenergic receptor. *Science*, **245**, 1118–21.

Fain, J. N. and Garcia-Sainz, J. A. (1980). Minireview. Role of phosphoinositol turnover in alpha₁- and of adenylate cyclase inhibition in alpha₂ effects of catecholamines. *Life Sci.*, **26**, 1183–94.

Fargin, A., Raymond, J. R., Lohse, M. J., Kobilka, B. K., Caron, M. G., and Lefkowitz, R. J. (1988). The genomic clone G-21 which resembles a β-adrenergic receptor sequence encodes the 5-HT₁ₐ receptor. *Nature*, **335**, 358–60.

Fish, D., Sperti, G., Colucci, W., and Clapham, D. (1988). Phorbol ester increases the dihydropiridine-sensitive calcium conductance in a vascular smooth muscle cell line. *Circ. Res.*, **62**, 1049–54.

Flavahan, N. A. and Vanhoutte, P. M. (1986). α₁-Adrenoceptor subclassification in vascular smooth muscle. *Trends Pharmacol. Sci.*, **7**, 347–9.

Fraser, C. M., Arakawa, S., McCombie, W. R., and Venter, J. C. (1989). Cloning, sequence analysis and permanent expression of a human α₂-adrenergic receptor in chinese hamster ovary cells. *J. Biol. Chem.*, **264**, 11754–61.

Frielle, T., Collins, S., Kiefer, W. D., Caron, M. G., Lefkowitz, R. J., and Kobilka, B. K. (1987). Cloning of the cDNA for the human β₁-adrenergic receptor. *Proc. Natl. Acad. Sci. USA*, **84**, 7920–4.

Frielle, T., Daniel, K. W., Caron, M. G., and Lefkowitz, R. J. (1988). Structural basis of β-adrenergic receptor subtype specificity studied with chimeric β₁/β₂ adrenoceptors. *Proc. Natl. Acad. Sci. USA*, **85**, 9494–8.

Furuichi, T., Yoshkawa, S., Miyawaki, A., Wada, K., Maeda, N., and Mikoshiba, K. (1992). Primary structure and functional expression of the inositol 1,4,5-trisphosphate-binding protein P₄₀₀. *Nature*, **342**, 32–8.

Gaddum, J. H. and Picarelli, Z. P. (1957). Two kinds of tryptamine receptors. *Br. J. Pharmacol., Chemother.*, **12**, 323–8.

Galzi, J.-L., Revah, F., Bessie, A., and Changeux, J.-P. (1991). Functional architecture of the nicotinic acetylcholine receptor: from electric organ to brain. *Annu. Rev. Pharmacol.*, **31**, 37–72.

Gantz, I., Schaffer, M., DelValle, J., Logsdon, C., Campbell, V., Uhler, M., *et al.* (1991). Molecular cloning of a gene encoding the histamine H₂ receptor. *Proc. Natl. Acad. Sci. USA*, **88**, 429–33.

Goldschmidt-Clermont, P. J. (1991). Regulation of phospholipase C-γ₁ by profilin and tyrosine phosphorylation. *Science*, **251**, 1231–3.

Goyal, R. K. and Rattan, S. (1978). Neurohumoral, hormonal and drug receptors of the lower esophageal shpincter. *Gastroenterology*, **74**, 598–619.

Granneman, J. G., Lahners, K. N., and Chaudry, A. (1991). Molecular cloning and expression of the rat β₃-adrenergic receptor. *Mol. Pharmacol.*, **40**, 895–9.

Guyer, C. A., Horstman, D. A., Wilson, A. L., Clark, J. D., and Cragoe, E. J. (1990). Cloning, sequencing and expression of the gene encoding the porcine α₂-adrenergic receptor. *J. Biol. Chem.*, **265**, 17307–17.

Haga, K. and Haga, T. (1992). Activation of G protein βγ subunits of agonist or light-dependent phosphorylation of muscarinic acetylcholine receptors or rhodopsin. *J. Biol. Chem.*, **267**, 2222–7.

Hamblin, M. and Metcalf, M. (1991). Primary structure and functional characterization of a human 5-HT$_{1D}$-type serotonin receptor. *Mol. Pharmacol.*, **40**, 143-8.

Hamblin, M. W., McGuffin, R. W., Metcalf, M. A., Dorsa, D. M., and Merchan, K. M. (1992). Distinct 5-HT$_{1B}$ and 5-HT$_{1D}$ receptors in rat: structure and pharmacological comparison of the two cloned receptors. *Mol. Cell. Neurosci.*, **3**, 578-87.

Hammer, R., Berrie, C., Birdsall, N., Burgen, A., and Hulme, E. (1980). Piperizeane distinguishes between different subclasses of muscarinic receptors. *Nature*, **283**, 90-2.

Han, C., Abel, P. W., and Minneman, K. P. (1987). Heterogeneity of α_1-adrenergic receptors revealed by chlorethylclonidine. *Mol. Pharmacol.*, **32**, 505-10.

Hanft, G., Gross, G., Beckeringh, J. J., and Korstanje, C. (1989). α_1-adrenoceptors: the ability of various agonists and antagonists to discriminate between two distinct [^{3}H]prazosin binding sites. *J. Pharm. Pharmacol.*, **41**, 714-16.

Hartig, P. R., Branchek, T. A., and Weinshank, R. L. (1992). A subfamily of 5-HT$_{1D}$ receptor genes. *Trends Pharmacol. Sci.*, **13**, 152-9.

Hartig, P. R. (1989). Molecular biology of 5-HT receptors. *Trends Pharmacol. Sci.*, **10**, 64-9.

Haudsdorff, W. P., Caron, M. G., and Lefkowitz, R. J. (1990). Turning off the signal: desensitisation of beta-adrenergic receptor function *FASEB J.*, **11**, 2881-9.

Hepler, J. R. and Gilman, A. G. (1992). G proteins. *Trends Biochem. Sci.*, **17**, 383-7.

Hicks, P. E. (1981). Antagonism of pre and postsynaptic α-adrenoceptors by BE2254 (HEAT) and prazosin. *J. Auton. Pharmacol.*, **1**, 391-7.

Hirata, M., Hayashi, Y., Ushikubi, F., Yokota, Y., Kageyama, R., Nakanishi, S., *et al.* (1991). Cloning and expression of cDNA for a human thromboxane A$_2$ receptor. *Nature*, **349**, 617-20.

Hollmann, M., O'Shea-Greefield, A., Rogers, S. W., and Heinemann, S. (1989). Cloning by functional expression of a member of the glutamate receptor family. *Nature*, **342**, 643-8.

Houslay, M. D. and Milligan, G. (ed.) (1990). *G Proteins as mediators of cellular signaling processes*. Wiley, New York.

Humphrey, P. P. A., Hartig, P., and Hoyer, D. (1993). A proposed new nomenclature for 5-HT receptors. *Trends Pharmacol. Sci.*, **14**, 233-6.

Inguez-Liuhi, J. A., Simon, M. I., Robishaw, J. D., and Gilman, A. G. (1992). G protein $\beta\gamma$ subunits synthesized in Sf9 cells: functional characterization and the significance of prenylation of γ. *J. Biol. Chem.*, **267**, 23409-17.

Jakobs, K. H. and Schultz, G. (1982). Signal transformation involving α-adrenoceptors. *J. Cardiovasc. Pharmacol.*, **4(suppl. 1)**, S63-7.

Jard, S. (1988). Mechanism of action of vasopressin and vasopressin antagonists. *Kidney Int.*, **34(suppl. 26)**, S38-42.

Jelsema, C. L. and Axelrod, J. (1987). Stimulation of phospholipase A$_2$ activity in bovine rod outer segments by the $\beta\gamma$ subunits of transducin and its inhibition by α subunits. *Proc. Natl. Acad. Sci. USA*, **84**, 3623-7.

Jin, H., Oksenberg, D., Ashkenazi, A., Peroutka, S. J., Duncan, A. M. V., Rozmahel, R., *et al.* (1992). Characterization of the human 5-hydroxytryptamine$_{1B}$ receptor. *J. Biol. Chem.*, **267**, 5735-8.

Julius, D., MacDermott, A. B., Axel, R., and Jessell, T. M. (1988). Molecular characterization of a functional cDNA encoding the serotonin 1C receptor. *Science*, **241**, 558-64.

Kamishima, T., Nelson, M. T., and Patlak, J. B. (1992). Carbachol modulates voltage sensitivity of calcium channels in bronchial smooth muscle of rats. *Am. J. Physiol.*, **263**, C69-77.

Katz, A., Wu, D., and Simon, M. I. (1992) Subunits $\beta\gamma$ of heterotrimeric G protein active β_2 isoform of phospholipase C. *Nature*, **360**, 686-9.

Kaupp, U. B. (1991). The cyclic nucleotide-gated channels of vertebrate photoreceptors and olfactory epithelium. *Trends Neurosci.*, **14**, 150–7.

Kaziro, Y., Hiroshi, I., Kozasa, T., Nakafuku, M., and Satoh, T. (1991). Structure and function of signal-transducing GTP-binding proteins. *Annu. Rev. Biochem.*, **60**, 349–400.

Kimura, T., Tanizawa, O., Mori, K., Brownstein, M. J., and Okayama, H. (1992). Structure and expression of a human oxytocin receptor. *Nature*, **366**, 526–9.

Kleuss, C., Scherubl, H., Hescheler, J., Schultz, G., and Wittig, B. (1993). Selectivity in signal transduction determined by gamma subunits of heterotrimeric G proteins. *Science*, **259**, 832–4.

Kobilka, B. K., Frielle, T., Collins, S., Yang-Feng, T., Kobilka, T. S., Francke, U., et al. (1987). An intronless gene encoding a potential member of the family of receptors to guanine nucleotide regulatory proteins. *Nature*, **329**, 75–8.

Kobilka, B. K., Kobilka, T. S., Daniel, K. W., Regan, J. W., Caron, M. G., and Lefkowitz, R. J. (1988). Chimeric α_2-, β_2-adrenergic receptors: delineation of domains involved in effector coupling and ligand binding specificity. *Science*, **240**, 1310–16.

Kubo, T., Fukuda, K., Mikami, A., Takahashi, H., Mishina, M., Haga, K., et al. (1986a). Cloning, sequencing and expression of complementary DNA encoding the muscarinic acetylcholine receptor. *Nature*, **323**, 411–16.

Kubo, T., Maeda, A., Sugimoto, K., Akiba, I., Mikami, A., Takahashi, T., et al. (1986b). Primary structure of porcine cardiac muscarinic acetylcholine receptor deduced from cDNA sequence. *FEBS Lett.*, **209**, 367–72.

Kursar, J. D., Nelson, D. L., Wainscott, D. B., Cohen, M. L., and Baez, M. (1992). Molecular cloning, functional expression and pharmacological characterization of a novel serotonin receptor (5-hydroxytryptamine$_{2F}$) from rat stomach fundus. *Mol. Pharmacol.*, **42**, 549–57.

Lands, A. M., Arnold, A., McAuliff, J. P., Luduena, T. P., and Braun, T. G. (1967). Differentiation of receptor systems activated by sympathomimetic amines. *Nature*, **214**, 597–8.

Langosch, D., Becker, C.-M., and Betz, H. (1990). The inhibitory glycine receptor: a ligand-gated chloride channel of the central nervous system. *Eur. J. Biochem.*, **194**, 1–8.

Lanier, S. M., Homey, C. J., Patenande, C., and Graham, R. M. (1988). Identification of structurally distinct α_2-adrenergic receptors. *J. Biol. Chem.*, **263**, 14491–6.

Lanier, S. M., Downing, S., Duzic, E., and Honey, C. J. (1991). Isolation of rat genomic clones encoding subtypes of the α_2-adrenergic receptor. *J. Biol. Chem.*, **266**, 10470–8.

Lefkowitz, R. J., Hausdorff, W. P., and Caron, M. G. (1990). The role of phosphorylation in desensitization of the β-adrenoceptor. *Trends Pharmacol. Sci.*, **11**, 190–4.

Leonhardt, S., Herrick-Davis, K., and Tietler, M. (1989). Detection of a novel serotonin receptor subtype (5-HT$_{1E}$) in human brain: Interaction with a GTP-binding protein. *J. Neurochem.*, **53**, 465–71.

Liard, J.-F. (1990). Interaction between V1 and V2 effects in hemodynamic response to vasopressin in dogs. *Am. J. Physiol.*, **258**, H482–9.

Libert, L., Parmentier, M., Lefort, A., Dinsart, C., van Sande, J., Maenhaut, C., et al. (1989). Selective amplification and cloning of four new members of the G protein-coupled receptor family. *Science*, **244**, 569–72.

Limbird, L. E. (ed.) (1988). *The alpha-2 adrenergic receptors*. Humana Press, New Jersey.

Logothetis, D. E., Kuracki, Y., Galper, J., and Neer, E. J. (1987). The $\beta\gamma$ subunits of GTP-binding proteins activate the muscarinic K$^+$ channel in heart. *Nature*, **325**, 321–6.

Lomasney, J. W., Lorenz, W., Allen, L. F., King, K., Regan, J. W., Yang-Feng, T. L., et al. (1990). Expansion of the α_2-adrenergic receptor family: Cloning and characterization of a human α_2-adrenergic receptor subtype, the gene for which is located on chromosome 2. *Proc. Natl. Acad. Sci. USA*, **87**, 5094–8.

Lomasney, J. W., Cotecchia, S., Lorenz, W., Leung, W.-Y., Schwinn, D. A., Yang-Feng,

T. L., et al. (1991). Molecular cloning and expression of the cDNA for the α_{1A}-adrenergic receptor. *J. Biol. Chem.*, **266**, 6365–9.

Lubbert, H., Snutch, T. P., Dascal, N., Lester, H. A., and Davidson, N. (1987a). Rat brain 5-HT$_{1C}$ receptors are encoded by a 5–6 Kbase mRNA size class and are functionally expressed in injected xenopus oocytes. *J. Neurosci.*, **7**, 1159–65.

Lubbert, H., Hoffman, B. J., Snutch, T. P., van Dyke, T., Levine, A. J., Hartig, P. R., et al. (1987b). cDNA cloning of a serotonin 5-HT$_{1C}$ receptor by electrophysiological assays of mRNA-injected xenopus oocytes. *Proc. Natl. Acad. Sci. USA*, **84**, 4332–6.

Maack, T. (1992). Receptors of atrial natriuretic factor. *Annu. Rev. Physiol.*, **54**, 11–27.

Machida, C. A., Bunzow, J. R., Searles, R. P., Van Tol, H., Tester, B., Neve, K. A., et al. (1990). Molecular cloning and expression of the rat β_1-adrenergic receptor. *J. Biol. Chem.*, **265**, 12960–5.

Maenhault, C., van Sande, J., Massart, C., Dinsart, C., Libert, F., Monferini, E., et al. (1991). The orphan receptor cDNA RDC4 encodes a 5-HT$_{1D}$ serotonin receptor. *Biochem. Biophys. Res. Commun.*, **180**, 1460–8.

Maricq, V. A., Peterson, A. S., Brake, A. J., Myers, R. M., and Julius, D. (1991). Primary structure and functional expression of the 5-HT$_3$ receptor, a serotonin-gated ion channel. *Science*, **254**, 432–7.

Maroteaux, L., Saudou, F., Amlaiky, N., Boschert, U., Plassat, J.-L., and Hen, R. (1992). Mouse 5-HT$_{1B}$ serotonin receptors: cloning, functional expression and localization in motor control centres. *Proc. Natl. Acad. Sci. USA*, **89**, 3020–4.

Marullo, S., Emorine, L. J., Strosberg, A. D., and Delavier-Klutchko, C. (1990). Selective binding of ligands to β_1/β_2 or chimeric β_1/β_2 adrenergic receptors. *EMBO J.*, **9**, 1471–6.

Matthes, H., Boschert, U., Amlaiky, N., Grailhe, R., Plassat, J.-P., Muscatelli, F., et al. (1993). Mouse 5-hydroxytryptamine$_{5A}$ and 5-hydroxytryptamine$_{5B}$ receptors define a new family of serotonin receptors: cloning, functional expression and chromosomal location. *Mol. Pharmacol.*, **43**, 313–19.

Maura, G., Gemignani, A., and Raiteri, M. (1985). α_2-adrenoceptors in rat hypothalamus and cerebral cortex: functional evidence for pharmacologically distinct subpopulations. *Eur. J. Pharmacol.*, **116**, 335–9.

McGrath, J. C. (1983). Ca^{2+}-free and Ca^{2+}-requiring α_1-responses in rat anococcygeus having differing agonist potency series. *Br. J. Pharmacol.*, **79**, 227P.

McGrath, J. C., Brown, C. M., and Wilson, V. G. (1989). Alpha-adrenoceptors a critical review. *Med. Res. Rev.*, **9**, 407–533.

McKernan, R. M., Dickinson, K. E. J., Miles, C. M. M., and Sever, P. S. (1986). Heterogeneity between soluble human and rabbit splenic α_2-adrenoceptors. *Biochem. Pharmacol.*, **35**, 3517–23.

Metcalf, M. A., McGuffen, R. W., and Hamblin, M. W. (1992). Conversion of the human 5-HT$_{1D}$ beta serotonin receptor to the rat 5-HT$_{1B}$ ligand-binding phenotype by Thr[355] Asn[351] site directed mutagenesis. *Biochem. Pharmacol.*, **44**, 1917–20.

Mikoshiba, K. (1993). Inositol 1,4,5-trisphosphate receptor. *Trends Pharmacol. Sci.*, **14**, 86–9.

Milligan, G. (1993). Mechanisms of multifunctional signalling by G protein-linked receptors. *Trends Pharmacol. Sci.*, **14**, 239–44.

Minneman, K. P. (1988). α_1 adrenergic receptor subtypes, inositol phosphates and sources of cell Ca^{2+}. *Pharmacol. Rev.*, **40**, 87–120.

Monsma, F. J., Yong Shen, J. R., Ward, R. P., Hamblin, H. W., and Sibley, D. R. (1993). Cloning and expression of a novel serotonin receptor with high affinity for tricyclic psychotropic drugs. *Mol. Pharmacol.*, **43**, 320–7.

Morel, A., O'Carrol, A.-M., Brownstein, M. J., and Lolait, S. L. (1992). Molecular cloning and expression of the rat V1α arginine vasopressin receptor. *Nature*, **356**, 523–6.

Morel, A., Lolait, S. J., and Brownstein, M. J. (1993). Molecular cloning and expression of rat V1α and V2 arginine vasopressin receptors. *Regul. Pept.*, **45**, 53-9.

Moriyoshi, K., Masu, M., Ishii, T., Shigemoto, R., Mizuno, N., and Nakanishi, S. (1991). Molecular cloning and characterization of the rat NMDA receptor. *Nature*, **354**, 31-7.

Morrow, A. L. and Creese, I. 1986). Characterization of α-adrenergic receptor subtypes in rat brain: a reevaluation of [^{3}H]WB4101 and [^{3}H]prazosin binding. *Mol. Pharmacol.*, **29**, 321-30.

Muntz, K. H., Sternweis, P. G., Gilman, A. G., and Mumby, S. M. (1992). Influence of gamma subunit prenylation on association of guanine nucleotide-binding regulatory proteins with membranes. *Mol. Biol. Cell.*, **3**, 49-61.

Murphy, T. J., Alexander, R. W., Griendling, K. K., Runge, M. S., and Bernstein, K. E. (1991). Isolation of a cDNA encoding the vascular type 1 angiotensin receptor. *Nature*, **351**, 233-6.

Nahmias, C., Blin, N., Elalouf, J.-M., Mattei, M. G., Strosberg, A. D., and Emorine, L. J. (1991). Molecular characterisation of the mouse β-adrenergic receptor: relationship with the atypical receptor of adipocytes. *EMBO J.*, **10**, 3721-7.

Namba, T., Sugimoto, Y., Hirata, M., Hayashi, Y., Honda, A., Watabe, A., et al. (1992). Mouse thromboxane A2 receptor: cDNA cloning, expression and northern blot analysis. *Biochem. Biophys. Res. Commun.*, **184**, 1197-203.

Nathanson, N. M. (1987). Molecular properties of the muscarinic acetylcholine receptor. *Annu. Rev. Neurosci.*, **10**, 195-236.

Nelson, M. T., Patlak, J. B., Worley, J. F., and Standen, N. B. (1990a). Calcium channels, potassium channels and voltage dependence of arterial smooth muscle. *Am. J. Physiol.*, **259**, C3-18.

Nelson, M. T., Huang, Y., Brayden, J. E., Hescheler, J., and Standen, N. B. (1990b). Arterial dilations in response to calcitonin gene-related peptide involves activation of K$^+$ channels. *Nature*, **344**, 770-3.

Ostrowski, J., Kjelsberg, M. A., Caron, M. G., and Lefkowitz, R. J. (1992). Mutagenesis of the β$_2$-adrenergic receptor: How structure elucidates function. *Annu. Rev. Pharmacol. Toxicol.*, **32**, 167-83.

Pandiella, A., Beguinot, L., Vicentini, L. M., and Meldolesi, J. (1989). Transmembrane signalling at the epidermal growth factor receptor. *Trends Pharmacol. Sci.*, **10**, 411-14.

Peralta, E. G., Ashkfnazi, A., Winslow, J. W., Smith, D. H., Ramachandran, J., and Capon, D. J. (1987). Distinct primary structures, ligand binding properties and tissue expression of four human acetylcholine receptors. *EMBO J.*, **6**, 3923-9.

Perez, D. M., Piascik, M. T., and Graham, R. M. (1991). Solution-phase library screening for the identification of rare clones: identification of an alpha 1D-adrenergic receptor cDNA. *Mol. Pharmacol.*, **40**, 876-83.

Peroutka, S. J. and Snyder, S. H. (1979). Multiple serotonin receptors: differential binding of [^{3}H]-5-hydroxytryptamine, [^{3}H]lysergic acid diethylamine and [^{3}H] — spiroperidol. *Mol. Pharmacol.*, **16**, 637-99.

Pritchett, D. B., Bach, A. W., Wozny, M., Taleb, O., Dal Toso, R., Shih, J. C., et al. (1988). Structure and functional expression of cloned rat serotonin 5-HT$_2$ receptor. *EMBO J.*, **7**, 4135-40.

Pronin, A. N. and Gautam, N. (1992). Interaction between G protein β and γ subunit types is selective. *Proc. Natl. Acad. Sci. USA*, **89**, 6220-4.

Raymond, J. R., Hnatowich, M., Lefkowitz, R. J., and Caron, M. G. (1990). Adrenergic receptors. Models for regulation of signal transduction processes. *Hypertension*, **15**, 119-31.

Regan, J. W., Kobilka, T. S., Yang-Feng, T. L., Caron, M. G., Lefkowitz, R. J., and

Kobilka, B. J. (1988). Cloning and expression of a human kidney cDNA for an α_2-adrenergic receptor subtype. *Proc. Natl. Acad. Sci. USA*, **85**, 6301-5.

Rhee, S. G. and Choi, K. D. (1992). Multiple forms of phospholipase C isoenzymes and their activation mechanisms. *Adv. Second Messenger Phosphoprotein Res.*, **26**, 35-61.

Rodbell, M., Birnbaumer, L., Pohl, S. L., and Krans, H. M. J. (1971). The glucagon-sensitive adenylate cyclase system in plasma membrane of rat liver. *J. Biol. Chem.*, **246**, 1877-82.

Rosen, O. M. (1987). After insulin binds. *Science*, **237**, 1452-8.

Rosenbaum, L. C., Malencik, D. A., Anderson, S. R., Tota, M. R., and Schimerlik, M. I. (1987). Phosphorylation of the porcine atrial muscarinic acetylcholine receptor by cyclic AMP-dependent protein kinase. *Biochemistry*, **26**, 8183-8.

Ruat, M., Traiffort, E., Arrang, J. M., Leurs, R., and Schwartz, J. C. (1991). Cloning and tissue expression of a rat histamine H_2 receptor gene. *Biochem. Biophys. Res. Commun.*, **179**, 1470-8.

Ruffolo, R. R., Sulpizio, A. C., Nichols, A. J., DeMarinins, R. M., and Hieble, J. P. (1987). Pharmacological differentiation between pre- and postjunctional α_2-adrenoceptors by SKF 104078. *Naunyn-Schmiedeberg's Arch. Pharmacol.*, **336**, 415-18.

Ruffolo, R. R., Nicols, A. J., Stadel, J. M., and Hieble, J. P. (1991). Structure and function of α-adrenoceptors. *Pharmacol. Rev.*, **43(4)**, 475-501.

Sasaki, K., Yamamo, Y., Bardhan, S., Iwai, N., Murray, J. J., Hasegawa, M., *et al.* (1991). Cloning and expression of a complementary DNA encoding a bovine adrenal andiotensin II type 1 receptor. *Nature*, **351**, 230-3.

Schmidt, C. J., Thomas, T. C., Levine, M. A., and Neer, E. J. (1992). Specificity of G protein $\beta$and γ subunit interactions. *J. Biol. Chem.*, **267**, 13807-10.

Schofield, P. R., Darlison, M. G., Fujita, N., Burt, D. R., Stephenson, F. A., Rodriguez, H., *et al.* (1987). Sequence and functional expression of the $GABA_A$ receptor shows ligand-gated receptor super-family. *Nature*, **328**, 221-7.

Schwinn, D. A. and Lomasney, J. W., (1992). Pharmacological characterization of cloned alpha 1-adrenoceptor subtype selective antagonists suggest the existence of a fourth subtype. *Eur. J. Pharmacol.*, **227**, 433-6.

Schwinn, D. A., Lomasney, J. W., Lorenz, W., Szklut, P. J., Fremeau, R. T., Yang-Feng, T. L., *et al.* (1990). Molecular cloning and expression of the cDNA for a novel α_1-adrenergic receptor subtype. *J. Biol. Chem.*, **265**, 8183-9.

Shearman, M. ., Sekiguchi, K., and Nishizuka, Y. (1989). Modulation of ion channel activity: A key function of the protein kinase C enzyme family. *Pharmacol. Rev.*, **41**, 212-31.

Simon, M. I., Strathmann, N. M. P., and Gautam, N. (1991). Diversity of G proteins in signal transduction. *Science*, **252**, 802-8.

Simonds, W. F., Butrynski, J. E., Gautam., N., Unson, C. B., and Spiegel, A. M. (1991). G protein $\beta\gamma$ dimers: Membrane targeting requires subunit coexpression and intact γ C-A-A-X domain. *J. Biol. Chem.*, **266**, 5363-6.

Spiegel, A. M., Backlund, P. S., Butrynski, J. E., Jones, T. L. Z., and Simonds, W. F. (1991). The G protein connection: molecular basis of membrane association. *Trends Biochem. Sci.*, **16**, 338-41.

Strader, C. D., Dixon, R. A. F., Cheung, A. H., Candelore, H. R., Blake, A. D., and Sigal, I. S. (1987). Mutations that uncouple the β-adrenergic receptor from Gs and increase agonist affinity. *J. Biol. Chem.*, **262**, 16439-43.

Strader, C. D., Sigal, I. S., and Dixon, R. A. F. (1989). Genetic approaches to the determination of structure-function relationships of G protein-coupled receptors. *Trends Pharmacol. Sci.*, **10** Suppl., 26-30.

Sugimoto, Y., Namba, T., Honda, A., Hayashi, Y., Negiski, M., Ichikawa, A., *et al.*

(1992). Cloning and expression of a cDNA for mouse prostaglandin E receptor EP3 subtype. *J. Biol. Chem.*, **267**, 6463–6.

Summers, R. J. and McMartin, L. R. (1993), Adrenoceptors and their second messenger systems. *J. Neurochem.*, **60**, 10–23.

Summers, R. J., Barnett, D. B., and Nahorski, S. R. (1983). The characteristics of adrenoceptors in homogenates of human cerebral cortex labelled by [^{3}H]rauwolscine. *Life Sci.*, **33**, 1105–12.

Tang, W. J. and Gillman, A. G. (1991). Type-specific regulation of adenylyl cyclase by G Protein $\beta\gamma$ subunits. *Science*, **254**, 1500–3.

Timmermann, P. B. M. W. M., Wong, P. C., Chiu, A. T., and Herblin, W. F. (1991). Nonpeptide angiotensin II receptor antagonists. *Trends Pharmacol. Sci.*, **12**, 55–61.

Tomita, T. (1988). Ionic channels in smooth muscle studied with patch-clamp methods. *Jap. J. Physiol.*, **38**, 1–18.

Tota, M. R., Candelore, M. R., Dixon, R. A. F., and Strader, C. D. (1991). Biophysical and genetic analysis of ligand-binding site of the β-adrenoceptor. *Trends Pharmacol. Sci.*, **12**, 4–6.

Tsien, R. W., Lipscombe, D., Madison, D. V., Bley, K. R., and Fox, A. P. (1990). Multiple types of neuronal calcium channels and their selective modulation. *Trends Neurosci.*, **11**, 413–30.

Tsien, R. W., Ellinor, P. T., and Horne, W. A. (1991). Molecular diversity of voltage-dependent Ca^{2+} channels. *Trends Pharmacol. Sci.*, **12**, 351–6.

Vivaudou, M. B., Clapp, L. H., Walsh, J. V., and Singer, J. J. (1988). Regulation of one type of Ca^{2+} current in smooth muscle cells by diacylglycerol ahd acetylcholine. *FASEB J.*, **2**, 2497–504.

Voight, M. M., Laurie, D. J., Seeburg, P. H., and Bach, A. (1991). Molecular cloning and characterization of a rat brain cDNA encoding a 5-hydroxytryptamine$_{1B}$ receptor. *EMBO J.*, **10**, 4017–23.

von Weizsacker, E., Strathmann, M. P., and Simon, M. I. (1992). Diversity among the beta subunits of heterotrimetic GTP-binding proteins: characterization of a novel beta-subunit cDNA. *Biochem. Biophys. Res. Commun.*, **183**, 350–6.

Weinshank, R. L., Zgombick, J. M., Macchi, M. J., Adham, N., Lichtblau, H., Branchek, T. A., et al. (1990). Cloning, expression and pharmacological characterization of a human α_{2B} adrenergic receptor. *Mol. Pharmacol.*, **38**, 681–8.

Weinshank, R. L., Zgombick, Macchi, M. J., Branchek, T. A., and Hartig, P. R. (1992). Human serotonin 1D recetor is encoded by a subfamily of two distinct genes: 5-HT$_{1D\alpha}$ and 5-HT$_{1D\beta}$. *Proc. Natl. Acad. Sci. USA*, **89**, 3630–4.

Weston, A. H. and Edwards, G. (1992). Recent progress in potassium channel opener pharmacology. *Biochem. Pharmacol.*, **43**, 47–54.

Worley, J. F., Quayle, J. M., Standen, N. B., and Nelson, M. T. (1991). Regulation of single calcium channels in cerebral arteries by voltage, serotonin and dihydropyridines. *Am. J. Physiol.*, **261**, H1951–60.

Yagaloff, K. A. and Hartig, P. R. (1985). [^{125}I]-lysergic acid diethylamide binds to a novel serotonergic site on rat choroid plexus epithelial cells. *J. Neurosci.*, **5**, 3178–83.

Yamashita, M., Fukui, H., Sugama, K., Horio, Y., Ito, S., Mizuguchi, H., et al. (1991). Expression and cloning of a cDNA encoding the bovine histamine H$_1$-receptor. *Proc. Natl. Acad. Sci. USA*, **88**, 11515–19.

Zeng, D., Harrison, J. K., D'Angelo, D. D., Barber, C. M., Tucker, A. L., Lu, Z., et al. (1990). Molecular characterization of the rat α_{2B}-adrenergic receptor. *Proc. Natl. Acad. Sci. USA*, **87**, 3102–6.

Zgombick, J. M., Wwinshank, R. L., Macchi, M., Schechter, L. E., Branchek, T. A., and Hartig, P. R. (1991). Expression and pharmacological characterization of a canine 5-hydroxytryptamine$_{1D}$ receptor subtype. *Mol. Pharmacol.*, **40**, 1036–42.

6. Membrane ion channels in vascular smooth muscle excitation–contraction coupling

Philip I. Aaronson and Sergey V. Smirnov

INTRODUCTION

The vascular smooth muscle cell (VSMC) plasma membrane is spanned by a number of types of ion channels which act in a co-ordinated fashion to regulate Ca^{2+} influx, thereby contributing to the control of the intracellular Ca^{2+} concentration ($[Ca^{2+}]_i$), and hence tension development and vascular constriction.

Vasoconstriction occurs in response to a variety of physiological stimuli, the most important of which include sympathetic neurotransmission, the binding of autacoids such as angiotensin II and endothelin to their receptors, and increases in transmural pressure. Endogenous vasorelaxants also make an important contribution to regulating vascular tone; these include substances such as nitric oxide and prostacyclin which are released by the endothelium, adrenaline acting on β-adrenoceptors, and peptides such as bradykinin, vasoactive intestinal polypeptide (VIP), and calcitonin gene-related peptide (CGRP). Unlike tension development in visceral smooth muscle and the heart, vasoconstriction is in many cases not obligatorily linked to membrane depolarization, although depolarization of a sufficient magnitude will always lead to vasoconstriction. Agonists such as noradrenaline may, for example, constrict arteries by releasing cellular stored Ca^{2+}; this process does not require depolarization. In arteries such as the rabbit pulmonary artery and ear artery, noradrenaline may also elicit Ca^{2+} influx in the apparent absence of depolarization (Bolton 1979). Vasoconstriction associated with sympathetic stimulation appears to involve both depolarization-dependent and independent components (Bolton and Large 1986).

Most vascular smooth muscles, especially in resistance arteries, are however depolarized beyond the threshold for contraction by bath-applied noradrenaline, locally released vasoconstricting agonists (Bolton 1979), and by increases in transmural pressure (Harder 1984). Similarly, vasodilating agonists often cause a membrane hyperpolarization which may contribute to relaxation. It is therefore clear that membrane potential plays an important, if not primary, role in regulating vascular tension.

Since the advent a decade ago of the use of the patch-clamp technique to investigate membrane ion channels in vascular smooth muscle, a detailed picture of the involvement of these channels in excitation–contraction coupling has begun to emerge. This picture may be summarized as follows: activation of their receptors by vasoconstricting agonists leads to the opening of non-specific cation channels (receptor-gated channels) which depolarize the cell membrane. These channels may also directly support a significant Ca^{2+} influx. Depolarization may also be elicited by the opening of chloride channels which are activated by the rise in $[Ca^{2+}]_i$ resulting from the release of cellular Ca^{2+} stores. Depolarization may be promoted by an agonist-mediated reduction of K^+ channel activity. Depolarization then leads to the opening of voltage-gated Ca^{2+} channels which probably make the primary contribution to Ca^{2+} influx. This influx may be enhanced by a further direct agonist-mediated potentiation of the activity of voltage-gated Ca^{2+} channels.

Several qualifications of this scheme must immediately be introduced. Firstly, ion channel-mediated events interact in a complex manner with changes in intracellular Ca^{2+} compartmentalization and second messenger-mediated effects on enzyme and ion pump activities. Secondly, the relative importance of the various elements of this scheme are likely to differ for different agonists, for individual blood vessels, and probably even at different sites within individual vessels. Thirdly, characterization of these processes is incomplete, and in certain respects, still controversial.

In this chapter, we attempt to organize the information obtained to date, concerning the properties and possible physiological roles of the various ion channels which contribute to maintaining the resting membrane potential, and to activating VSMCs as summarized above. Effects of vasodilators are discussed in less detail due to space limitations. Emphasis is placed upon electrophysiological studies at the cellular or single channel level.

POTASSIUM CHANNELS

Most vascular smooth muscles have a stable resting potential between -60 and -70 mV and either do not freely generate action potentials or generate only small regenerative responses in response to membrane depolarization (reviewed by Bolton 1979; Bolton and Large 1986; Hirst and Edwards 1989). The nearness of the resting potential to the equilibrium K^+ potential (between -82 and -84 mV with a physiological K^+ gradient of 130–140 mM intracellular K^+ and 5 mM extracellular K^+) means that the K^+ permeability is mainly responsible for setting the resting potential.

Three major classes of K^+ channels/currents have been distinguished in VSMCs. These are the large conductance Ca^{2+}- and voltage-sensitive K^+ (K_{Ca}) channels, the delayed rectifier (K_{DR}) K^+ channels, and the ATP-sensitive K^+ (K_{ATP}) channels. Although detailed comparative studies of different vascular beds have not been carried out, it is likely that most types of VSMCs exhibit each of these types of channel. In addition, there are several reports of A-type K^+ currents, inwardly rectifying K^+ currents, and other types of Ca^{2+}-sensitive currents. The activities of both K_{Ca} and K_{ATP} channels have been shown to be modulated by endogenous agonists. It is noteworthy, however, that the characteristics of each of these types appear to vary to some extent from tissue to tissue; it is not obvious whether this variation reflects real differences in channel characteristics, or in methodology. K^+ conductances which have been identified on the single channel level are listed with their salient characteristics in Table 6.1.

K^+ currents are typically characterized in isolated, voltage-clamped cells, with the K^+ gradient set to a 'physiological' level. Upon depolarization from a holding potential of -60 to -80 mV, two distinct components of K^+ current could be distinguished in single VSMCs isolated from rabbit portal vein (Beech and Bolton 1989*b*; Hume and Leblanc 1989) and pulmonary artery (Clapp and Gurney 1991*a*), canine renal artery (Gelband and Hume 1992), human mesenteric artery (Smirnov and Aaronson 1992*a*), and cultured rat pulmonary arterial cells (Yuan *et al*. 1993*a*). One component became apparent positive of -40 or -30 mV, and its activation accelerated with increasing membrane depolarization. This component, which has been termed the delayed rectifier (K_{DR}) on the basis of its similarity to analogous voltage-gated currents in other tissues (reviewed by Rudy 1988), can be visualized pharmacologically by its relatively high sensitivity to the blockers 4-aminopyridine (4-AP) and phencyclidine, and its lower sensitivity to tetraethylammonium (TEA). K_{DR} is also distinguished by its inactivation, which although relatively slow compared to that of A-like currents, limits its availability at holding potentials positive -30 mV (although see Gelband and Hume 1992). Beech and Bolton (1989*b*) estimated the unitary conductance of K_{DR} in a physiological K^+ gradient as 5 pS in rabbit portal vein, while Gelband and Hume (1992) measured a conductance of 57 pS. This divergence, as well as additional differences in current characteristics at the whole-cell level, suggest that the various currents which are lumped together as 'delayed rectifiers' are in fact mediated by somewhat diverse channels.

The physiological role of the K_{DR} channel has not been extensively evaluated in single cell studies. Although the appearance of a measurable K_{DR} requires some depolarization in isolated cells, channel activation is known to be a continuous function of membrane potential, so that some K_{DR} channels are doubtless open at the resting potential. In agreement with this possibility, 4-AP markedly depolarized isolated canine renal arterial cells (Gelband *et al*. 1993). Similarly, a low concentration of 4-AP caused depolarization, an increased membrane resistance, and a suppression of outward rectification in isolated guinea-pig pulmonary artery; the frequency of spontaneous action potentials was also increased in guinea-pig portal vein (Hara *et al*. 1980). It is also very likely that the activation of K_{DR} plays some part in attenuating depolarization during excitation. There is presently little known concerning the regulation of K_{DR} by second messenger systems in VSMCs. It is interesting, however, that 4-AP sensitive currents have been shown to be activated by small reductions of pH in cerebral arterial cells (Bonnet *et al*. 1991), and to be attenuated by hypoxia in cells cultured from rat pulmonary, but not mesenteric, artery (Yuan *et al*. 1993*b*). K_{DR} is also inhibited by increased intracellular Mg^{2+} in canine renal, pulmonary, and

Table 6.1 Potassium channels in vascular smooth muscle cells[a]

Tissue	Conductance (pS)	$[K^+]_o/[K^+]_i$ (mM)	Properties (pharmacology, selectivity, activation)	References
			I. Ca^{2+}-activated K^+ channels	
Rabbit portal vein: large conductance	130 273	6.2/142 142/142	K_L channels (according to authors classification), blocked by 0.1–1 mM external TEA.	Inoue et al. 1985
small conductance	50 92	6.2/142 142/142	K_S channels, TEA resistant.	
Rabbit aorta	337	250/250	50% open probability at $[Ca^{2+}]_i$ between 75–100 μM at -60 mV.	Gelband et al. 1990
Rabbit aorta (primary culture)	230	145/145	Blocked by external TEA (1–10 mM) or charybdotoxin (0.5 nM), and by 1–100 μM internal Ba^{2+}. Quinine, quinidine (0.01–1 mM), and lidocaine (5 mM) blocked channels from both sides.	Pavenstädt et al. 1991
Rabbit cerebral artery	213	120/140	Blocked by external TEA (IC_{50} 190 μM at 0 mV and 215 μM at $+50$ mV), and by 16 μM charybdotoxin.	Brayden and Nelson 1992

Tissue	pS	Ionic conditions	Description	Reference
Guinea-pig mesenteric artery	99 / 183	6/126 126/126	Approximately 60% open probability at 1 μM $[Ca^{2+}]_i$ at -60 mV; selectivity: $Tl^+ > K^+ > Rb^+ \gg Na^+, Cs^+$.	Benham et al. 1986
Human aorta (cell culture)	125 / 242	2.8/140 140/140	Blocked by 1 mM TEA and 0.1 mM quinine; selectivity: $K^+ > Rb^+ > Li^+ Na^+ \gg Tris^{+b} = NH_4^+$.	Bregestovski et al. 1988
Canine renal artery	130 / 232	5.4/140 140/140	Blocked by 0.25 mM external TEA.	Gelband and Hume 1992
Porcine coronary artery (incorporated into lipid bilayer)[c]	245 / 295	250/250[d] 250/250[d]	50% open probability of 245 pS channels at $[Ca^{2+}]_i = 2$ μM at -60 mV, blocked by external TEA ($IC_{50} = 180$ μM at -40 mV and 466 μM at $+80$ mV), and 5–50 nM charybdotoxin. 295 pS channels started to activate at $[Ca^{2+}]_i > 10$ μM at -60 mV.	Toro et al. 1991

II. Voltage-gated K$^+$ channels (delayed rectifier)

Tissue	pS	Ionic conditions	Description	Reference
Rabbit portal vein	≈5	6/126	—	Beech and Bolton 1989b
Rabbit coronary artery	8.5 / ≈15	5.4/140 140/140	—	Volk and Shibata 1993
Canine renal artery	57–59 / 104	5.4/140 140/140	Blocked by intracellular Mg^{2+} (10 mM) and Ca^{2+}.	Gelband and Hume 1992; Gelband2 et al. 1993

III. ATP-sensitive K⁺ channels

Rabbit mesenteric artery	135	60/120	Activated by 1 μM cromakalim and blocked by 1 mM ATP and 20 μM glibenclimide.	Standen et al. 1989
Rabbit mesenteric artery	20	6/120	Activated by 1 μM cromakalim and 5 nM CGRP, and blocked by 30 μM glibenclimide.	Nelson et al. 1990a
Rabbit portal vein	15	6/140	Activity required pinacidil (100 μM), blocked by 100 μM glibenclimide and ≥ 10 μM ATP; GDP (> 100 μM) and GTP (1 mM) reactivate channels after 'run-down' in excised patch.	Kajioka et al. 1991a

IV. Extracellular Ca²⁺-sensitive K⁺ channels

Rabbit portal vein	93 180	6.2/142 142/142	K_M channels, activated by external [Ca²⁺] (threshold ≈ 7.5 μM), potential-independent, and sensitive to intracellular TEA (1–3 mM).	Inoue et al. 1986
Porcine coronary artery	30	2.7/145	Activated by ≈ 10 μM external [Ca²⁺] and by 30 nM nicorandil or SITS[e] at [Ca²⁺]$_o$ < 10⁻⁷ M. Blocked by 5 mM 4-AP.	Inoue et al. 1989

[a] Table represents only results of investigations of single channels in vascular smooth muscle cells where specific K⁺ channels were identified and characterized.
[b] Tris⁺ is tris[hydroxymethyl]aminomethane.
[c] Two populations of large conductance Ca²⁺-activated K⁺ channels were observed.
[d] In this case the ratio represents cis/trans K⁺ concentrations.
[e] SITS is 4-acetamide-4′-isothiocyanostilbene-2,2′-disulphonic acid.

coronary VSMCs; elevations of $[Ca^{2+}]_i$ also suppressed K_{DR} in the coronary cells (Gelband et al. 1993).

Superimposed upon K_{DR} in the cells referred to above was a second component of current, which tended to become obvious at more positive potentials, and which could be distinguished by its noticeably noisy appearance and its apparent lack of inactivation. This current was characterized pharmacologically by its sensitivity to TEA and charybdotoxin, and to drugs or multivalent cations that block Ca^{2+} influx through voltage-gated channels. This current (K_{Ca}) is mediated by large conductance channels, the open probability of which strongly depends both upon $[Ca^{2+}]_i$ and upon membrane potential. K_{Ca} channels (also called maxi-K or BK channels) have a unitary conductance between 70–125 pS in physiological K^+ gradients and between 135 and 270 pS in symmetrical (126–142 mM) KCl solutions (Inoue et al. 1985; Benham et al. 1986; Bregestovski et al. 1988; Sadoshima et al. 1988; Gelband and Hume 1992).

A number of observations suggest that the K_{Ca} channel is involved in setting and modulating the VSMC membrane potential. Bath application of 2–15 mM TEA caused depolarization in a variety of arteries and arterioles, and generation of action potentials (see reviews by Bolton 1979; Hirst and Edwards 1989). It is now known from experiments performed on single VSMCs that TEA, externally applied at millimolar concentrations, is a relatively selective blocker of K_{Ca} channels, apparently having little effect on delayed rectifier and K_{ATP} currents (Benham and Bolton 1986; Okabe et al. 1987; Beech and Bolton 1989b; Gelband and Hume 1992; Russell et al. 1992; Smirnov and Aaronson 1992a). In rabbit cerebral arteries, elevation of luminal pressure caused vasoconstriction and depolarization, which could be prevented by blocking the influx of extracellular Ca^{2+}. Under these conditions TEA, and the highly selective K_{Ca} channel blocker charybdotoxin, caused further depolarization and tension development, which were not seen at low pressure. Brayden and Nelson (1992) therefore argued that K_{Ca} channels served as a negative feedback mechanism to control myogenic tone in these arteries. The possibility that K_{Ca} channels are involved in attenuating the action of vasoconstricting stimuli is supported by analyses of the Ca^{2+} and voltage-dependencies of K_{Ca} channel activation. Channel opening was observed at membrane potentials between -60 and -50 mV when $[Ca^{2+}]_i$ was between 10^{-8} and 10^{-7} M, and open probability increased steeply with membrane depolarization. At $[Ca^{2+}]_i$ higher than 10^{-6} M the channel was mainly in the open state over a wide range of the membrane potentials (Inoue et al. 1985; Benham et al. 1986). Therefore, increases in $[Ca^{2+}]_i$ caused Ca^{2+} entry through voltage-gated Ca channels during cell depolarization, or by Ca^{2+} release from internal stores without depolarization, could lead to activation of K_{Ca} channels.

It is thought that spontaneous and stochastic Ca^{2+} release from submembrane elements of the sarcoplasmic reticulum results in a membrane activity unique to smooth muscle cells, the generation of spontaneous transient outward currents (STOCs) caused by the simultaneous activation of up to 100 K_{Ca} channels (Benham and Bolton 1986; Beech and Bolton 1989b; Hume and Leblanc 1989; Ganitkevich and Isenberg 1990a). It has been shown that at least some of the submembrane elements of the sarcoplasmic reticulum are associated closely enough with the cell membrane so that they may be excised during the formation of inside out patches, and may activate K_{Ca} channels in the patch when stimulated to release Ca^{2+} by inositol trisphosphate or caffeine (Xiong et al. 1992). STOCs were observed at membrane potentials of -50 and -60 mV in rabbit ear artery (Benham and Bolton 1986), guinea-pig coronary artery (Ganitkevich and Isenberg 1990a), and human mesenteric artery (Smirnov and Aaronson 1992a). Recently, spikelike hyperpolarizations (SLHs) of up to -20 mV were described in guinea-pig coronary arterial cells. The SLHs were associated with STOCs which could be measured in these cells under voltage-clamp (Ganitkevich and Isenberg 1990a). Summation of these stochastic SLHs from different cells could cause a net stable hyperpolarization due to the syncytial nature of vascular smooth muscle and thus contribute to the resting potential at least in some arterial cells.

ATP-sensitive K^+ channels, inhibited by intracellular ATP, are considered to be a link between cellular metabolism and electrical events in pancreatic β-cells (for review see Ashcroft and Ashcroft 1990). K_{ATP} channels in vascular smooth muscle are also proposed as the main target for the novel class of vasodilators, called K^+ channel activators or openers, which include pinacidil and cromakalim. These substances cause hyperpolarization of vascular smooth muscle, and thus its relaxation, via activation of these K^+ channels (Weston 1989; Nelson et al. 1990a,b; Kajioka et al. 1991b). The hyperpolarization can be blocked by micromolar concentrations of external Ba^{2+}, phentolamine, and the sulfonylurea compounds glibenclamide and tolbutamide (Standen et al. 1989), which are proposed to be a selective blockers of K_{ATP} channels. A role for K_{ATP} channels in setting the membrane potential was suggested in rabbit pulmonary artery, where the resting potential was -55 mV when the pipette solution contained 1 mM ATP, but shifted to -70 mV when ATP was absent. 1-5 μM glibenclamide in the external solution depolarized these cells in the absence, but not in the presence of 3 mM internal ATP (Clapp and Gurney 1992). K^+ channel openers and depletion of cellular ATP elicit a sustained, voltage-independent current in cells from rabbit pulmonary artery, mesenteric artery, and portal vein, rat portal vein, and human mesenteric artery (Clapp and Gurney 1992; Noack et al. 1992; Russell et al. 1992; Silberberg and van Breeman 1992) which underlies the hyperpolarization.

K^+ channels blocked by ATP, or with the pharmacological profile of K_{ATP} channels, have also been characterized at the single channel level, and a variety of unitary conductance amplitudes have been observed. With a physiological K^+ gradient, conductance values ranged from 25 pS in rabbit mesenteric artery (Standen et al. 1989) to 15 pS in portal vein (Kajioka et al. 1991a); Noack et al. (1992) used noise analysis to estimate a conductance of 17 pS in rat portal vein. Guanine nucleotides (GDP and to a lesser extent GTP) have been shown to be a necessary factor for regulation of these channels in the rabbit portal vein (Kajioka et al. 1991a).

Activation of K_{ATP} channels is possible over a wide range of membrane potentials, and gives rise to a time-independent current, thus in principle making physiological regulation of the resting potential by these channels feasible. It is clear that pharmacological activation of these channels by K^+ channel agonists is capable of hyperpolarizing blood vessels. The question arises, however, as to whether these channels would normally exhibit a significant open probability at the physiological intracellular ATP concentration, which has been measured to be close to 1.5 mM (Post and Jones 1991). Clapp and Gurney (1992) have shown, however, that glibenclamide causes a significant depolarization of rabbit pulmonary arterial cells at an intracellular ATP concentration of 1 mM, and Nelson *et al.* (1990*a*) have demonstrated a similar depolarization to glibenclamide in intact mesenteric artery. K^+ channels sensitive to the extracellular Ca^{2+} concentration, and also to intracellular ATP, were recorded in membrane patches from coronary arterial cells (Wakatsuki *et al.* 1992). These channels were active in cell attached patches held near the resting potential at physiological concentrations of extracellular Ca^{2+}, suggesting that they might contribute to the resting potential. Evidence was also presented, however, to suggest that these channels were completely blocked in excised patches by 1 mM internal ATP. It is possible that the physiological regulation of K_{ATP} channels in smooth muscle involves factors other than ATP, such that they are to some extent open under normal conditions. Observations that the activity of K_{ATP} channels can be modified by agonists suggest strongly that this is the case (see below).

In addition to the major classes of K^+ channels described above, several other types of K^+ currents have been observed in various vascular smooth muscles. A transient K^+ current elicited by depolarization from quite negative potentials was found in rabbit portal vein (Beech and Bolton 1989*a*) and pulmonary artery (Clapp and Gurney 1991*a*), and human mesenteric artery (Smirnov and Aaronson 1992*a*). This current was characterized by the rapidity of both its activation and subsequent decay, and the relatively negative potential range over which it inactivates (half-inactivation potential ranged from -78 mV in rabbit portal vein to -38 mV in human mesenteric artery). The transient outward currents were effectively blocked by 4-aminopyridine and were classified as A-currents (Beech and Bolton 1989*a*) or A-like current (Clapp and Gurney 1991*a*; Smirnov and Aaronson 1992*a*).

An inwardly rectifying K^+ current has been identified in isolated cells from a cerebral artery (Quayle *et al.* 1993), as well as in short segments of submucosal and cerebral arterioles which were voltage-clamped using a microelectrode technique (Hirst and Edwards 1988). The possible physiological role of this current has recently been reviewed (Hirst and Edwards 1989). Both the potential-dependency of current activation, and the amplitude of this current were sensitive to the extracellular K^+ concentration. It was also shown that the inward rectifier current is more prominent in proximal segments of cerebral arterioles than in distal ones (Edwards *et al.* 1988). Therefore, it is possible that this current is absent in larger arteries in contrast to arterioles.

Finally, there have been several reports of Ca^{2+}-sensitive K^+ currents or unitary conductances which appear not to be due to K_{Ca} channels. For example, Wilde and Lee (1989) observed an instantaneous K^+ current in canine coronary artery which was dependent upon internal Ca^{2+} but which was relatively insensitive to TEA. Hume and Leblanc (1989) characterized an instantaneous K^+ current in rabbit portal vein cells which was sensitive to external, but not internal, Ca^{2+}. This current may have corresponded to a voltage-independent, but external Ca^{2+}-activated K^+ channel, designated the K_M channel, earlier recorded in membrane patches from these cells (Inoue et al. 1986). A smaller conductance K^+ channel, K_S, was also found in these cells, which was activated by a rise in $[Ca^{2+}]_i$, and, unlike the K_{Ca} channel, was insensitive to externally applied TEA (Inoue et al. 1985). The ATP-sensitive K^+ channel present in porcine coronary artery cells has also been found to be sensitive to extracellular Ca^{2+} (Miyoshi et al. 1992); the physiological significance of this property is unknown.

CALCIUM CHANNELS

The activation of vascular smooth muscle differs from that of most visceral smooth muscle, and from that of myocardial cells, in that Ca^{2+} influx usually occurs with relatively small membrane depolarizations and in the absence of action potentials, and can be sustained over many seconds or minutes. Controlled depolarization of isolated blood vessels using high K^+ solutions has shown that Ca^{2+} influx and tension development usually occur when the membrane potential becomes more positive than -50 or -45 mV (e.g. Nelson et al. 1988). Arterial smooth muscle cells, which have been of primary interest owing to their central role in regulating the total and local peripheral resistances of the cardiovascular system, are unlikely to become depolarized beyond -20 mV. These factors imply that the behaviour of the Ca^{2+} channels is most interesting in a relatively negative range of membrane potentials, where channel openings are infrequent and therefore most difficult to observe.

Two types of Ca^{2+} channels, high-threshold-activated or L-type and low-threshold-activated or T-type, have been described in a variety of vascular smooth muscle cells (Sturek and Hermsmeyer 1986; Benham et al. 1987; Yatani et al. 1987; Aaronson et al. 1988; Bean 1989; Loirand et al. 1989). The L-type Ca^{2+} channel has been found in all arterial and venous cells studied with the patch-clamp technique. Currents through this class of Ca^{2+} channel are characterized by a relatively slow inactivation, a greater permeability to Ba^{2+} than to Ca^{2+}, a high sensitivity to dihydropyridines (Bean 1989), and a unitary conductance of 15–28 pS in 80–110 mM Ba^{2+} (Benham et al. 1987; Yatani et al. 1987; Ganitkevich and Isenberg 1990b; Nelson et al. 1990b). This conductance was reduced to 5.5 pS in 2 mM Ca^{2+} (Gollasch et al. 1992). A subconductance level approximately half that of the more common conductance has also been observed in several types of VSMC (Worley et al. 1991). In near-physiological Ca^{2+} concentrations (1.5–2.5 mM) an inward Ca^{2+} current(I_{Ca}) through L-type Ca^{2+}

channels could be detected in the voltage range between −50 and −30 mV. The current reached its peak between −10 and +10 mV and had an average maximal amplitude of between 15 and 50 pA in different arteries studied at room temperature (Benham *et al.* 1987; Aaronson *et al.* 1988; Matsuda *et al.* 1990; Smirnov and Aaronson 1992*b*). This may underestimate Ca^{2+} influx *in vivo*, since increasing the temperature resulted in an increase of I_{Ca} peak with a Q_{10} equal to 1.6 in rabbit coronary artery (Matsuda *et al.* 1990), and the current reached an amplitude of up to 500–600 pA at 37 °C in rat portal vein cells (Loirand *et al.* 1989).

The amount of Ca^{2+} entering rabbit ear artery cells during the first 500 msec of a depolarization to −24 mV was estimated to be enough to increase $[Ca^{2+}]_i$ by up to 30 μM at room temperature, assuming that no binding or extrusion of Ca^{2+} occurred (Aaronson *et al.* 1988). Determination of the Ca^{2+} influx which might develop during the smaller and more sustained depolarizations occurring during normal functioning requires, however, consideration of the effects of potential on both activation and inactivation of I_{Ca}. In vascular smooth muscle, as in many other types of tissue, the L-type Ca^{2+} channel possesses two main mechanisms of inactivation. The first type, Ca^{2+}-dependent inactivation, can be caused either by the Ca^{2+} entering the cell during the development of I_{Ca}, or by Ca^{2+} released from cellular stores, and is characterized by a U-shaped dependency of current availability and kinetics on the membrane potential. This type of inactivation can be minimized by the replacement of external Ca^{2+} by Ba^{2+} (Loirand *et al.* 1989; Matsuda *et al.* 1990; Ganitkevich *et al.* 1991; Giannattasio *et al.* 1991; Smirnov and Aaronson 1992*b*). With an increasing duration of the membrane depolarization, or in the presence of Ba^{2+} instead of Ca^{2+}, another component of Ca^{2+} channel inactivation which is potential-dependent becomes more significant (Smirnov and Aaronson 1992*b*). Potential-dependent inactivation tends to occur in a potential range which is somewhat more negative than the range of current activation, although these processes overlap over a voltage range where a sustained I_{Ca}, or 'window current' can exist. Such a sustained I_{Ca} was measured in rabbit portal vein and femoral artery (Imaizumi *et al.* 1989). In human mesenteric arterial cells, I_{Ca} activation and inactivation curves were fitted by Boltzmann functions (Fig. 6.1A), allowing the Ca^{2+} influx mediated by the window current to be calculated to be $2.4 \times 10^5 \, Ca^{2+}$ ions/sec at −60 mV at room temperature (Smirnov and Aaronson 1992*b*). An I_{Ca} of this magnitude would be difficult to resolve experimentally. In rabbit ear artery cells, however, a measurable I_{Ca} was detected positive of −56 mV (Aaronson *et al.* 1988) suggesting that the probability of opening of L-type Ca^{2+} channels near the resting potential may differ greatly between blood vessels. Measurement of single channel activity under near-physiological conditions showed that L-type calcium channel openings could be detected at −50 mV in arterial cells (Ganitkevich and Isenberg 1990*b*; Nelson *et al.* 1990*b*). The steady state open probability was steeply dependent on voltage in this voltage range (e-fold change per 6–8 mV (Nelson *et al.* 1990*b*). A similar voltage-dependency was calculated for the sustained whole-cell I_{Ca} in human mesenteric artery (Smirnov and Aaronson 1992*b*), and is illustrated in Fig. 6.1B. Small changes in the membrane potential

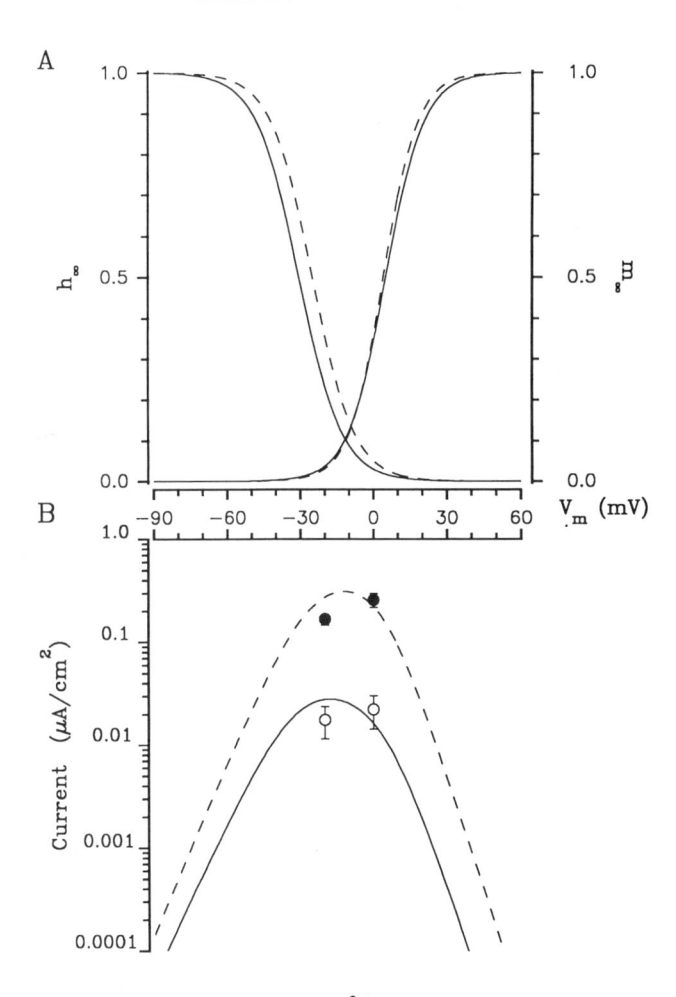

Fig. 6.1 Voltage-sensitivity of sustained Ca^{2+} current in human mesenteric artery cells. (A) Boltzmann functions representing the voltage-dependencies of steady state inactivation (h_∞) and activation (m_∞) in a bathing solution containing 1.5 mM Ca^{2+} (solid line) and 10 mM Ba^{2+} (used to increase the current amplitude, dashed line). (B) The theoretical 'window current' calculated by multiplying the functions for activation and inactivation, on a logarithmic scale, for both 1.5 mM Ca^{2+} and 10 mM Ba^{2+}. The open and solid circles superimposed on these lines represent the actual amplitude of the sustained current measured at two potentials under these conditions. The ordinate represents the absolute value of current density. Note the steep dependency of the current upon membrane potential over its physiological range (−75 to −35 mV). See Smirnov and Aaronson (1992*b*), from which this figure has been slightly modified, for additional discussion.

would therefore be expected to strongly affect Ca^{2+} influx. A recent, elegant characterization of single Ca^{2+} channel activity in rabbit basilar artery demonstrated that unitary Ca^{2+} currents could be detected over the physiologically interesting range potentials at a normal (2 mM) Ca^{2+} concentration (Gollasch *et al.* 1992). The flux through a single open Ca^{2+} channel at -50 mV was calculated to be 7.5×10^5 ions/sec at room temperature. Considering a channel open probability of 0.002 and the presence of 1000 Ca^{2+} channels per cell (Nelson *et al.* 1990*b*), Ca^{2+} influx would be approximately 1.5×10^6 ions/sec at -60 mV. Taking into account a Q_{10} for the Ca^{2+} current of 1.6, and an estimate of the volume of a single cell as 10^{-12} litres, the data from whole cell (Smirnov and Aaronson 1992*b*) and single channel (Gollasch *et al.* 1992) studies suggest that Ca^{2+} influx even at -60 mV is enough to raise $[Ca^{2+}]_i$ by 0.8 to 5 μM/sec if Ca^{2+} buffering and extrusion are neglected. These estimates, although indirect, suggest that L-type Ca^{2+} channels contribute a considerable basal Ca^{2+} influx which can then be modulated by small changes in the membrane potential.

Low-threshold-activated or T-type Ca^{2+} channels in VSMCs are characterized by rapid inactivation, a small (6–8 pS) unitary conductance, and voltage ranges of activation and inactivation which are more negative than those of the L-type channels. A low sensitivity of T-type channels to dihydropyridines has usually been reported (Sturek and Hermsmeyer 1986; Benham *et al.* 1987; Yatani *et al.* 1987; Aaronson *et al.* 1988; Bean 1989; Ganitkevich and Isenberg 1990*b*; Smirnov and Aaronson 1992*b*). Conversely, T-type Ca^{2+} channels which are highly sensitive to dihydropyridines have also been reported in cells from cultured rat aorta (Akaike *et al.* 1989) and portal vein (Loirand *et al.* 1989). The physiological role of T-type Ca^{2+} channels in VSMCs is still unclear. It is possible that they are more important during cell proliferation (Richard *et al.* 1992) and at early stages of postnatal development, as they have been found to be more prominent during this period in rat ileal cells (Smirnov *et al.* 1992). Also T-type channels might take part in the generation of spontaneous activity in venous cells and arterial cells which fire action potentials. In most types of arterial cells, which lack this activity, T-type currents are very small and can be detected only by using elevated Ca^{2+} or Ba^{2+} concentrations. In addition, only L-type Ca^{2+} channels were found in rabbit coronary artery (Matsuda *et al.* 1990) and human cystic artery (Akbarali *et al.* 1992). T-type Ca^{2+} channels are likely to be mostly inactivated at the resting potential under normal conditions, and would certainly become inactivated very rapidly during depolarization; we believe that their physiological role in most VSMCs is at best minor.

VOLTAGE-GATED SODIUM CHANNELS

Potential-dependent Na^+ channels have not been widely observed in VSMCs. A tetrodotoxin-sensitive sodium current has however been described in rat azygous vein (Sturek and Hermsmeyer 1986) and rabbit pulmonary artery (Okabe *et al.*

1988), where it was suggested to take part in the generation of spontaneous activity. It does not appear, however, that all VSMCs which exhibit spontaneous activity have Na^+ channels.

EFFECTS OF AGONISTS

Individual excitatory and inhibitory agonists exert multiple effects upon VSMCs. Information regarding effects of agonists upon membrane transport processes is incomplete, but several common themes appear to be emerging, especially with regard to vasoconstrictors. First, vasoconstrictors directly or indirectly activate depolarizing currents, which are carried by non-specific cation channels and/or Ca^{2+}-activated Cl^- channels. Secondly, vasoconstrictors may inhibit K^+ channels, thus promoting depolarization. Thirdly, such agonists may augment the open probability of voltage-gated Ca^{2+} channels, thereby potentiating Ca^{2+} entry stimulated by depolarization.

RECEPTOR-GATED CHANNELS

The existence in smooth muscle cells of receptor-gated ion channels, responsible for causing both direct Ca^{2+} influx, and depolarization leading to indirect Ca^{2+} influx via voltage-gated Ca^{2+} channels, was proposed by Bolton (1979), and later confirmed for acetylcholine in electrophysiological studies of intestinal smooth muscle cells (Benham et al. 1985). Complementary work by van Breemen and co-workers (van Breemen et al. 1979; Meisheri et al. 1981) focused upon the role of receptor-gated channels in causing a direct $^{45}Ca^{2+}$ influx which could be differentiated from that induced by depolarization, in that it was less sensitive to inhibition by organic Ca^{2+} channel antagonists. A similar scheme for parallel activation of tension development by voltage- and receptor-gated Ca^{2+} channels was also proposed by Shuba (1981).

The conductances gated by noradrenaline in vascular smooth muscle fall into several categories (e.g. Byrne and Large 1988; Amédée et al. 1990; Loirand et al. 1990; Wang and Large 1991). First, noradrenaline (acting on α-adrenoceptors) opens a non-specific cation channel, which appears to be permeable enough to divalent cations to sustain a significant Ca^{2+} influx. Secondly, noradrenaline, by causing a G protein-mediated release of intracellular Ca^{2+} stores, induces the opening of a Ca^{2+}-dependent Cl^- channel. The coexistence of these two mechanisms has been proposed to contribute to the biphasic depolarization induced by exogenous noradrenaline, or stimulation of sympathetic nerve endings, in several types of smooth muscle (Byrne and Large 1988). Thirdly, noradrenaline and other agonists, by increasing $[Ca^{2+}]_i$, causes an outward current in single cells dialysed with a normal K^+ concentration which is due to the opening of K_{Ca} channels (Byrne and Large 1988; Ganitkevich and Isenberg 1990a). The presence of both depolarizing and hyperpolarizing conductances which are apt to be activated by noradrenaline may provide part of the explanation as to why relatively slow contractions caused by sympathetic neurotransmission are not obligatorily linked to membrane depolarization (Bolton and Large 1986).

A number of other vasoconstrictors, including ATP, endothelin, histamine, vasopressin (AVP), angiotensin II, and 5-hydroxytryptamine (5-HT), have also been shown to induce inward currents in VSMCs. ATP elicits the opening of both non-specific cation channels (which are also permeable to Ca^{2+}) and Ca^{2+}-activated Cl^- channels. Evidence has been presented that the cation channel is coupled to the ATP receptor by a pertussis toxin-sensitive G protein (Benham and Tsien 1987; Benham 1989; Xiong et al. 1991). Endothelin activates a Ca^{2+}-dependent Cl^- current in porcine coronary and human mesenteric arterial cells by releasing intracellular Ca^{2+} (Klöckner and Isenberg 1991); histamine has a similar action in rabbit pulmonary artery (Wang and Large 1993). Endothelin may also open a non-selective cation channel (van Renterghem et al. 1988b; Chen and Wagoner 1991). AVP has been observed to open a non-selective (Ca^{2+}-permeable) cation channel in A7r5 cells (van Renterghem et al. 1988a). Angiotensin II and 5-HT have a similar effect in isolated rabbit ear artery cells, which can be mimicked by the inclusion of GTPγS in the patch pipette solution (Hughes and Bolton 1991).

AGONIST MODULATION OF VOLTAGE-GATED Ca^{2+} AND K^+ CHANNELS

As described above, Ca^{2+} influx is increased by vasoconstricting agonists both directly, through receptor-gated cation channels which admit Ca^{2+}, and indirectly, through depolarization and the opening of voltage-gated Ca^{2+} channels. In addition, there is evidence that several agonists may further promote electromechanical coupling by potentiating Ca^{2+} channel activation and/or inhibiting K^+ channel activation, as initially suggested by Shuba (1981).

An enhancement of L-type I_{Ca} activation by noradrenaline has been observed in several types of VSMCs. The precise nature of this effect remains controversial. Benham and Tsien (1988) showed initially that noradrenaline increased the amplitude of I_{Ca} without shifting the voltage-dependence of its activation. This action, however, did not appear to be mediated by either α- or β-adrenoceptors. Loirand et al. (1990) also found a similar action of noradrenaline in rat portal vein cells; this action was however mediated by α-adrenoceptors. Conversely, Droogmans et al. (1987) observed that noradrenaline acted on α-adrenoceptors to *decrease* I_{Ca} in rabbit ear artery cells. It has subsequently been shown that vasoconstrictors can decrease I_{Ca} indirectly by releasing Ca^{2+} from cellular stores. This results in Ca^{2+}-induced current inactivation, and can be eliminated by depleting these Ca^{2+} stores, or by preventing Ca^{2+} release (Pacaud et al. 1987; Klöckner and Isenberg 1991). It is not known whether an effect of this type was responsible for the results of Droogmans et al. (1987).

Nelson et al. (1988.) demonstrated a potentiating effect of noradrenaline on single Ca^{2+} channel activity in rabbit mesenteric artery cells. This was characterized by a hyperpolarizing shift of the activation of this current. The possibility that such a shift in the gating of the Ca^{2+} channel might occur is significant, since this type of response could not only lead to potentiation of the effect of depolarization upon Ca^{2+} influx, but could lead to a rise in Ca^{2+} entry through voltage-gated channels in the absence of any depolarization.

Histamine, angiotensin II, endothelin, and 5-HT have also been demonstrated to increase I_{Ca} or single Ca^{2+} channel open probability in VSMCs (Inoue et al. 1990; Ohya and Sperelakis 1991; Worley et al. 1991; Oike et al. 1992), although conflicting evidence has been presented for endothelin (van Renterghem et al. 1988b; Klöckner and Isenberg 1991). There is general agreement that the enhancement of I_{Ca} by the excitatory agonists involves a pertussis toxin-insensitive G protein, although the details of this process appear to differ between agonists, and/or particular blood vessels. For example, the stimulation of I_{Ca} by noradrenaline can be mimicked by phorbol-12,13-dibutyrate (PDBu; which mimics diacylglycerol in stimulating protein kinase C) in rat portal vein, suggesting that noradrenaline is acting via protein kinase C (Loirand et al. 1990). Conversely, a similar compound, phorbol 12-myristate 13-acetate, diminishes I_{Ca} in the A7r5 line of cultured rat aortic cells (van Renterghem et al. 1988a).

The role in excitation–contraction coupling of agonist-induced enhancement of I_{Ca} remains unclear, although it has been claimed to be of predominant importance, (Nelson et al. 1988, 1990b). Agonists tend to cause only a modest enhancement of the whole-cell I_{Ca}, although a more impressive enhancement of single channel open probability has been measured when recordings are made from cell attached patches, where second messenger systems which may mediate this effect are presumably intact (e.g. Worley et al. 1991). It should also not be overlooked that β-receptor agonists cause a marked increase in I_{Ca} in porcine coronary artery smooth muscle cells (Fukumitsu et al. 1990), even though this artery is relaxed by such agonists. It is likely, however, that agonist-induced enhancement of I_{Ca} is of great importance in the process of contraction for some agonists and vascular beds.

Information regarding the regulation of I_{Ca} by endogenous vascular relaxants is presently sparse. It is worth noting that although β-agonists apparently increase I_{Ca} in porcine coronary artery, they have been shown to either decrease, or not to affect, I_{Ca} in cells of the rabbit ear artery (Droogmans et al. 1987). It is not clear whether this disparity is due to real tissue or species variability, or to differences in methodology. Sodium nitroprusside, which is thought to act ultimately via the production of nitric oxide and an elevation of cGMP, decreases the amplitude of I_{Ca} in rabbit pulmonary artery (Clapp and Gurney 1991b) although this response is likely to be only one factor leading to the vasodilation by this compound.

As discussed above, it is thought that the membrane potential of vascular smooth muscle cells is dependent mainly upon the K^+ conductance of the cell membrane. Excitatory agonists such as noradrenaline and angiotensin II, which act to cause a rise in $[Ca^{2+}]_i$, should therefore cause the opening of K_{Ca} channels, thereby causing a hyperpolarization which would attenuate excitation. In addition, the opening of K_{DR} and A-type K^+ channels might also serve to blunt depolarization. Observations of this type therefore implied that vasoconstrictors might act to suppress outward currents, thereby assuring depolarization. This concept has recently been substantiated by a number of reports that the vasoconstrictors endothelin (Miyoshi et al. 1992), vasopressin (Wakatsuki et al. 1992), and angiotensin II (Miyoshi and Nakaya, 1991) inhibit an ATP-sensitive K^+ channel in porcine coronary artery. In addition, angiotensin II and the stable thromboxane A_2 analogue U46619 have been shown to reduce the open probability of large conductance Ca^{2+}-activated K^+ channels in cells from this artery (Scornik and Toro 1992). These effects may have been mediated by activation of protein kinase C, which has been shown to inhibit K_{Ca} channels in these cells (Minami et al. 1993). Elevation of $[Ca^{2+}]_i$ induced by Ca^{2+} release from the sarcoplasmic reticulum partially suppressed K_{DR} in canine coronary arterial cells, mainly by decreasing the open time of the channel (Gelband et al. 1993).

Several endogenous vasodilators, which are thought to act, at least in part, by hyperpolarizing vascular smooth muscle, appear to do so by opening K^+ channels. The β-adrenoceptor agonist isoprenaline increased the open probability of large conductance K_{Ca} channels in cultured aortic cells. It was suggested that this response, which could explain the ability of β-agonists to hyperpolarize vascular smooth muscle, was due to a cAMP-dependent protein kinase-mediated phosphorylation of the channel (Sadoshima et al. 1988). The hyperpolarization and associated relaxation of rabbit mesenteric artery by the potent vasodilator CGRP was reversed by glibenclamide; CGRP also dramatically increased the open probability of a glibenclamide-sensitive K^+ channel (Nelson et al. 1990a). Hyperpolarizations of rabbit middle cerebral artery to VIP, and to acetylcholine (presumably acting via an endothelium-derived factor) are also reversed by glibenclamide (Standen et al. 1989). Conversely, nitroglycerine, a source of nitric oxide, activated K_{Ca} channels in porcine coronary arterial cells, a response that was mimicked by cGMP (Fujino et al. 1991). Epoxyeicosatrienoic acids, vasodilating metabolites of arachadonic acid, increased the open probability of a 98 pS K^+ channel in feline cerebral arteries. The corresponding arterial hyperpolarization was reduced by TEA, again suggesting the involvement of K_{Ca} channels (Gebremedhin et al. 1992). It therefore appears likely that activation of both K_{Ca} and K_{ATP} channels plays an important role in the action of a number of endogenous vasodilators.

SUMMARY

A simplified scheme relating ion channel activity to the control of VSMC tone which reflects the recent observations described above is presented in Fig. 6.2. At least four mechanisms exist which should promote vasoconstrictor-induced depolarization: the activation of non-specific cation (NSC) and chloride channels, and the inhibition of K_{Ca} and K_{ATP} channels. Depolarization would then lead to

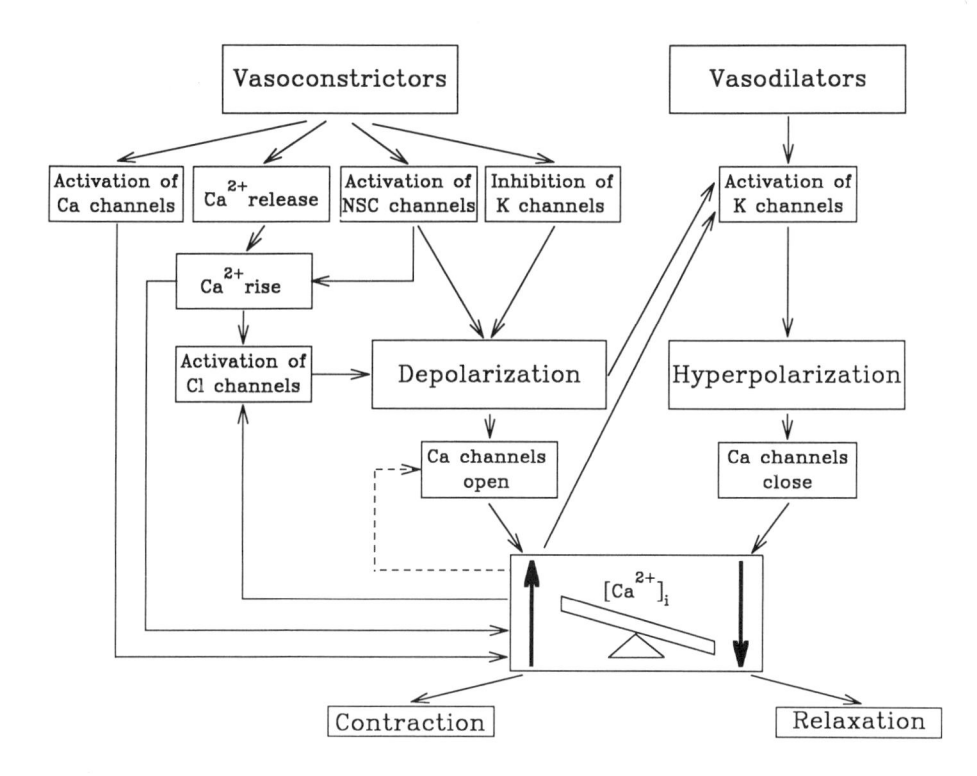

Fig. 6.2 Schematic representation of the involvement of ion channels in the actions of vasoactive agonists. Solid lines represent stimulation and dashed line represents inhibition. See text for discussion.

an increased opening probability of voltage-gated Ca^{2+} channels, and consequently a rise in $[Ca^{2+}]_i$ and tension development. In addition, the permeation of Ca^{2+} through NSC channels, and a direct (or G protein-mediated) effect of agonists to increase the opening probability of voltage-gated Ca^{2+} channels would allow Ca^{2+} influx without depolarization. Putative Ca^{2+} channels which open as a result of depletion of intracellular Ca^{2+} stores (Missiaen et al. 1990) might also contribute a component of Ca^{2+} influx which would not require depolarization (not shown).

Several mechanisms exist which would allow the rise in $[Ca^{2+}]_i$ during activation to be self-regulating. The most important of these are likely to be the negative feedback pathways represented by the opening of K_{Ca} channels and the inactivation of voltage-gated Ca^{2+} channels. The activation of Ca^{2+}-sensitive Cl^- channels, and the suppression of K_{DR} channel activity, by an increase in $[Ca^{2+}]_i$ represent possible positive feedback pathways.

Finally, vasodilators such as CGRP and endothelium-derived hyperpolarizing factor (Garland and McPherson 1992) may act as endogenous K^+ channel agonists, thereby causing membrane hyperpolarization and the closing of voltage-gated Ca^{2+} channels.

Determination of the relative importance of these, and other as yet unknown, mechanisms in the overall actions of individual vasoconstricting and vasodilating agonists is an important future goal, as is an elucidation of the differences and similarities in channel distributions in various types of blood vessels. The identification and sequencing of ion channels in vascular smooth muscle cells which is now in progress seems likely to present an entirely new perspective from which to attack these and other complex questions dealing with how multiple mechanisms are integrated in vascular cells.

REFERENCES

Aaronson, P. I., Bolton, T. B., Lang, R. J., and MacKenzie, I. (1988). Calcium currents in single isolated smooth muscle cells from the rabbit ear artery in normal-calcium and high-barium solutions. *J. Physiol.*, **405**, 57-75.

Akaike, N., Kanaide, H., Kuga, T., Nakamura, M., Sadoshima, J., and Tomoike, H. (1989). Low-voltage-activated calcium current in rat aorta smooth muscle cells in primary culrure. *J. Physiol.*, **416**, 141-60.

Akbarali, H. I., Wyse, D. G., and Giles, W. R. (1992). Ionic currents in single cells from human cystic artery. *Circ. Res.*, **70**, 536-45.

Amédée, T., Benham, C. D., Bolton, T. B., Byrne, N. G., and Large, W. A. (1990). Potassium, chloride and non-selective cation conductances opened by noradrenaline in rabbit ear artery cells. *J. Physiol.*, **423**, 551-68.

Ashcroft, S. J. H. and Ashcroft, F. M. (1990). Properties and functions of ATP-sensistive K-channels. *Cell Signal*, **2**, 197-214.

Bean, B. P. (1989). Classes of calcium channels in vertebrate cells. *Annu. Rev. Physiol.*, **51**, 367-84.

Beech, D. J. and Bolton, T. B. (1989a). A voltage-dependent outward current with fast kinetics in single smooth muscle cells isolated from rabbit portal vein. *J. Physiol.*, **412**, 397-414.

Beech, D. J. and Bolton, T. B. (1989b). Two components of potassium current activated by depolarization of single smooth muscle cells from the rabbit portal vein. *J. Physiol.*, **418**, 293-309.

Benham, C. D. (1989). ATP-activated channels gate calcium entry in single smooth muscle cells dissociated from rabbit ear artery. *J. Physiol.*, **419**, 689-701.

Benham, C. D. and Bolton, T. B. (1986). Spontaneous transient outward currents in single visceral and vascular smooth muscle cells of the rabbit. *J. Physiol.*, **381**, 385-406.

Benham, C. D. and Tsien, R. W. (1987). ATP receptor-operated channels permeable to calcium in arterial smooth muscle. *Nature*, **328**, 275-8.

Benham, C. D. and Tsien, R. W. (1988). Noradrenaline modulation of calcium channels in single smooth muscle cells from rabbit ear artery. *J. Physiol.*, **404**, 767-84.

Benham, C. D., Bolton, T. B., and Lang, R. J. (1985). Acetylcholine activates an inward current in single mammalian smooth muscle cells. *Nature*, **316**, 345-7.

Benham, C. D., Bolton, T. B., Lang, R. J., and Takewaki, T. (1986). Calcium-activated potassium channels in single smooth muscle cells of rabbit jejunum and guinea-pig mesenteric artery. *J. Physiol.*, **371**, 45-67.

Benham, C. D., Hess, P., and Tsien, R. W. (1987). Two types of calcium channels in single smooth muscle cells from rabbit ear artery studied with whole-cell and single-channel recordings. *Circ. Res.*, **61 (suppl. 1)**, 10-16.

Bolton, T. B. (1979). Mechanisms of action of transmitters and other substances on smooth muscle. *Physiol. Rev.*, **59**, 606-718.

Bolton, T. B. and Large, W. A. (1986). Are junction potentials essential? Dual mechanism of smooth muscle cell activation by transmitter released from autonomic nerves. *Q. J. Exp. Physiol.*, **71**, 1-28.

Bonnet, P., Rusch, N. S., and Harder, D. R. (1991). Characterization of an outward K^+ current in freshly dispersed cerebral arterial muscle cells. *Pflügers Arch.*, **418**, 292-6.

Brayden, J. E. and Nelson, M. T. (1992). Regulation of arterial tone by activation of calcium-dependent potassium channels. *Science*, **256**, 532-5.

Bregestovski, P. D., Printseva, O. Yu., Serebryakov, V., Stinnakre, J., Turmin, A., and Zamoyski, V. (1988). Comparison of Ca^{2+}-dependent K^+ channels in the membrane of smooth muscle cells isolated from adult and foetal human aorta. *Pflügers Arch.*, **413**, 8-13.

Byrne, N. G. and Large, W. A. (1988). Mechanism of action of α-adrenoceptor activation in single cells freshly dissociated from the rabbit portal vein. *Br. J. Pharmacol.*, **94**, 475-82.

Chen, C. and Wagoner, P. K. (1991). Endothelin induces a nonselective cation current in vascular smooth muscle cells. *Circ. Res.*, **69**, 447-54.

Clapp, L. H. and Gurney, A. M. (1991a). Outward currents in rabbit pulmonary artery cells dissociated with a new technique. *Exp. Physiol.*, **76**, 677-93.

Clapp, L. H. and Gurney, A. M. (1991b). Modulation of calcium movements by nitroprusside in isolated vascular smooth muscle cells. *Pflügers Arch.*, **418**, 462-70.

Clapp, L. H. and Gurney, A. M. (1992). ATP-sensitive K^+ channels regulate resting potential of pulmonary arterial smooth muscle cells. *Am. J. Physiol.*, **262**, H916-20.

Droogmans, G., Declerck, I., and Casteels, R. (1987). Effect of adrenergic agonists on Ca^{2+}-channel currents in single vascular smooth muscle cells. *Pflügers Arch.*, **409**, 7-12.

Edwards, F. R., Hirst, G. D., and Silverberg, G. D. (1988). Inward rectification in rat cerebral arterioles; involvement of potassium ions in autoregulation. *J. Physiol.*, **404**, 455-66.

Fujino, K., Nakaya, S., Wakatsuki, T., Miyoshi, Y., Nakaya, Y., Mori H., *et al.* (1991). Effects of nitroglycerin on ATP-induced Ca(++)-mobilization, Ca(++)-activated K channels and contraction of cultured smooth muscle cells of porcine coronary artery. *J. Pharmacol. Exp. Ther.*, **256(1)**, 371-7.

Fukumitsu, T., Hayashi, H., Tokuno, H., and Tomita, T. (1990). Increase in calcium channel current by β-adrenoceptor agonists in single smooth muscle cells isolated from porcine coronary artery. *Br. J. Pharmacol.*, **100**, 593-9.

Ganitkevich, V. and Isenberg, G. (1990a). Isolated guinea-pig coronary smooth muscle cells. Acetylcholine induces hyperpolarization due to sarcoplasmic reticulum calcium release activating tassium channels. *Circ. Res.*, **67**, 525-8.

Ganitkevich, V. Ya. and Isenberg, G. (1990b). Contribution of two types of calcium channels to membrane conductance of single myocytes from guinea-pig coronary artery. *J. Physiol.*, **426**, 19-42.

Ganitkevich, V. Ya., Shuba, M. F., and Smirnov, S. V. (1991). Inactivation of calcium channels in single vascular and visceral smooth muscle cells of the guinea-pig. *Gen. Physiol. Biophys.*, **10**, 137-61.

Garland, C. J. and McPherson, G. A. (1992). Evidence that nitric oxide does not mediate the hyperpolarization and relaxation to acetylcholine in the rat small mesenteric artery. *Br. J. Pharmacol.*, **105**, 429-35.

Gebremedhin, D., Ma, Y. H., Falck, J. R., Roman, R. J., VanRollins, M., and Harder D. R. (1992). Mechanism of action of cerebral epoxyeicosatrienoic acids on cerebral arterial smooth muscle. *Am. J. Physiol.*, **263**, H519-25.

Gelband, C. H. and Hume, J. R. (1992). Ionic currents in single smooth muscle cells of the canine renal artery. *Circ. Res.*, **71**, 745-58.

Gelband, C. H., Ishikawa, T., Post, J. M., Keef, K. D., and Hume, J. R. (1993). Intracellular divalent cations block smooth muscle K⁺ channels. *Circ. Res.*, **73**, 24-34.

Gelband, C. H., Silberberg, S. D., Groschner, K., and van Breemen, C. (1990). ATP inhibits smooth muscle Ca²⁺-activated K⁺ channels. *Proc. Royal Soc. (Lond.) Series B*, **242**, 23-8.

Giannattasio, B., Jones, S. W., and Scarpa, A. (1991). Calcium currents in the A7r5 smooth muscle-derived cell line. Calcium-dependent and voltage-dependent inactivation. *J. Gen. Physiol.*, **98**, 987-1003.

Gollasch, M., Hescheler, J., Quayle, J. M., Patlak, J. B., and Nelson, M. T. (1992). Single calcium channel currents of arterial smooth muscle at physiological calcium concentrations. *Am. J. Physiol.*, **263**, C948-52.

Hara, Y., Kitamura, K., and Kuriyama, H. (1980). Actions of 4-aminopyridine on vascular smooth muscle tissues of the guinea-pig. *Br. J. Pharmacol.*, **68**, 99-106.

Harder, D. R. (1984). Pressure-dependent membrane depolarization in cat middle cerebral artery. *Circ. Res.*, **55**, 197-202.

Hirst, G. D. and Edwards, F. R. (1989). Sympathetic neuroeffector transmission in arteries and arterioles. *Physiol. Rev.*, **69**, 546-604.

Hughes, A. D. and Bolton, T. B. (1991). Receptor-operated conductances in isolated rabbit ear artery cells. In *Resistance arteries, structure and function* (ed. M. J. Mulvany, C. Aalkjaer, A. M. Heagerty, N. C. B. Nyborg, and S. Strandgaard, pp. 115-20. Excerpta Medica, Amsterdam, New York, Oxford.

Hume, J. R. and Leblanc, N. (1989). Macroscopic K⁺ currents in single smooth muscle cells of the rabbit portal vein. *J. Physiol.*, **413**, 49-73.

Imaizumi, Y., Muraki, K., Takeda, M., and Watanabe, M. (1989). Measurement and simulation of noninactivating Ca current in smooth muscle cells. *Am. J. Physiol.*, **256**, C880-5.

Inoue, R., Kitamura, K., and Kuriyama, H. (1985). Two Ca-dependent K-channels classified by the application of tetraethylammonium distribute to smooth muscle membranes of the rabbit portal vein. *Pflügers Arch.* **405**, 173-9.

Inoue, R., Okabe, K., Kitamura, K., and Kuriyama, H. (1986). A newly identified Ca²⁺ dependent K⁺ channel in the smooth muscle membrane of single cells dispersed from the rabbit portal vein. *Pflügers Arch.*, **406**, 138-43.

Inoue, I., Nakaya, Y., Nakaya, S., and Mori, H. (1989). Extracellular Ca²⁺-activated K channel in coronary artery smooth muscle cells and its role in vasodilation. *FEBS Lett.*, **255**, 281-4.

Inoue, Y., Oike, M., Nakao, K., Kitamura, K., and Kuriyama, H. (1990). Endothelin augments unitary calcium channel currents on the smooth muscle cell membrane of guinea-pig portal vein. *J. Physiol.*, **423**, 171-91.

Kajioka, S., Kitamura, K., and Kuriyama, H. (1991a). Guanosine diphosphate activates an adenosine 5'-triphosphate-sensitive K⁺ channel in the rabbit portal vein. *J. Physiol.*, **444**, 397-418.

Kajioka, S., Nakashima, M., Kitamura, K., and Kuriyama, H. (1991b). Mechanisms of vasodilatation induced by potassium-channel activators. *Clin. Sci.*, **81**, 129-39.

Klöckner, U. and Isenberg, G. (1991). Endothelin depolarizes myocytes from porcine coronary and human mesenteric arteries through a Ca-activated chloride current. *Pflügers Arch.*, **418**, 168-75.

Loirand, G., Mironneau, C., Mironneau, J., and Pacaud, P. (1989). Two types of calcium currents in single smooth muscle cells from rat portal vein. *J. Physiol.*, **412**, 333-49.

Loirand, G., Pacaud, P., Mironneau, C., and Mironneau, J. (1990). GTP-binding proteins mediate noradrenaline effects on calcium and chloride currents in rat portal vein myocytes. *J. Physiol.*, **428**, 517-29.

Matsuda, J. J., Volk, K. A., and Shibata, E. F. (1990). Calcium currents in isolated rabbit coronary arterial smooth muscle myocytes. *J. Physiol.*, **427**, 657–80.

Meisheri, K. D., Hwang, O., and van Breemen, C. (1981). Evidence for two separate Ca^{2+} pathways in smooth muscle plasmalemma. *J. Memb. Biol.*, **59**, 19–25.

Minami, K. Fukuzawa, K., and Nakaya, Y. (1993). Protein kinase C inhibits the Ca(2+)-activated K+ channel of cultured porcine coronary artery smooth muscle cells. *Biochem. Biophys. Res. Commun.*, **190(1)**, 263–9.

Missiaen, L., Declerck, I., Droogmans, G., Plessers, L., De Smedt, H., Raeymaekers, L. et al. (1990). Agonist-dependent Ca^{2+} and Mn^{2+} entry dependent on state of filling of Ca^{2+} stores in aortic smooth muscle cells of the rat. *J. Physiol.*, **427**, 171–86.

Miyoshi, Y. and Nakaya, Y. (1991). Angiotensin II blocks ATP-sensitive K+ channels in porcine coronary artery smooth muscle cells. *Biochem. Biophys. Res. Commun.*, **181(2)**, 700–6.

Miyoshi, Y., Nakaya, Y., Wakatsuki, T., Nakaya, S., Fujino, K., Saito, et al. (1992). Endothelin blocks ATP-sensitive K^+ channels and depolarizes smooth muscle cells of porcine coronary artery. *Circ. Res.*, **70**, 612–16.

Nelson, M. T., Standen, N. B., Brayden, J. E., and Worley, J. F. III. (1988). Noradrenaline contracts arteries by activating voltage-dependent calcium channels. *Nature*, **336**, 382–5.

Nelson, M. T., Huang, Y., Brayden, J. E., Hescheler, J., and Standen, N. B. (1990a). Arterial dilations in response to calcitonin gene-related peptide involve activation of K^+ channels. *Nature*, **344**, 770–3.

Nelson, M. T., Patlak, J. B., Worley, J. F., and Standen, N. B. (1990b). Calcium channels, potassium channels, and voltage dependence of arterial smooth muscle tone. *Am. J. Physiol.*, **259**, C3–18.

Noack, T., Deitmer, P., Edwards, G., and Weston, A. H. (1992). Characterization of potassium currents modulated by BRL 38227 in rat portal vein. *Br. J. Pharmacol.*, **106**, 717–26.

Ohya, Y. and Sperelakis, N. (1991). Involvement of a GTP-binding protein in stimulating action of angiotensin II on calcium channels in vascular smooth muscle cells. *Circ. Res.*, **68**, 763–71.

Oike, M., Kitamura, K., and Kuriyama, H. (1992). Histamine H₃-receptor activation augments voltage-dependent Ca^{2+} current via GTP hydrolysis in rabbit saphenous artery. *J. Physiol.*, **448**, 133–52.

Okabe, K., Kitamura, K., and Kuriyama, H. (1987). Features of 4-aminopyridine sensitive outward current observed in single smooth muscle cells from the rabbit pulmonary artery. *Pflügers Arch.*, **409**, 561–8.

Okabe, K., Kitamura, K., and Kuriyama, H. (1988). The existence of a highly tetrodotoxin sensitive Na channel in freshly dispersed smooth muscle cells of the rabbit main pulmonary artery. *Pflügers Arch.*, **411**, 423–8.

Pacaud, P., Loirand, G., Mironneau, C., and Mironneau, J. (1987). Opposing effects of noradrenaline on the two classes of voltage-dependent calcium channels of single vascular smooth muscle cells in short-term primary culture. *Pflügers Arch.*, **410**, 557–9.

Pavenstädt, H., Lindeman, S., Lindeman, V., Spath, M., Kunzelmann, K., and Greger, R. (1991). Potassium conductance of smooth muscle cells from rabbit aorta in primary culture. *Pflugers Arch.*, **419**, 57–68.

Post, J. M. and Jones, A. W. (1991). Stimulation of arterial ⁴²K efflux by ATP depletion and cromakalim is antagonized by glyburide. *Am. J. Physiol.*, **260**, H848–54.

Quayle, J. M., McCarron, J. G., Brayden, J. E., and Nelson, M. T. (1993). Inward rectifier K^+ currents in smooth muscle cells from rat resistance-sized cerebral arteries. *Am. J. Physiol.*, **265**, C1363–70.

Richard, S., Neveu, D., Carnac, G., Bodin, P., Travo, P., and Nargeot, J. (1992). Differential expression of voltage-gated Ca^{2+}-currents in cultivated aortic myocytes. *Biochim. Biophys. Acta.*, **1160**, 95–104.

Rudy, B. (1988). Diversity and ubiquity of K channels. *Neuroscience*, **25**, 729–49.
Russell, S. N., Smirnov, S. V., and Aaronson, P. I. (1992). Effects of BRL 38227 on potassium currents in smooth muscle cells isolated from rabbit portal vein and human mesenteric artery. *Br. J. Pharmacol.*, **105**, 549–56.
Sadoshima, J., Akaike, N., Kanaide, H., and Nakamura, M. (1988). Cyclic AMP modulates Ca-activated K channel in cultured smooth muscle cells of rat aortas. *Am. J. Physiol.*, **255**, H754–9.
Scornik, F. S. and Toro, L. (1992). U46619, a thromboxane A_2 agonist, inhibits K_{Ca} channel activity from pig coronary artery. *Am. J. Physiol.*, **262**, C708–13.
Shuba, M. F. (1981). The transport mechanisms by which contraction activating extracellular Ca^{2+} ions enter smooth muscle cells. In *Advances in physiological sciences Vol. 5, Molecular and cellular aspects of muscle function* (ed. E. Varga, A. Köver, T. Kovacs, and L. Kovacs), pp. 83–94. Pergamon Press, Akadémiai Kiadó, Budapest.
Silberberg, S. D. and van Breemen, C. (1992). A potassium current activated by lemakalim and metabolic inhibition in rabbit mesenteric artery. *Pflügers Arch.*, **420**, 118–20.
Smirnov, S. V. and Aaronson, P. I. (1992a). Ca^{2+}-activated and voltage-gated K^+ currents in smooth muscle cells isolated from human mesenteric arteries. *J. Physiol.*, **457**, 431–54.
Smirnov, S. V. and Aaronson, P. I. (1992b). Ca^{2+} currents in single myocytes from human mesenteric arteries: evidence for a physiological role of L-type channels. *J. Physiol.*, **457**, 455–75.
Smirnov, S. V., Zholos, A. V., and Shuba, M. F. (1992). Potential-dependent inward currents in single isolated smooth muscle cells of the rat ileum. *J. Physiol.*, **454**, 549–71.
Standen, N. B., Quayle, J. M., Davies, N. W., Brayden, J. E., Huang, Y., and Nelson, M. T. (1989). Hyperpolarizing vasodilators activate ATP-sensitive K^+ channels in arterial smooth muscle. *Science*, **245**, 177–80.
Sturek, M. and Hermsmeyer, K. (1986). Calcium and sodium channels in spontaneously contracting vascular muscle cells. *Science*, **233**, 475–8.
Toro, L., Vaca, L., and Stefani, E. (1991). Calcium-activated potassium channels from coronary smooth muscle reconstituted in lipid bilayers. *Am. J. Physiol.*, **260**, H1779–89.
Van Breemen, C., Aaronson, P., and Loutzenhiser, R. (1979). Na-Ca interactions in mammalian smooth muscle. *Pharma. Rev.*, **30**, 167–208.
Van Renterghem, C., Romey, G., and Lazdunski, M. (1988a). Vasopressin modulates the spontaneous electrical activity in aortic cells (line A7r5) by acting on three different types of ionic channels. *Proc. Natl. Acad. Sci. USA*, **85**, 9365–9.
Van Renterghem, C., Vigne, P., Barhanin, J., Schmid-Alliana, A., Frelin, C., and Lazdunski, M. (1988b). Molecular mechanism of action of the vasoconstrictor peptide endothelin. *Biochem. Biophys. Res. Commun.*, **157**, 977–85.
Volk, K. A. and Shibata, E. F. (1993). Single delayed rectifier potassium channels from rabbit coronary artery myocytes. *Am. J. Physiol.*, **264**, H1146–53.
Wakatsuki, T., Nakaya, Y., and Inoue, I. (1992). Vasopressin modulates K^+-channel activities of cultured smooth muscle cells from porcine coronary artery. *Am. J. Physiol.*, **263**, H491–6.
Wang, Q. and Large, W. A. (1991). Noradrenaline-evoked cation conductance recorded with the nystatin whole-cell method in rabbit portal vein cells. *J. Physiol.*, **435**, 21–39.
Wang, Q. and Large, W. A. (1993). Action of histamine on single smooth muscle cells dispersed from the rabbit pulmonary artery. *J. Physiol.*, **468**, 125–39.
Weston, A. H. (1989). Smooth muscle K^+ channel openers; their pharmacology and clinical potential. *Pflügers Arch.*, **414 (Suppl. 1)**, S99–105.
Wilde, D. W. and Lee, K. S. (1989). Outward potassium currents in freshly isolated smooth muscle cell of dog coronary arteries. *Circ. Res.*, **65**, 1718–34.

Worley, J. F., Quayle, J. M., Standen, N. B., and Nelson, M. T. (1991). Regulation of single calcium channels in cerebral arteries by voltage, serotonin, and dihydropyridines. *Am. J. Physiol.*, **261**, H1951-60.

Xiong, Z., Kitamura, K., and Kuriyama, H. (1991). ATP activates cationic currents and modulates the calcium current through GTP-binding protein in rabbit portal vein. *J. Physiol.*, **440**, 143-65.

Xiong, Z., Kitamura, K., and Kuriyama, H. (1992). Evidence for contribution of Ca^{2+} storage sites on unitary K^+ channel currents in inside-out membrane of rabbit portal vein. *Pflügers Arch.*, **420**, 112-14.

Yatani, A., Seidel, C. L., Allen, J., and Brown, A. M. (1987). Whole-cell and single-channel calcium currents of isolated smooth muscle cells from saphenous vein. *Circ. Res.*, **60**, 523-33.

Yuan, X.-J., Goldman, W. F., Tod, M. L., Rubin, L. J., and Blaustein, M. P. (1993a). Ionic currents in rat pulmonary and mesenteric arterial myocytes in primary culture and subculture. *Am. J. Physiol.*, **264**, L107-15.

Yuan, X.-J., Goldman, W. F., Tod, M. L., Rubin, L. J., and Blaustein, M. P. (1993b). Hypoxia reduces potassium currents in cultured rat pulmonary but not mesenteric arterial myocytes. *Am. J. Physiol.*, **264**, L116-23.

7. Cell signalling pathways involved in the regulation of vascular smooth muscle contraction and relaxation

Kevin Malarkey, Dorothy Aidulis, Christopher M. Belham, Anne Graham, Angela McLees, Andrew Paul, and Robin Plevin

INTRODUCTION

A vast array of agonists regulate smooth muscle function by interacting with specific receptors located upon the cell membrane. This results in the activation of intracellular signalling pathways and the formation of a number of key second messengers. In this chapter we will review recent studies implicating a role for protein kinase C (PKC) and tyrosine kinase pathways in regulating smooth muscle contraction and the involvement of cyclic nucleotide generating systems in relaxation.

THE ROLE OF PHOSPHOLIPID HYDROLYSIS IN THE REGULATION OF SMOOTH MUSCLE CONTRACTION

Agonist-stimulated phosphoinositide hydrolysis in vascular smooth muscle cells

The seminal work of Berridge, Irvine, Michell and co-workers in the late 70s and early 80s identified the hydrolysis of inositol-containing phospholipids as a universal signalling pathway activated in response to calcium mobilizing agonists (Berridge and Irvine 1989). In vascular smooth muscle cells this pathway is activated in response to vasoconstrictors such as angiotensin II (AII), endothelin-1 (ET-1), and vasopressin, and growth factors such as platelet-derived growth factor (PDGF) (Doyle and Ruegg 1985; Araki *et al.* 1989; Block *et al.* 1989; Lyall *et al.* 1992). Following receptor activation, phosphatidylinositol 4,5-bisphosphate (PtdIns $(4,5)P_2$) is hydrolysed by a phosphoinositide-specific phospholipase C (PLC) to generate two second messengers, inositol 1,4,5-trisphosphate ($InsP_3$) and *sn*-1,2 diacylglycerol (DAG) (see Fig. 7.1).

In the case of vasoconstrictors, whose receptors comprise seven transmembrane spanning domains, stimulation of PLC by the agonist receptor complex is transduced via the activation of a heterotrimeric guanine nucleotide binding protein (G protein). This has been demonstrated in a number of cell systems, including

Cell signalling pathways

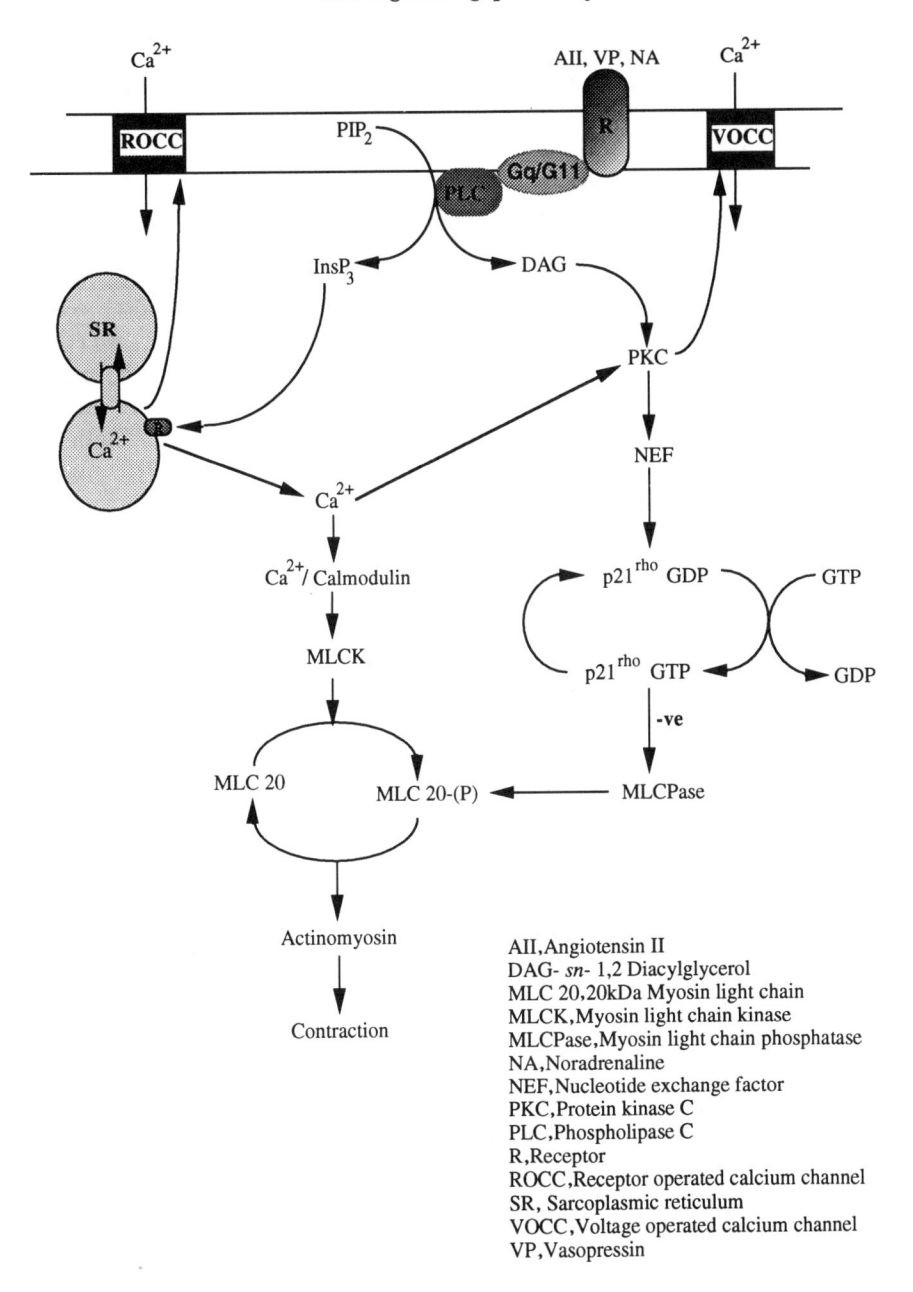

Fig. 7.1 Inositol lipid hydrolysis and calcium mobilization in the initiation of vascular smooth muscle contraction.

smooth muscle cells, where it was found that non-hydrolysable analogues of GTP potentiated agonist-stimulated inositol phosphate production (Huang and Ives 1989). Recent studies have implicated the involvement of a pertussis toxin-insensitive G protein, Gq/G11, in InsP$_3$ formation (Strathmann and Simon 1990) as antibodies against the α-subunit of this protein have been demonstrated to inhibit agonist-stimulated inositol phosphate formation in neuronal and hepatocyte cell membranes (Gutowski et al. 1991). To date several PLC isoforms have been identified in mammalian tissues (Meldrum et al. 1991), but reconstitution experiments indicate that PLCβ1 is preferentially activated by α-Gq/G11 *in vitro* (Smrcka et al. 1991). In vascular smooth muscle cells Gq/G11 is expressed (Clark et al. 1992), however, PLCβ1 is absent (Marrero et al. 1994), suggesting the involvement of another PLC isoform in the hydrolysis of PtdIns(4,5)P$_2$ in this system.

In addition for a number of agonists, in particular thrombin, formation of InsP$_3$ is reduced by pertussis toxin pre-treatment (Huang and Ives 1989) suggesting the involvement of a G protein which is susceptible to ADP-ribosylation. Recently, it has been shown that $\beta\gamma$ subunits of pertussis toxin-sensitive G proteins can activate other isoforms of PLC such as PLCβ2 (Katz et al. 1992), although it remains to be determined if this mechanism of activation of PLC is a universal one. As vasoconstrictor-stimulated InsP$_3$ formation is also dependent upon extracellular Ca^{2+} (Block et al. 1989; Morimoto et al. 1990; Dickenson et al. 1993) these results suggest that indirect routes may also be involved in the activation of PLC in smooth muscle.

InsP$_3$-induced intracellular calcium mobilization in vascular smooth muscle cells

It is generally accepted that InsP$_3$ stimulates the release of calcium from intracellular calcium stores through interaction with specific InsP$_3$ receptors located upon the sarcoplasmic reticulum (Berridge 1993). After release in response to InsP$_3$, Ca^{2+} binds to calmodulin and this complex activates myosin light chain kinase (MLCK). MLCK phosphorylates the 20 kDa fragment of myosin light chain (MLC$_{20}$) which in turn stimulates actin/myosin ATPase, actin/myosin cross-bridging, and the development of force (Somlyo and Himpens 1989) (see Fig. 7.1). In permeabilized vascular smooth muscle preparations, exogenous InsP$_3$ is able to stimulate intracellular calcium release and induce contraction (Somlyo et al. 1985; Hashimoto et al. 1986; Seager et al. 1994), implicating a central role for the phosphoinositide-PLC catalytic pathway in pharmacomechanical coupling.

The release of calcium from intracellular stores by InsP$_3$ may also be influenced by a number of regulatory mechanisms (Berridge 1993). A large body of evidence suggests that not all intracellular stores of Ca^{2+} are sensitive to InsP$_3$ yet are still involved in intracellular Ca^{2+} mobilization in response to agonist stimulation. In smooth muscle there is evidence to suggest the presence of interconnected Ca^{2+} stores, one of which is InsP$_3$-sensitive and a second which is InsP$_3$-insensitive (Wong and Klassen 1993; Berman et al. 1994), implicated by the differing sensitivities of intracellular Ca^{2+} release to $InsP_3$, caffeine and ryanodine (Kanaide *et al.* 1987; Iino *et al.* 1988). However, the degree of overlap can be considerable and a single pool may be present in some cells (Blatter and Weir 1992). Release of Ca^{2+} from the $InsP_3$-sensitive store is thought to promote movement of calcium from the $InsP_3$-insensitive store by an undefined mechanism possibly involving a pertussis toxin-sensitive G protein (Neylon *et al.* 1992). Ca^{2+} released from $InsP_3$-sensitive stores has both positive and negative feedback effects on its own release through altering the affinity of the $InsP_3$ receptor (Iino 1990). These mechanisms acting in concert give rise to calcium oscillations inside the cells with a defined spatio-temporal pattern (Simpson and Ashley 1989; Blatter and Weir 1992). However, it should be noted that individual smooth muscle cells may exhibit differences in the types of Ca^{2+} stores present and regulatory mechanisms involved in the release process (Shin *et al.* 1991; see also Chapter 3). Therefore, each smooth muscle preparation may contain different elements of the pathways described above.

The emptying of calcium from the $InsP_3$-sensitive Ca^{2+} pool has also been proposed to promote calcium influx from extracellular sources thereby sustaining contraction (Putney 1986). In smooth muscle, this process appears to be both tissue- and agonist-dependent (Xuan *et al.* 1992; Noguera and D'Ocon 1993). The mechanism by which influx is initiated is unknown, however, inositol-(1,3,4,5)-tetrakisphosphate ($InsP_4$), a small molecular weight G protein and a peptide influx factor have been implicated (Fasolato *et al.* 1994). It is also unclear in smooth muscle which type of channel regulates calcium influx (Xuan *et al.* 1992; Noguera and D'Ocon 1993; Fasolato *et al.* 1994) and if calcium enters the cytosol directly or is sequestered in the $InsP_3$-sensitive store before release into the cytoplasm.

A role for Ca^{2+} influx through the activation of specific plasma membrane Ca^{2+} channels in the initiation of smooth muscle contraction has also been established. See Chapter 3 and 6.

Phosphatidylcholine hydrolysis and sustained DAG formation in vascular smooth muscle cells

In vascular smooth muscle cells it is recognized that agonist-stimulated formation of $InsP_3$ does not always correlate with the formation of DAG. In AII or vasopressin-stimulated smooth muscle cells, $InsP_3$ formation is transient whilst DAG formation is sustained (Griendling *et al.* 1986; Sunako *et al.* 1990; Plevin and Wakelam 1992; Lassegue *et al.* 1993). The transient nature of the $InsP_3$ signal is not due to enhanced phosphatase or kinase activity but reflects a rapid desensitization of phosphoinositide hydrolysis (Plevin and Wakelam 1992), and suggests a source other than $PtdIns(4,5)P_2$ provides the source of sustained DAG in vascular smooth muscle cells.

Initial investigations implicated phosphatidylinositol in sustained DAG formation in vascular smooth muscle cells (Griendling *et al.* 1986; Plevin and Wakelam 1992). However, recently it has been established using HPLC analysis that phosphatidylcholine (PC) hydrolysis provides the majority of DAG species formed at later times (Lassegue et al. 1993). DAG may be derived from PC by two main routes, a phospholipase D (PLD) catalysed pathway which generates phosphatidic acid (PA) which can then be converted to DAG by phosphatidic acid phosphohydrolase, and a second route generating DAG directly via a putative PC-PLC enzyme, which is distinct from phosphoinositide-specific PLC.

A third, PLA$_2$- catalysed pathway which generates arachidonic acid (Wakelam 1992) may also contribute to DAG formation in vascular smooth muscle cells. The regulation of smooth muscle PLA$_2$ activity is not examined in detail in this chapter although many of the mechanisms of activation are similar to those outlined for PLD. Arachidonic acid has been suggested to play a role in the regulation of smooth muscle contraction indirectly through the formation of vasoactive prostaglandin and leukotriene products (Morimoto et al. 1990), and directly by regulating myosin light chain phosphorylation (see below).

Regulation of agonist-stimulated PC hydrolysis in vascular smooth muscle cells

A number of studies have demonstrated agonist-stimulated PLD activation in vascular smooth muscle cells (Lassegue et al. 1991; Gu et al. 1992; Plevin et al. 1992). In the majority of receptor/cell systems, activation of PLD is kinetically downstream of phosphoinositide hydrolysis and requires the intermediate activation of PKC. This is consistent with studies which show that following PKC inhibition or down-regulation using chronic phorbol ester pre-treatment, agonist-stimulated PLD activity is abolished (Plevin et al. 1992; Pfeilschifter and Merriweather 1993). A number of different PKC isoforms have been identified with differing function (Hug and Sarre 1993; see below) and experiments using chronic PMA pre-treatment to selectively down-regulate specific PKC isoforms implicate PKCϵ in the regulation of agonist-stimulated PLD activity in mesangial cells (Pfeilschifter and Merriweather 1993).

A number of PKC-independent mechanisms are also involved in the regulation of PC hydrolysis in smooth muscle. Agonist-mediated calcium influx may result in the formation of DAG via direct activation of PLD or PC-PLC under conditions where no phosphoinositide hydrolysis is observed or where PKC is inhibited (Clark and Garland 1991; Lassegue et al. 1991; Gu et al. 1992). Recent studies have also implicated a small molecular weight G protein, designated as ADP-ribosylation factor (ARF), in receptor/PLD coupling in granulocytes (Brown et al. 1993). It remains to be determined if a similar G protein is involved in regulating PLD activity in vascular smooth muscle.

Growth factors such as PDGF, also stimulate PC hydrolysis in vascular smooth muscle cells. This mechanism is believed to be indirect since activation is PKC-dependent (Kondo et al. 1992), and it is likely that tyrosine phosphorylation of an isoform of PLC, PLCγ, is the primary signalling event in this cascade (see below). However, in response to some growth factors, PLD may be activated in the absence of InsP$_3$ formation (Ahmed et al. 1994), also providing evidence that PLD can be regulated in a manner independent of phosphoinositide PLC activation. Tyrosine kinases have also been implicated in the regulation of PLD in vascular smooth muscle in response to certain G protein coupled receptor agonists such as ET-1 (Wilkes et al. 1993).

In smooth muscle cells, as in other systems, the contention that PLD catalysed hydrolysis of PC provides the source of sustained DAG remains controversial. PLD-derived DAG contributes varying proportions of the prolonged DAG signal observed in response to different agonists (Plevin and Wakelam 1992; Lassegue et al. 1993). Indeed PA may not be converted to DAG in smooth muscle cells but may have a bona fide second messenger function (Pyne and Pyne 1993). Activation of PC-PLC by vasopressin, noradrenaline and phorbol esters has also been demonstrated in vascular smooth muscle cells (Grillone et al. 1988; Huang and Cabot 1990; Gu et al. 1992), and may thus contribute to sustained formation of DAG.

Activation of protein kinase C in vascular smooth muscle

The main physiological target of DAG is a family of phosphatidyl serine-dependent serine/threonine-directed kinases collectively called protein kinase C. Since their discovery by Nishizuka and co-workers, at least ten isoforms have been identified by purification and molecular cloning and these can be divided into two main groups based on structural and regulatory properties (Nishizuka 1988; Parker et al. 1989; Hug and Sarre 1993). Group 1 consisting of α, β_i, β_{ii}, and γ isoforms are activated by both DAG and Ca^{2+}. Group 2 isoforms (δ, ϵ, ν, and θ), which lack the C2 domain that is necessary for Ca^{2+} binding, are activated by DAG but are Ca^{2+}-independent. Isoforms from both groups are known to translocate to the plasma membrane following agonist stimulation. A third group, lacking both V1 and C2 domains and consisting of the ζ and λ isoforms, have recently been identified. Isoforms of this class are not activated by either DAG or Ca^{2+} and do not translocate to the plasma membrane following agonist stimulation (Hug and Sarre 1993). These PKC isoforms do not appear to be down-regulated by chronic phorbol ester pre-treatment (Ways et al. 1992).

In smooth muscle cells the α, β, ϵ, and ζ isoforms of PKC are expressed (Andrea and Walsh 1992; K. Malarkey, A. M'Lees, A. Paul, G. W. Gould, and R. Plevin, submitted), thus total PKC activity will necessarily be a composite of the activation of several different isoforms with differing Ca^{2+} and DAG dependencies. Vasoconstrictors such as AII, Et-1, and histamine, which hydrolyse membrane phospholipids and stimulate the formation of DAG, have been shown to activate protein kinase C in vascular smooth muscle cells and in smooth muscle strips (Lang and Vallotton, 1989; Haller et al. 1990). Within these preparations, a large number of intracellular proteins have been identified as potential targets for PKC-mediated phosphorylation. These include MLC_{20}, MLCK, VOCCs, phospholipases A_2 and D, and Na^+/Ca^{2+} exchange pumps (Andrea and Walsh 1992). As a result of these findings a role for PKC has been implicated in both the initial phase of vascular smooth muscle contraction, where tension develops rapidly, and in the second sustained phase of contraction, where tension is maintained over time.

Protein kinase C isoforms in the regulation of smooth muscle contraction

Sensitization of vascular smooth muscle contraction by G proteins

A rise in $[Ca^{2+}]_i$ is not the only mechanism by which maximal contraction is obtained following vasoconstrictor stimulation. During contraction, MLC_{20} phosphorylation is greater than the corresponding increase in intracellular Ca^{2+} concentration and subsequent activation of MLCK would predict, resulting in an enhanced contraction at a given Ca^{2+} concentration. One mechanism by which sensitization of contractile elements is achieved is through an inhibition of myosin light chain phosphatase (Somlyo and Himpens 1989) and involves the activation of a G protein (Kitazawa et al. 1991). Sensitization induced by non-hydrolysable analogues of GTP such as GTPγS, is still observed in the presence of neomycin, which binds PtdIns(4,5)P$_2$ and prevents agonist-stimulated phosphoinositide hydrolysis (Itoh et al. 1994). This excludes an involvement of the heterotrimeric G protein Gq/G11, and suggests a role for a small molecular weight G protein such as p21^{rho} or p21^{ras} in the sensitization process (Hirata et al. 1992; Satoh et al. 1993) (see Fig. 7.1).

PKC appears to play a role in the G protein-mediated sensitization of smooth muscle contraction. Agents such as Et-1 and PMA are able to enhance contraction at a given $[Ca^{2+}]_i$ (Nishimura et al. 1992) or potentiate contraction induced by other vasoconstrictors (Henrion et al. 1992). This correlates with a PKC-mediated inhibition of myosin light chain phosphatase (Itoh et al. 1993). Furthermore, in permeabilized smooth muscle cells sensitization induced by agonist and GTP in combination is reduced by PKC inhibition (Seager et al. 1994).

The mechanisms underlying the regulation of p21^{rho} function by contractile agonists have not been elucidated. However, since the stimulation of a G protein requires the exchange of GTP for GDP, the activation of a nucleotide exchange factor or a GTPase inhibitor protein is implicated (see Fig. 7.1). PKC has been shown to be involved in the regulation of nucleotide exchange on other small molecular weight G proteins (Antonietta De Matteis et al. 1993) and it is possible that PKC acts in this manner rather than via direct phosphorylation of contractile proteins. This would explain why in some studies no effect of PKC inhibition is observed upon direct GTPγS-induced sensitization but is apparent following PMA or agonist stimulation (Itoh et al. 1994; Seager et al. 1994).

A number of other events have been proposed to play a role regulating Ca^{2+} sensitization. In rat aorta, agonist-mediated enhancement of contraction is still observed following PKC down-regulation (Hori et al. 1993) while in skinned smooth muscle strips, arachidonic acid inhibits MLC phosphatase directly without intermediate involvement of PKC or a G protein (Gong et al. 1992). Further studies are required to elucidate the complex mechanisms underlying this phenomenon.

The role of protein kinase C in sustained contraction

It is now recognized that the phosphorylation of MLC_{20} does not correlate with the kinetics of smooth muscle contraction. Following the initial development of force, MLCK-mediated phosphorylation of MLC_{20} declines, however, contraction is maintained through the formation of actinomyosin 'latch bridges' (Hai and Murphy 1989). It has been postulated that PKC may function to maintain tension at low $[Ca^{2+}]_i$ through the phosphorylation of a number of contractile proteins associated with the actin and myosin filaments (Rasmussen *et al.* 1987). Tonic contraction is likely to be regulated through the sustained formation of DAG species which can selectively activate PKC isoforms which are Ca^{2+}-independent (Andrea and Walsh 1992). It has been proposed that PA may directly activate a PA-dependent kinase or an isoform of PKC which is both DAG and Ca^{2+}-independent, such as PKCζ (Pyne and Pyne 1993). Thus contraction could be maintained at low $[Ca^{2+}]_i$ through activation of PC hydrolysis (see Fig. 7.2).

The evidence currently available partially supports this hypothesis. A number of agonists, including Et-1 and $PGF_{2\alpha}$ are able to sustain smooth muscle contraction in the absence of extracellular Ca^{2+} (Itoh *et al.* 1991; Hori *et al.* 1992; Shimamoto *et al.* 1992). Phorbol esters or analogues of DAG have been demonstrated to initiate a slow, prolonged contraction in a large number of tissues, and although in A7r5 smooth muscle cells this is associated with an increase in intracellular Ca^{2+} (Nakajima *et al.* 1993), in rabbit aorta bathed in Ca^{2+}-free solution, this action is not associated with intracellular Ca^{2+} mobilization nor with MLCK phosphorylation (Sato *et al.* 1992). Furthermore, the translocation and activation of PKC in smooth muscle in response to Et-1, AII, histamine, and KCl display kinetics which closely correlate with sustained contraction (Haller *et al.* 1990; Singer *et al.* 1992). Significantly, in noradrenaline-stimulated ferret aorta, the Ca^{2+} independent PKC isoform, PKCε, is translocated to the plasma membrane under conditions where Ca^{2+}-independent contraction is induced (Khalil *et al.* 1992).

Studies using PKC inhibitors have been unable to provide unequivocal support for a role for protein kinase C in the maintenance of contraction. Although in rat aortic strips, H-7 subtantially reduces Ca^{2+}-independent contraction in responce to phorbol ester, Et-1, and $PGF_{2\alpha}$ (Sugiura *et al.* 1989; Morimoto *et al.* 1990), such compounds, inhibitors at the ATP binding domain of PKC, may act non-specifically to inhibit other protein kinases. A recent study using calphostin C, a PKC inhibitor specific for the DAG binding site (Shimamoto *et al.* 1992), has suggested that the role of PKC in regulating sustained contraction has been overestimated. In addition, the effects of PKC inhibitors are dependent upon a number of factors including extracellular Ca^{2+} levels (Shimamoto *et al.* 1992), the agonist employed, and the tissue under study, suggesting that PKC-dependent and -independent mechansims are in operation within a single cell and within different vessels.

Phosphorylation of contractile proteins by PKC has been examined in detail

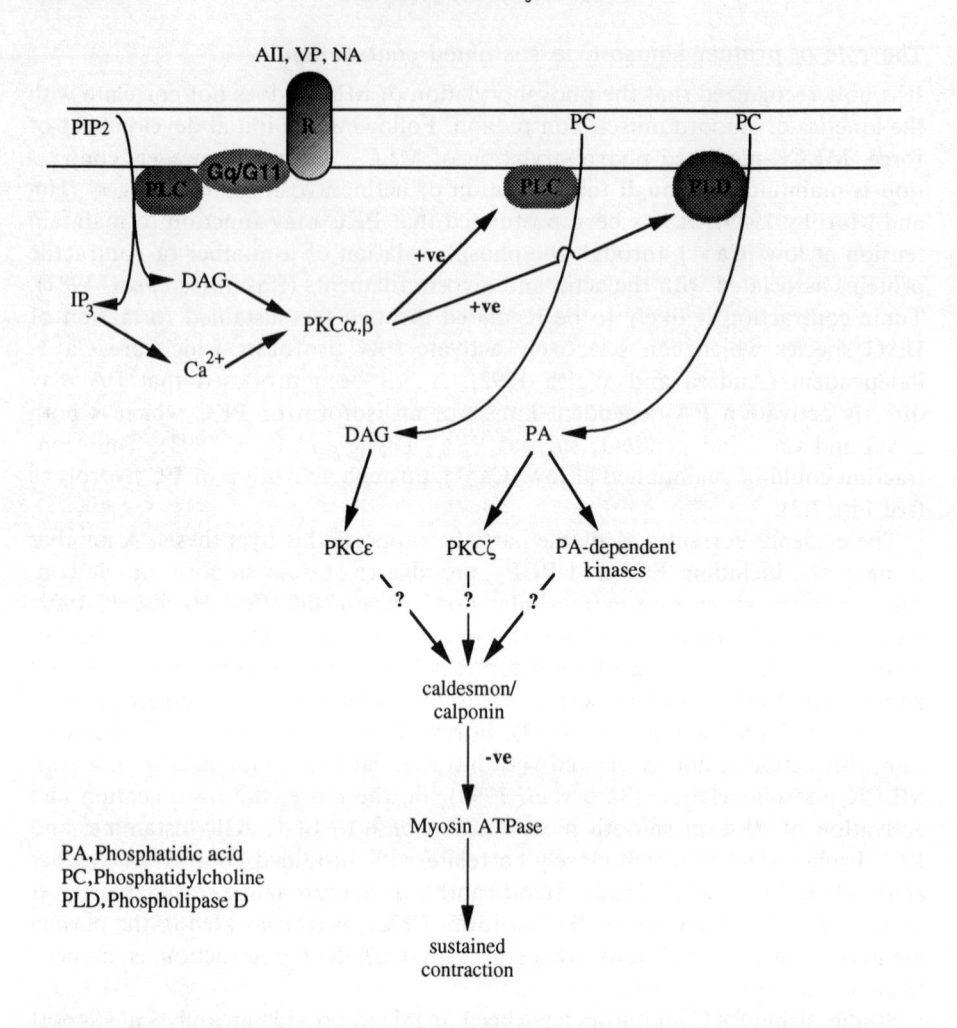

Fig. 7.2 Proposed model for the role of PKC isoforms involved in the regulation of sustained contraction.

in smooth muscle preparations. Partially purified PKC is able directly to phosphorylate myosin upon specific serine residues *in vitro* (Ikebe *et al.* 1987) and this reduces actin-activated Mg^{2+}-ATPase activity of myosin previously phosphorylated by MLCK (Nishikawa *et al.* 1984). These findings do not however, correlate with studies in intact strips or in cells in culture where a very low level of phosphorylation at sites corresponding to *in vitro* studies occurs following agonist or phorbol ester stimulation (Singer *et al.* 1989).

Two other proteins associated with actin and myosin regulate vascular smooth muscle tone. The high molecular weight form of caldesmon (*h*-caldesmon) is a major vascular smooth muscle protein which regulates contraction by binding to actin and inhibiting actin-activated myosin Mg^{2+}-ATPase (Sobue and Sellers

1991). Peptides containing the Gly^{651}–Ser^{667} sequence of h-caldesmon are functional antagonists of caldesmon and induce a dose-dependent contraction (Katsuyama et al. 1992) implicating a functional role for caldesmon in the inhibition of vascular smooth muscle tone. However, although PKC is able to phosphorylate the h-caldesmon in the region of the carboxy terminus in vitro, which reduces both the affinity of the protein for actin and inhibition of myosin ATPase, phosphopeptide mapping of immunoprecipitated h-caldesmon is not consistent with the phosphorylation being PKC-mediated in vivo (Adam et al. 1989). Another protein associated with thin filaments, calponin, has also been implicated in the regulation of smooth muscle contraction (Winder and Walsh 1990; Willis et al. 1994). Once again, contradictory evidence has emerged regarding the significance in vivo of the PKC-mediated phosphorylation observed in vitro (Barany et al. 1991).

With regards to PA-mediated contraction, although it has previously been shown that the formation of PA correlates closely with noradrenaline-induced contraction in isolated strips (Ohanian et al. 1990), and that PA activates PKCζ in vitro (Nakanishi and Exton 1992), there has been no direct demonstration of a role for PKCζ or a PA-dependent kinase in the regulation of myosin Mg^{2+}-ATPase or cross-linkage of actin and myosin filaments. Indeed, in ferret aorta vasoconstrictor stimulation results in the translocation of PKCζ to the nucleus suggesting role for this particular isoform in gene expression rather than contraction (Khalil et al. 1992).

The role of protein kinase C in smooth muscle relaxation

The putative role of PKC in the regulation of smooth muscle contraction is further complicated by studies which implicate a role for PKC in relaxation. Activated PKC relaxes contracted smooth muscle, an effect which is associated with the in vivo phosphorylation of MLC$_{20}$ by a catalytically active fragment of PKC (Inaki et al. 1987; Andrea and Walsh 1992). Phosphorylation of MLCK resulting in a decrease in the affinity of the enzyme for the Ca^{2+}/CaM complex may also be mediated by PKC, directly or possibly indirectly, through calmodulin-dependent protein kinase II (CaM kinase II) (Tansey et al. 1994).

PKC also stimulates Ca^{2+} extrusion in intact smooth muscle cells (Furukawa et al. 1989), uncouples agonist-activation of phosphoinositide hydolysis (Huang and Ives 1989), and is involved in regulating adenylyl cyclase activity (see below) in response to contractile agonists such as AII and phorbol esters (Nabika et al. 1985; Phaneuf et al. 1988). Further studies are required to confirm the physiological relevance of these observations in whole tissues.

TYROSINE PHOSPHORYLATION AND SMOOTH MUSCLE CONTRACTION

In recent years major advances have been achieved in defining cell signalling pathways which involve the activation of proteins by phosphorylation upon tyrosine residues (Fantl et al. 1993). Although this cascade has been most closely examined in response to growth factor stimulation in fibroblast cell lines, tyrosine phosphorylation has recently been implicated in the regulation of smooth muscle contraction in response to vasoconstrictors and growth factors (Hollenberg 1994).

Growth factor receptors and the activation of tyrosine kinase pathways

Following activation of the growth factor receptor, autophosphorylation occurs upon specific tyrosine residues within the kinase insert domain of the receptor. Phosphorylation allows interaction with a number of cell signalling molecules including PLCγ, phosphatidylinositol 3 kinase (PI 3-kinase) and GTPase activating protein (GAP) (Fig. 7.3). These interactions are possible by virtue of the presence of *src* homology (SH) domains within the target enzyme or protein (Pawson and Gish 1992). A large number of proteins have been shown to be activated by growth factor directly or indirectly through SH-2 and SH-3 containing proteins and this is a key mechanism underlying growth factor-mediated responses.

An example of a kinase pathway initiated by growth factor activation involves the activation of a family of kinases called mitogen-activated protein (MAP) kinases (Davis 1993). Activation of MAP kinase is achieved by a complex mechanism involving a series of protein/protein interactions (Fig. 7.3). Growth factor receptor activation allows the interaction of the receptor with a growth factor receptor binding protein (GRB2), composed solely of SH-2 and SH-3 domains. GRB2 interacts with mSos (mammalian son of sevenless), a nucleotide exchange factor which was originally found in drosophila encoded by the son of sevenless gene. mSos promotes GTP loading on the small molecular weight G protein p21^{ras} (Egan et al. 1993). Activated GTP bound p21^{ras} stimulates the serine/threonine kinase Raf-1 which in turn activates the immediate upstream activator of MAP kinase, MAP kinase kinase (Schlessinger 1993).

Vasoconstrictor activation of MAP kinase in vascular smooth muscle cells

It was quickly recognized that a number of agonists whose receptors were coupled to G proteins were also able to stimulate the tyrosine phosphorylation of MAP kinase in a number of systems including vascular smooth muscle cells. In response to AII or vasopressin, a rapid phosphorylation of MAP kinase is observed which is dependent upon the activation of PKC (Kribben et al. 1993). PKCα has recently been shown to phosphorylate Raf-1 *in vitro* (Kolch et al. 1993), implicating this mechanism as the major pathway for the activation of MAP kinase by vasoconstrictors (Fig. 7.4). Indeed, hyperphosphorylation of Raf-1 is observed in vascular smooth muscle cells following stimulation with AII (Molloy et al. 1993). However, it has also been shown that for some agonists including thrombin and lysophosphatidic acid, the activation of MAP kinase is pertussis toxin-sensitive

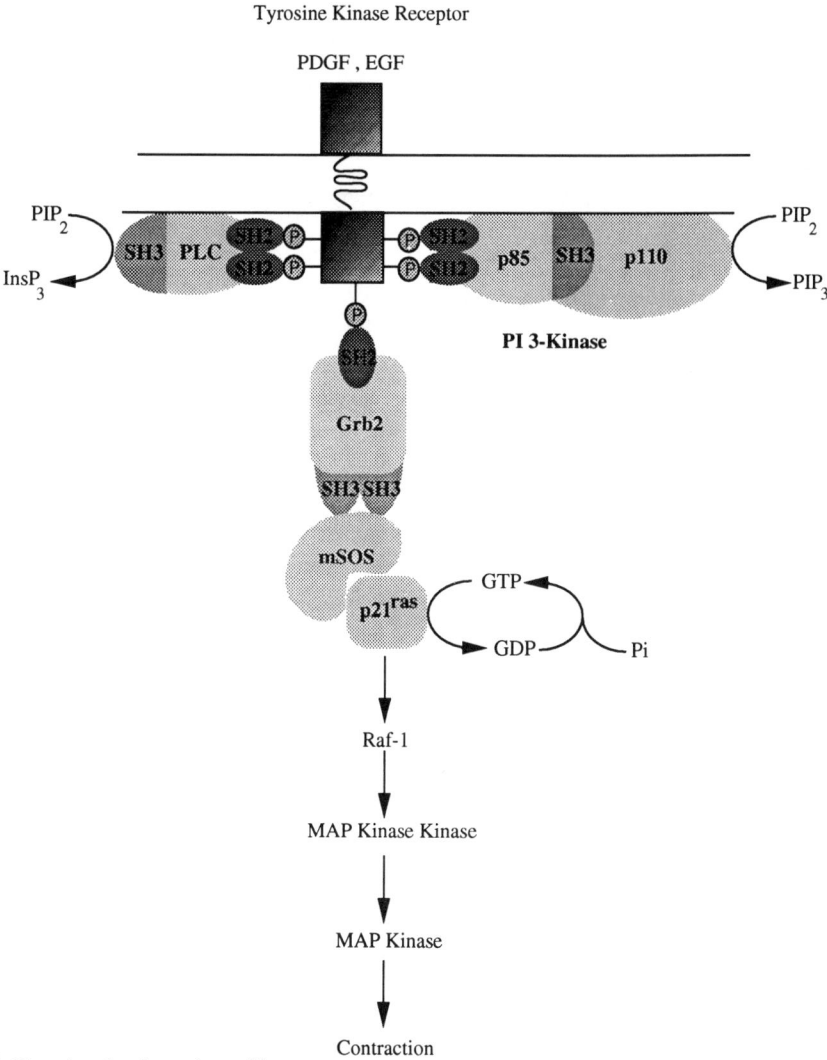

Cell signalling pathways

Fig. 7.3 Growth factor activation of tyrosine kinase pathways.

Ⓟ, Phosphorylated tyrosine residue
EGF, Epidermal growth factor
Grb2, Growth factor receptor binding protein 2
PDGF, Platelet derived growth factor
PI 3-Kinase, Phosphatidylinositol 3-kinase
mSOS, Mammalian homologue of son of sevenless
SH2/SH3, SRC homology domains

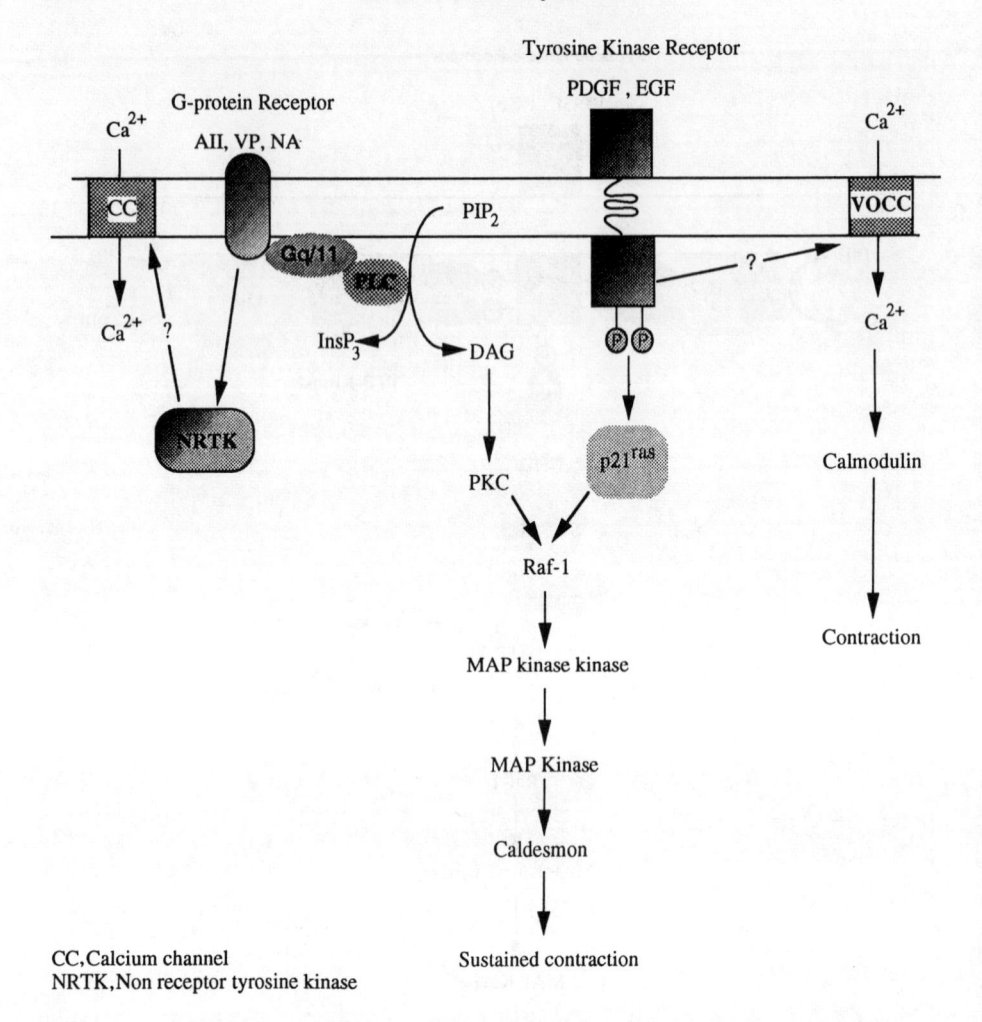

Fig. 7.4 Activation of smooth muscle contraction through tyrosine kinase pathways by both growth factor and G protein coupled agonists acting as vasoconstrictors.

and that stimulation of p21^{ras} is also involved in the activation cascade (van Corven *et al.* 1993). In addition, a third pathway which is both p21^{ras}- and Raf-independent has been implicated in the regulation of MAP kinase by G protein coupled receptors. This involves the activation of another kinase, MEK kinase (Lange-Carter *et al.* 1993), an upstream activator of MAP kinase kinase which is distinct from Raf-1.

Tyrosine kinase pathways in the regulation of smooth muscle contraction

Although a great deal of attention has focused upon the role for MAP kinase in the regulation of proliferation, recent evidence has accumulated to suggest a role for MAP kinase in vasoconstrictor stimulated contraction. Purified pp44 MAP kinase has been shown to phosphorylate smooth muscle caldesmon *in vitro* (Childs *et al.* 1992) at a site identical to that observed following PMA stimulation *in vivo* (Adam *et al.* 1992). This finding therefore satisfies a role for PKC in sustained smooth muscle contraction through the indirect activation of MAP kinase. However, PKC may also be involved in another aspect of MAP kinase activation. In ferret aorta, vasoconstrictor stimulation in Ca^{2+}-free conditions results in the PKC-dependent translocation of MAP kinase to the plasma membrane (Khalil and Morgan 1993). Since both vasoconstrictor activation of MAP kinase and Ca^{2+}-independent contraction are associated with PKCε (Khalil *et al.* 1992; Malarkey *et al.* 1995) this isoform may play a central role in the sustained contractile response by regulating MAP kinase distribution and activity.

PDGF and EGF also stimulate contraction in a number of smooth muscle preparations (Berk *et al.* 1986; Hollenberg 1994). This may be due to activation of MAP kinase as described above (Malarkey *et al.* 1995), however, it is likely that a number of other tyrosine phosphorylation events are involved. Growth factors are able to stimulate calcium influx (Block *et al.* 1989) and PLA_2 activation (Margolis *et al.* 1988; Goldberg *et al.* 1990), events which may be critical in regulating contraction (Hollenberg 1994). How this is achieved is unclear but may involve a direct interaction of the receptor with the target protein or the activation of intermediate non-receptor associated tyrosine kinase (see Fig. 7.4). This also would explain the relative sensitivity of each growth factor-mediated contractile response to different types of tyrosine kinase inhibitors (Merkel *et al.* 1993; Sauro and Thomas 1993; Hollenberg 1994).

Other tyrosine phosphorylation events critical in the regulation of contraction may be activated by G protein coupled receptor agonists through a similar recruitment of non-receptor tyrosine kinases to the receptor (see Fig. 7.4). This type of mechanism could be involved in vasoconstrictor activation of calcium channels (Lee *et al.* 1993) and PLD (Wilkes *et al.* 1993).

CYCLIC NUCLEOTIDE FORMATION AND VASCULAR SMOOTH MUSCLE RELAXATION

It is now generally accepted that cAMP and cGMP are intimately involved in initiating relaxation in vascular smooth muscle. The intracellular levels of cAMP and cGMP are regulated by the synthetic enzymes, adenylyl cyclase and guanylyl cyclase respectively, as well as by the cyclic nucleotide phosphodiesterases (PDEs), a family of isoenzymes which degrade cyclic nucleotides.

Adenylyl cyclase

A major role for the adenylyl cyclase/cAMP signalling system in relaxation is implicated by agonists such as isoprenaline, adrenaline, prostacylin, and VIP, which raise intracellular cAMP levels and evoke relaxation of vascular smooth muscle.

At least six forms of adenylyl cyclase exist in mammalian cell systems and are classified by structural homology, tissue expression, and regulatory properties (Tang and Gilman 1992). Adenylyl cyclase is positively regulated by the α-subunit of Gs activated by agonist receptor occupation or directly by compounds such as forskolin. In addition, types I and III are regulated by Ca^{2+}/calmodulin and types I, II, and IV by $\beta\gamma$ subunits of heterotrimeric G proteins. At present it is unknown which isotypes of adenylyl cyclase are expressed in vascular smooth muscle cells but these are likely to include the type II and type IV isoforms which are regulated by PKC (Yoshimura and Cooper 1993). As outlined previously, interaction with PKC makes smooth muscle adenylyl cyclase a potential target for regulation by vasoconstrictors (Nabika et al. 1985).

The effects of cAMP are thought to be mediated through the activation of a family of cAMP-dependent protein kinases designated as PKA (Taylor et al. 1990). PKA appears to cause vascular relaxation by lowering both $[Ca^{2+}]_i$ and the sensitivity of the contractile elements to Ca^{2+}. It has been shown that PKA diphosphorylates MLCK at specific sites (A and B), increasing the Ca^{2+} requirement for MLC_{20} phosphorylation (Adelstein et al. 1978; Nishikawa et al. 1984). However, in rat aorta, forskolin reduces agonist-induced increases in $[Ca^{2+}]_i$ at concentrations which do not affect Ca^{2+}/tension relationships (Abe and Karaki 1989) and thus it is possible that the latter effect is more important in initiating relaxation.

PKA can reduce $[Ca^{2+}]_i$ through a number of mechanisms including the inactivation of the $InsP_3$ receptor or inhibition of phosphoinositide hydrolysis (Supattapone et al. 1988). However, in rabbit mesenteric artery, neither dibutyryl-cAMP nor a forskolin derivative affected noradrenaline stimulated $InsP_3$ production or $InsP_3$-induced calcium release despite lowering $[Ca^{2+}]_i$ and reducing contraction (Ito et al. 1993). Experiments using thapsigargin, a sarcoplasmic Ca^{2+}-ATPase inhibitor, suggests stimulation of Ca^{2+} uptake as the most likely mechanism involved. Raising cAMP has been shown to inhibit agonist-stimulated [^{3}H]inositol phosphate accumulation in a number of other smooth muscle cell systems, however, this is achieved via an indirect effect at the level of Ca^{2+} mobilization (Dickenson et al. 1993; Berman et al. 1994).

Guanylyl cyclase

Both particulate and soluble forms of guanylyl cyclase are present in vascular smooth muscle cells and activation of these enzymes promotes the formation of cGMP and induces relaxation (Ignarro and Kadowitz 1985; Fujitani et al. 1993). At least three forms of particulate guanylyl cyclase (GC A-C) have been isolated and cloned and consist of a single transmembrane domain, an intracellular kinase-like domain, and a cyclase catalytic domain (Garbers 1992). In smooth muscle particulate guanylyl cyclase is activated by atrial natriuretic peptide and related peptides, in a manner analogous to tyrosine kinase receptor activation. Soluble forms of guanylyl cyclase contain only the catalytic domain and are activated by nitric oxide (NO) through interaction with the haem moiety. This is achieved *in vivo* by the release of NO from adjacent endothelial cells by calcium-mobilizing agonists (Fujitani *et al.* 1993) (see Chapter 10).

A major intracellular target for cGMP is cyclic GMP-dependent protein kinase (PKG) (Lincoln and Cornwell 1993) which mediates cGMP-stimulated vascular relaxation. Consistent with this hypothesis is the observation that analogues of cGMP which activate purified PKG *in vitro* stimulate relaxation in smooth muscle tissues (Francis *et al.* 1988).

Like cAMP, cGMP has effects on both Ca^{2+} mobilization and contractile protein function. In vascular smooth muscle raising cGMP reduces phosphorylation of MLC_{20}, possibly via PKG-mediated phosphorylation and inactivation of MLCK (Rapoport *et al.* 1983; Nishikawa *et al.* 1984). However, the extent to which phosphorylation of MLCK by PKG is involved in mediating relaxation is unclear. In rat aorta vascular smooth muscle cells, non-hydrolysable analogues of cGMP lower agonist or K^+-induced increases in intracellular Ca^{2+} through activation of smooth muscle particulate Ca^{2+}-ATPase (Rashatwar *et al.* 1987). This is associated with the PKG-mediated phosphorylation of a number of proteins which regulate Ca^{2+}-ATPase function including phospholamban (Cornwell *et al.* 1991; Yoshida *et al.* 1991). In rat vascular smooth muscle, PKG may also have direct inhibitory effects upon agonist activation of phosphoinositide hydrolysis via an action on G protein/PLC coupling (Hirata *et al.* 1990), although in rabbit aortic smooth muscle cells, cGMP affects smooth muscle function without changes in calcium mobilization (Assender *et al.* 1992). This suggests tissue specificity in the involvement of mechanisms described above.

Clearly, cAMP and cGMP have many similar intracellular effects in vascular smooth muscle. An increasing body of evidence suggests that the activation of PKG underlies the relaxation mediated by both cAMP and cGMP. For example, in permeabilized smooth muscle cells, purified PKG can stimulate a decrease in $[Ca^{2+}]_i$ and relaxation whilst PKA is ineffective. However, under these conditions forskolin is still able to cause relaxation and reduce $[Ca^{2+}]_i$ (Francis *et al.* 1988; Lincoln *et al.* 1990; Lincoln and Cornwell 1993). The physiological relevance of these observations is unclear since *in vitro*, the K_a values for the activation of each α and β isozyme of PKG by cAMP is 20 and 100 times greater than that for PKG (Landgraf *et al.* 1992). The suprapharmacological generation of cAMP in smooth muscle by forskolin may not be easily mimicked by agonists *in vivo*.

Cyclic nucleotide phosphodiesterases

Three main isoforms of PDE, types I, II, and III are present in vascular smooth muscle. These isoforms have been further subdivided on the basis of substrate specificity, and regulation by Ca^{2+}/CaM or by cGMP itself (Beavo and Reifsnyder 1990). Types IA and II hydrolyse both cAMP and cGMP, and type IIB is specific for cAMP. In addition, type II is stimulated by cGMP whereas type IIIB is inhibited by cGMP. Furthermore, types IA and IB are activated by Ca^{2+}/CaM, but the other PDE isoforms are Ca^{2+}/CaM-insensitive (Weishaar et al. 1991).

The relative roles of each isoform in the removal of cyclic nucleotide from the cell is unknown but will necessarily be dependent upon the relative expression of each subtype and the mode of cell activation. However, relaxation of vascular smooth muscle by PDE inhibitors has been well documented (Weishaar et al. 1991) and provides further evidence of a role for cyclic nucleotides in vascular relaxation.

REFERENCES

Abe, A. and Karaki, H. (1989). Effect of forskolin on cytosolic Ca^{2+} level and contraction in vascular smooth muscle. J. Pharmacol. Exp. Ther., 249, 895-900.

Adam, L. P., Haeberle, J. R., and Hathaway, D. R. (1989). Phosphorylation of caldesmon in arterial smooth muscle. J. Biol. Chem., 264, 7698-703.

Adam, L. P., Gapinski, C. J., and Hathaway, D. R. (1992). Phosphorylation sequences in h-caldesmon from phorbol ester stimulated canine aortas. FEBS Lett., 302, 223-6.

Adlestein, R. S., Conti, M. A., Hathaway, D. R., and Klee, C. B. (1978). Phosphorylation of smooth muscle myosin light chain kinase by the catalytic subunit of adenosine 3,5,-monophosphate-dependent protein kinase. J. Biol. Chem., 253, 8347-50.

Ahmed, A., Plevin, R., Mahmood, S. A., Shoaibi, M. A., Fountain, S. A., Ferriani, R. A., et al. (1994). Basic FGF activates phospholipase D in endothelial cells in the absence of inositol lipid hydrolysis. Am. J. Physiol., 266, C206-12.

Andrea, J. E. and Walsh, M. P. (1992). Protein kinase C of smooth muscle. Hypertension, 20, 585-95.

Antonietta De Matteis, M., Santini, G., Kahn, R. A., Di Tullio, G., and Luini, A. (1993). Receptor and protein kinase C-mediated regulation of ARF binding to the golgi complex. Nature, 364, 818-21.

Araki, S., Kawahara, Y., Kariya, K., Sunako, M., and Fukuzaki, H. (1989). Stimulation of phospholipase C-mediated hydrolysis of phosphoinositides by endothelin in cultured rabbit aortic smooth muscle cells. Biochem. Biophys. Res. Commun., 159, 1072-9.

Assender, J. W., Southgate, K. M., Hallett, M. B., and Newby, A. C. (1992). Inhibition of proliferation, but not of Ca^{2+} mobilisation, by cyclic AMP and GMP in rabbit aortic smooth muscle cells. Biochem. J., 288, 527-32.

Barany, M., Rokolya, A., and Barany, K. (1991). Absence of calponin phosphorylation in contracting or resting arterial smooth muscle. FEBS Lett., 279, 65-8.

Beavo, J. A. and Reifsnyder, D. H. (1990). Primary sequence of cyclic nucleotide phosphodiesterase isozymes and the design of selective inhibitors. Trends Pharmacol. Sci., 11, 150-5.

Berk, B. C., Alexander, R. W., Brock, T. A., Gimbrone, M. A. Jr, and Webb, R. C. (1986). Vasoconstriction: A new activity for platelet-derived growth factor. Science, 232, 87-90.

Berman, D. M., Sugiyama, T., and Goldman, W. F. (1994). Ca^{2+} stores in smooth muscle cells: Ca^{2+} buffering and coupling to AVP-evoked inositol phosphate synthesis. Am. J. Physiol., 266, C276-83.

Berridge, M. J. (1993). Inositol trisphosphate and calcium signalling. *Nature*, 361, 315–25.
Berridge, M. J. and Irvine, R. F. (1989). Inositol phosphates and cell signalling. *Nature*, 341, 197–205.
Blatter, L. and Wier, W. P. (1992). Agonist-induced $[Ca^{2+}]_i$ waves and Ca^{2+}-induced Ca^{2+} release in mammalian vascular smooth muscle cells. *Am. J. Physiol.*, 263, H576–86.
Block, L. H., Emmons, L. R., Vogt, E., Sachinidis, A., Vetter, W., and Hoppe, J. (1989). Ca^{2+}-channel blockers inhibit the action of recombinant platelet-derived growth factor in vascular smooth muscle cells. *Proc. Natl. Acad. Sci. USA*, 86, 2388–92.
Brown, H. A., Gutowski, S., Moomaw, C. R., Slaughter, C., and Sternweis, P. C. (1993). ADP-ribosylation factor, a small GTP-dependent regulatory protein, stimulates phospholipase D activity. *Cell*, 75, 1137–44.
Childs, T. J. Watson, M. H., Sanghera, J. S., Campbell, D. L., Pelech, S. L., and Mak, A. S. (1992). Phosphorylation of smooth muscle caldesmon by mitogen-activated protein kinase and expression of MAP kinase in differentiated smooth muscle cells. *J. Biol. Chem.*, 267, 22853–9.
Clark, A. H. and Garland, C. J. (1991). 5-hydroxytryptamine-stimulated accumulation of 1,2-diacylglycerol in the rabbit basilar artery: a role for protein kinase C in smooth muscle contraction. *Br. J. Pharmacol.*, 102, 415–21.
Clark, C. J., Milligan, G., McLellan, A. R., and Connell, J. M. C. (1992). Guanine nucleotide regulatory protein levels and function in spontaneously hypertensive rat vascular smooth muscle cells. *Biochem. Biophys Acta*, 1136, 290–6.
Cornwell, T. L., Pryzwansky, K. B., Wyatt, T. A., and Lincoln, T. M. (1991). Regulation of sarcoplasmic reticulum protein phosphorylation localised by cyclic-GMP-dependent protein kinase in vascular smooth muscle cells. *J. Pharmacol. Exp. Ther.*, 40, 923–31.
Davis, R. J. (1993). The mitogen activated protein kinase signal transduction pathways. *J. Biol. Chem.*, 268, 14553–6.
Dickenson, J. M., White, T. E., and Hill, S. J. (1993). The effects of elevated cyclic AMP levels on histamine-H1-receptor-stimulated inositol phospholipid hydrolysis and calcium mobilisation in the smooth-muscle cell line DTT1MF-2. *Biochem. J.*, 292, 409–17.
Doyle, V. M. and Ruegg, U. T. (1985). Vasopressin induced production of inositol trisphosphate and calcium efflux in a smooth muscle cell line. *Biochem. Biophys. Res. Commun.*, 131, 469–76.
Egan, S. E., Giddings, B. W., Brooks, M. W., Buday, L., Sizeland, A. M., and Weinberg, R. A. (1993). Association of Sos Ras exchange protein with Grb2 is implicated in tyrosine kinase signal transduction and transformation. *Nature*, 363, 45–51.
Fantl, W. J., Johnson, D. E., and Williams, L. T. (1993). Signalling by receptor tyrosine kinases. *Annu. Rev. Biochem.*, 62, 453–81.
Fasolato, C., Innocenti, B., and Pozzan, T. (1994). Receptor operated Ca^{2+} influx: How many mechanisms for how many channels? *Trends Pharmacol. Sci.*, 15, 77–83.
Francis, S. H., Noblett, B. D., Todd, B. W., Wells, J. N., and Corbin, J. D. (1988). Relaxation of vascular and tracheal smooth muscle by cyclic nucleotide analogues that preferentially activate purified cGMP dependent protein kinase. *Mol. Pharmacol.*, 34, 506–17.
Fujitani, Y., Ueda, H., Okada, T., Urade, Y., and Karaki, H. (1993). A selective agonist of endothelin type B receptor, IRL, 1620, stimulates cyclic GMP increase via nitric oxide formation in rat aorta. *J. Pharmacol. Exp. Ther.*, 267, 683–9.
Furukawa, K.-I., Tawada, Y., and Shigekawa, M. (1989). Protein kinase C activation stimulates plasma membrane Ca^{2+} pump in cultured vascular smooth muscle cells. *J. Biol. Chem.*, 264, 4844–9.

Garbers, D. L. (1992). Guanylyl cyclase receptors and their endocrine, paracrine and autocrine ligands. *Cell*, **71**, 1-4.

Goldberg, H. J., Viegas, M. M., Margolis, B. L., Schlessinger, J., and Skorecki, K. L. (1990). The tyrosine kinase activity of the epidermal-growth-factor receptor is necessary for phospholipase A_2 activation. *Biochem. J.*, **267**, 461-5.

Gong, M. C., Fugslang, A., Alessi, D., Kobayashi, S., Cohen, P., Somylo, A. V., et al. (1992). Arachidonic acid inhibits myosin light chain phosphatase and sensitizes smooth muscle to calcium. *J. Biol. Chem.*, **267**, 21492-8.

Griendling, K. K., Rittenhouse, S. E., Brock, T. A., Ekstein, L. S., Gimbrone, M. A. Jr, and Alexander, R. W. (1986). Sustained diacylglycerol formation from inositol phospholipids in angiotensin II-stimulated vascular smooth muscle cells. *J. Biol. Chem.*, **261**, 5901-6.

Grillone, L. R., Clark, M. A., Godfrey, R. W., Stassen, F., and Crooke, S. T. (1988). Vasopressin induces V_1 receptors to activate phosphatidylinositol and phosphatidylcholine-specific phospholipase C and stimulates release of arachidonic acid by at least two pathways in the smooth muscle cell line A-10. *J. Biol. Chem.*, **263**, 2658-63.

Gu, H., Trajkovic, S., and LaBelle, E. P. (1992). Norepinephrine-induced phosphatidylcholine hydrolysis by phospholipases D and C in rat tail artery. *Am. J. Physiol.*, **262**, C1376-83.

Gutowski, S., Smrcka, A., Nowak, L., Wu, D., Simon, M., and Sternweis, P. C. (1991). Antibodies to the aq subfamily of guanine nucleotide-binding regulatory protein α-subunits attenuate activation of phosphatidylinositol 4,5-bisphosphate hydrolysis by hormones. *J. Biol. Chem.*, **266**, 20519-24.

Hai, C.-M. and Murphy, R. A. (1989). Ca^{2+}, Crossbridge phosphorylation and contraction. *Annu. Rev. Physiol.*, **51**, 285-98.

Haller, H., Smallwood, J. I., and Rasmussen, H. (1990). Protein kinase C translocation in intact vascular smooth muscle strips. *Biochem. J.*, **270**, 375-81.

Hashimoto, T., Hirata, M., Itoh, T., Kanmura, Y., and Kuriyama, H. (1986). Inositol 1,4,5-trisphosphate activates pharmacomechanical coupling in smooth muscle of the rabbit mesenteric artery. *J. Physiol.*, **370**, 605-18.

Henrion, D., Laher, I., Laporte, R., and Bevan, J. A. (1992). Angiotensin II amplifies arterial contractile responses without increasing Ca^{2+} influx: role of protein kinase C. *J. Pharmacol. Exp. Ther.*, **261**, 835-40.

Hirata, M., Kohse, K. P., Chang, C.-H., Ikebe, T., and Murad, F. (1990). Mechanism of cyclic GMP inhibition of inositol phosphate formation in rat aorta segments and cultured bovine aortic smooth muscle cells. *J. Biol. Chem.*, **265**, 1268-73.

Hirata, K.-I., Kikuchi, A., Sasaki, T., Kuroda, S., Kaibuch, K., Matsuura, Y., et al. (1992). Involvement of rho p21 in the GTP-enhanced calcium ion sensitivity of smooth muscle contraction. *J. Biol. Chem.*, **267**, 8719-22.

Hollenberg, M. D. (1994). Tyrosine kinase pathways and the regulation of smooth muscle contractility. *Trends Pharmacol. Sci.*, **15**, 108-14.

Hori, M., Sato, K., Sakata, K., Ozaki, H., Takano-Ohmuro, H., Tsuchiya, T., et al. (1992). Receptor agonists induce myosin phosphorylation-dependent and phosphorylation-independent contractions in vascular smooth muscle. *J. Pharmacol. Exp. Ther.*, **261**, 506-12.

Hori, M., Sato, K., Miyamoto, S., Ozaki, H., and Karaki, H. (1993). Different pathways of calcium sensitization activated by receptor agonists and phorbol esters in vascular smooth muscle. *Br. J. Pharmacol.*, **110**, 1527-31.

Huang, C. and Cabot, M. C. (1990). Phorbol diesters stimulate the accumulation of phosphatidate, phosphatidylethanol and diacylglycerol in three cell types. *J. Biol. Chem.*, **265**, 14858-63.

Huang, C.-L. and Ives, H. E. (1989). Guanosine 5'-O-(3-thiotrisphosphate) potentiates both thrombin- and platelet derived growth factor-induced inositol phosphate release in permeabilized vascular smooth muscle cells. *J. Biol. Chem.*, **264**, 4391-7.

Hug, H. and Sarre, T. F. (1993). Protein kinase C isoenzymes divergence in signal transduction. *Biochem. J.*, **291**, 329-43.

Ignarro, L. J. and Kadowitz, P. J. (1985). The pharmacological and physiological role of cyclic GMP in vascular smooth muscle relaxation. *Annu. Rev. Pharmacol. Toxicol.*, **25**, 171-91.

Iino, M. (1990). Biphasic Ca^{2+} dependence of inositol 1,4,5-trisphosphate-induced Ca^{2+} release in smooth muscle cells of the guinea pig taeni caeci. *J. Gen. Physiol.*, **95**, 1103-22.

Iino, M., Kobayashi, T., and Endo, M. (1988). Use of ryanodine for functional removal of the calcium store in smooth muscle cells of the guinea-pig. *Biochem. Biophys. Res. Commun.*, **152**, 417-22.

Ikebe, M., Hartshorne, D. J., and Elzinga, M. (1987). Phosphorylation of the 20,000 dalton light chain of smooth muscle myosin by the calcium-activated phospholipid dependent protein kinase. *J. Biol. Chem.*, **262**, 7613-17.

Inaki, M., Yokokura, H., Itoh, T., Kanmura, Y., Kuriyama, H., and Hidaka, H. (1987). Purified rabbit brain protein kinase C relaxes skinned vascular smooth muscle and phosphorylates myosin light chain. *Arch. Biochem. Biophys.*, **254**, 136-41.

Ito, S., Suzuki, S., and Itoh, T. (1993). Effects of a water-soluble forskolin derivative (NKH477) and a membrane permeable cyclic AMP anlogue on noradrenaline-induced Ca^{2+} mobilization in smooth muscle of rabbit mesenteric artery. *Br. J. Pharmacol.*, **110**, 1117-25.

Itoh, H., Higuchi, H., Hiraoka, N., Ito, M., Konishi, T., Nakano, T., et al. (1991). Contraction of rat thoracic aorta strips by endothelin-1 in the absence of extracellular Ca^{2+}. *Brit. J. Pharmacol.*, **104**, 847-52.

Itoh, H., Shimomura, A., Okubo, S., Ichikawa, K., Ito, M., Konishi, T., et al. (1993). Inhibition of myosin light chain phosphatase during Ca^{2+}-independent vasocontraction. *Am. J. Physiol.*, **265**, C1319-24.

Itoh, T., Suzuki, A., and Watanabe, Y. (1994). Effect of a peptide inhibitor of protein kinase C on G protein increase in myofilament Ca^{2+}-sensitivity in rabbit arterial skinned muscle. *Br. J. Pharmacol.*, **111**, 311-17.

Kanaide, H., Shogakiuchi, Y., and Nakamura, M. (1987). The norepinephrine-sensitive Ca^{2+}-storage site differs from the caffeine-sensitive site in vascular smooth muscle of the rat aorta. *FEBS Lett.*, **214**, 130-4.

Kasuya, Y., Takuwa, Y., Yanagisawa, M., Masaki, T., and Goto, K. (1992). A pertussis toxin-sensitive mechanism of endothelin action in porcine coronary artery smooth muscle. *Br. J. Pharmacol.*, **107**, 456-62.

Katsuyama, H., Wang, C.-L. A., and Morgan, K. G. (1992). Regulation of vascular smooth muscle tone by caldesmon. *J. Biol. Chem.*, **267**, 14555-8.

Katz, A., Wu, D., and Simon, M. I. (1992). Subunits βγ of heterotrimeric G protein activate β2 isoform of phospholipase C. *Nature*, **360**, 687-9.

Khalil, R. A. and Morgan, K. G. (1993). PKC-mediated redistribution of mitogen-activated protein kinase during smooth muscle cell activation. *Am. J. Physiol.*, **265**, C406-11.

Khalil, R. A., Lajoie, C., Resnick, M. S., and Morgan, K. G. (1992). Ca^{2+}-independent isoforms of protein kinase C differentially translocate in smooth muscle. *Am. J. Physiol.*, **263**, C714-19.

Kitazawa, T., Gaylinn, B. D., Denney, G. H., and Somlyo, A. P. (1991). G protein mediated Ca^{2+} sensitization of smooth muscle contraction through myosin light chain phosphorylation. *J. Biol. Chem.*, **266**, 1708-15.

Kolch, W., Heidecker, G., Kochs, G., Hummel, R., Vahidi, H., Mischak, H., et al. (1993). Protein kinase Cα-activates Raf-1 by direct phosphorylation. *Nature*, **364**, 249–52.

Kondo, T., Inui, H., Konishi, F., and Inagami, T. (1992). Phospholipase D mimics platelet-derived growth factor as a competence factor in vascular smooth muscle cells. *J. Biol Chem.*, **267**, 23609–16.

Kribben, A., Wieder, E. D., Li, X., Van-Putten, V., Granot, Y., Schrier, R. W., et al. (1993). AVP-induced activation of MAP kinase in vascular smooth muscle cells is mediated through protein kinase C. *Am. J. physiol.*, **265**, C939–45.

Landgraf, W., Ruth, P., Keilbach, A., May, B., Welling, A., and Hofmann, F. (1992). Cyclic GMP-dependent protein kinase and smooth muscle relaxation. *J. Cardiovasc. Pharmacol.*, **20 (Supp. 1)**, S18–22.

Lang, U. and Vallotton, M. B. (1989). Effects of angiotensin II and of phorbol ester on protein kinase C activity and on prostacyclin production in cultured rat aortic smooth-muscle cells. *Biochem. J.*, **259**, 477–84.

Lange-Carter, C. A., Pleiman, C. M., Gardner, A. M., Blumer, K. J., and Johnson, G. L. (1993). A divergence in the MAP kinase regulatory cascade defined by MEK kinase and raf. *Science*, **260**, 315–19.

Lassegue, B., Alexander, R. W., Clark, M., and Griendling, K. K. (1991). Angiotensin II-induced phosphatidylcholine hydrolysis in cultured vascular smooth muscle cells. *Biochem. J.*, **276**, 19–25.

Lassegue, B., Alexander, R. W., Clark, M., Akers, M., and Griendling, K. K. (1993). Phosphatidylcholine is a major source of phosphatidic acid and diacylglycerol in angiotensin II-stimulated vascular smooth muscle cells. *Biochem. J.*, **292**, 509–17.

Lee, K.-M., Toscas, K., and Villereal, M. T. (1993). Inhibition of bradykinin and thapsigargin-induced Ca^{2+} entry by tyrosine kinase inhibitors. *J. Biol. Chem.*, **268**, 9945–8.

Lincoln, T. M. and Cornwell, T. L. (1993). Intracellular cyclic GMP receptor proteins. *FASEB J.*, **7**, 328–38.

Lincoln, T. M., Cornwell, T. L., and Taylor, A. E. (1990). cGMP-dependent protein kinase mediates the reduction of Ca^{2+} by cAMP in vascular smooth muscle cells. *Am. J. Physiol.*, **258**, C399–407.

Lyall, F., Dornan, E. S., McQueen, J., Boswell, F., and Kelly, M. (1992). Angiotensin II increases proto-oncogene expression and phosphoinositide turnover in vascular smooth muscle cells via the activation of the angiotensin II AT1 receptor. *J. Hypertens.*, **10**, 1463–9.

Malarkey, K., Aidulis, D., Paul, A., McLees, A., Gould, G. W., and Plevin, R. (1995). Regulation of vasoconstrictor stimulated tyrosine phosphorylation of mitogen activated protein kinase by multiple protein kinase C dependent pathways. *Cell Signalling* (In press).

Margolis, B. L., Bonventre, J. V., Kremer, S. G., Kudlow, J. E., and Skorecki, K. L. (1988). Epidermal growth factor is synergistic with phorbol esters and vasopressin in stimulating arachidonate release and prostaglandin production in renal glomerular mesangial cells. *Biochem. J.*, **249**, 587–92.

Marrero, M. B., Paxton, W. G., Duff, J. L., and Berk, B. C. (1994). Angiotensin II stimulates tyrosine phosphorylation of phospholipase Cγ 1 in vascular smooth muscle cells. *J. Biol. Chem.*, **269**, 10935–9.

Meldrum, E., Parker, P. J., and Carozzi, A. (1991). The PtdIns-PLC superfamily and signal transduction. *Biochem. Biophys. Acta.*, **1092**, 49–71.

Merkel, L. X., Rivera, L. M., Colussi, D. J., and Perrone, M. H. (1993). Inhibition of EGF-induced vasoconstriction in isolated rabbit aortic rings with the tyrosine kinase inhibitor RG50864. *Biochem. Biophys. Res. Commun.*, **192**, 1319–26.

Molloy, C. J., Taylor, D. S., and Weber, H. (1993). Angiotensin II-stimulation of rapid protein tyrosine phosphorylation and protein kinase activation in rat aortic smooth muscle cells. *J. Biol. Chem.*, **268**, 7338–45.

Morimoto, S., Kim, S., Fukuo, K., Koh, E., Morita, R., Kitano, S., et al. (1990). Participation of both intracellular free Ca^{2+} and protein kinase C in tonic vasoconstriction induced by prostaglandin $F_{2\alpha}$. *Eur. J. Pharmacol.*, **188**, 369–78.

Nabika, T., Nara, Y., Yamori, Y., Lovenberg, W., and Endo, J. (1985). Angiotensin II and phobol ester enhance isoproterenol- and vasoactive intestinal peptide (VIP)-induced cyclic AMP accumlation in vascular smooth muscle cells. *Biochem. Biophys. Res. Commun.*, **131**, 30–6.

Nakajima, S., Fujimoto, M., and Ueda, M. (1993). Spatial changes of $[Ca^{2+}]_i$ and contraction caused by phorbol esters in vascular smooth muscle cells. *Am. J. Physiol.*, **265**, C1138–45.

Nakanishi, H. and Exton, J. H. (1992). Purification and characterisation of the z isoform of protein kinase C from bovine kidney. *J. Biol. Chem.*, **267**, 16347–54.

Neylon, C. B., Nickashin, A., Little, P. J., Tkachuk, V. A., and Bobik, A. (1992). Thrombin-induced Ca^{2+} mobilization in vascular smooth muscle utilizes a slowly ribosylating pertussis toxin-sensitive G protein. *J. Biol Chem.*, **267**, 7295–302.

Nishikawa, M., Hidaka, H., and Adelstein, R. S. (1983). Phosphorylation of a smooth muscle heavy meromyosin by calcium-activated, phospholipid-dependent protein kinase. *J. Biol. Chem.*, **258**, 14069–72.

Nishikawa, M., De Lanerolle, P., Lincoln, T. M., and Adelstein, R. S. (1984). Phosphorylation of mammalian myosin light chain kinases by the catalytic subunit of cyclic AMP-dependent protein kinase and by cyclic GMP-dependent protein kinase. *J. Biol. Chem.*, **259**, 8429–36.

Nishimura, J., Moreland, S., Ahn, H. Y., Kawase, T., Moreland, R. S., and van Bremen, C. (1992). Endothelin increases myofilament sensitivity in a toxin-permeabilized rabbit mesenteric artery. *Circ. Res.*, **71**, 951–9.

Nishizuka, Y. (1988). The molecular heterogeneity of protein kinase C and its implications for cellular regulation. *Nature*, **334**, 661–5.

Noguera, M. A. and D'Ocon, M. P. (1993). Evidence that depletion of internal calcium stores sensitive to noradrenaline elicits a contractile response dependent on extracellular calcium in rat aorta. *Br. J. Pharmacol.*, **110**, 861–7.

Ohanian, J., Ollerenshaw, J., Collins, P., and Heagerty, A. (1990). Agonist-induced production of 1,2 diacyglycerol and phosphatidic acid in intact resistance arteries. *J. Biol. Chem.*, **265**, 8921–8.

Parker, P. J., Kaur, G., Marais, R. M., Mitchell, F., Pears, C., Schaap, D., et al. (1989). Protein kinase C- a family affair. *Mol. Cell. Endocrinol.*, **6S**, 1–11.

Pawson, T. and Gish, G. D. (1992). SH2 and SH3 domains; From structure to function. *Cell*, **71**, 359–62.

Pfeilschifter, J. and Merriweather, C. (1993). Extracellular ATP and UTP activation of phospholipase D is mediated by protein kinase Cε in rat renal mesangial cells. *Br. J. Pharmacol.*, **110**, 847–53.

Phaneuf, S., Berta, P., Le Peuch, C., Haiech, J., and Cavadore, J.-C. (1988). Phorbol ester modulation of cyclic AMP accumulation in a primary culture of rat aortic smooth muscle cells. *J. Pharmacol. Exp. Ther.*, **245**, 1042–7.

Plevin, R. and Wakelam, M. J. O. (1992). Rapid desensitization of vasopressin-stimulated phosphatidylinositol 4,5-bisphosphate and phosphatidycholine hydrolysis questions the role of these pathways in sustained diacylglycerol formation in A10 vascular smooth muscle cells. *Biochem J.*, **285**, 759–66.

Plevin, R., Stewart, A., Paul, A., and Wakelam, M. J. O. (1992). Vasopressin-stimulated

[^{3}H]-inositol phosphate and [^{3}H]-phosphatidylbutanol accumulation in A10 vascular smooth muscle cells. *Br. J. Pharmacol.*, **107**, 109-15.

Putney, J. W. (1986). A model for receptor-regulated calcium entry. *Cell Calcium*, **7**, 1-12.

Pyne, N. J. and Pyne, S. (1993). Cellular signalling pathways in tracheal smooth muscle. *Cell Signal*, **5**, 401-9.

Rapoport, R. M., Draznin, M. P., and Murad, F. (1983). Endothelium-dependent relaxation in rat aorta may be mediated through cyclic GMP-dependent protein phosphorylation. *Nature*, **306**, 174-6.

Rashatwar, S. S., Cornwell, T. L., and Lincoln, T. L. (1987). Effects of 8-bromo-cGMP on Ca^{2+} levels in vascular smooth muscle cells: Possible regulation of Ca^{2+}-ATPase by cGMP-dependent protein kinase. *Proc. Natl. Acad. Sci. USA*, **84**, 5685-9.

Rasmussen, H., Takuwa, Y., and Park, S. (1987). Protein kinase C in the regulation of smooth muscle contraction. *FASEB J.*, **1**, 177-85.

Sato, K., Hori, M., Ozaki, H., Takano-Ohmuro, H., Tsuchiya, T., Sugi, H., *et al.* (1992). Myosin phosphorylation-independent contraction induced by phorbol ester in vascular smooth muscle. *J. Pharmacol. Exp. Ther.*, **261**, 497-505.

Satoh, S., Rensland, H., and Pfitzer, G. (1993). Ras proteins increase Ca^{2+} responsiveness of smooth muscle contraction. *FEBS Lett.*, **324**, 211-15.

Sauro, M. D. and Thomas, B. (1993). Tryphostin attenuates platelet-derived growth factor-induced contraction in aortic smooth muscle through inhibition of protein tyrosine kinase. *J. Pharmacol. Exp. Ther.*, **267**, 1119-23.

Schlessinger, J. (1993). How receptor tyrosine kinases activate Ras. *Trends Biochem. Sci.*, **18**, 273-5.

Seager, J. M., Murphy, T. V., and Garland, C. J. (1994). Importance of inositol (1,4,5)-trisphosphate, intracellular Ca^{2+} release and myofilament Ca^{2+} sensitization in 5-hydroxytryptamine-evoked contraction of rabbit mesenteric artery. *Br. J. Pharmacol.*, **111**, 525-32.

Shimamoto, H., Shimamoto, Y., Kwan, C.-Y., and Daniel, E. E. (1992). Participation of protein kinase C in endothelin-1 induced contraction in rat aorta: studies with a new tool, calphostin C. *Br. J. Pharmacol.*, **107**, 282-7.

Shin, W. S., Toyo-oka, T., Masuo, M., Okai, Y., Fujita, H., and Sugimoto, T. (1991). Subpopulations of rat vascular smooth muscle cells as discriminated by calcium release mechanisms from internal stores. *Circ. Res.*, **69**, 551-6.

Simpson, A. W. M. and Ashley, C. C. (1989). Spontaneous oscillations and agonist evoked changes in Ca^{2+} in cultured smooth muscle cells. *J. Cardio. Pharmacol.*, **14**, S59-62.

Singer, H. A., Oren, J. W., and Benscoter, H. A. (1989). Myosin light chain phosphorylation in ^{32}P rabbit aorta stimulated by phorbol, 12, 13, dibutyrate and phenylephrine. *J. Biol. Chem.*, **264**, 21215-22.

Singer, H. A., Schworer, C. M., Sweeley, C., and Benscoter, H. (1992). Activation of protein kinase C isozymes by contractile stimuli in arterial smooth muscle. *Arch. Biochem. Biophys.*, **299**, 320-9.

Smrcka, A. V., Hepler, J. R., Brown, K. O., and Sternweis, P. C. (1991). Regulation of polyphosphoinositide-specific phospholipase C activity by purified Gq. *Science*, **251**, 804-7.

Sobue, K. and Sellers, J. R. (1991). Caldesmon, A novel regulatory protein in smooth muscle and nonmuscle actinomysin systems. *J. Biol. Chem.*, **266**, 12115-18.

Somlyo, A. P. and Himpens, B. (1989). Cell calcium and its regulation in smooth muscle. *FASEB J.*, **3**, 2266-76.

Somlyo, A. V., Bond, M., Somlyo, A. P., and Scarpa, A. (1985). Inositol trisphosphate induced calcium release and contraction in vascular smooth muscle. *Proc. Natl. Acad. Sci. USA*, **82**, 5231-5.

Strathmann, M. and Simon, M. I. (1990). G protein diversity: A distinct class of α subunit present in vertebrates and invertebrates. *Proc. Natl. Acad. Sci. USA*, **87**, 9113-17.
Sugiura, M., Inagami, T., Hare, M. T., and Johns, J. A. (1989). Endothelin action: inhibition by a protein kinase C inhibitor and involvement of phosphoinositols. *Biochem. Biophys. Res. Commun.*, **158**, 170-6.
Sunako, M., Kawahara, Y., Hirata, K.-I., Tsuda, T., Yokoyama, M., Fukuzaki, H., et al. (1990). Mass analysis of 1,2-diacylglycerol in cultured rabbit vascular smooth muscle cells. *Hypertension*, **15**, 84-8.
Supattapone, S., Danoff, S. K., Theibert, A., Joseph, S. K., Steiner, J., and Snyder, S. H. (1988). Cyclic-AMP dependent phosphorylation of a brain inositol trisphosphate receptor decreases its release of calcium. *Proc. Natl. Acad. Sci. USA*, **85**, 8747-50.
Tang, W. J. and Gilman, A. G. (1992). Adenylyl cyclases. *Cell*, **70**, 869-72.
Tansey, M. G., Luby-Phelps, K., Kamm, K. E., and Stull, J. T. (1994). Ca^{2+} dependent phosphorylation of myosin light chain kinase decreases the Ca^{2+} sensitivity of light chain phosphorylation within smooth muscle cells. *J. Biol. Chem.*, **269**, 9912-20.
Taylor, S. S., Buechler, J. A., and Yonemoto, W. (1990). cAMP-dependent protein kinase: framework for a diverse family of regulatory enzymes. *Annu. Rev. Biochem.*, **59**, 971-1005.
van Corven, E. J., Hordijk, P. L., Medema, R. H., Bos, J. L., and Moolenaar, W. H. (1993). Pertussis toxin-sensitive activation of $p21^{ras}$ by G protein-coupled receptor agonists in fibroblasts. *Proc. Natl. Acad. Sci. USA*, **90**, 1257-61.
Wakelam, M. J. O. (1992). Phosphatidycholine hydrolysis: a multiple messenger generating system. In *Advances in second messenger and phosphoprotein research*, Vol. 28 (ed. B. L. Brown and P. R. M. Dobson), pp. 73-81. Raven Press, NY.
Ways, D. K., Cook, P. P., Webster, C., and Parker, P. J. (1992). Effect of phorbol esters on protein kinase Cz. *J. Biol. Chem.*, **267**, 4799-805.
Weishaar, R. E., Kobylarz-Singer, D., Keiser, J. A., Wright, C. D., Cornicelli, J., and Panek, R. (1991). Cyclic nucleotide phosphodiesterases in the circulatory system: biochemical, pharmacological and functional characteristics. In *Advances in second messenger and phosphoprotein Research*, Vol. 24 (ed. S. J. Strada and H. Hidaka), pp. 249-71. Raven Press, NY.
Wilkes, L. C., Patel, V., Purkiss, J. R., and Boarder, M. R. (1993). Endothelin-1 stimulated phospholipase D in A10 vascular smooth muscle derived cells is dependent on tyrosine kinase. *FEBS Lett.*, **322**, 147-50.
Willis, F. L., McCubbin, W. D., and Kay, C. M. (1994). Smooth muscle calponin-caltropin interaction: Effect on biological activity and stability of calponin. *Biochemistry*, **33**, 5562-9.
Winder, S. J. and Walsh, M. P. (1990). Smooth muscle calponin. Inhibition of actinomyosin MgATPase and regulation by phosphorylation. *J. Biol. Chem.*, **265**, 10148-55.
Wong, A. Y. K. and Klassen, G. A. (1993). A model of calcium regulation in smooth muscle. *Cell Calcium*, **14**, 227-43.
Xuan, Y.-T., Wang, O.-L., and Whorton, A. R. (1992). Thapsigargin stimulates Ca^{2+} entry in vascular smooth muscle cells; nicardipine-sensitive and -insensitive pathways. *Am. J. Physiol.*, **262**, C1258-65.
Yoshida, Y., Sun, H.-T., Cai, J.-Q., and Imai, S. (1991). Cyclic GMP-dependent protein kinase stimulates the plasma membrane Ca^{2+} pump ATPase of vascular smooth muscle via phosphorylation of a 240 kDa protein. *J. Biol. Chem.*, **266**, 19819-25.
Yoshimura, M. and Cooper, D. M. (1993). Type-specific stimulation of adenylylcyclase by protein kinase C. *J. Biol. Chem.*, **268**, 4604-7.

8. Neuroeffector transmission in arteries, arterioles, and veins

Susan E. Luff, G. D. S. Hirst, and T. C. Cunnane

INTRODUCTION

Sympathetic nerve stimulation causes most arteries, arterioles, and veins to contract. This results from an increase in free concentration of calcium ions, $[Ca^{2+}]_i$, inside the smooth muscle cells which make up a part of the walls of arteries, veins, and arterioles. Sympathetic nerve activity can increase $[Ca^{2+}]_i$ in several ways. When a constriction occurs because neurally released noradrenaline activates vascular α-adrenoceptors, $[Ca^{2+}]_i$ is increased by a mechanism that does not rely on the entry of Ca^{2+}, rather Ca^{2+} is released from internal stores (van Helden 1991). This mechanism does not rely on a change in the membrane potential of the vascular smooth muscle cells. Alternatively, sympathetic nerve stimulation may activate a pathway which does not involve α-adrenoceptors (Hirst and Lew 1987). It seems that the sympathetic nerves release a cotransmitter, probably ATP (Sneddon and Burnstock 1984; Kügelgen and Starke 1985). ATP then activates a set of purinoceptors which are linked to cation-selective channels, so producing a membrane depolarization. This depolarization in turn triggers the opening of the voltage-dependent Ca^{2+} channels present in the membranes of vascular smooth muscle cells (see Hirst and Edwards 1989). Thirdly, sympathetic nerves may release vasoactive peptides which produce persistent vasoconstrictions (Wharton and Gulbenkian 1987) by mechanisms which are not well understood. The actions of peptides will not be considered further in this section.

The importance of the membrane potential-dependent and membrane potential-independent mechanisms varies from vascular bed to vascular bed and from species to species. As a generalization, in blood vessels which are normally subjected to low perfusion pressures, i.e. pulmonary arteries and veins the responses to sympathetic nerve stimulation are entirely dependent upon the activation of α-adrenoceptors. In contrast, in fine arterioles of the systemic circulation the sympathetic vasoconstrictor responses are largely resistant to α-adrenoceptor blockade; thus the contractile response appears to result only from the activation of purinoceptors and the subsequent activation of voltage-dependent Ca^{2+} channels. In larger systemic vessels, the responses result from the concurrent activation of purinoceptors and α-adrenoceptors but the proportions vary from vessel to vessel. For example, the contractile responses of isolated rabbit saphenous arteries persist after α-adrenoreceptor blockade (Burnstock and Warland 1987).

Neuroeffector transmission in arteries, arterioles, and veins 185

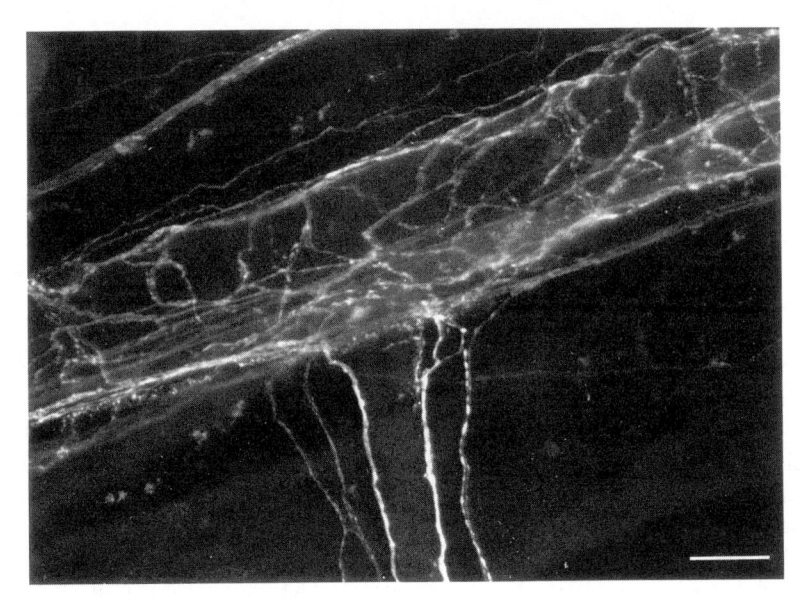

Fig. 8.1 Micrograph of two arterioles from the guinea pig submucosa showing the branching plexus of varicose catecholaminergic axons around the larger vessel but not around the smaller branch. The smaller branch has two non varicose paravascular axon bundles extending along the length of the vessel. The vessels were prepared for fluorescence microscopy using aldehyde fixation after which the axons containing catecholamines fluorescence when illuminated with UV light. Calibration bar 25 μm.

In contrast, α-antagonists block the responses of rabbit isolated ear arteries under most conditions (Kennedy *et al.* 1986). As another example, in dog mesenteric arteries sympathetic nerve responses are barely affected by the addition of α-adrenoceptor antagonists (Murumatsu *et al.* 1984) whilst in the rat they are largely abolished (Angus *et al.* 1988).

This chapter will deal with the structure of sympathetic neuroeffector junctions, the pathways activated by the transmitters released at these junctions, and finally with our understanding of how transmitter is released at individual junctions.

STRUCTURE OF SYMPATHETIC AXONS INNERVATING VASCULAR SMOOTH MUSCLE

The nerves supplying blood vessels are unmyelinated and form a plexus of branching varicose axons (Fig. 8.1) (Hillarp 1946, 1959; Caesar *et al.* 1957; Richardson 1962; Thaemert 1963, 1966; Taxi 1965). The plexus in most blood vessels is situated in the outermost layer of the vessel wall, the adventitia, outside of the layer of contractile smooth muscle cells (the media) (Devine and Simpson 1967; Burnstock and Costa 1975; Bevan 1979). Hence, in vessels with several layers of smooth muscle cells only the muscle cells at the medio-adventitial border can be in direct contact with the axons. There are some exceptions where axons have been reported to ramify the outer two or three layers of smooth muscle cells of some arteries and veins (Keatinge 1966; Fillenz 1967; Tsunekawa et al. 1967; Morhri et al. 1969). The axons innervating the facial vein of the rabbit have been reported to reach the endothelium (Pergram et al. 1976).

The axon plexus around blood vessels is predominantly composed of sympathetic postganglionic axons which are almost all noradrenergic and vasoconstrictor in function. There are a small proportion of cholinergic synthetic fibres which are thought to be vasodilatory and which mainly innervate the larger arterial vessels supplying blood to skeletal muscle (Bülbring and Burn 1936) and muscle of the tongue (Erici et al. 1952). There are some cholinergic parasympathetic axons and sensory axons. The number of non-sympathetic axons around blood vessels varies considerably in different vessels and most of them contain neuropeptides (for recent reviews on this topic see Morris and Gibbins (1992) and Owman (1988)).

Although sympathetic axons occur singly, most are grouped in bundles (Burnstock and Costa 1975; Luff et al. 1987). The axons are usually associated with Schwann cells which wrap around individual axons, or groups of axons within the bundles (Figs 8.2 and 8.3). Each individual axon has a proximal non-varicose region and a distal region with numerous varicosities arranged in series along its length. There are two types of axon bundles; those which contain the more proximal non-varicose region of the axon which is often referred to as the preterminal region and those which contain the more distal varicose or terminal region of the axon. The bundles of preterminal axons are located some distance away from the media and may even occur outside the adventital layer running along the outside of the vessel (i.e. paravascular bundles). These preterminal axon bundles may contain from a few to tens or even hundreds of axons in the case of the paravascular bundles. Some of these axons are presumably travelling down the vessel to innervate more distal regions of the vessel. However, in some tissues, vessels are used by axons as routes to innervate more distal segments of the vascular tree (Bevan et al. 1980; Gabella 1992) and some cases non-vascular effectors. The bundles containing varicose axons are predominantly located close, within 1-2 mm, to the medio-adventitial border. The size of these bundles varies in different vessels ranging from 2-15 axons (Devine and Simpson 1967; Luff et al. 1987, 1991; Klemm et al. 1993). The terminal region of the axon undergoes extensive branching (Luff and McLachlan 1988; Gabella 1992) and it is possible that some branching may also occur in the preterminal regions, though this has not been confirmed.

Each axon bundle is surrounded by a layer of basal lamina which is produced by the Schwann cell and consists of types IV and V collagens, laminin, entactin, and heparan sulfate (Bunge et al. 1986). Although the axons enclosed by Schwann cell are not surrounded by basal lamina, where they become exposed, the exposed regions of plasmalemma are usually covered by basal lamina (Merrillees et al. 1963; Devine and Simpson 1967).

The preterminal axon segments predominantly contain microtubules, neurofilaments with some mitochondria, large dense-core vesicles, occasional small vesicles, and smooth endoplasmic reticulum (Burnstock and Costa 1975). The swellings or varicosities of the distal segment are arranged in series along the length of the axon and are separated by narrow intervaricose regions (intervaricosities) (Merrillees 1968). The varicosities are irregularly distributed along the axon with separations between individual varicosities ranging from almost nothing to >7μm (Luff et al. 1987). The varicosities of axons within individual bundles frequently are clustered together which in fluorescent micrographs, would appear as a single spot. Hence, estimations of varicosity number made from such micrographs may be grossly inaccurate.

The length of the terminal segment and the number of varicosities along individual axons are not known and neither is the extent of the region of vessel that they innervate. However, there is evidence from experiments on the rat tail artery in which a region of the tail was denervated, that axons innervate a few millimetres of this vessel at the most (Sittiracha et al. 1987).

Intervaricosities predominantly contain microtubules, neurofilaments, and occasional mitochondria. The diameter of the intervaricosities varies along the length of individual axons and between axons (Luff and McLachlan 1988). In most vessels they range from 0.1–0.5 μm in diameter and from almost nothing to 10 μm (Devine and Simpson 1967; Burnstock 1986; Luff et al. 1987; Gabella 1992). A recent serial section study of the sympathetic innervation of the cortical arterioles in the kidney has identified two structurally distinct types (I and II) of axon. The type I axons have larger intervaricosity diameters (range 0.15–0.86 μm) than the type II axons (range 0.05–0.13 μm). Type I axons are predominantly located on afferent arterioles whereas type II occur with similar densities on both afferent and efferent arterioles (Luff et al. 1991). This suggests that the two types of axons may have different functions.

Sympathetic varicosities contain numerous vesicles, one or two mitochondria, and some smooth endoplasmic reticulum. They also contain neurofilaments and microtubules. Microtubules enter the varicosities from the intervaricose segments, but do not usually extend across an entire varicosity (Devine and Simpson 1967; Luff et al. 1987; Gabella 1992). Vesicles within the varicosities contain neurotransmitter and consequently are believed to be sites for neurotransmitter release (Bennett and Burnstock 1968; Furness 1970; Geffen and Livett 1971). Varicosities have generally been regarded as having a fusiform shape (Devine et al. 1971; Burnstock and Costa 1975) however more recent studies involving reconstructions of varicosities from serial sections have shown that they can be complex in shape (Luff et al. 1987; Luff and McLachlan 1988). This is commonly observed for axons contained in bundles where varicosities of adjacent axons are twisted around one another whereas, varicosities of axons occurring singly (Luff et al. 1991; Klemm et al. 1993) are more likely to be fusiform in shape. The size of varicosities has been variably reported as 1–3 μm in diameter and up to 4 μm in length (Gabella 1992), and 0.4–2 μm in diameter and 0.5–3 μm in length (Burnstock and Costa 1975), and 0.25–3 μm (Luff et al. 1987, 1991). There is some evidence that the mean size of varicosities is different in different tissues and may become smaller towards the distal end of the axon (Klemm *et al.* 1993; Luff unpublished data).

Three types of vesicles are found in sympathetic varicosities, many granular and agranular small vesicles (30–60 nm in diameter) and a few dense-cored vesicles (60–150 nm in diameter) (Geffen and Livett 1971). Noradrenaline is contained in both large and small vesicles. In addition both large and small vesicles contain adenosine 5'-triphosphate (ATP) (Klein and Lagercrantz 1981); in many vessels ATP appears to act as the major neurotransmitter released by sympathetic nerve stimulation. It has recently been postulated that the relative quantities of ATP and noradrenaline contained within a single small synaptic vesicle may vary in different vessels (Burnstock 1990). There are suggestions that the presence of small granular vesicles indicates that axons contain catecholamines, whereas those containing small agranular vesicles are cholinergic. This differentiation seems unlikely, the preservation of granules in vesicles and the proportion of agranular vesicles is significantly affected by different fixatives, and by drugs that increase the levels of noradrenaline in the nerves (Hökfelt and Jonasson 1968; Tranzer *et al.* 1969). (For a fixation method to preserve the granular nature of vesicles in varicosities of catecholaminergic axons, see Tranzer and Richards 1976.) Other methods for identifying adrenergic axons are those using 5- and 6-hydroxydopamine (Furness and Costa 1975), glyoxylic acid (Axelsson *et al.* 1973), and immunohistochemical methods (e.g. using antibodies to tyrosine hydroxylase). The number of vesicles contained in a varicosity is variable and again can be affected by fixation procedures (Burnstock and Costa 1975) although there appears to be a direct correlation between the size of varicosities and the number of vesicles (Luff *et al.* 1987).

Although noradrenaline in sympathetic varicosities is predominantly located in vesicles it also exists in the cytosol (Tranzer 1972). It is generally agreed that the neurotransmitter released by sympathetic nerve activity originates from the vesicular stores rather than the cytosol (Iversen *et al.* 1965; Potter 1967; Häggendal and Malmfors 1969; Smith *et al.* 1970; Smith and Winkler 1972). Transmitter release is thought to result from exocytosis involving specific phosphoproteins located on the membrane surface of the vesicle and the membrane. A number of proteins have been identified on the membranes of synaptic vesicles which are thought to regulate the number of vesicles available for exocytosis. These include synapsins I and II, synaptogamin, syntaxin, synaptophysin, symnaptoporin, and p29 protein. For recent reviews on this topic see Bennett *et al.* (1992), Greengard *et al.* (1993). An alternative proposal to exocytosis for the release of neurotransmitter from axon terminals is a cation exchange process across the varicosity membrane at points where vesicles are attached (Uvnäs and Åborg 1980).

Neuropeptides are stored in the larger vesicles from which they are believed to be released, particularly during trains of stimuli. Neuropeptides are manufactured in the perikaryon and stored in the large granular vesicles (Fried and Lundberg 1985; De Deyn *et al.* 1989) which are then transported via the axoplasm to the varicosities (Geffen and Ostberg 1969). Conversely, small synaptic vesicles are predominantly manufactured in the varicosity (Hökfelt 1973).

STRUCTURE OF SYMPATHETIC NEUROVASCULAR JUNCTIONS

Organized neuromuscular junctions have been described in a large number of muscular arteries and veins (Luff *et al.* 1987, 1991; Luff and McLachan 1989; Klemm *et al.* 1993). Each of these vessels readily respond to sympathetic nerve stimulation. Organized neuroeffector junctions have not been detected in elastic arteries and a few cerebral arteries; conversely these only respond to high frequency repetitive nerve stimulation (for further discussion see Luff and McLachlan 1989).

Early studies on the relationship between varicosities and vascular smooth muscle cells conducted on single random sections reported that although some varicosities were observed to oppose smooth muscle cells closely, the majority were not. The closest appositions found were between 50 and 100 nm, always with a single intervening layer of basal lamina (Appenzeller 1964; Lever *et al.* 1965a,b; Devine and Simpson 1967; Rhodin 1967; Iwayama *et al.*, 1970; Nelson and Rennels 1970; Burnstock and Iwayama 1971; Govyrin 1976; Bevan *et al.* 1980; Lee 1981a,b; Moffat 1981; Osswald and Guimaraes 1983; Rowan and Bevan 1983; Cowen 1984; Matsuyama *et al.* 1985). However, even in small arteriolar vessels, fewer than 4% of varicosities were reported to be less than 100 nm from smooth muscle membranes (Devine and Simpson 1967). In addition, these studies on single random sections did not identify any consistent association of vesicles with the presynaptic membrane or structural specialization of the pre- and postsynaptic membrane. From this it was concluded that specialized neuromuscular junctions do not exist on blood vessels. This view was supported by reports of the existence of 'close contacts' on smooth muscle cells of some non-vascular smooth muscle cells such as the guinea-pig vas deferens (Merrillees 1968), sphincter pupillae (Uehara and Burnstock 1972; Gabella 1974), rabbit iris (Richardson 1964), and the nictitating membrane of the cat (Evans and Evans 1964), where the width of the synaptic cleft was 20 nm with no intervening basal lamina. Such close neuromuscular contacts have rarely been found in blood vessels. However, these 'close contacts' were observed infrequently in most of these tissues, whereas neuromuscular contacts with a junctional cleft of the order of 50-100 nm and containing a single layer of basal lamina (i.e. similar to those found on blood vessels) were more frequently encountered although Gabella (1974) reported that ~50% of varicosities formed close (20 nm) contacts in the guinea-pig sphincter pupillae.

More recent quantitative serial section ultrastructural studies investigating the structure of axons around a number of different vessels in serial sections using computer assisted reconstruction (Luff *et al.* 1987, 1991, 1992; Luff and McLachlan, 1988; Klemm *et al.* 1993) have changed our views on the fine structure of the innervation of blood vessels and in particular the structural relationship between axons and vascular smooth muscle cells and the structure of neurovascular junctions. In guinea-pig submucous arterioles it has been found that most varicosities (i.e. 83% and 92%) form neuromuscular junctions with 50-100 nm neuromuscular cleft widths (Luff *et al.* 1987). These results concur with the physiological results of Hirst and Neild (1981) on the same tissue which suggest that in these vessels neuromuscular transmission occurs predominantly at these junctions. Three-dimensional reconstructions of individual varicosities forming junctions with smooth muscle cells also showed that the varicosities have specialized features with many of the characteristics of axon terminals on skeletal muscle. Additional serial section studies on rat and rabbit renal cortical arterioles (Luff *et al.* 1992) and guinea-pig mesenteric vein (Klemm *et al.* 1993) have confirmed that at least in these vessels, most varicosities form neuromuscular junctions.

The structure of sympathetic neuroeffector junctions has been found to be essentially similar in all vessels (Figs 8.2 and 8.3). The synaptic cleft is always less than 100 nm wide and contains a single layer of basal lamina which appears to be formed by the fusion of the basal lamina around the axon with that around the smooth muscle. The small synaptic vesicles are clustered at the presynaptic membrane. Some junctions also have a small region of the presynaptic membrane which appears thickened and electron dense, at which vesicles are clustered (Fig. 8.3). Such a structure can usually be seen in two or more successive sections (Luff and McLachlan 1988). However, a consistent postsynaptic structural specialization has not been found in any electron microscopical studies of vascular smooth muscle. Consequently, it has been questioned as to whether sympathetic neuromuscular junctions constitute a true specialized junction (Burnstock 1986; Gabella 1992). There has only been one freeze-fracture study on intramembrane ultrastructure (Devine *et al.* 1971) and the authors found 'no clear modification of the smooth muscle membrane at the site of neuromuscular contact'. However, it is probable that the authors did not fracture through a vascular neuromuscular junction as the membrane separation was greater than 100 nm. It remains to be determined if any intramembrane particles exist at sympathetic neuromuscular junctions or if sympathetic neuromuscular junctions have postsynaptic receptor or ion channel specialization as is found at skeletal neuromuscular junctions (Burden 1985; Magill *et al.* 1987).

The size of varicosities and area of neuromuscular contact varies considerably, the latter ranging from 0.02–$3\,\mu m^2$. Similarly the number of small (50 nm) synaptic vesicles per junction also varies but is generally directly proportional to the size of the varicosity (Luff *et al.* 1987). Presynaptic membrane specializations have only been observed at a proportion of neuromuscular junctions but in the vessels in which these have been quantified the value is similar, i.e. 15, 15, and 24% in guinea-pig submucous arterioles, rabbit renal arterioles, and guinea-pig mesenteric veins respectively (Luff and McLachlan 1988; Luff *et al.* 1992; Klemm *et al.* 1993). The functional significance of their presence or absence and the differences in their size (range 0.006–$0.8\,\mu m^2$) is not known. Since it appears that the probability of release of transmitter from individual varicosities is very low (Hirst and Neild 1981; Åstrand and Stjärne 1989*a,b*; Brock and Cunnane 1993) and that the probability may be greater at some varicosities than at others (Lavidis and Bennett 1992), it is possible that those junctions with specializations have a higher probability of release.

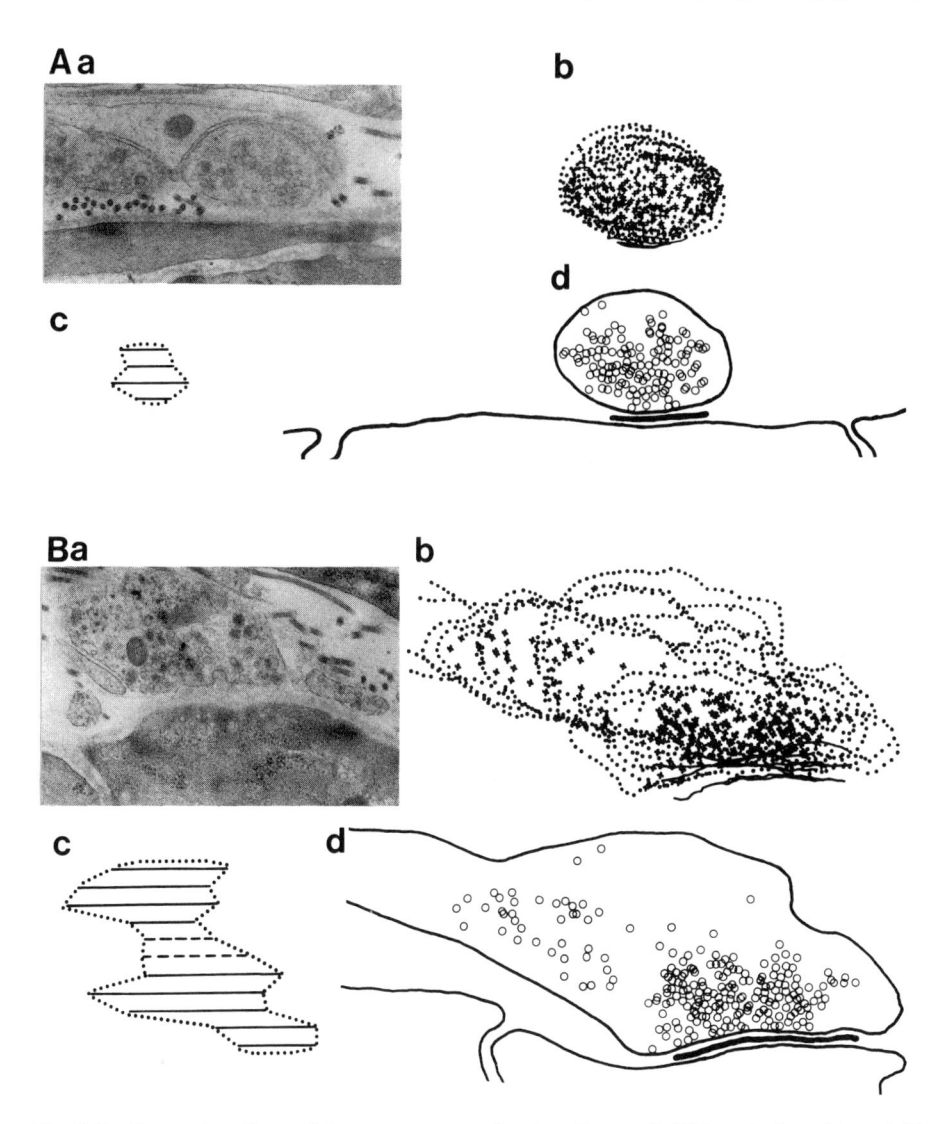

Neuroeffector transmission in arteries, arterioles, and veins 191

Fig. 8.2 Reconstruction of two neuromuscular junctions of different sizes (A and B) showing the main structural characteristics. In each set of figures for each junction, (a) shows a micrograph through the middle of the contact regions of two varicosities; (b) shows the superimposition of all of the axon profiles obtained in each series of sections (dotted lines), the small diameter synaptic vesicles (crosses) and the regions of fused basal lamina (solid lines); (c) shows the outlines of each contact region, viewed perpedicular to the sections shown in (b); and (d) presents diagrammatic representations of the two reconstructed varicosities. Calibration bar of 1 μm applies throughout figure. From Luff *et al.* (1987), reprinted by permission.

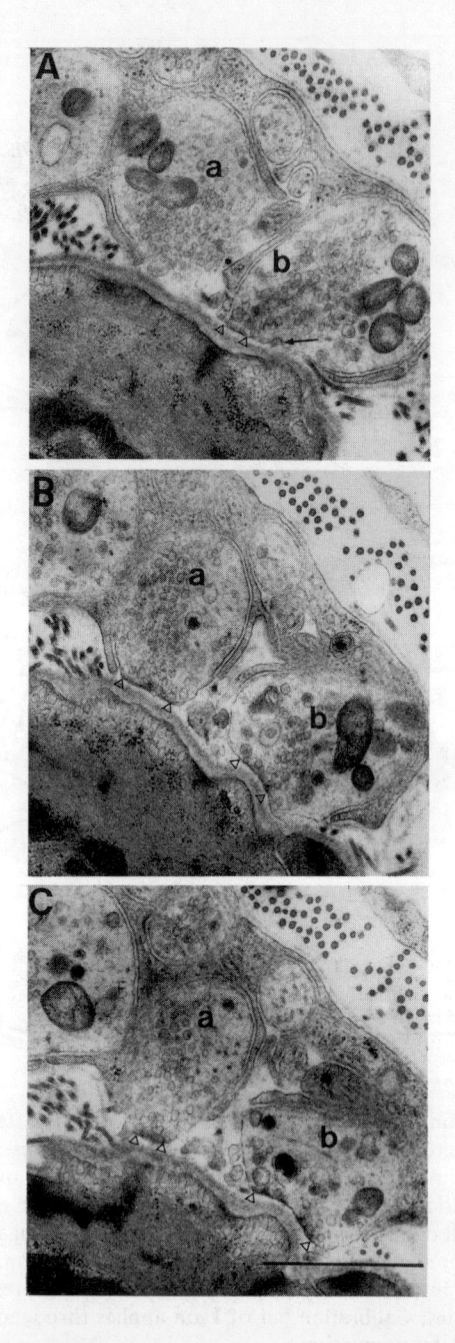

Fig. 8.3 Serial sections through two neuromuscular junctions formed by varcosities (a and b) with a single smooth muscle cell of a small submucous arteriole of the guinea-pig. Prejunctional membrane specializations, seen as electron dense membrane thickenings associated with clusters of synaptic vesicles, are indicated by Δ. The plates A, B, and C,

DISTRIBUTION OF NEUROMUSCULAR JUNCTIONS ALONG BLOOD VESSELS

Neuromuscular junctions are not evenly distributed but commonly occur in clusters. Hence, a single muscle cell frequently has more than one adjacent junction. The physiological significance of this arrangement of junctions is not clear but it is possible that juxtaposition of neuromuscular junctions may be important in modulating the release of neurotransmitter from adjacent varicosities. However, physiological studies have failed to demonstrate that exogenous noradrenaline regulates it own release locally in the guinea-pig vas deferens (Brock and Cunnane 1990). In addition a single varicosity may also form a junction across two adjacent smooth muscle cells.

The density of neurovascular junctions is different in different vessels. In general, the density is inversely related to vessel diameter (Luff and McLachlan 1989). However in some arterial beds the terminal arterioles become devoid of innervation (e.g. cerebral arterioles, Hill *et al.* 1986) or the innervation is restricted to the vessel branch points (e.g. submucous arterioles, Luff and McLachlan 1988). A further exception to this generalization is found in large thermoregulatory arteries, such as the rat tail and rabbit ear arteries which have a very high density of junctions when compared to systemic arteries of similar size (Luff and McLachlan 1989). Studies of larger (50 μm diameter) gut arterioles and the renal afferent arteriole suggest that in these vessels all smooth muscle cells receive at least one junction (Luff *et al.* 1987, 1991), whereas in the small gut terminal arterioles only the smooth muscle cells at the vessel branch points receive neuromuscular junctions (Luff and McLachlan 1988). Obviously, in vessels with more than one layer of smooth muscle cells, where the innervation is restricted to the medio-adventitial border, only the outer layer of cells can receive neuromuscular junctions.

NEUROMUSCULAR TRANSMISSION INVOLVING THE ACTIVATION OF α-ADRENOCEPTORS

In pulmonary arteries and veins, sympathetic nerve stimulation produces membrane depolarizations that last for many tens of seconds (Suzuki 1981, 1983; van Helden 1988*a*). When triggered by only a few stimuli, the membrane potential changes occur after a long latency, 1-2 sec and are of small amplitude, some 2-3 mV. Repetitive nerve stimulation causes larger more sustained depolarizations but the latency to onset remains unchanged. In both types of vessels the potential change becomes complex, often a transient component occurs at the

---

are successive sections at 0.2 μm intervals. The *arrow* in (A) points to a coated vesicle that is open to the junctional cleft. Calibration bar of 1 μm applies throughout the figure. From Luff and Mclachlan, (1988), reprinted by permission.

start of the response and it is followed by the sustained component. Both components are blocked by α-adrenoceptor antagonists (Suzuki 1981, 1983; van Helden 1988b). The process of neuromuscular transmission has been analysed in detail in mesenteric veins (van Helden 1988a,b, 1991). In these vessels an ongoing discharge of spontaneous transient depolarizations, s.t.ds, is detected. S.t.ds increase in frequency shortly after a period of sympathetic nerve stimulation, thus summing to give the slow excitatory junction potential. However s.t.ds do not result from the spontaneous release of quanta of transmitter from sympathetic nerve terminals, rather they appear to result from the irregular pulsatile release of Ca^{2+} from internal stores (van Helden 1991). After release from the internal stores, as well as activating contractile proteins, Ca^{2+} activates a set of Cl^- selective channels present in the membranes of these cells (van Helden 1991). It is not clear whether the resulting depolarization contributes to venoconstriction.

It is of interest to note that this form of transmission is the first to occur in systemic arteries, before the innervation is mature. A few days after the sympathetic innervation has first appeared, repetitive sympathetic nerve stimulation produces a slow membrane depolarization that is blocked by α-adrenoceptor antagonists. A few days later single stimuli initiate depolarizations which are not blocked by α-adrenoceptor antagonists (Hill *et al.* 1983). The period over which this developmental change occurs corresponds to the period over which the mean systemic blood pressure of rats rises towards the value recorded in adult animals.

NEUROMUSCULAR TRANSMISSION INVOLVING THE ACTIVATION OF PURINOCEPTORS

In all mammalian arteries sympathetic nerve stimulation triggers a sequence of membrane potential changes quite different to those recorded from veins (Hottenstein and Kreulen 1987). A single sympathetic nerve stimulus initiates a membrane depolarization, termed an excitatory junction potential or e.j.p. E.j.ps by themselves do no initiate contraction, rather several e.j.ps must sum to give a depolarization of some 15-20 mV before threshold is reached for voltage-dependent Ca^{2+} channels to be activated (Hirst 1977; Blakely *et al.* 1981; Hirst and Edwards 1989). When this occurs a contraction ensues. Unlike the slow responses detected in veins, the rapid e.j.ps recorded from arterial preparations (and vas deferens) are resistant to α-adrenoceptor blockade (Burnstock and Holman 1964; Holman and Surprenant 1980a; Angus *et al.* 1988).

If the stimulus is applied close to the recording point, e.j.ps are seen to have short latencies, 10-20 ms. Typically such e.j.ps have total durations of about 1 s. For example, an e.j.p. recorded from a submucosal arteriole has a time to peak potential of 100 ms and then decays with a time constant of 500 ms (Hirst and Neild 1978). E.j.ps with very similar time courses have been recorded from many different systemic arteries and arterioles taken from a wide variety of species (Bell 1969; Holman and Surprenant 1980b; Cheung 1982b; Hill *et al.* 1983; Itoh *et al.* 1983; Ishikawa 1985; Cheung and Fujikoa 1987; Hottenstein and Kreulen 1987;

Kajiwara *et al.* 1987). Sympathetic nerve stimulation evokes e.j.ps, very similar to those recorded from arteries, in vas deferens of many species (Burnstock and Holman 1961; Bennett 1972). Since it seems likely that the same sequence of events underlies the generation of e.j.ps in these different tissues, reference to results on vas deferens, where relevant, will be included in this chapter. In passing it should be noted that even though the e.j.ps of either tissue have slow time courses compared to those of most other excitatory synaptic potentials recorded from neuronal or skeletal synapses, their time courses are faster than those of junction potentials recorded from any other autonomic organs.

The time course of the excitatory junctional current, e.j.c., underlying an e.j.p. is brief. When measured directly from submucosal arterioles using a single electrode voltage-clamp technique (Finkel *et al.* 1984) the peak current occurred after 10 ms and current had a total duration of about 200 ms. After the peak, the decay of current could be described by a single exponential with a time constant of 50 ms. These observations indicate that the long time course of an e.j.p. reflects the long membrane time constant of arteriolar smooth muscle. Clearly since one frequently has to sum together successive e.j.ps to reach threshold for the initiation of voltage-dependent Ca^{2+} entry, any agent which makes the membranes of arteries more leaky will make it more unlikely that this threshold is reached.

An alternative way of determining the duration of junctional current flow relies on the application of the extracellular recording technique (Brock and Cunnane 1988). With this technique a large electrode is placed near a varicosity. When transmitter causes current to flow across the membrane of the cell under the electrode, a voltage change is detected which has the same time course as that of the junctional current. Using this method to record e.j.cs in arteries (and in the vas deferens), it has been found that sympathetic nerve stimulation causes a brief current flow (Åstrand *et al.* 1988). An indirect way in which the time course of e.j.cs can be determined is to record an e.j.p. from a particular artery and then to determine the membrane time constant of the vessel. The time course of the e.j.c. can then be calculated (see Hirst and Neild 1978). When this was done with submucosal arterioles, rabbit saphenous arteries or rat tail arteries, the calculated e.j.cs were again found to be brief (Hirst and Neild 1978; Holman and Surprenant 1979, 1980*b*; Cassell *et al.* 1988). The time constants of decay of the e.j.ps were the same as the resting membrane time constants (Hirst and Neild 1978; Holman and Surprenant 1980*b*; Cassell *et al.* 1988), indicating that the membrane time constant determines the duration of the e.j.p. Little is known about the processes responsible for the inactivation of current flowing during an e.j.c. Although the time course of an e.j.c. is very brief when compared to that resulting from the activation of α-adrenoceptors, it is long when compared with the synaptic currents found at the skeletal neuromuscular junction (Katz 1969), at autonomic ganglia (Rang 1981), or central nervous system synapses (Jack *et al.* 1975). The rapid onset of current suggests that the sympathetic transmitter is activating a ligand-gated channel. Presumably the decay phase reflects a slow rate of closure of such ligand-gated channels.

The amplitudes of e.j.cs depend upon the membrane potential at which they are recorded. They increase linearly with hyperpolarization and decrease linearly with depolarization (Finkel *et al.* 1984). Their reversal potential, the membrane potential where inward current just equals outward current, is about 0 mV; thus the ligand-gated channels must resemble the cation-selective channels activated by acetylcholine at the skeletal neuromuscular junction.

Most muscle cells in an arteriole are directly innervated and hence may be directly activated by transmitters. However in larger vessels most cells are not directly innervated with the innervation being restricted to the medio-adventitial border. For the membrane potentials of all cells to be changed during sympathetic neuromuscular transmission, some of the junctional current generated on the outer most layer of muscle cells must flow to the deeper non-innervated cells. This occurs because individual vascular smooth muscle cells are electrically connected to their neighbouring cells. Such electrical coupling has been demonstrated in many preparations. The analyses show that many arterial preparations behave as simple linear cables with electrical length constants in the range 0.3–1.5 mm (Bolton 1974; Mekata 1974; Casteels *et al.* 1977; Holman and Surprenant 1980; Kajiwara *et al.* 1981; Cassel *et al.* 1988). Electrical coupling between arterioler cells has been demonstrated more directly using two independent intracellular electrodes, one to pass current and the other to record potential changes (Hirst and Neild 1978, 1980). As individual cells have a circumferential organization, the two electrodes could not have been in the same cell. When a small current was passed through one electrode, it caused a membrane potential change at the second electrode. Again some of the injected current must have flowed to the recording point via low resistance pathways between cells.

In vessels where purinergic e.j.ps are detected, in the absence of stimulation and ongoing discharge of spontaneous excitatory junction potentials, s.e.j.ps are detected (Hirst 1977; Hirst and Neild 1980; Cheung 1982*b*). These are thought to reflect the spontaneous release of individual quanta of transmitter. In a complex structure such as a thick walled artery (and vas deferens) their shapes and their contribution to evoked potentials is difficult to analyse. However in short isopotential segments of arteriole, many of these complications are avoided. When s.e.j.ps were examined in short arteriolar segments they were found to have mean amplitudes of some 2–3 mV (Hirst and Neild 1980). A calculation, using the measured resting membrane properties of the arteriolar segments, suggested that the underlying spontaneous excitatory junctional currents (s.e.j.cs) had peak amplitudes of some 0.1–0.2 nA (Hirst and Neild 1980). This was subsequently confirmed by direct measurement with a voltage-clamp; the underlying peak conductance change was found to be 1.5–3.0 nS (Finkel *et al.* 1984). The peak amplitude of an s.e.j.c. is small when compared to that of a miniature end-plate current recorded from skeletal muscle (Gage 1976) but is similar to that of spontaneous excitatory synaptic currents (s.e.s.c.) recorded from autonomic ganglion cells (Rang 1981). At ganglionic synapses, fewer acetylcholine channels are activated during a s.e.s.c. than the number of molecules of acetylcholine in a vesicle. This suggests that there are only about 100 subsynaptic acetylcholine receptors present to be activated (Hirst and McLachlan 1984). Presumably a similar number of receptor operated channels must be present at each arteriolar neuroeffector junction.

The responses produced by arterioles during sympathetic nerve activity are modified by metabolic products released from the organ to which they supply blood. Metabolic products which participate in the process of autoregulatory control include:

(a) Changes in pH resulting from variations in tissue production of carbon dioxide. A reduction in pH increases the threshold for voltage-dependent Ca^{2+} entry into vascular smooth muscle; conversely an increase in pH lowers the threshold for Ca^{2+} entry to such an extent that rhythmic myogenic activity may occur. Thus as a tissue increases its carbon dioxide production, the local pH will fall and Ca^{2+} entry will be reduced. Conversely during hypocapnia, arteries will become more excitable (Hirst et al. 1992).

(b) The resting membrane potential and membrane resistance of arterioles is largely determined by the activity of inward rectifier K^+ channels in their membranes (Edwards and Hirst 1988; Edward et al. 1988). The activation potential of these channels is very sensitive to $[K^+]_o$. An increase in $[K^+]_o$ moves the activation potential of arteriolar inward rectifier K channels to more positive potentials so making the cells more leaky. The most obvious consequence is that at potentials near rest, the duration of e.j.ps are dramatically reduced; the ability of such potentials to sum to the threshold for voltage-dependent Ca^{2+} entry to occur is reduced. Since many nerve and muscle cells release small amounts of K^+ during electrical activity, the resulting changes in $[K^+]_o$ will act to reduce arteriolar excitability.

(c) Many cells release nucleotides during metabolic activity. The major product of nucleotide breakdown is adenosine which inhibits the release of transmitter from sympathetic nerves (Kuriyama and Makita 1983). Adenosine also suppresses Ca^{2+} entry into arterial smooth muscle (Harder et al. 1979).

Thus the accumulation of these three metabolic products will oppose the effects of sympathetic nerve stimulation and so enhance the blood supply to the organ.

IDENTITY OF TRANSMITTER PRODUCING α-ANTAGONIST RESISTANT e.j.ps IN ARTERIES AND ARTERIOLES

There are many lines of evidence that support the idea that e.j.ps in arterioles and arteries result from the release of ATP and subsequent activation of purinoceptors. However a few problems remain before this hypothesis can be fully accepted. The basis of the purinergic hypothesis lies with the finding that ATP causes an α-adrenoceptor antagonist resistant depolarization in a wide variety of blood vessels (Suzuki 1985; Benham et al. 1987; Hirst and Jobling 1989).

Furthermore each of the ATP analogues, α-β-methylene ATP and ANAPP$_3$, prevents both the α-adrenoceptor antagonist resistant neuronally-mediated responses and the contractions that follow P$_2$ purinoceptor activation (Fedan *et al.* 1981; Sneddon and Burnstock 1984; Burnstock and Warland 1987; Cheung and Fujioka 1987; Hirst and Jobling 1989). Arguments against the ATP hypothesis relate to the ability of sympathetic nerves to release ATP from sympathetically innervated preparations. Although release undoubtably occurs (Lew and White 1987) the majority is released by muscle cells (Kügelgen and Starke 1991) and it is not clear whether sufficient ATP is released from varicosities to initiate e.j.ps. Furthermore isolated small granular vesicles, the vesicles which are held to contain noradrenaline and ATP in peripheral sympathetic nerve, contain only about 50 molecules of ATP and 3000 molecules of noradrenaline (Fried 1980; Fried *et al.* 1984). When ATP acts on single isolated arterial cells it activates channels of small conductance, about 5 pS (Benham and Tsei 1987). Since the conductance change underlying an s.e.j.p. is about 2 nS some 400 ATP-gated channels must be opened (Finkel *et al.* 1984). Thus there are insufficient ATP molecules in a single vesicle to cause a s.e.j.p. unless as suggested earlier that some vesicles are devoid of ATP whereas others contain high concentrations. In the vas deferens it has been recently shown that although suramin is an effective blocker of e.j.ps, it is ineffective at blocking the effects of applied ATP in this tissue (Reilly and Hirst 1995). Finally the channels opened by ATP in vascular smooth muscle show a high selectivity for Ca^{2+} (Benham 1989), they only open after a latency of about 50 msec and display rectification (Benham *et al.* 1987). E.j.ps occur with latencies much less than this and appear by themselves not to cause a contraction (Hirst 1977); there is no evidence that the underlying current shows membrane potential-dependent rectification (Finkel *et al.* 1984). One explanation for each of these observations would be that ATP activates a specialized junctional purinoceptor. These receptors must be coupled to channels that have a high conductance, little selectivity towards [Ca^{2+}]$_i$, be blocked by suramin, fail to rectify, and open rapidly on the application of ATP. Such channels have not yet been identified in vascular smooth muscle. Furthermore it has been pointed out that veins and pulmonary arteries only generate α-antagonist sensitive responses following sympathetic nerve stimulation (Suzuki 1981, 1983; van Helden 1988*a*). These types of vessel respond to ATP (Burnstock and Brown 1981) and the sympathetic nerves innervating these vessels have been shown to release labelled nucleotides (Su 1975). Some explanation is required as to why these vessels do not produce α-adrenoceptor antagonist resistant e.j.ps.

THE RELEASE OF TRANSMITTER FROM INDIVIDUAL SYMPATHETIC VARICOSITIES

At the outset it should be stated that we can only discuss the release of sympathetic transmitter from the sympathetic varicosities that innervate arteries, arterioles, and vas deferens. To be able to describe the release of transmitter from single, or a group of varicosities, it is necessary that a quantum of transmitter is able to produce a detectable response. At this stage, quantal responses produced when sympathetic nerves release noradrenaline cannot be detected: either they produce too small a potential change or they simply do not exist. The following discussion will therefore be limited to transmission at junctions where an α-adrenoceptor antagonist resistant e.j.p. is detected. There is now uniform acceptance that the likelihood of a sympathetic varicosity releasing transmitter with each nerve impulse is very low. That is, release is considered to be intermittent.

The idea that sympathetic varicosities might only release transmitter intermittently first came from the pioneering studies of Burnstock and Holman (1961). They pointed out that although most e.j.ps recorded during a single impalement had smooth rising phases, during a sequence of stimuli, a few e.j.ps had briefer rising phases. They commented that if these resulted from the local release of a packet of transmitter, that event was rare. This idea was taken up and analysed in more detail by Blakeley and Cunnane (1979). They differentiated the rising phases of many successive e.j.ps and confirmed that the likelihood that a quantum of transmitter would be released near the recording electrode was extremely low. At the same time the properties of s.e.j.ps and e.j.ps were compared in short isopotential segments of arteriole (Hirst and Neild 1980). It was found that under these conditions, s.e.j.ps and e.j.ps had identical shapes. S.e.j.ps were found to have a tight unimodal amplitude distribution. It was also noted that the size of an evoked potential was either the same as, or a small multiple, of that of an s.e.j.p. Since the preparations were found to contain some 100 to 200 individual varicosities these observations suggested that:

(a) S.e.j.ps must arise from similarly organized neuroeffector junctions.

(b) Either the probability of release from an individual varicosity per nerve impulse must be very low or that most varicosities must not release transmitter.

This ambiguity was resolved when it became possible to simultaneously record the arrival of the nerve impulse in a pool of varicosities and the output of transmitter from that pool of varicosities (Cunnane and Stjärne 1982; Brock and Cunnane 1988). This was done by placing an extracellular recording pipette on the surface of the vas deferens. The arrival of a nerve impulse was signalled by a brief diphasic potential. A few milliseconds after this, if a quantum of transmitter was released from one of the varicosities under the pipette, a long lasting monophasic potential change was detected. Histological studies suggested that the pipettes might cover an area containing some 50 to 100 individual varicosities. Using this technique it was shown that:

(a) With each stimulus a nerve impulse invariably invaded the nerve terminal.

(b) At low frequencies of stimulation, the release of a quantum of transmitter was a very rare event.

(c) Quantal responses often had characteristic shapes that corresponded to those that occurred spontaneously.

(d) The output of transmitter per nerve impulse was dramatically increased when the frequency of nerve stimulation was increased.

(e) The interval between the arrival of the nerve impulse and the release of transmitter was very short, some 1–3 ms.

(f) The duration of transmitter action was brief when compared to the time course of an e.j.p. recorded in the same preparation.

(g) Release only occurred if an action potential spread actively into a varicosity: the depolarization produced by the passive spread of depolarization into a pool of varicosities was inadequate to evoke release.

(h) The release of transmitter was prevented by activation of prejunctional α-adrenoceptors.

More recently this technique has been further refined so that the release of transmitter from only a few or a single varicosity was detected. Essentially the same observations were made (Lavidis and Bennett 1992). Release was found to be monoquantal but it was found that there was considerable variation in the probability of release from various release points. Each of these points has been subsequently reconfirmed on arterial and arteriolar smooth muscle preparations (Astrand and Stjärne 1989*a,b*; Brock and Cunnane 1993).

Thus in summary at purinergic sympathetic nerve junctions, the probability of release of transmitter is very low. When release occurs it appears to result from the release of a single quantum of transmitter at an individual neuroeffector junction. Since there is little variance in the shape of quantal responses recorded from a pool of varicosities, one might expect release to occur at the structured neuroeffector junctions found in arteriolar tissues. Presumably this is the same for arterial (and vas deferens) sympathetic neuroeffector junctions.

TROPHIC EFFECTS OF SYMPATHETIC NERVES

In some arterial beds the electrical properties of arterioles appear to change as the density of sympathetic innervation changes. In the cerebral circulation (Hill *et al.* 1986), the innervation density falls as the arterioles branch to give rise to vessels of smaller diameter. As the vessels became smaller, and hence less densely innervated, the muscle action potentials, initiated by direct stimulation, had slower rates of rise and less marked plateau components. When the amplitudes of the voltage-dependent Ca^{2+} currents were measured in segments of different diameter, this was found to result from a fall in current density along the arteriolar tree. No obvious differences in the thresholds of the Ca^{2+} currents was detected (Hill *et al.* 1986). Presumably the density of Ca channels in a region of a vascular bed is influenced by the density of sympathetic innervation received by that region.

As has been pointed out the resting membrane potential of arterioles is largely determined by the activity of a set of inward rectifier K channels. The properties of the inward rectifier in fine non-innervated cerebral arterioles differ from those of innervated arterioles. Innervated segments of arteriole have stable membrane potentials of about −70 mV in solutions containing normal $[K^+]_o$, with inward rectifier K channels contributing an outward current at resting potential. In contrast, segments of non-innervated arteriole had unstable low resting membrane potentials of about −40 mV in control solutions and their rectifier K channels were closed. When $[K^+]_o$ was increased, in the range 7-10 mM, the inward rectifier K channels were opened and the arterioles hyperpolarized. Clearly the decrease in E_K had been more than offset by the increase in g_K. Thus the $[K^+]_o$ requirement for activation of inward rectifier K channels varied with innervation pattern (Edwards et al. 1988). A similar change in the properties of inward rectifier K channels was detected during the postnatal development of rat basilar arteries. At birth, when there were few sympathetic axons, the arteries had low unstable membrane potentials: these arteries were hyperpolarized when $[K^+]_o$ was increased. By postnatal age 21 days, a dense innervation was present. At this time the membrane potential was stable, more negative, and was depolarized when $[K^+]_o$ was increased (Clarke et al. 1991).

Together these observations suggest that sympathetic nerves may exert a trophic effect on the properties of both inward rectifier K channels and voltage-dependent Ca^{2+} channels in some arterial beds.

SUMMARY

After surveying a number of blood vessels, it is apparent that sympathetic nerves form organized neuroeffector junctions with nearby vascular muscle cells. Typically a part of the sympathetic varcosity that is devoid of Schwann cell wrap lies within 100 nm of the muscle cell membrane. Small synaptic vesicles accumulate at these points of close apposition. It seems likely that transmitter release occurs at these points. At this stage it appears likely that all sympathetic varicosities release transmitter only very intermittently. When transmitter is released it acts locally to trigger contraction. There appears to be two distinct ways in which sympathetic nerve stimulation can cause a blood vessels to constrict. One relies on the activation of α-adrenoceptors and involves the activation of a second messenger; Ca^{2+} is released from an internal store. In the other pathway sympathetic transmitter activates a ligand-gated channel and membrane depolarization ensues. Voltage-dependent Ca^{2+} channels are opened and Ca^{2+} entry occurs.

REFERENCES

Angus, J. A., Broughton, A., and Mulvany, M. J. (1988). Role of α-adrenoceptors in constrictor responses of rat, guinea-pig and rabbit small arteries to neural activation. J. Physiol., **403**, 495-510.

Appenzeller, O. (1964). Electron microscopic study of the innervation of the auricular artery in the rat. J. Anat., **98**, 87-91.

Åstrand, P. and Stjärne, L. (1989a). On the secretory activity of single varicosities in the sympathetic nerves innervating rat tail artery. *J. Physiol.*, **409**, 207-20.

Åstrand, P. and Stjärne, L. (1989b). ATP as a sympathetic co-transmitter in rat vasomotor nerves — further evidence that individual release sites respond to nerve impulses by intermittent release of single quanta. *Acta Physiol. Scand.*, **136**, 355-65.

Åstrand, P., Brock, J. A., and Cunnane, T. C. (1988). Time course of transmitter action at the sympathetic neuroeffector junction in vascular and non-vascular smooth muscle. *J. Physiol.*, **401**, 657-70.

Axelsson, S., Bjorklund, A., Falck, B., Lindvall, O., and Svensson, L. A. (1973). Glyoxylic acid condensation: a new fluorescence method for the histochemical demonstration of biogenic monoamines. *Acta Physiol. Scand.*, **87**, 57-62.

Barajas, M. D. (1964). The innervation of the juxtaglomendar apparatus. *Lab. Invest.*, **13**, 917-29.

Bell, C. (1969). Transmission from vasoconstrictor and vasodilator nerves to single smooth muscle cells of the guinea-pig uterine artery. *J. Physiol.*, **205**, 695-708.

Benham, C. D. (1989). ATP activated channels gate calcium entry in single smooth muscle cells from rabbit ear artery. *J. Physiol.*, **419**, 689-701.

Benham, C. D. and Tsei, R. W. (1987). A novel receptor operated Ca^{2+}-permeable channel activated by ATP in smooth muscle. *Nature*, **328**, 275-8.

Benham, C. D., Bolton, T. B., Byrne, N. G., and Large, W. A. (1987). Action of externally applied adenosine triphosphate in single smooth muscle cells dispersed from rabbit ear artery. *J. Physiol.*, **387**, 473-88.

Bennett, M. R. (1972). *Autonomic neurotransmission.* Cambridge University Press, Cambridge.

Bennett, M. R. and Burnstock, G. (1968). Electrophysiology of the innervation of intestinal smooth muscle. In *Handbook of physiology. Section 6. Alimentary canal IV motility*, pp. 1709-32. American Physiological Society, Washington.

Bennett, M. K., Calakos, N., and Scheller, R. H. (1992). Syntaxin: a synaptic protein implicated in docking of synaptic vesicles at presynaptic active zones. *Science*, **257**, 255-9.

Bevan, J. A., Bevan, R. D., and Duckles, S. P. (1980). Adrenergic regulation of vascular smooth muscle. In *Handbook of physiology. The cardiovascular system. Vascular smooth muscle. Section 2* (ed. D. F., Bohr, A. P., Somlyo and H. V., Sparks), pp. 515-66. American Physiological Society, Bethesda.

Blakeley, A. G. H. and Cunnane, T. C. (1979). The packeted release of transmitter from the sympathetic nerves of the guinea-pig vas deferens; an electrophysiological study. *J. Physiol.*, **296**, 85-96.

Blakeley, A. G. H., Brown, D. A., Cunnane, T. C., French, A. M., McGrath, J. C., and Scott, N. C. (1981). Effects of nifedipine on electrical and mechanical responses of rat and guinea-pig vas deferens. *Nature*, **294**, 759-61.

Bolton, T. B. (1974). Electrical properties and constants of longitudinal muscle from the avian anterior mesenteric artery. *Blood Vessels*, **11**, 65-78.

Brock, J. A. and Cunnane, T. C. (1988). Electrical activity at the sympathetic neuroeffector junction in the guinea-pig vas deferens. *J. Physiol.*, **399**, 607-32.

Brock, J. A. and Cunnane, T. C. (1990). Transmitter release from sympathetic nerve terminals on an impulse-by-impulse basis and presynaptic receptors. *Ann. N.Y. Acad. Sci.*, **604**, 176-86.

Brock, J. A. and Cunnane, T. C. (1993). Neurotransmitter release mechanisms at the sympathetic neuroeffector junction. *Exp. Physiol.*, **78**, 591-614.

Bülbring, E. and Burn, J. H. (1936). Sympathetic vasodilatation in the skin and the intestine of the dog. *J. Physiol.*, **87**, 254-74.

Bunge, R. P., Bunge, M. B., and Eldridge, C. F. (1986). Linkage between axonal ensheathment and basal lamina production by schwann cells. *Annu. Rev. of Neurosci.*, **9**, 305-28.
Burden, S. J. (1985). The subsynaptic 43-kDa protein is concentrated at developing nerve-muscle synapses *in vitro*. *Proc. Natl. Acad. Sci. USA*, **82**, 8270-3.
Burnstock, G. (1986). Autonomic neuromuscular juctions: current developments and future directions. *J. Anat.*, **146**, 1-30.
Burnstock, G. (1990). Local mechanisms of blood flow control by perivascular nerves and endothelium. *J. Hypertens.*, **8**, S95-106.
Burnstock, G. and Brown, M. (1981). An introduction to purinergic receptors. In: *Receptors and recognition* (ed. G. Burnstock), Vol. B12; pp. 1-45. Chapman and Hall, London.
Burnstock, G. and Costa, M. (1975). *Adrenergic neurons*. Chapman and Hall, London.
Burnstock, G. and Holman, M. E. (1961). The transmission of excitation from autonomic nerve to smooth muscle. *J. Physiol.*, **155**, 115-33.
Burnstock, G. and Holman, M. E. (1964). An electrophysiological investigation of the actions of some autonomic blocking drugs on transmission in the guinea-pig vas deferens. *Br. J. Pharmacol.*, **23**, 600-12.
Burnstock, G. and Iwayama, T. (1971). Fine-structural identification of autonomic nerves and their relation to smooth muscle. *Prog. Brain Res.*, **34**, 389-404.
Burnstock, G. and Warland, J. J. I. (1987). A pharmacological study of the rabbit saphenous artery *in vitro*: a vessel with a large purinergic contractile response to sympathetic nerve stimulation. *Br. J. Pharmacol.*, **90**, 111-20.
Caesar, R., Edwards, G. A., and Ruska, H. (1957). Architecture and nerve supply of mammalian smooth muscle tissue. *J. Biophys. Biochem. Cytol.*, **3**, 867-91.
Cassell, J. F., McLachlan, E. M., and Sittiracha, T. (1988). The effect of temperature on neuromuscular transmission in the main caudal artery of the rat. *J. Physiol.*, **397**, 31-49.
Casteels, R., Kitamura, K., Kuriyama, H., and Suzuki, H. (1977). The membrane properties of the smooth muscle cells of the rabbit main pulmonary artery. *J. Physiol.*, **271**, 41-61.
Clarke, A., Edwards, F. R., Hirst, G. D. S., and Silverberg, G. D. (1991). Developmental changes in the resting membrane potential of rat cerebral arteries. In *Resistance arteries, structure and function* (ed. M. J. Mulvany, C. Aalkjaer, A. M., Heagerty, N. C. B. Nyborg, and S. Strandgaard, pp. 147-51. Excerpta Medica, Amsterdam.
Cheung, D. W. (1982*a*). Spontaneous and evoked excitatory junction potentials in rat tail arteries. *J. Physiol.*, **328**, 449-59.
Cheung, D. W. (1982*b*). Two components in the cellular response of the rat tail artery to nerve stimulation. *J. Physiol.*, **328**, 461-8.
Cheung, D. W. and Fujioka, M. (1987). Inhibition of the junction potential in the guinea-pig saphenous artery by ANAPP$_3$. *Br. J. Pharmacol.*, **89**, 3-5.
Cowen, T. (1984). An ultrastructural comparison of neuromuscular relationships in blood vessels with functional and "non functional" neuromuscular transmission. *J. Neurocytol.*, **13**, 369-92.
Cunnane, T. C. and Stjärne, L. (1982). Secretion of transmitter from individual varicosities of guinea-pig and mouse vas deferens: all-or-none and extremely intermittent. *Neuroscience*, **7**, 2565-76.
De Deyn, P. P., Pickut, B. A., Verzwijvelen, A., and D'Hooge, R. (1989). Subcellular distribution and axonal transport of noradrenaline, dopamine-β-hydroxylase and neuropeptide Y in dog splenic nerve. *Neurochem. Int.*, **15**, 39-47.
Devine, C. E. and Simpson, F. O. (1967). The fine structure of vascular sympathetic neuromuscular contacts in the rat. *Am. J. Anat.*, **121**, 153-74.

Devine, C. E., Simpson, F. O., and Bertaud, W. S. (1971). Freeze-etch studies on the innervation of mesenteric arteries and vas deferens. *J. Cell Sci.*, **9**, 411-25.

Edwards, F. R. and Hirst, G. D. S. (1988). Inward rectification in submucosal arterioles of guinea pig ileum. *J. Physiol.*, **404**, 437-54.

Edwards, F. R., Hirst, G. D. S., and Silverberg, G. D. (1988). Inward rectification in rat cerebral arterioles; involvement of potassium ions in auto regulation. *J. Physiol.*, **404**, 455-66.

Erici, I., Folkow, B., and Uvnäs, B. (1952). Sympathetic vasodilator nerves to the tongue of the cat. *Acta Physiol. Scand.*, **25**, 1-9.

Evans, D. H. L. and Evans, E. M. (1964). The membrane relationship of smooth muscle cells: an electron microscope study. *J. Anat.*, **98**, 37-46.

Fedan, J. S., Hogaboom, G. K., O'Donnell, J. P., Colby, J. and Westfall, D. P. (1981). Contribution by purines to the neurogenic response of the vas deferens of the guinea-pig. *Eur. J. Pharmacol.*, **69**, 41-53.

Fillenz, M. (1967). Innervation of blood vessels of lung and spleen. *Bibl. Anat.*, **8**, 56-9.

Fillenz, M. (1970). Innervation of pulmonary bronchial blood vessels of the dog. *J. Anat.*, **106**, 449-61.

Finkel, A. S., Hirst, G. D. S., and van Helden, D. F. (1984). Some properties of excitatory junction currents recorded from arterioles of the submucosa of guinea pig ileum. *J. Physiol.*, **351**, 87-98.

Fried, G. (1980). Small noradrenergic storage vesicles isolated from rat vas deferens — biochemical and morphological characterization. *Acta Physiol. Scand.*, *Suppl* **493**, 1-23.

Fried, G. and Lundberg, J. M. (1985). Subcellular storage and axonal transport of neuropeptide Y (NPY) in relation to catecholamines in the cat. *Acta Physiol. Scand.*, **125**, 145-54.

Fried, G., Lagercrantz, H., Klein, R., and Thureson-Klein, A. (1984). Large and small noradrenergic vesicles — origin, contents and functional significance. In *Catecholamines: basic and peripheral mechanisms* (ed. B. Usdin, A. Carlsson, S. Dahlstrom, and M. Eagel), pp. 45-53. Liss: New York.

Furness, J. B. and Costa, M. (1975). The use of glyoxylic acid for the fluorescence histochemical demonstration of peripheral stores of noradrenaline and 5-hydroxytryptamine in whole mounts. *Histochemistry*, **41**, 335-52.

Furness, J. B., McLean, J. R., and Burnstock, G. (1970). Distribution of adrenergic nerves and changes in neuromuscular transmission in the mouse vas deferens during postnatal development. *Dev. Biol.*, **21**, 491-505.

Gabella, G. (1974). The sphincter pupillae of the guinea pig: structure of muscle cells, intercellular relations and density of innervation. *Proc. R. Soc. Lond. (Biol.)* **186**, 369-86.

Gabella, G. (1992). Fine structure of post-ganglionic nerve fibres and autonomic neuroeffector junctions. In *Autonomic neuroeffector mechanisms* (ed. G. Burnstock and C. H. V. Hoyle), pp. 1-31. Harwood Academic, Chur.

Gage, P. W. (1976). Generation of end-plate potentials. *Physiol. Rev.*, **56**, 177-247.

Geffen, L. B. and Livett, B. G. (1971). Synaptic vesicles in sympathetic neurons. *Physiol. Rev.*, **51**, 98-157.

Geffen, L. B. and Ostberg, A. (1969). Distribution of granular vesicles in normal and constricted sympathetic neurones. *J. Physiol.*, **204**, 583-92.

Gorgas, K. (1978). Structure and innervation of the juxtaglomerular apparatus of the rat. *Adv. Anat. Embryol. Cell Biol.*, **54**, 5-84.

Greengard, P., Valtorta, F., Czernik, A. J., and Benfenati, F. (1993). Synaptic vesicle phosphoproteins and regulation of synaptic function. *Science*, **259**, 780-5.

Häggendal, J. and Malmfors, T. (1969). The effect of nerve stimulation on adrenergic nerves after reserpine pretreatment. *Acta Physiol. Scand.*, **75**, 33-8.

Harder, D. R., Belardinelli, L., Sperelakis, N., Rubio, R., and Berne, R. M. (1979). Differential effects of adenosine and nitroglycerine on the action potentials of large and small coronary arteries. *Circ. Res.*, **44**, 176-82.

Hill, C. E., Hirst, G. D. S., and van Helden, D. F. (1983). Development of the sympathetic innervation of proximal and distal arteries of the rat mesentery. *J. Physiol.*, **338**, 129-47.

Hill, C. E., Hirst, G. D. S., Silverberg, G. D., and van Helden, D. F. (1986). Sympathetic innervation and excitability of arterioles originating from the rat middle cerebral artery. *J. Physiol.*, **371**, 305-16.

Hillarp, N.-Å. (1946). Structure of the synapse and the peripheral innervation apparatus of the autonomic nervous system. *Acta Anat.*, **2 (Suppl. 4)**, 1-153.

Hillarp, N.-Å. (1959). The construction and functional organization of the autonomic innervation apparatus. *Acta Physiol. Scand.*, **46 (Suppl. 157)**, 1-38.

Hirst, G. D. S. (1977). Neuromuscular transmission in arterioles of guinea pig submucosa. *J. Physiol.*, **273**, 263-75.

Hirst, G. D. S. and Edwards, F. R. (1989). Sympathetic neuroeffector transmission in arteries and arterioles. *Physiol. Rev.*, **69**, 546-604.

Hirst, G. D. S. and Jobling, P. (1989). Distribution of gamma adrenoceptors and P_2 purinoceptors in mesenteric arteries and veins of the guinea-pig. *Br. J. Pharmacol.*, **96**, 993-9.

Hirst, G. D. S. and Lew, M. J. (1987). Lack of involvement of α-adrenoceptors in sympathetic neural vasoconstriction in the hindquarters of the rabbit. *Br. J. Pharmacol.*, **90**, 51-60.

Hirst, G. D. S. and McLachlan, E. M. (1984). Post-natal development of synaptic connections in the lower lumbar sympathetic chain of the rat. *J. Physiol.*, **349**, 119-34.

Hirst, G. D. S. and Neild, T. O. (1978). An analysis of excitatory junction potentials recorded from arterioles. *J. Physiol.*, **280**, 87-104.

Hirst, G. D. S. and Neild, T. O. (1980). Some properties of spontaneous excitatory junction potentials recorded from arterioles of guinea pig. *J. Physiol.;* **303**, 43-60.

Hirst, G. D. S. and Neild, T. O. (1981). Localization of specialized noradrenaline receptors at neuromuscular juctions on arterioles of the guinea-pig. *J. Physiol.*, **313**, 343-50.

Hirst, G. D. S., Edwards, F. R., and Silverberg, G. D. (1992). Control of arteriolar excitability by neural and metabolic factors. *Jap. J. Pharmacol.*, **58, Suppl. II**, 174-8.

Hökfelt, T. (1973). On the origin of small adrenergic storage vesicles: Evidence for local formation in nerve endings after chronic reserpine treatment. *Experientia*, **29**, 580-2.

Hökfelt, T. and Jonasson, G. (1968). Studies on the reaction and binding of monamines after fixation and processing for electron microscopy with potassium permanganate. *Histochemie*, **16**, 45-67.

Holman, M. E. and Surprenant, A. M. (1979). Some properties of the excitatory junction potentials recorded from saphenous arteries of rabbit. *J. Physiol.*, **287**, 337-51.

Holman, M. E. and Surprenant, A. M. (1980). An electrophysiological analysis of the effects of noradrenaline and receptor antagonists on neuromuscular transmssion in mammalian muscular arteries. *Br. J. Pharmacol.*, **71**, 337-51.

Hottenstein, O. D. and Kreulen, D. L. (1987). Comparison of the frequency dependence of venous and arterial responses to sympathetic nerve stimulation in guinea-pigs. *J. Physiol.*, **384**, 153-67.

Ishikawa, S. (1985). Actions of ATP and α,β,-methylene ATP on neuromuscular transmission in smooth muscle membrane of rabbit and guinea-pig mesenteric arteries. *Br. J. Pharmacol.*, **86**, 777-87.

Itoh, T., Kitamura, K., and Kuriyama, H. (1983). Roles of extra-junctional receptors in the response of guinea-pig mesenteric and rat tail arteries to adrenergic nerves. *J. Physiol.*, **345**, 409–22.

Iversen, L. L., Glowinsky, J., and Axelrod, J. (1965). The uptake and storage of ^{3}H-norepinephrine in the reserpine-treated rat heart. *J. Pharmocal. Exp. Ther.*, **150**, 173–83.

Iwayama, T., Furness, J. B., and Burnstock, G. (1970). Dual adrenergic and cholinergic innervation of the cerebral arteries of the rat. *Circ. Res.*, **26**, 635–46.

Jack, J. J. B., Noble, D., and Tsien, R. W. (1975). *Electrical current flow in excitable cells.* Claredon Oxford, UK.

Kajiwara, M., Kitamura, K., and Kuriyama, H. (1981). Neuromuscular transmission and smooth muscle membrane properties in the guinea-pig ear artery. *J. Physiol.*, **315**, 283–302.

Katz, B. (1969). *The release of neural transmitter substances.* Liverpool University Press (Sherrington Lectures X), Liverpool, UK.

Keatinge, W. R. (1966). Electrical and mechanical responses of arteries to stimulation of sympathetic nerves. *J. Physiol.*, **185**, 710–15.

Kennedy, C., Seville, V. L., and Burnstock, G. (1986). The contributions of noradrenaline and ATP to the responses of the rabbit central ear artery to sympathetic nerve stimulation depend on the parameters of stimulation. *Eur. J. Pharmacol.*, **122**, 291–300.

Klein, R. L. and Lagercrantz, H. (1981). Noradrenergic vesicles: composition and function. In *Chemical neurotransmission 75 years* (ed. L. Stjärne, P. Hedqvist, H. Lagercrantz, and A. Wennmalm), pp. 69–83. Academic Press, London.

Klemm, M. F., Van Helden, D. F., and Luff, S. E. (1993). Ultrastructural analysis of sympathetic neuromuscular junctions on mesenteric veins of the guinea pig. *J. Comp. Neurol.*, **334**, 159–67.

Kügelgen, I. V. and Starke, K. (1985). Noradrenaline and adenosine triphosphate as co-transmitters of neurogenic vasoconstriction in rabbit mesenteric arteries. *J. Physiol.*, **367**, 435–55.

Kügelgen, I. V. and Starke, K. (1991). Release of noradrenaline and ATP by electrical stimulation and nicotine in the guinea-pig vas deferens. *Naunyn-Schmiederberg's Arch. Pharmakol.*, **344**, 419–29.

Kuriyama, H. and Makita, Y. (1983). Modulation of noradrenergic transmission in the guinea-pig mesenteric artery: an electrophysiological study. *J. Physiol.*, **335**, 609–27.

Lavidis, N. A. and Bennett, M. R. (1992). Probabilistic secretion of quanta from visualized sympathetic nerve varicosities in mouse vas deferens. *J. Physiol.*, **454**, 9–26.

Lee, J. T.-F. (1981a). Ultrastructural distribution of vasodilator and constrictor nerves in cat cerebral arteries. *Circ. Res.*, **49**, 971–9.

Lee, J. T.-F. (1981b). Nerve relationships in cerebral arteries. *Blood Vessels*, **18**, 218.

Lever, J. D., Ahmed, M., and Irvine, G. (1965a). Neuromuscular and intercellular relationships in the coronary arterioles. A morphological and quantitative study by light and electron microscopy. *J. Anat.*, **99**, 829–40.

Lever, J. D., Graham, J. D. P., Irvine, G., and Chick, W. J. (1965b). The vesiculated axons in relation to arteriolar smooth muscle in the pancreas. A fine structural and quantitative study. *J. Anat.*, **99**, 299–313.

Lew, M. and White, T. D. (1987). Release of endogenous ATP during sympathetic nerve stimulation. *Br. J. Pharmacol.*, **92**, 349–55.

Luff, S. E. and McLachlan, E. M. (1988). The form of sympathetic postganglionic axons at clustered neuromuscular junctions near branch points of arterioles in the submucosa of the guinea pig ileum. *J. Neurocytol.*, **17**, 451–63.

Luff, S. E. and McLachlan, E. M. (1989). Frequency of neuromuscular junctions on arteries of different dimensions in the rabbit, guinea pig and rat. *Blood Vessels*, **26**, 95–106.

Luff, S. E., McLachlan, E. M., and Hirst, G. D. S. (1987). An ultrastructural analysis of the sympathetic neuromuscular junctions of arterioles of the submucosa of the guinea pig ileum. *J. Comp. Neurobiol.*, **257**, 578–94.

Luff, S. E., Hengstberger, S. G., McLachlan, E. M., and Anderson, W. P. (1991). Two types of sympathetic axon innervating the juxtaglomerular arterioles of the rabbit and rat kidney differ structurally from those supplying other arteries. *J. Neurocytol.*, **20**, 781–95.

Luff, S. E., Hengstberger, S. G., McLachlan, E. M., and Anderson, W. P. (1992). Distribution of sympathetic neuroeffector junctions in the juxtaglomerular region of the rabbit kidney. *J. Auton. Nerv. Syst.*, **40**, 239–54.

Magill, C., Reist, N. E., Fallon, J. R., Nitkin, R. M., Wallace, R. M., and McMahon, U. J. (1987). Agrin. *Prog. Brain Res.*, **71**, 391–6.

Matsuyama, T., Shiosaka, S., Wanaka, A., Yoneda, S., Kimura, K., Hayakawa, T., *et al.* (1985). Fine structure of peptidergic and catecholaminergic nerve fibers in the anterior cerebral artery and their interelationship: an immunoelectron microscopic study. *J. Comp. Neurol.*, **235**, 268–76.

Mekata, F. (1974). Current spread in the smooth muscle of the rabbit aorta. *J. Physiol.*, **242**, 143–55.

Merrillees, N. C. R. (1968). The nervous environment of individual smooth muscle cells of the guinea pig vas deferens. *J. Cell Biol.*, **37**, 794–817.

Merrillees, N. C. R., Burnstock, G., and Holman, M. E. (1963). Correlation of fine structure and physiology of the innervation of smooth muscle in the guinea pig vas deferens. *J. Cell Biol.*, **19**, 529–50.

Morhri, K., Ohgushi, N., Ikeda, M., Yamamoto, K., and Tsunekawa, T. (1969). Histochemical demonstration of adrenergic fibres in the smooth muscle layers of media of arteries supplying abdominal organs. *Arch. Jpn. Chir.*, **38**, 236–48.

Morris, J. L. and Gibbins, I. L. (1992). Con-transmission and neuromodulation. In *Autonomic neuroeffector mechanisms* (ed. G. Burnstock and C. H. V. Hoyle), pp. 33–119. Harwood Academic, Chur.

Murumatsu, I., Kigoshi, S., and Oshita, M. (1984). Non-adrenergic nature of prazosin resistant sympathetic contraction in dog mesenteric artery. *J. Pharmacol. Exp. Ther.*, **229**, 532–8.

Nelson, E. and Rennels, M. (1970). Innervation of intracranial arteries. *Brain*, **93**, 475–90.

Osswald, W. and Guimarães, S. (1983). Adrenergic mechanisms in blood vessels: morphological and pharmacological aspects. *Rev. Physiol. Biochem. Pharmacol.*, **96**, 53–122.

Owman, C. (1988). Autonomic innervation of the cardiovascular system. In *Handbook of chemical neuroanatomy. The peripheral nervous system* (ed. A. Björklund, T. Hökfelt, and C. Owman), pp. 327–89. Elsevier Publishers, Amsterdam.

Pergram, B. L., Bevan, R. D., and Bevan, J. A. (1976). Facial vein of the rabbit: neurogenic vasodilation mediated by β-adrenergic receptors. *Circ. Res.*, **39**, 854–60.

Potter, L. T. (1967). Role of intraneuronal vesicles in the synthesis, storage and release of noradrenaline. *Circ. Res.*, **21 (Suppl 3)**, 13–24.

Rang, H. P. (1981). The characteristics of synaptic current and responses to acetylcholine of rat submandibular ganglion cells. *J. Physiol.*, **311**, 23–55.

Reilly, M. and Hirst, G. D. S. (1995). Purinergic nerve stimulation and applied ATP in the guinea pig vas deferens. *J. Auton. Nerv. Syst.* (in press)

Rhodin, J. A. G. (1967). The ultrastructure of mammalian arterioles and precapillary sphincters. *J. Ultrastruct. Res.*, **18**, 181–223.

Richardson, K. C. (1962). The fine structure of autonomic nerve endings in smooth muscle of the rat vas deferens. *J. Anat.*, **96**, 427-42.

Richardson, K. C. (1964). The fine structure of the albino rabbit iris with special reference to the identification of adrenergic and cholinergic nerves and nerve endings in its intrinsic muscles. *Am. J. Anat.*, **114**, 173-205.

Rowan, R. A. and Bevan, J. A. (1983). Distribution of adrenergic synaptic cleft width in vascular and nonvascular smooth muscle. In *Vascular neuroeffector mechanisms: 4th international symposium* (ed. J. A. Bevan), pp. 75-83. Raven Press, New York.

Rowan, R. A., Bevan, R. D., and Bevan, J. A. (1981). Ultrastructural features of the innervation and smooth muscle of the rabbit facial vein and their relationship to function. *Circ. Res.*, **49**, 1140-51.

Sittiracha, T., McLachlan, E. M., and Bell, C. (1987). The innervation of the caudal artery of the rat. *Neuroscience*, **21**, 647-59.

Smith, A. D. and Winkler, H. (1972). Fundamental mechanisms of the release of catacholamines. In *Handbook of experimental pharmacology* (ed. H. Blaschko and E. Muscholl), pp. 538-617. Springer-Verlag, Berlin.

Smith, A. D., De Potter, W. P., Moerman, E. J., and Schaepdryver, A. F. (1970). Release of dopamine β-hydroxylase and chromogranin A upon stimulation of the splenic nerve. *Tissue Cell*, **2**, 547-68.

Sneddon, P. and Burnstock, G. (1984). ATP as a co-transmitter in rat tail artery. *Eur. J. Pharmacol.*, **106**, 149-52.

Sneddon, P. and Westfall, D. P. (1984). Pharmacological evidence that adenosine triphosphate and noradredaline are co-transmitters in the guinea-pig vas deferens. *J. Physiol.*, **347**, 561-80.

Su, C. (1975). Neurogenic release of purine compounds in blood vessels. *J. Pharmacol. Ther.* **195**, 159-66.

Suzuki, H. (1981). Effects of endogenous and exogenous noradrenaline on the smooth muscle of guinea-pig mesenteric vein. *J. Physiol.*, **321**, 495-512.

Suzuki, H. (1983). An electrophysiological study of excitatory neuromuscular transmission in the guinea-pig main pulmonary artery. *J. Physiol.*, **336**, 47-59.

Suzuki, H. (1985). Electrical responses of smooth muscle cells of the rabbit ear artery to adenosine triphosphate. *J. Physiol.*, **359**, 401-16.

Taxi, P. J. (1965). Contribution a l'étude des connexions des neurones moteurs du système nerveux autonome. *Ann. Sci. Nat. Zool. (Paris)*, **7**, 413-674.

Thaemert, J. C. (1963). The ultrastructure and disposition of vesiculated nerve processes in smooth muscle. *J. Cell Biol.*, **16**, 361-77.

Thaemert, J. C. (1966). Ultrastructural interrelationships of nerve processes and smooth muscle cells in three dimensions. *J. Cell Biol.*, **28**, 37-49.

Tranzer, J. P. (1972). A new amine storing compartment in adrenergic axons. *Nature*, **237**, 57-8.

Tranzer, J.-P. and Richards, J. G. (1976). Ultrastructural cytochemistry of biogenic amines in nervous tissue: Methodologic improvements. *J. Histochem. Cytochem.*, **24**, 1178-93.

Tranzer, J. P., Thoenen, H., Snipes, R. L., and Richards, J. G. (1969). Recent developments on the ultrastructural aspect of adrenergic nerve endings in various experimental conditions. *Prog. Brain Res.*, **31**, 33-46.

Tsunekawa, K., Morhri, K., Ikeda, M., Ohgushi, N., and Fujiwara, M. (1967). Histochemical demonstration of adrenergic fibres in the smooth muscle layer of media of dorsal pedal artery in dog. *Experientia*, **23**, 842-3.

Uehara, Y. and Burnstock, G. (1972). Postsynaptic specialization of smooth muscle at close neuromuscular junctions in the guinea pig spincter pupillae. *J. Cell Biol.*, **53**, 849-53.

Uvnäs, B. and Åborg, C.-H. (1980). Possible role of nerve impulse induced sodium ion flux in a proposed multivesicular fractional release of adrenaline and noradrenaline from the chromaffin cell. *Acta Physiol. Scand.*, **109**, 363-8.

van Helden, D. F. (1988a). Electrophysiology of neuromuscular transmission in guinea-pig mesenteric veins. *J. Physiol.*, **401**, 469-88.

van Helden, D. F. (1988b). An α-mediated chloride conductance in mesenteric veins of the guinea-pig. *J. Physiol.*, **401**, 489-501.

van Helden, D. F. (1991). Spontaneous and noradrenaline induced transient depolarizations in the smooth muscle of guinea-pig mesenteric vein. *J. Physiol.*, **437**, 543-62.

Wharton, J. and Gulbenkian, S. (1987). Peptides in the mammalian cardiovacular system. *Experientia Basel*, **43**, 821-32.

9. Cotransmission

G. Burnstock and V. Ralevic

GENERAL INTRODUCTION

For many years our understanding of neurotransmission has been dominated by the concept that one neurone releases only a single transmitter, known as 'Dale's Principle'. This idea arose from a widely adopted misinterpretation of Dale's suggestion in 1935 that the same neurotransmitter was stored in and released from all terminals of a single neurone, a suggestion which did not specifically preclude the possibility that more than one transmitter may be associated with the same neurone. Several lines of evidence emerged which were inconsistent with the single transmitter concept and it is now known that individual neurones contain and can release a large number and variety of substances which are capable of influencing target cells — this phenomenon of 'cotransmission' is widespread involving virtually all known transmitter systems. Hence, our concept of neural vascular control must incorporate cotransmission, the simultaneous release from the same neurone of two or more postjunctionally-acting transmitters, together with an appreciation of pre- and/or postjunctional mechanisms involved in the control of transmitter release or action, 'neuromodulation'.

Early hints of cotransmission began in the 1950s with evidence for the involvement of both noradrenaline (NA) and acetylcholine (ACh) in sympathetic transmission. Koelle (1955) identified acetylcholinesterase in some adrenergic neurones, while Burn and Rand (1959) introduced the concept of a 'cholinergic' link in adrenergic transmission. Abrahams *et al.* (1957) suggested that impulses conducted along the hypothalamoneurohypophysial neurosecretory fibres might liberate ACh at their terminals to provide the stimulus for the release of oxytocin and vasopressin from the same nerve terminals. Another line of evidence concerned the coexistence of adenosine 5'-triphosphate (ATP) with catecholamines, first in adrenal chromaffin cells (Hillarp *et al.* 1955; Blaschko *et al.* 1956; von Euler *et al.* 1963; Douglas and Poisner 1966) and later in sympathetic nerves (Schumann 1958; Stjärne and Lishajko 1966; Geffen and Livett 1971). Also contributing to the forced recognition of the concept of cotransmission were the increasing number of studies which showed that in addition to the classical transmitters NA and ACh, nerves store and release many other biologically active 'transmitter' substances. Inconsistencies in the single transmitter hypothesis provided by these and other studies from the early literature were rationalized in an article with the provocative title: 'Do some nerve cells release more than one transmitter?' (Burnstock 1976). Today, it is widely accepted that cotransmission is an integral feature of neurotransmission (see Potter *et al.* 1981; Cuello 1982; Osborne 1983; Chan-Palay and Palay 1984; Hökfelt *et al.* 1986; Campbell 1987; Bartfai *et al.* 1988; Furness *et al.* 1989; Burnstock 1990; Kupfermann 1990).

Some commonly recurring themes appear when looking at the coexistence and co-release of transmitters from nerves. For instance, despite the large number and variety of transmitter substances not all combinations occur in coexistence within specific classes of neurones. In this respect, some progress has been made in establishing the patterns of favoured packaging of transmitter substances in certain specific combinations, otherwise known as 'chemical coding'. Another common feature is the differential storage of cotransmitters in characteristic vesicles that can be categorized ultrastructurally according to size, shape, and electron density which may hold a clue as to the differential proportional release of cotransmitters at different frequencies of stimulation. These patterns of cotransmission and their functional significance will be discussed for particular combinations of cotransmitters as they occur.

A pharmacological consequence of cotransmission is the resistance to total blockade of some neurogenic vasoconstrictor or vasodilator responses by single specific antagonists. A combination of antagonists against each of the coexisting transmitters, however, exposes these responses as a composite of postjunctional actions mediated by multiple neuronal messengers. For instance, stimulation of sympathetic nerves produces a vasoconstrictor response which in many vessels is only partially blocked by antagonists selective for either of the sympathetic cotransmitters NA or ATP, but which is abolished by a combination of antagonists to both NA and ATP. Pharmacological studies of pre- and postjunctional neuromodulation provide evidence which is complementary to the concept of cotransmission. For example, parallel presynaptic modulation of transmitter overflow supports the concept of closely associated co-release, while postjunctional synergism between co-localized transmitters provides justification of cotransmission in terms of transmitter economy. The fact that opposite actions between co-released transmitters have also been shown depending on the tone of the effector muscle cell (Morris *et al.* 1985) indicates that there is much that is still not understood about the physiological relevance of cotransmission. It may be that a better understanding of the complex interplay between co-released transmitter substances may be gained by looking at neurotransmitter vascular control mechanisms after changes in the balance of cotransmission such as may occur in various pathophysiological conditions.

VASCULAR NEUROEFFECTOR JUNCTION

Perivascular nerves at the adventitial–medial border of most blood vessels form a plexus consisting of an extensive network of branching terminal fibres. These terminal axons are devoid of Schwann cell covering and are rich in varicosities (1–2 μm diameter) separated by intervaricose regions (0.1–0.3 μm diameter) (Burnstock 1986). The varicosities are the main sites of storage of neurotransmitters which are released 'en passage' by the depolarizing effect of nerve impulses passing along the axons. Unlike the classical synapse of the skeletal neuromuscular junction and those present in ganglia, a fixed relationship between varicosities and smooth muscle cells is not a feature of the autonomic neuroeffector junction. In addition, while prejunctional varicosity membranes sometimes show thickenings, there are no postjunctional specializations. The junctional cleft can vary between 50 to 2000 nm (but see also Chapter 8, pp. 189–92), depending on the size of the vessel and it has been suggested that the often wide cleft predisposes the autonomic neuroeffector junction to both pre- and postjunctional modulatory influences from locally released transmitters from the same or adjacent nerve terminals or from circulating substances.

Neuromodulation

A neuromodulator is defined as a substance that modifies the process of neurotransmission. Neuromodulation may take place prejunctionally, acting to increase or decrease the amount of transmitter from the nerve terminal, or postjunctionally, altering the time course or extent of action of the neurotransmitter. Neuromodulators may be transmitters released from the same nerve terminal or from adjacent terminals of neighbouring perivascular nerves. Circulating neurohormones and local agents such as prostanoids, bradykinin, or histamine can also act as nuromodulators.

Cotransmission

Cotransmission is broadly defined as the process involving the simultaneous release of two or more transmitters from the same neurone and their postjunctional actions on the same target tissue. According to this definition a substance co-released from a nerve terminal and not having direct actions on effector cells, but which pre- or postjunctionally modulates the effects of the main transmitter(s) is a neuromodulator but not a cotransmitter. A cotransmitter is often (but not always) a neuromodulator.

SYMPATHETIC NERVE COTRANSMISSION

There is now substantial evidence to show that NA, ATP, and neuropeptide Y (NPY) are cotransmitters in sympathetic nerves, having differentially important roles as transmitters and neuromodulators depending on the tissue, the species, and on the parameters of stimulation (see Burnstock 1990; Ralevic and Burnstock 1991) (Fig. 9.1). Most of the early studies establishing the model of cotransmission of NA and ATP were made on the vas deferens, a tissue with a high density of sympathetic nerves (see Stjärne 1989; Burnstock 1990). Subsequently, numerous studies demonstrated that cotransmission of NA and ATP also occurs in many different blood vessels in a variety of species (see Burnstock 1990).

SYMPATHETIC NEUROTRANSMISSION

Vas deferens
many blood vessels

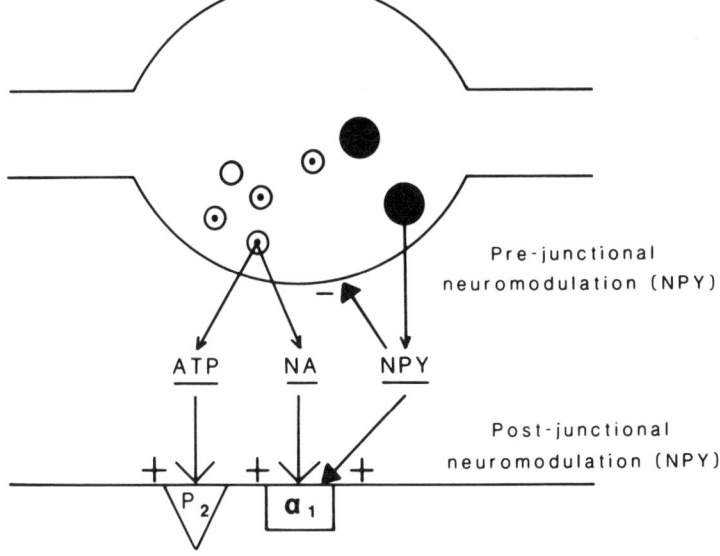

Fig. 9.1 Schematic representation showing that noradrenaline (NA), adenosine 5'-triphosphate (ATP), and neuropeptide Y (NPY) are released as cotransmitters from single nerve varicosities of sympathetic nerves supplying the vas deferens and many blood vessels. NA and ATP, released from small (and large) granular vesicles, act on the smooth muscle to elicit contraction (+) via α_1-adrenoceptors and P_2-purinoceptors, respectively. NPY, preferentially released from large vesicles, generally has little direct action on the muscle cell, but exerts potent neuromodulatory actions: both prejunctional inhibition (−) of the release of NA (and ATP) and postjunctional enhancement of the action of NA. (From Burnstock 1987.)

Several lines of evidence support the concept of cotransmission of NA and ATP in perivascular sympathetic nerves. Su (1975) took advantage of purine catabolic pathways to prime tissues with tritiated [^{3}H] adenosine and then using tritium efflux as a measure of ATP release showed that electrical stimulation of the rabbit aorta and portal vein evokes the release of [^{3}H] purine together with NA and that this release was tetrodotoxin- and guanethidine-sensitive (Su 1975). The same technique was later used to show cotransmission of NA and ATP in the dog basilar artery (Muramatsu *et al.* 1981), rabbit pulmonary artery (Katsuragi and Su 1982), and rabbit mesenteric artery (von Kügelgen and Starke 1985).

Following release from sympathetic nerve terminals NA and ATP elicit vasoconstriction of the smooth muscle via an action at α-adrenoceptors and P_{2x}-purinoceptors respectively. The rabbit saphenous artery provides a classic example

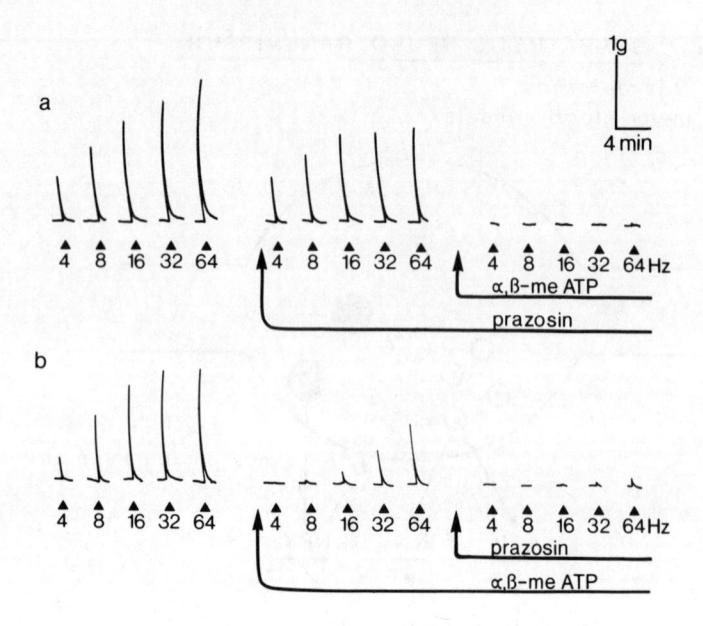

Fig. 9.2 Contractions produced in the isolated saphenous artery of the rabbit on neurogenic transmural stimulation (0.08–0.1 ms; supramaximal voltage) for 1 s (a,b) at the frequencies (Hz) indicated (▲). Nerve stimulations were repeated in the presence of 10 μM prazosin added before (a) or after (b) desensitizaton of the P_2-purinoceptor with α,β-methylene ATP (α,β-me ATP) as indicated on the figure by the arrowed lines. The horizontal bar signifies 4 min and the vertical bar 1 g. (From Burnstock and Warland 1987.)

of a vessel in which pharmacological manipulations have been used to identify the relative contribution of NA and ATP to sympathetic transmission (Burnstock and Warland 1987; Warland and Burnstock 1987). In this vessel, sympathetic nerve stimulation produces a contractile response less than 30% of which is blocked by the α-adrenoceptor antagonist prazosin, whereas the remainder, the purinergic component, is abolished following desensitization of the P_{2x}-purinoceptor with α,β-methylene ATP (Burnstock and Warland 1987) (Fig. 9.2). The sympathetic origin of the purinergic response is confirmed by the fact that reserpine treatment, which depletes sympathetic nerves of their catecholamine content, failed to abolish nerve-mediated contractions, whereas after destruction of sympathetic nerves with 6-hydroxydopamine, no nerve-mediated responses were observed (Warland and Burnstock 1987) (Fig. 9.3). The P_2-purinoceptor antagonists arylazido aminoproprionyl ATP (White et al. 1985) and suramin (Leff et al. 1990; Bultmann et al. 1991; Evans and Surprenant 1992) have also been used to identify a purinergic component of the sympathetic vasoconstrictor response.

Electrophysiological studies have shown that in a number of vessels the electrical response to stimulation of sympathetic nerves is biphasic; an initial fast, transient depolarization or 'excitatory junction potential' (e.j.p.) of the vascular smooth muscle is followed by a slow, prolonged depolarization. The e.j.p. and

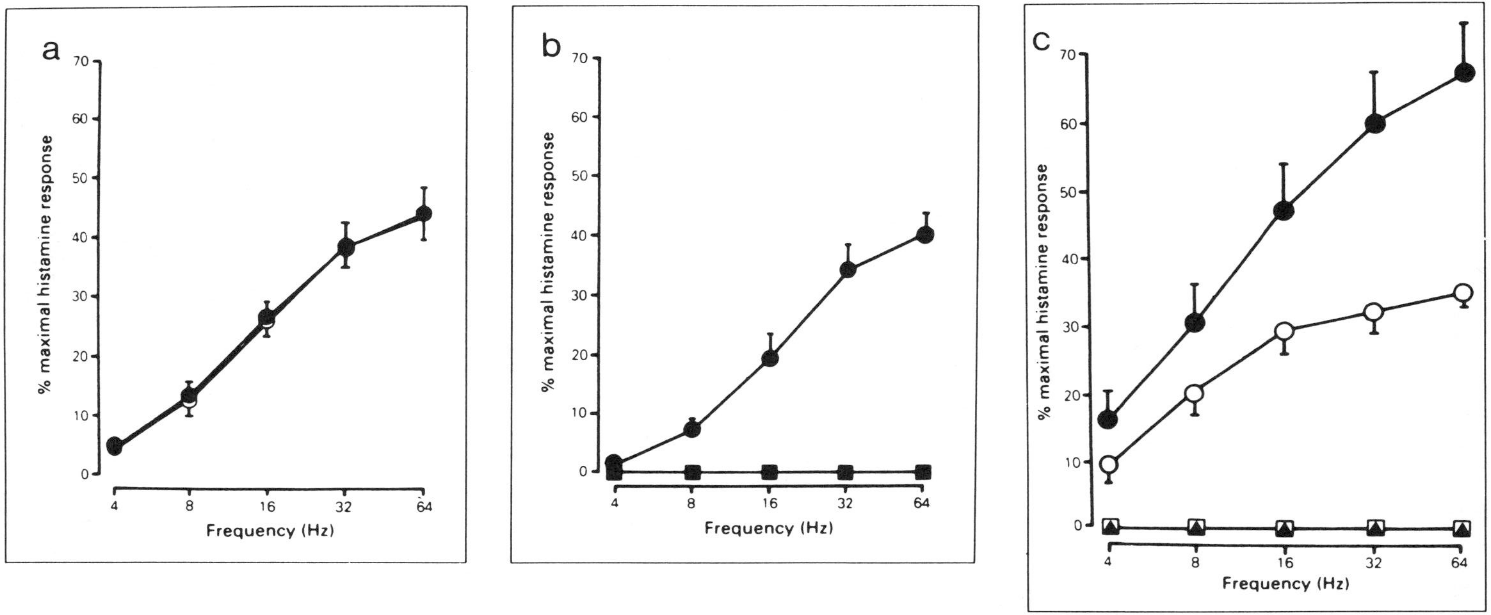

Fig. 9.3 (a,b) Contractions of isolated saphenous artery from rabbits treated with reserpine (n = 8). Responses to 1 s periods of stimulation (0.1 ms submaximal voltage, 4–64 Hz) are expressed as a percentage of the maximal histamine contraction. The response to each frequency of stimulation was measured in the absence of α,β-methylene ATP and prazosin (●) and in the presence of 10 μM prazosin (○) (a) or 10 μM α,β-methylene ATP (■) (b). Note that in reserpine treated vessels α,β-methylene ATP completely inhibited the contractile response while prazosin had no significant effect. (c) Neurogenic responses of rabbit isolated saphenous artery treated *in vitro* in Krebs solution containing 6-hydroxydopamine and 0.1% ascorbic acid for 4 h, and untreated control arteries incubated for 4 h in Krebs containing 0.1% ascorbic acid. Responses to 1 s periods of stimulation (0.1 ms, submaximal voltage, 4–64 Hz) are expressed as a percentage of the maximal histamine contraction. In the control preparations the responses to each frequency of stimulation were measured in the absence of prazosin and α,β-methylene ATP (●), in the presence of 10 μM prazosin (○), and in the presence of prazosin and 10 μM α,β-methylene ATP (□). In the 6-hydroxydopamine treated vessels in the absence of prazosin and α,β-methylene ATP no neurogenic response was observed (n = 7) (▲). Symbols represent mean response and vertical lines denote s.e. (From Warland and Burnstock 1987.)

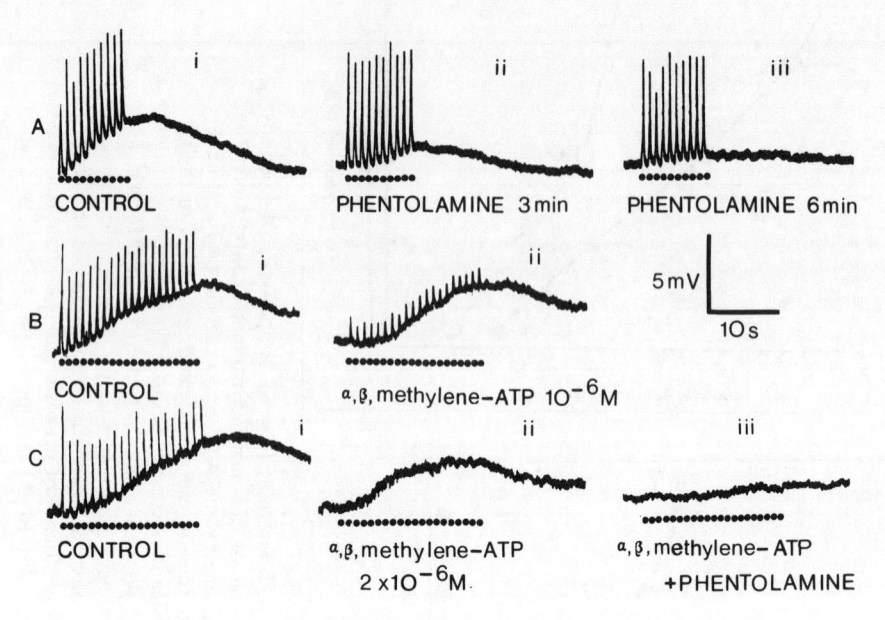

Fig. 9.4 Intracellular recording of the electrical responses of single smooth muscle cells of the rat tail artery to field stimulation of the sympathetic motor nerves (the pulse width was 0.1 ms at 0.5 Hz, indicated by ●). (Ai) Control response of the muscle. Note that to each individual stimulus there was a rapid depolarization, and as the train of pulses progressed, a slow depolarization developed. Similar responses were obtained in (Bi) and (Ci), which are also control responses in Krebs solution. (Aii) and (Aiii) show the effect of phentolamine (2×10^{-6}M, added to the bathing solution). The fast depolarizations produced by each stimulus were not reduced, but there was a progressive reduction in the size of the slow depolarization, which was almost abolished after 6 min. In (Bii) the tissues have been in the presence of 10^{-6} M α,β-methylene ATP for over 15 min. The fast depolarizations produced by each stimulus were greatly reduced, but the slow depolarization persisted. (Cii) shows the effect of a higher concentration of α,β-methylene ATP. Here the fast depolarization was totally abolished, whilst the slow depolarization persisted, although reduced to some extent. Subsequent addition of phentolamine (2×10^{-6}M), together with α,β-methylene ATP, abolished the neurogenic response completely (Ciii). (From Sneddon and Burnstock 1984.)

slow depolarization are mimicked by the effects of ATP and NA respectively. Furthermore, the e.j.p. is resistant to α-adrenoceptor blockade with prazosin or phentolamine but is blocked by α,β-methylene ATP and abolished by guanethidine or tetrodotoxin (Sneddon and Burnstock 1984; Suzuki 1985; Vidal et al. 1986; Ramme et al. 1987; Angus et al. 1988), while the slow depolarization is abolished by α-adrenoceptor antagonists (Fig. 9.4). These results are consistent with ATP and NA acting as sympathetic cotransmitter mediators of the e.j.p. and slow depolarization respectively.

Considerable variation exists in the proportions of NA and ATP utilized by sympathetic nerves. For example, in guinea-pig submucosal arterioles both vasoconstriction and e.j.p.s evoked in response to electrical stimulation of sympathetic nerves are mediated exclusively by ATP with NA assuming the role of a neuromodulator by acting through prejunctional α_2-adrenoceptors to depress transmitter release (Evans and Surprenant 1992). At the other extreme, in rat mesenteric arteries the purinergic component is relatively small. In addition, it has been noted that the purinergic component is optimal with short bursts of low frequency stimulation, whereas longer durations of higher frequency favour adrenergic transmission (Kennedy et al. 1986; Burnstock and Warland 1987; Ramme et al. 1987; Evans and Cunnane 1992). The reason for this variation is not known but may in part be a reflection of the differential storage and release of NA and ATP in sympathetic vesicles. ATP is co-stored with NA in small and large sympathetic vesicles; the NA:ATP ratio is three to five times higher in small than in large vesicles (von Kügelgen and Starke 1991). It is possible that there may be selectivity in the choice of vesicle involved in transmitter release during different stimuli. Differential prejunctional modulation of the release of NA and ATP by various agents has been shown in the vas deferens and has interesting implications for prejunctional modulation of sympathetic neurotransmission in blood vessels (see Stjärne 1989; Burnstock 1990; von Kügelgen and Starke 1991).

Some of the functional implications of cotransmission are evidenced by studies of the pre- and postjunctional actions of co-released transmitter substances. Both NA and ATP can prejunctionally modulate sympathetic transmission, NA via prejunctional α_2-adrenoceptors and ATP via P_1-purinoceptors following breakdown to adenosine. Postjunctionally, the effects of NA and ATP released as sympathetic cotransmitters are generally co-operative since both typically act as vasoconstrictors following release from sympathetic nerves. Postjunctional synergism may occur having been described in the rat femoral artery, guinea-pig and rat portal vein, and the rat mesenteric arterial bed (see Burnstock 1990; Ralevic and Burnstock 1991). Atypically of most blood vessels, precontracted strips or segments of coronary arteries relax in response to NA following its action on β-adrenoceptors (Cohen et al. 1984). It is interesting that ATP, which constricts most blood vessels, has been shown to relax rabbit coronary arteries via P_{2y}-purinoceptors located on the vascular smooth muscle (Corr and Burnstock 1991; Keefe et al. 1992), consistent with the general caveat that co-released transmitters act in concord to produce a response.

NPY has been found to be present as a cotransmitter in almost all perivascular sympathetic nerves examined so far. In these nerves, the release of both NPY and NA due to electrical stimulation of sympathetic nerve terminals is prevented by guanethidine, while surgical removal of the stellate ganglion, or of the superior cervical ganglion, or 6-hydroxydopamine treatment, attenuate levels of NPY in the cardiovascular system (see Lundberg et al. 1990; Mione et al. 1990). Electron microscopy and fractionation studies carried out in some non-vascular tissues have demonstrated that NPY is preferentially localized, along with NA and ATP, in large dense-cored vesicles (80–90 nm), while no NPY is found in the small dense-cored vesicles which are the major storage sites for NA and ATP (Stjärne et al. 1986). Again, the pattern of stimulation appears to be an important determinant of the release of coexisting sympathetic transmitters. For example, in the spleen NPY release is optimal at high frequency intermittent bursts of stimulation (Lundberg *et al.* 1986). It has commonly been suggested that frequency and duration of stimulation may be important in relation to synthesis of transmitters and hence for the supply/depletion of transmitter content of the nerve terminal; classical transmitters are synthesized in the nerve terminal, thus re-supply is rapid being by local synthesis and re-uptake, while re-supply of peptides is a longer process being by axonal transport.

The major role of NPY in the vasculature, and in the vas deferens, appears to be that of a pre- and/or postjunctional modulator of sympathetic transmission since it has little direct postjunctional action or causes contraction only at high concentrations. Direct vasoconstrictor actions of NPY have, however, been demonstrated in some vessels. At the prejunctional level, NPY has potent inhibitory effects, reducing the release of NA and ATP from sympathetic nerves. Postjunctionally, NPY generally acts to enhance the actions of sympathetic nerve stimulation, NA and ATP (see Edvinsson 1988; Lundberg *et al.* 1990; Mione *et al.* 1990). Interestingly, it has been reported that in the guinea-pig saphenous artery NPY potentiates sympathetic constriction by a selective action on the purinergic component without modifying the noradrenergic component of the response (Cheung 1991). Postjunctional inhibitory effects of NPY have been demonstrated in canine cerebral arteries, where NPY was shown to suppress the contractile action of exogenously applied NA (Suzuki *et al.* 1988).

5-Hydroxytryptamine (5-HT) immunofluorescent nerves have been localized in a number of vessels, however, it seems that for the most part, 5-HT is not synthesized and stored in separate nerves, but is taken up, stored in, and released as a 'false transmitter' from sympathetic nerves (Kawasaki and Takasaki 1984; Jackowski *et al.* 1989). Accordingly, 5-HT immunostaining is lost after surgical and/or chemical sympathectomy (Cowen *et al.* 1986; Gale and Cowen 1988). 5-HT has direct effects on the vascular smooth muscle (usually vasoconstriction) and can act as a pre- or postjunctional neuromodulator of sympathetic transmission; it inhibits the release of NA from sympathetic nerve terminals and postjunctionally potentiates the vasoconstrictor effects of NA (Seabrook and Nolan 1983; Medgett *et al.* 1984).

Enkephalins have been shown to coexist with NA in cell bodies and fibres of postganglionic sympathetic neurones. In bovine splenic nerve, NA is found in both small and large dense-cored vesicles, whereas [met]enkephalin is co-localized only in the large vesicles (Fried *et al.* 1986). Similarly, in bovine vas deferens, immunoelectron microscopy and density gradient separations have shown co-localization of peptide and amine exclusively within the large dense-cored vesicles (De Potter *et al.* 1987). Furthermore, both NA and [met]enkephalin were co-released by transmural stimulation in a guanethidine-sensitive manner (De Potter *et al.* 1987). In the pig cerebral artery a population of large dense-cored sympathetic vesicles were found to contain dopamine β-hydroxylase, NPY, and enkephalin (Kong *et al.* 1990). The functional significance of sympathetic coexistence of opioids is likely to be related to their prejunctional inhibitory effects on sympathetic transmission.

SENSORY MOTOR NERVE COTRANSMISSION

The neuropeptides substance P and calcitonin gene-related peptide (CGRP) are the principal transmitters of primary afferent nerves and have been shown to coexist in the same perivascular terminals (Gibbins *et al.* 1985; Lee *et al.* 1985; Uddman *et al.* 1985). Furthermore, with the use of colloidal gold particles of different sizes, they have been shown to coexist in the same large granular vesicles (Gulbenkian *et al.* 1986; Wharton and Gulbenkian 1987). The motor (efferent) function of sensory nerves has been demonstrated in rat mesenteric arteries where overwhelming evidence exists for a role for CGRP as the mediator of vasodilatation following release from sensory motor nerves (Kawasaki *et al.* 1988; Fujimori *et al.* 1990). In contrast, despite the extensive co-localization of substance P-like immunoreactivity (-LI) with CGRP-LI in sensory nerve fibres in rat mesenteric arteries, substance P is not co-released with CGRP by electrical stimulation at parameters causing release of CGRP and subsequent profound vasodilatation (Fujimori *et al.* 1990) and substance P has little or no vasodilator action on rat mesenteric arteries (Kawasaki *et al.* 1988). The role of substance P co-localized with CGRP in sensory motor nerves is problematical. In most vessels substance P does not appear to act directly on receptors on the vascular smooth muscle to produce vasodilatation. It does however produce potent vasodilatation via receptors on endothelial cells which leads to the release of nitric oxide (NO). While it is possible that substance P released from nerves supplying the microvasculature could produce vasodilatation via endothelial cells, it is most unlikely to reach the endothelium without degradation in larger blood vessels. This raises the possibility that differential release of coexisting transmitters can occur from the same vesicle and emphasizes the importance of ascertaining co-release, and not just coexistence when identifying cotransmission. In this case it may be that the role of the coexisting substance P is either trophic or sensory (and not motor).

Many other peptide and non-peptide substances including neurokinin A, somatostatin, and VIP have been described in capsaicin-sensitive sensory neurones (see Maggi and Meli 1988). Unmyelinated sensory neurones containing cholecystokinin (CCK)/CGRP/dynorphin (DYN)/substance P have been shown to project to cutaneous arterioles in guinea-pig skin (Gibbins *et al.* 1987). Neurones from the same ganglia which contain CCK/CGRP/substance P innovate arterioles of skeletal muscle, CGRP/DYN/substance P nerve fibres mostly supply the pelvic viscera, and CGRP/substance P fibres run mainly to the heart, large arteries, and veins (Gibbins *et al.* 1987). There is also evidence for a sensory role for ATP and it has been proposed that ATP may coexist in sensory nerve terminals with substance P and CGRP (Burnstock 1990).

In addition to their direct effects, pre- and postjunctional neuromodulatory actions have been described for substance P and CGRP. When substance P is injected with CGRP into human skin, it is able to convert the CGRP-mediated long lasting vasodilatation into a transient response by a mechanism which is dependent on the action of proteases released from mast cells by substance P

(Brain and Williams 1988). On the other hand, CGRP potentiates tachykinin-induced plasma protein extravasation in rat and rabbit skin (Gamse and Saria 1985). CGRP has been shown to potentiate substance P transmission in the spinal cord by inhibiting a specific substance P endopeptidase and by increasing the release of substance P from capsaicin-superfused slices of dorsal spinal cord *in vitro* (see Mione *et al.* 1990). By analogy with other systems, it seems likely that modulatory interactions between substance P, CGRP, ATP, and other putative sensory cotransmitters will increasingly be described in the periphery.

PARASYMPATHETIC NERVE COTRANSMISSION

The classical evidence for cotransmission of ACh and VIP in certain postganglionic parasympathetic neurones comes from pharmacological studies performed on cat salivary glands (Lundberg 1981). ACh and VIP are released from the same parasympathetic nerve terminals in response to transmural nerve stimulation. During low frequency stimulation ACh is released to cause an increase in salivary secretion from acinar cells and also to elicit some minor dilatation of blood vessels in the gland. VIP is preferentially released at high frequencies to cause marked vasodilatation of blood vessels and, while it has no direct effect on acinar cells, it acts as a neuromodulator to enhance substantially both the postjunctional effect of ACh on acinar cell secretion and the release of ACh from nerve varicosities via prejunctional receptors (Fig. 9.5). The differential release of ACh and VIP at different frequencies of stimulation may be related to the preferential storage of ACh and VIP in small clear vesicles and in large dense-cored vesicles respectively, with the latter apparently needing stronger frequencies of stimulation to release their transmitter content (Lundberg 1981).

Peptide histidine isoleucine (PHI) and VIP are fragments of the same precursor molecule, prepro-VIP, and certain of their amino acid sequences are identical. PHI has been shown to be released in addition to VIP and ACh from parasympathetic neurones supplying the submandibular salivary gland (Lundberg *et al.* 1984). Double immunostaining has revealed coexistence of VIP and PHI in cerebrovascular nerve fibres (Edvinsson and McCulloch 1985). VIP/PHI-LI nerve fibres have also been demonstrated in the rabbit uterine artery but the physiological significance of this coexistence is not clear since the two peptides are equipotent and their effects are additive. Vasodilator nerves to the uterine arteries in the guinea-pig contain immunoreactivity to VIP which coexists with DYN, NPY, and somatostatin (Morris *et al.* 1985, 1987). NPY-LI has been reported in some of the choline acetyltransferase-/VIP-containing neurones of the parasympathetic ciliary, sphenopalatine, otic (Leblanc *et al.* 1987; Leblanc and Landis 1988), and pterygopalatine ganglia (Kuwayama *et al.* 1988; Cavanagh *et al.* 1989) with targets including the iris and cerebral vessels. Double immunostaining has revealed a population of fibres which contain NPY co-localized with VIP in guinea-pig cerebral arteries (Gibbins and Morris 1988). CGRP-LI has been reported in parasympathetic cholinergic neurones located in the pontine and sacral parasympathetic

PARASYMPATHETIC NEUROTRANSMISSION

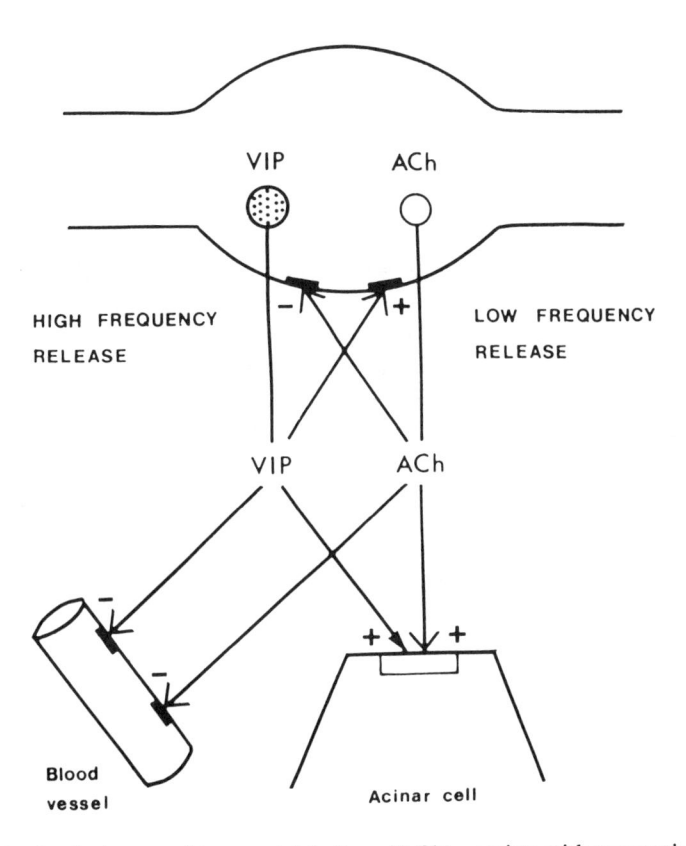

Fig. 9.5 A classical transmitter, acetylcholine, (ACh) coexists with vasoactive intestinal polypeptide (VIP) in parasympathetic nerves supplying the cat salivary gland. ACh and VIP are stored in separate vesicles; they can be released differentially at different stimulation frequencies to act on acinar cells and glandular blood vessels. Co-operation is achieved by the selective release of ACh at low impulse frequencies and of VIP at high frequencies. Pre- and postjunctional modulation is indicated. (From Burnstock 1983.)

nuclei and in the ventral horn (see Mione *et al.* 1990). The functional significance of these examples of co-localization remains to be determined.

Autonomic control of penile erection, involving relaxation of the smooth muscle of the corpus cavernosum as well as dilatation of other penile vascular beds, has traditionally been attributed to the vasodilator effects of ACh and VIP released from parasympathetic nerves. Recent evidence suggests that NO released from nerves may have an important role in smooth muscle relaxation leading to penile erection. In the rat penis all of the parasympathetic neurones projecting to the penis are found in the major pelvic ganglion. Positive staining for nitric oxide synthase (NOS) and nicotinamide adenine dinucleotide phosphate-diaphorase

(NADPH-d) (now regarded as a marker for NOS) has been shown in many of the neurones of the major pelvic ganglion, axons of the penile cavernous nerve, varicose terminals associated with various tissues of the rat penis, and neuronal plexuses in the adventitial layer of penile arteries (Burnett et al. 1992; Keast 1992). A functional correlate for this evidence for the presence of NO in nerves has been provided by demonstrations of a role for NO as a vasodilator transmitter of isolated strips of rabbit and human corpus cavernosum and in the bovine penile artery (see Rand 1992).

Recently NOS-containing fibres, shown by lesion studies to arise from parasympathetic cell bodies in the sphenopalatine ganglia, have been localized in the adventitia of cerebral arteries and many of these also contain VIP (see Bredt and Snyder 1992). A functional role for perivascular neuronal NO in cerebral arteries has been identified in studies showing that stimulation of adventitial nerve fibres causes vascular relaxation which is attenuated by inhibitors of NOS (Toda et al. 1990). VIP/NO co-localization has been identified; it is likely that NO also coexists with other transmitters in other nerve profiles which raises the question as to which other combinations are possible and what is their functional significance?

INTRAMURAL NERVE COTRANSMISSION

Perivascular substance P-LI fibres which are insensitive to capsaicin treatment have been found supplying arterioles of the distal colon and rectum of rats (Holzer et al. 1980; Cuello et al. 1981) and are likely to have arisen from enteric substance P neurones in the gut. Hence the combinations of coexisting substances in neurones of the gut are of relevance in considering the innervation of these and other local vessels. Extensive and detailed studies have allowed a very complete mapping of the complex neuronal markers and projections of enteric neurones (Costa et al. 1986; Furness and Costa 1987). Several peptidergic substances including NPY, VIP, PHI, substance P, and CGRP have been identified in enteric neurones, often coexisting (up to six peptides in the same neurone) with the classical neurotransmitters NA and ACh (Furness and Costa 1987). The precise roles of the coexisting substances, however, have not for the most part been established, except for the proposed combinations of ACh and substance P in the excitatory nerves and ATP and VIP in the non-adrenergic, non-cholinergic (NANC) inhibitory neurones involved in peristaltic reflexes. The co-localization of NOS and NADPH-d in cultured myenteric neurones of the guinea-pig (Saffrey et al. 1992) together with evidence for a role for NO in the inhibitory control of some intestinal smooth muscle, and the co-localization of NOS and VIP in neurones of the myenteric plexus (Rand 1992) raises the possibility of cotransmission of NO/ATP/VIP.

Studies of intrinsic cardiac neurones in culture have shown that some of these neurones show immunofluorescence for mixtures of both NPY and 5-HT in different proportions (Hassall and Burnstock 1987). A clue to the physiological significance of this coexistence is that both 5-HT and NPY are potent vasoconstrictors of coronary vessels and may have synergistic actions. ACh and ATP may also be utilized as neurotransmitters by intracardiac neurones (Crowe and Burnstock 1982). In addition, the presence of NOS immunoreactivity and positive staining for NADPH-d has recently been detected in a subpopulation of intrinsic neurones of the guinea-pig heart (Hassall *et al.* 1992), suggesting that complex patterns of coexistence and interactions between a variety of neurotransmitters and NO are likely to occur.

Recently, NO together with ATP have been shown to be the mediators of NANC vasodilatation of the rabbit portal vein suggesting the possibility of cotransmission of NO/ATP (Brizzolara *et al.* 1993) (Fig. 9.6).

PLASTICITY OF PERIVASCULAR NERVES AND INTERACTIONS BETWEEN PERIVASCULAR NERVE COTRANSMITTERS AND ENDOTHELIAL VASOACTIVE AGENTS

The plasticity of perivascular nerves in development, ageing, and pathophysiological conditions is well established (see Burnstock 1991). Less well recognized is the fact that this plasticity may encompass changes in the proportions of coexisting transmitters. For example, despite the co-localization of certain transmitters there is no apparent correlation between their expression during development. Hence, CGRP-like immunoreactivity was found earlier than substance P-like immunoreactivity in cerebrovascular nerves, and increased in old age, while the density of substance P-like immunoreactive fibres did not change (Dhital *et al.* 1988; Mione *et al.* 1988). NA and NPY also underwent different expression in cerebrovascular nerves during development (Dhital *et al.* 1988; Mione *et al.* 1988). Direct evidence for changes in transmitter ratio in disease comes from a study of hypertension where the purinergic component of sympathetic cotransmission has been claimed to be enhanced to the extent that it is the dominant component of the sympathetic response (Vidal *et al.* 1986).

To put perivascular nerve cotransmission into a physiological context of local vascular control mechanisms it should be recognized that a dynamic balance involving both short- and long-term interactions exists beween perivascular nerves and the endothelial cells that form the innermost cell layer of the vessel wall. Reciprocal interactions between these two systems potentially have an important impact on patterns of cotransmission. In many isolated blood vessels, contractions produced by sympathetic nerve stimulation or due to vasoconstrictors including catecholamines and 5-HT, are greater after the endothelium is removed, or during antagonism of endothelium-derived relaxing factor (EDRF). While part of this effect is likely to involve postjunctional mechanisms evidence has been presented that substances released from the endothelium may act prejunctionally to influence neurotransmitter release from nerves (Cohen and Weisbrod 1988; Greenberg *et al.* 1989; Tesfamariam *et al.* 1989). This may or may not involve endothelial-derived

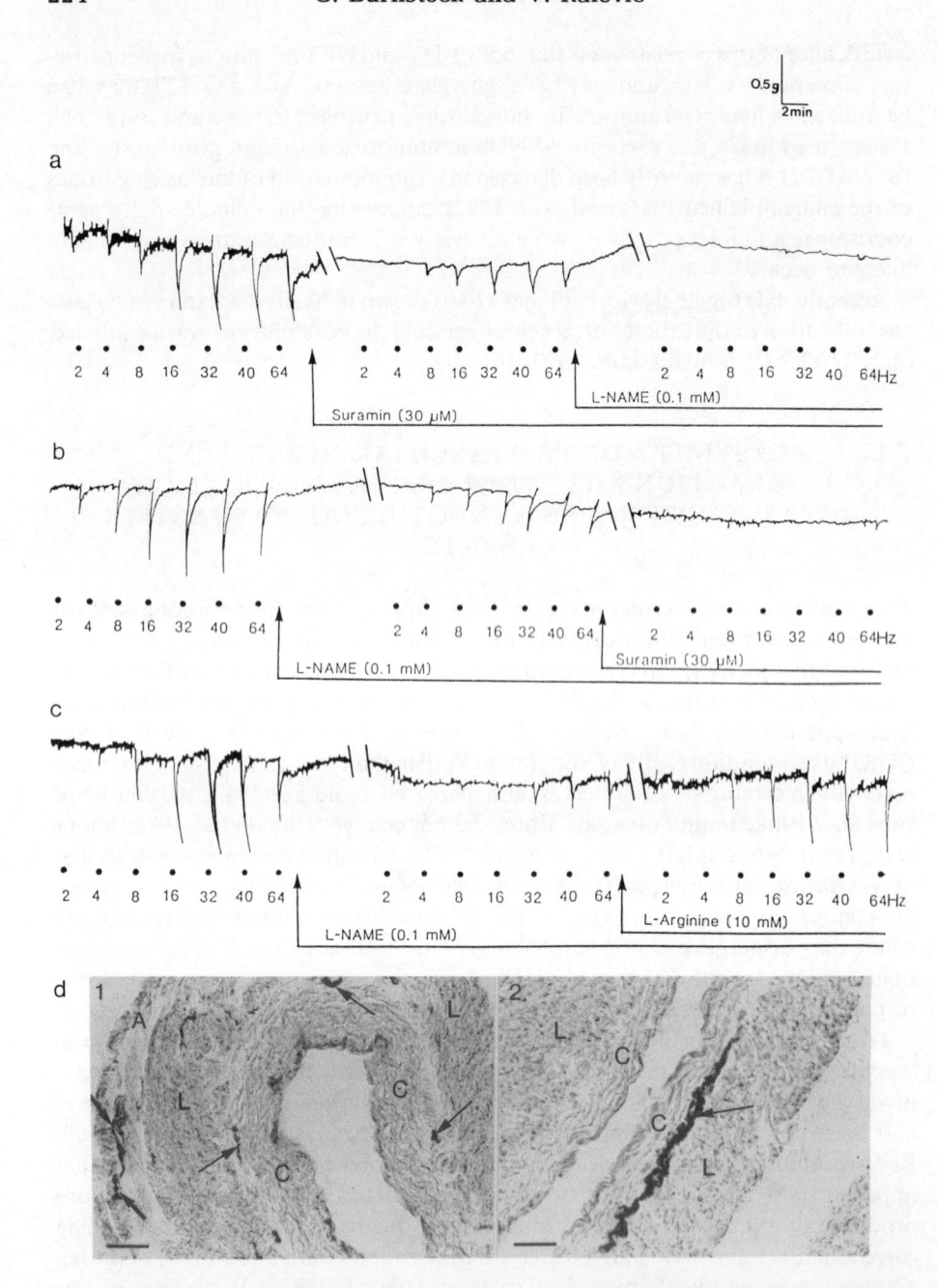

Fig. 9.6 Relaxations of the rabbit portal vein to neurogenic transmural stimulation for 10 s. (2–64 Hz. 0.7 ms, 100 V) at 5 min intervals. Guanethidine (3.4 µM) and atropine (0.114 µM) were present throughout to block adrenergic and cholinergic neurotransmission respectively. Tone was induced with ergotamine (8.6 µM). Panel (a) shows that

NO. ATP is also released from endothelial cells in response to physiological stimuli such as hypoxia or shear stress and may thus modulate the activity of perivascular nerves via prejunctional P_1 purinoceptors following breakdown to adenosine and diffusion through the vessel wall (Burnstock 1988). Conversely, in the microvasculature, where neural-endothelial separation is small, cotransmitters released from nerves could act directly on endothelial cells to influence the release of endothelium-derived factors.

Long-term (trophic) changes in the amount or balance of cotransmitters released from perivascular nerves can lead to changes in endothelial cells. For instance in the rabbit ear artery selective denervation has been associated with impaired endothelial function (Mangiarua and Bevan 1986), while long-term stimulation of perivascular nerves induced structural changes and the appearance of CGRP- and NPY-like immunoreactivity in a subpopulation of endothelial cells (Loesch et al. 1992). Selective denervation (of sensory motor nerves) also resulted in impaired endothelium-dependent relaxation in the rat mesenteric arterial bed (Miller and Scott 1990). CGRP has been shown to have a proliferative effect on endothelial cells in culture (Haegerstrand et al. 1990) and trophic effects of cotransmitters on other cell types have also been described for VIP (George and Ojeda 1987), NPY (Rebuffet et al. 1988), and substance P (Nilsson et al. 1985). Conversely, sustained changes in the release of endothelial vasoactive factors can influence the development of perivascular nerves and hence patterns of cotransmission. In this respect, it is possible that the impaired sympathetic function seen in mesenteric, hepatic, and ear arteries of Watanabe heritable hyperlipidaemic rabbits (Burnstock et al. 1991) and cholesterol fed rats (Panek et al. 1985) may be a consequence of the long-term endothelial damage that is characteristic of atherosclerosis.

---

pre-incubation with suramin (30 μM) for 20 min reduced the nerve-mediated relaxations compared with controls and that suramin-resistant neurogenic relaxations were abolished 20 min after the addition of the nitric oxide synthase inhibitor, N^G-nitro-L-arginine methyl ester (L-NAME, 0.1 mM). Panel (b) shows that neurogenic relaxations remaining after 20 min pre-treatment of the tissue with L-NAME (0.1 mM) were abolished 20 min after the addition of suramin (30 μM). In (c), the effect of adding L-NAME (0.1 mM) to the tissue is shown; there was an additional rise in tone and inhibition of the response to nerve stimulation after a 20 min incubation period. The subsequent treatment of tissues with L-arginine (10 mM) for 20 min reversed this effect. Panel (d) shows the histochemical localization of reduced nicotinamide adenine dinucleotide phosphate (NADPH)-diaphorase in the rabbit portal vein. (d1) NADPH-diaphorase reaction seen in nerve fibres between the inner circular (C) and outer longitudinal muscle coats (thin black *arrows*). Note also the NADPH-diaphorase positive nerves in adventitia (A) (thick black *arrows*). Tangentional section. (d2) NADPH-diaphorase reaction seen in a dense nerve plexus between the inner circular (C) and outer longitudinal muscle coats of the portal vein (thin black *arrow*). Transverse section. Calibration bar for d1 and d2 is 30 μm. Each of the traces in (a), (b), and (c) is representative of similar results in six separate experiments. (From Brizzolara et al. 1993.)

CONCLUSIONS

The ability to release more than one transmitter substance serves to increase the amount and variety of information imparted by a single neurone thus greatly increasing the sophistication and complexity of local control mechanisms. This is achieved via pre- and/or postjunctional neuromodulation as well as by variation in the proportions of co-released transmitter substances with different patterns of neural discharges. Plasticity and long-term (trophic) interactions between perivascular nerves and endothelial cells should also be considered, where changes in expression of transmitters can occur in development and ageing as well as in pathophysiological conditions.

REFERENCES

Abrahams, V. C., Koelle, G. B., and Smart, P. (1957). Histochemical demonstration of cholinesterases in the hypothalamus of the dog. *J. Physiol.*, **139**, 137-44.

Angus, J. A., Broughton, A., and Mulvany, M. J. (1988). Role of α-adrenoceptors in constrictor responses of rat, guinea-pig and rabbit small arteries to neural activation. *J. Physiol.*, **403**, 495-510.

Bartfai, T., Iverfeldt, K., and Fisone, G. (1988). Regulation of the release of coexisting neurotransmitters. *Annu. Rev. Pharmacol. Toxicol.*, **28**, 285-310.

Blaschko, H., Born, G. V. R., D'Lorio, A., and Eade, N. R. (1956). Observations on the distribution of catecholamines and adenosine triphosphate in the bovine adrenal medulla. *J. Physiol.*, **133**, 548-57.

Brain, S. D. and Williams, T. J. (1988). Substance P regulates the vasodilator activity of calcitonin gene-related peptide. *Nature*, **355**, 73-5.

Bredt, D. S. and Snyder, S. H. (1992). Nitric oxide, a novel neuronal messenger. *Neuron*, **8**, 3-11.

Brizzolara, A. L., Crowe, R., and Burnstock, G. (1993). Evidence for the involvement of both ATP and nitric oxide in non-adrenergic, non-cholinergic inhibitory neurotransmission in the rabbit portal vein. *Br. J. Pharmacol.*, **109**, 606-8.

Bultmann, R., von Kügelgen, I., and Starke, K. (1991). Adrenergic and purinergic cotransmission in nicotine-evoked vasoconstriction in rabbit ileocolic arteries. *Naunyn-Schmiedeberg's Arch. Pharmacol.*, **344**, 174-82.

Burn, J. H. and Rand, M. J. (1959). Sympathetic postganglionic mechanism. *Nature*, **184**, 163-5.

Burnett, A. L., Lowenstein, C. J., Bredt, D. S., Chang, T. S. K., and Snyder, S. H. (1992). Nitric oxide: a physiologic mediator of penile erection. *Science*, **257**, 401-3.

Burnstock, G. (1976). Do some nerve cells release more than one transmitter? *Neuroscience*, **1**, 239-48.

Burnstock, G. (1983). Recent concepts of chemical communication between excitable cells. In *Dale's principle and communication between neurones*. (ed. N. N. Osborne), pp. 7-35. Pergamon Press, Oxford.

Burnstock, G. (1986). Autonomic neuromuscular junctions: Current developments and future directions. (The Anatomical Society Review Lecture). *J. Anat.*, **146**, 1-30.

Burnstock, G. (1987). Mechanisms of interaction of peptide and nonpeptide vascular neurotransmitter systems. *J. Cardiovasc. Pharmacol.*, **10 (Suppl. 12)**, S74-81.

Burnstock, G. (1988). Regulation of local blood flow by neurohumoral substances

released from perivascular nerves and endothelial cells. *Acta Physiol. Scand.*, **133** (**Suppl. 571**), 53-9.
Burnstock, G. (1990). Co-transmission. (The Fifth Heymans Memorial Lecture). *Arch. Int. Pharmacodyn. Ther.*, **304**, 7-33.
Burnstock, G. (1991). Plasticity in expression of co-transmitters and autonomic nerves in aging and disease. In *Plasticity and regeneration of the nervous system* (ed. P. S. Timiras and A. Privat), pp. 291-301. Plenum Press, New York.
Burnstock, G. and Warland, J. J. I. (1987). A pharmacological study of the rabbit saphenous artery *in vitro*: A vessel with a large purinergic contractile response to sympathetic nerve stimulation. *Br. J. Pharmacol.*, **90**, 111-20.
Burnstock, G., Stewart-Lee, A., Brizzolara, A., Tomlinson, A., and Corr, L. (1991). Dual control by nerves and endothelial cells of arterial blood flow in atherosclerosis. In *Atherosclerotic plaques* (ed. R. W. Wissler, M. G. Bond, M. Mercuri, and P. Tanganelli), pp. 285-92. Plenum Press, New York.
Campbell, G. (1987). Cotransmission. *Annu. Rev. Pharmacol. Toxicol.*, **27**, 51-70.
Cavanagh, J. F. R., Mione, M. C., and Burnstock, G. (1989). Colocalization of NPY and VIP in the cerebrovascular nerves originating from the pterygopalatine ganglion in the rat. *J. Cereb. Blood Flow Metab.*, **9 (Suppl. 1)**, S34.
Chan-Palay, V., and Palay, S. L. (ed.) (1984). *Co-existence of neuroactive substances in neurones*. Wiley, New York.
Cheung, D. W. (1991). Neuropeptide Y potentiates specifically the purinergic component of the neural responses in the guinea pig saphenous artery. *Circ. Res.*, **68**, 1401-7.
Cohen, R. A. and Weisbrod, R. M. (1988). The endothelium inhibits norepinephrine release from adrenergic nerves of the rabbit carotid artery. *Am. J. Physiol.*, **254**, H871-8.
Cohen, R. A., Shepherd, J. T., and Vanhoutte, P. M. (1984). Effects of the adrenergic transmitter on epicardial coronary arteries. *Fed. Proc.*, **43**, 2862-70.
Corr, L. and Burnstock, G. (1991). Vasodilator response of coronary smooth muscle to the sympathetic co-transmitters noradrenaline and adenosine 5'-triphosphate. *Br. J. Pharmacol.*, **104**, 337-42.
Costa, M., Furness, J. B., and Gibbins, I. L. (1986). Chemical coding of enteric neurones. In *Coexistence of neuronal messengers: A new principle in chemical transmission* (ed. T. Hökfelt, K. Fuxe, and B. Pernow), pp. 217-39. Elsevier, Amsterdam.
Cowen, T., Alafaci, C., Crockard, H. A., and Burnstock, G. (1986). 5-HT-containing nerves to major cerebral arteries of the gerbil originate in the superior cervical ganglia. *Brain Res.*, **384**, 51-9.
Crowe, R. and Burnstock, G. (1982). Fluorescence histochemical localisation of quinacrine-positive neurones in the guinea-pig and rabbit atrium. *Cardiovasc. Res.*, **16**, 384-90.
Cuello, A. C. (ed.) (1982). *Co-transmission*. Proceedings of the symposium 50th anniversary meeting of the British Pharmacological Society, Oxford. Macmillan Press, London.
Cuello, A. C., Gamse, R., Holzer, P., and Lembeck, F. (1981). Substance P immunoreactive neurons following neonatal administration of capsaicin. *Naunyn-Schmiedeberg's Arch. Pharmacol.*, **315**, 185-94.
Dale, H. (1935). Pharmacology and nerve endings. *Proc. R. Soc. Med.*, **28**, 319-32.
De Potter, W. P., Coen, E. P., and De Potter, R. W. (1987). Evidence for the co-existence and co-release of [MET]enkephalin and noradrenaline from sympathetic nerves of the bovine vas deferens. *Neuroscience*, **20**, 855-66.
Dhital, K. K., Gerli, R., Lincoln, J., Milner, P., Tanganelli, P., Weber, G., *et al.* (1988). Increased density of perivascular nerves to the major cerebral vessels of the spontaneously

hypertensive rat: differential changes in noradrenaline and neuropeptide Y during development. *Brain Res.*, **444**, 33–45.

Douglas, W. W. and Poisner, A. M. (1966). Evidence that the secreting adrenal chromaffin cell releases catecholamines directly from ATP-rich granules. *J. Physiol.*, **183**, 236–48.

Edvinsson, L. (1988). The effects of neuropeptide Y on the circulation. *ISI Atlas of Science: Pharmacology*, 357–61.

Edvinsson, L. and McCulloch, J. (1985). Distribution and vasomotor effects of peptide HI (PHI) in feline cerebral blood vessels *in vitro* and *in situ*. *Reg. Peptides*, **10**, 345–56.

Evans, R. J. and Cunnane, T. C. (1992). Relative contributions of ATP and noradrenaline to the nerve evoked contraction of the rabbit jejunal artery. *Naunyn-Schmiedeberg's Arch. Pharmacol.*, **345**, 424–30.

Evans, R. J., and Surprenant, A. (1992). Vasoconstriction of guinea-pig submucosal arterioles following sympathetic nerve stimulation is mediated by the release of ATP. *Br. J. Pharmacol.*, **106**, 242–9.

Fried, G., Terenius, L., Brodin, E., Efendic, S., Dockray, G., Fahrenkrug, J., *et al.* (1986). Neuropeptide Y, enkephalin and noradrenaline coexist in sympathetic neurons innervating the bovine spleen. *Cell Tissue Res.*, **243**, 495–508.

Fujimori, A., Saito, A., Kimura, S., and Goto, K. (1990). Release of calcitonin gene-related peptide (CGRP) from capsaicin-sensitive vasodilator nerves in the rat mesenteric artery. *Neurosci. Lett.*, **112**, 173–8.

Furness, J. B. and Costa, M. (ed.) (1987). *The enteric nervous system*. Churchill Livingstone, Edinburgh.

Furness, J. B., Morris, J. L., Gibbins, I. L., and Costa, M. (1989). Chemical coding of neurons and plurichemical transmission. *Annu. Rev. Pharmacol. Toxicol.*, **29**, 289–306.

Gale, J. D. and Cowen, T. (1988). The origin and distribution of 5-hydroxytryptamine-like immunoreactive nerve fibres to major mesenteric vessels of the rat. *Neuroscience*, **24**, 1051–9.

Gamse, R. and Saria, A. (1985). Potentiation of tachykinin-induced protein extravasation by calcitonin gene-related peptide. *Eur. J. Pharmacol.*, **114**, 61–6.

Geffen, L. B. and Livett, B. G. (1971). Synaptic vesicles in sympathetic neurons. *Physiol. Rev.*, **51**, 98–157.

George, F. W. and Ojeda, S. R. (1987). Vasoactive intestinal peptide enhances aromatase activity in the neonatal rat ovary before development of primary follicles or responsiveness to follicle-stimulating hormone. *Proc. Natl Acad. Sci. USA*, **84**, 5803–7.

Gibbins, I. L. and Morris, J. L. (1988). Co-existence of immunoreactivity to neuropeptide Y and vasoactive intestinal polypeptide in non-noradrenergic axons innervating guinea-pig cerebral arteries after sympathectomy. *Brain Res.*, **444**, 402–6.

Gibbins, I. L., Furness, J. B., Costa, M., MacIntyre, I., Hillyard, C. J., and Girgis, S. (1985). Colocalization of calcitonin gene-related peptide-like immunoreactivity with substance P in cutaneous, vascular and visceral sensory neurons of guinea pigs. *Neurosci. Lett.*, **57**, 125–30.

Gibbins, I. L., Furness, J. B., and Costa, M. (1987). Pathway-specific patterns of coexistence of substance P, calcitonin gene-related peptide, cholecystokinin and dynorphin in neurons of the dorsal root ganglia of the guinea-pig. *Cell Tissue Res.*, **248**, 417–37.

Greenberg, S., Diecke, F. P. J., Peevy, K., and Tanaka, T. P. (1989). The endothelium modulates adrenergic neurotransmission to canine pulmonary arteries and veins. *Eur. J. Pharmacol.*, **162**, 67–80.

Gulbenkian, S., Merighi, A., Wharton, J., Varndell, I. M., and Polak, J. M. (1986). Ultrastructural evidence for the coexistence of calcitonin gene-related peptide and substance P in secretory vesicles of peripheral nerves in the guinea-pig. *J. Neurocytol.*, **15**, 535–42.

Haegerstrand, A., Dalsgaard, C.-J., Jonzon, B., Larsson, O., and Nilsson, J. (1990).

Calcitonin gene-related peptide stimulates proliferation of human endothelial cells. *Proc. Natl Acad. Sci. USA*, **87**, 3299-303.
Hassall, C. J. S. and Burnstock, G. (1987) Immunocytochemical localisation of neuropeptide Y and 5-hydroxytryptamine in a subpopulation of amine-handling intracardiac neurones that do not contain dopamine β-hydroxylase in tissue culture. *Brain Res.*, **422**, 74-82.
Hassall, C. J. S., Saffrey, M. J., Belai, A., Hoyle, C. H. V., Moules, E. W., Moss, J., *et al.* (1992). Nitric oxide synthase immunoreactivity and NADPH-diaphorase activity in a subpopulation of intrinsic neurones of the guinea-pig heart. *Neurosci. Lett.*, **143**, 65-8.
Hillarp, N.-A., Hogberg, B., and Nilson, B. (1955). Adenosine triphosphate in the adrenal medulla of the cow. *Nature*, **176**, 1032-3.
Hökfelt, T., Fuxe, K., and Pernow, B. (ed.) (1986). Coexistence of neuronal messengers: A new principle in chemical transmission. *Progress in Brain Research*, Vol. 68. Elsevier, Amsterdam.
Holzer, P., Gamse, R., and Lembeck, F. (1980). Distribution of substance P in the rat gastrointestinal tract — lack of effect of capsaicin pretreatment. *Eur. J. Pharmacol.*, **61**, 303-7.
Jackowski, A., Crockard, A., and Burnstock, G. (1989). 5-Hydroxytryptamine demonstrated immunohistochemically in rat cerebrovascular nerves largely represents 5-hydroxytryptamine uptake into sympathetic nerve fibres. *Neuroscience*, **29**, 453-62.
Katsuragi, T. and Su, C. (1982). Augmentation by theophylline of [^{3}]purine release from vascular adrenergic nerves: Evidence for presynaptic autoinhibition. *J. Pharmacol. Exp. Ther.*, **220**, 152-6.
Kawasaki, H. and Takasaki, K. (1984). Vasoconstrictor responses induced by 5-hydroxytryptamine released from vascular adrenergic nerves by periarterial nerve stimulation. *J. Pharmacol. Exp. Ther.*, **28**, 255-72.
Kawasaki, H., Takasaki, K., Saito, A., and Goto, K. (1988). Calcitonin gene-related peptide (CGRP) from capsaicin-sensitive vasodilator nerves in the rat mesenteric artery. *Nature*, **335**, 165-7.
Keast, J. R. (1992). A possible neural source of nitric oxide in the rat penis. *Neurosci. Lett.*, **143**, 69-73.
Keefe, K. D., Pasco, J. S., and Eckman, D. M. (1992). Purinergic relaxation and hyperpolarization in guinea pig and rabbit coronary artery: role of the endothelium. *J. Pharmacol. Exp. Ther.*, **260**, 592-600.
Kennedy, C., Saville, V. L., and Burnstock, G. (1986). The contributions of noradrenaline and ATP to the responses of the rabbit central ear artery to sympathetic nerve stimulation depend on the parameters of stimulation. *Eur. J. Pharmacol.*, **122**, 291-300.
Koelle, G. B. (1955). The histochemical identification of acetyl-cholinesterase in cholinergic, adrenergic and sensory neurons. *J. Pharmacol. Exp. Ther.*, **114**, 167-84.
Kong, J. Y., Thureson-Klein, A. K., and Klein, R. L. (1990). Are NPY and enkephalins costored in the same noradrenergic neurons and vesicles? *Peptides*, **11**, 565-75.
Kupfermann, I. (1990). Functional studies of cotransmission. *Physiol. Rev.*, **71**, 683-732.
Kuwayama, Y., Emson, P. C., and Stone, R. A. (1988). Pterygopalatine ganglion cells contain neuropeptide Y. *Brain Res.*, **446**, 219-24.
Leblanc, G. G. and Landis, S. C. (1988). Target specificity of neuropeptide Y-immunoreactive cranial parasympathetic neurones. *J. Neurosci.*, **8**, 146-55.
Leblanc, G. C., Trimmer, B. A., and Landis, S. C. (1987). Neuropeptide Y-like immunoreactivity in rat cranial parasympathetic neurons: coexistence with vasoactive intestinal peptide and choline acetyltransferase. *Proc. Natl Acad. Sci. USA*, **84**, 3511-15.
Lee, Y., Takami, K., Kawai, Y., Girgis, S., Hillyard, C. J., MacIntyre, I., *et al.* (1985). Distribution of calcitonin gene-related peptide in the rat with special reference to coexistence with substance P. *Neuroscience*, **15**, 1227-37.

Leff, P., Wood, B. E., and O'Connor, S. E. (1990). Suramin is a slowly-equilibrating but competitive antagonist at P_{2x}-receptors in the rabbit isolated ear artery. *Br. J. Pharmacol.*, **101**, 645-9.

Loesch, A., Maynard, K. I., and Burnstock, G. (1992). CGRP- and NPY-like immunoreactivity in endothelial cells after long-term stimulation of perivascular nerves. *Neuroscience*, **48**, 723-36.

Lundberg, J. M. (1981). Evidence for coexistence of vasoactive intestinal polypeptide (VIP) and acetylcholine in neurons of cat exocrine glands. Morphological, biochemical and functional studies. *Acta Physiol. Scand.*, **112 (Suppl. 496)**, 1-57.

Lundberg, J. M., Fahrenkrug, J., Larsson, O., and Anggard, A. (1984). Corelease of vasoactive intestinal polypeptide and peptide histidine isoleucine in relation to atropine resistant vasodilatation in cat submandibular salivary gland. *Neurosci. Lett.*, **52**, 37-45.

Lundberg, J. M., Rudehill, A., Sollevi, A., Theodorsson-Norheim, E., and Hamberger, B. (1986). Frequency- and reserpine-dependent chemical coding of sympathetic transmission. Differential release of noradrenaline and neuropeptide Y from pig spleen. *Neurosci. Lett.*, **63**, 96-100.

Lundberg, J. M., Franco-Cereceda, A., Hemsen, A., Lacroix, J. S., and Pernow, J. (1990). Pharmacology of noradrenaline and neuropeptide tyrosine (NPY)-mediated sympathetic cotransmission. *Fundam. Clin. Pharmacol.*, **4**, 373-91.

Maggi, C. A. and Meli, A. (1988). The sensory-efferent function of capsaicin-sensitive sensory neurons. *Gen. Pharmacol.*, **19**, 1-43.

Mangiarua, E. I. and Bevan, R. O. (1986). Altered endothelium-mediated relaxation after denervation of growing rabbit ear artery. *Eur. J. Pharmacol.*, **122**, 149-52.

Medgett, I. C., Fearn, H. J., and Rand, M. J. (1984). Serotonin enhances sympathetic vasoconstrictor responses in rat isolated perfused tail artery by activation of postjunctional serotonin-2 receptors. *Clin. Exp. Pharmacol. Physiol.*, **11**, 343-6.

Miller, M. E. and Scott, T. W. (1990). The effect of perivascular denervation on endothelium-dependent relaxation to acetylcholine. *Artery*, **17**, 233-47.

Mione, M. C., Dhital, K. K., Amenta, F., and Burnstock, G. (1988). An increase in expression of neuropeptidergic vasodilator, but not vasoconstrictor nerves in aging rats. *Brain Res.*, **460**, 103-13.

Mione, M. C., Ralevic, V., and Burnstock, G. (1990). Peptides and vasomotor mechanisms. *Pharmacol. Ther.*, **46**, 429-68.

Morris, J. L., Gibbins, I. L., Furness, J. B., Costa, M., and Murphy, R. (1985). Colocalization of neuropeptide Y, vasoactive intestinal polypeptide and dynorphin in non-noradrenergic axons of the guinea-pig uterine artery. *Neurosci. Lett.*, **62**, 31-7.

Morris, J. L., Gibbins, I. L., and Furness, J. B. (1987). Increased dopamine-β-hydroxylase-like immunoreactivity in non-noradrenergic axons supplying the guinea-pig uterine artery after 6-hydroxydopamine treatment. *J. Auton. Nerv. Syst.*, **21**, 15-27.

Muramatsu, I., Fujiwara, M., Miura, A., and Sakakibara, Y. (1981). Possible involvement of adenine nucleotides in sympathetic neuroeffector mechanisms of dog basilar artery. *J. Pharmacol. Exp. Ther.*, **216**, 401-9.

Nilsson, J., von Fuler, A. M., and Dalsgaard, C. (1985). Stimulation of tissue cell growth by substance P and substance K. *Nature*, **315**, 61-3.

Osborne, N. N. (ed.) (1983). *Dale's principle and communication between neurones.* Pergamon Press, Oxford.

Panek, R. L., Dixon, W. R., and Rutledge, C. O. (1985). Modification of sympathetic neuronal function in the rat tail artery by dietary lipid treatment. *J. Pharmacol. Exp. Ther.*, **233**, 578-83.

Potter, D. D., Furshpan, E. J., and Landis, S. C. (1981). Multiple transmitter status and "Dale's Principle". *Neurosci. Commun.*, **1**, 1-9.

Ralevic, V. and Burnstock, G. (1991). Roles of P_2-purinoceptors in the cardiovascular system. *Circulation*, **84**, 1-14.
Ramme, D., Regenold, J. T., Starke, K., Busse, R., and Illes, P. (1987). Identification of the neuroeffector transmitter in jejunal branches of the rabbit mesenteric artery. *Naunyn-Schmiedeberg's Arch. Pharmacol.*, **336**, 267-73.
Rand, M. J. (1992). Nitrergic transmission: nitric oxide as a mediator of non-adrenergic, non-cholinergic neuro-effector transmission. *Clin. Exp. Pharmacol. Physiol.*, **19**, 147-69.
Rebuffet, P., Malendowica, L. K., Beloni, A. S., Mazzochi, G., and Nussdorfer, G. G. (1988). Long-term stimulatory effect of neuropeptide Y on the growth and steroidogenic capacity of rat adrenal zona glomerulosa. *Neuropeptides*, **11**, 133-6.
Saffrey, M. J., Hassall, C. J. S., Hoyle, C. H. V., Belai, A., Moss, J., Schmidt, H. H. H. W., et al. (1992). Colocalization of nitric oxide synthase and NADPH-diaphorase in cultured myenteric neurons. *NeuroReport*, **3**, 333-6.
Schumann, H. J. (1958). Uber den noradrenalin und ATP-Gehalt sympathetischer nerven. *Naunyn-Schmiedeberg's Arch. Pharmacol.*, **233**, 296-300.
Seabrook, J. M. and Nolan, P. L. (1983). The vascular interaction of noradrenaline and 5-hydroxytryptamine. *Eur. J. Pharmacol.*, **89**, 131-5.
Sneddon, P. and Burnstock, G. (1984). Inhibition of excitatory junction potentials in guinea-pig vas deferens by α,β-methylene ATP: Further evidence for ATP and noradrenaline as cotransmitters. *Eur. J. Pharmacol.*, **100**, 85-90.
Stjärne, L. (1989). Basic mechanisms and local modulation of nerve-impulse-induced secretion of neurotransmitters from individual sympathetic nerve varicosities. *Rev. Physiol. Biochem. Pharmacol.*, **112**, 1-137.
Stjärne, L. and Lishajko, F. (1966). Comparison of spontaneous loss of catecholamines and ATP *in vitro* from isolated bovine adrenomedullary, vesicular gland, vas deferens and splenic nerve granules. *J. Neurocytochem.*, **13**, 1213-16.
Stjärne, L., Lundberg, J. M., and Astrand, P. (1986). Neuropeptide Y — a cotransmitter with noradrenaline and adenosine 5′-triphosphate in the sympathetic nerves of the mouse vas deferens? A biochemical, physiological and electropharmacological study. *Neuroscience*, **18**, 151-66.
Su, C. (1975). Neurogenic release of purine compounds in blood vessels. *J. Pharmacol. Exp. Ther.*, **195**, 159-66.
Suzuki, H. (1985). Electrical responses of smooth muscle cells of the rabbit ear artery to adenosine triphosphate. *J. Physiol.*, **359**, 401-15.
Suzuki, Y., Shihuya, M., Ikegaki, I., Satoh, S., Takayasu, M., and Asona, T. (1988). Effects of neuropeptide Y on canine cerebral circulation. *Eur. J. Pharmacol.*, **146**, 271-7.
Tesfamariam, B., Weisbrod, R. M., and Cohen, R. A. (1989). The endothelium inhibits activation by calcium of vascular neurotransmission. *Am. J. Physiol.*, **257**, H1871-7.
Toda, N., Minami, Y., and Okamura, T. (1990). Inhibitory effect of L-N^G-nitro-arginine on the synthesis of EDRF and the cerebroarterial response to vasodilator nerve stimulation. *Life Sci.*, **47**, 345-51.
Uddman, R., Edvinsson, L., Ekman, R., Kingman, T., and McCulloch, J. (1985). Innervation of the feline cerebral vasculature by nerve fibres containing calcitonin gene-related peptide: Trigeminal origin and coexistence with substance P. *Neurosci. Lett.*, **62**, 131-6.
Vidal, M., Hicks, P. E., and Langer, S. Z. (1986). Differential effects of α,β-methylene ATP on responses to nerve stimulation in SHR and WKY tail arteries. *Naunyn-Schmiedeberg's Arch. Pharmacol.*, **332**, 384-90.
von Euler, U. S., Lishajko, F., and Stjärne, L. (1963). Catecholamines and adenosine

triphosphate in isolated adrenergic nerve granules. *Acta Physiol. Scand.*, **59**, 495-6.

von Kügelgen, I. and Starke, K. (1985). Noradrenaline and adenosine triphosphate as cotransmitters of neurogenic vasoconstriction in rabbit mesenteric artery. *J. Physiol.*, **367**, 435-55.

von Kügelgen, I. and Starke, K (1991). Noradrenaline-ATP cotransmission in the sympathetic nervous system. *Trends Pharmacol. Sci.*, **12**, 319-24.

Warland, J. J. I. and Burnstock, G. (1987). Effects of reserpine and 6-hydroxydopamine on the adrenergic and purinergic components of sympathetic responses of the rabbit saphenous artery. *Br. J. Pharmacol.*, **92**, 871-80.

Wharton, J. and Gulbenkian, S. (1987). Peptides in the mammalian cardiovascular system. *Experientia*, **43**, 821-32.

White, T. D., Chaudry, A., Vohra, M. M., Webb, D., and Leslie, R. A. (1985). Characteristics of P_2-nucleotide receptors mediating contraction and relaxation of rat aortic strips: possible physiological relevance. *Eur. J. Pharmacol.*, **118**, 37-44.

10. Endothelium-dependent vasodilator mechanisms

T. M. Cocks

INTRODUCTION

The endothelium is a crucial organ in terms of control of the vascular system. It not only provides an important permeability barrier between the blood and the surrounding tissues, particularly in the brain, but it also presents a non-thrombogenic surface to the blood, inactivates many bioactive substances, regulates vascular tone, and signals immune cells to extravasate in response to inflammatory stimuli. This chapter will concentrate on possible roles for endothelium-dependent vasodilator mechanisms in the control of vascular tone. The main focus will be how multiple endothelium-dependent dilator systems, like nitric oxide (NO) (Moncada et al. 1991), membrane hyperpolarization, or K^+ channel-dependent mechanisms (Taylor and Weston 1988) and possibly archidonic acid-derived factors like prostacyclin and various lipoxygenase-derived products (Vane et al. 1987) interact to regulate smooth muscle relaxation. The generic term endothelium-derived relaxing factor or EDRF (Furchgott 1981, 1984; Cherry et al. 1982; Angus and Cocks 1989) will be used throughout, since it describes mediators of endothelium-dependent relaxation in general, rather than any one particular EDRF, like NO. Whilst Furchgott's (1981) definition of EDRF was initially only used to describe endothelium-dependent vascular relaxations to acetylcholine, the term was quickly used in a much broader sense to include all endothelium-dependent relaxation responses not mediated by prostanoids (see below). Therefore, although EDRF is used to describe a factor, it effectively describes a vascular smooth muscle relaxation response to endothelial cell stimulation both *in vitro* and *in vivo*.

Just how important endothelium-dependent dilator mechanisms may be in terms of cardiovasular control is encapsulated in the provocative proposal of Moncada et al. (1991) that 'the cardiovascular system is in a constant state of active vasodilatation dependent on the generation of NO'. Regardless of whether all the endothelium-dependent vasodilator capacity is due to NO (see below), constant, or basal, release of relaxing factors (EDRFs) from the endothelium probably tonically inhibits smooth muscle tone and therefore exerts an inhibitory input on blood pressure. This is not necessarily an alternative to the dogma of constant sympathetic drive and tonically high vascular tone. Rather, it implies that the vasculature is fine tuned by both short-acting constrictor (noradrenaline, angiotensin II, neuropeptide Y, ATP, etc.) and dilator (EDRF, PGI_2) factors from nerves and the endothelium respectively. The challenge now is not only to elucidate the relative contributions of these factors to the maintenance of basal vascular tone, but also to ascertain to what extremes the balance can be tipped when either major opposing controllers are abolished.

ENDOTHELIUM-DEPENDENT RELAXATION OF VASCULAR SMOOTH MUSCLE

History

In 1980, Furchgott and Zawadzki discovered that the well known vasodilator, acetylcholine (ACh) potently relaxed isolated ring segments of rabbit aorta only if the endothelium was present. If the endothelium was removed mechanically or enzymatically, the artery either failed to relax or contracted. From simple, yet elegant sandwich bioassay experiments which demonstrated transfer of a highly labile factor from endothelial to smooth muscle cells, as well as exploratory pharmacological studies with relatively crude drugs, Furchgott and Zawadzki (1980) proposed:

that ACh acting on the muscarinic receptor of the endothelial cells somehow activates a reaction sequence in which arachidonic (or some other unsaturated fatty acid) is liberated and then oxidized by lipoxygenase to a product that is responsible for the relaxation of the smooth muscle cells.

The following year, Furchgott (1981) expanded the list of vasoactive factors (e.g. substance P, bradykinin, ATP, and the calcium ionophore A23187) that caused endothelium-dependent relaxation in isolated blood vessels and further speculated:

that the relaxing substance is a labile hydroperoxide or free radical that activates guanylate cyclase in the smooth cells of the artery.

The unidentified endothelium-derived vasodilator was subsequently termed endothelium-derived relaxing factor or EDRF (Furchgott 1981, 1984; Cherry *et al.*1982; Angus and Cocks 1989). It was quickly discovered that relaxation responses in many isolated blood vessel preparations were dependent on the endothelium and that even more compounds like noradrenaline and 5-HT (Cocks and Angus 1983) were able to stimulate endothelial cells to release EDRF in some vascular beds. The convergent point for all stimuli appeared to be an increase in endothelial cell Ca^{2+}. Otherwise, little was known of the synthesis and the chemical nature of EDRF except that it was labile in artificial salt solutions.

EDRF

Two aspects of the discovery of EDRF are worthy of mention. First, the relatively old-fashioned method of bioassay used to determine how molecules interact with cells to produce alterations in their function remains a powerful part of any pharmacologist's 'kit bag'. Whilst other techniques like receptor binding, electrophysiology, enzyme kinetics, and molecular biology are essential to understand how cellular events are processed and integrated, at some stage such information needs to be tested in an intact, multicellular tissue or better still, a conscious animal. Until then, the fragmented data from the other techniques remains interesting but relatively meaningless. For unidentified substances like EDRF, bioassay provided not only the necessary sensitivity (vascular smooth muscle relaxation) to detect low levels of the active factor, but also some degree of specificity when combined with drugs with known effects against possible synthetic pathways. Bioassay also allowed an accurate estimation of the half-life of EDRF (Angus and Cocks 1987), as well as describing some important chemical properties such as its breakdown by superoxide (O_2^-) radicals, that it was highly labile under *in vitro* assay conditions, hydrophilic and possibly negatively charged (Cocks *et al*. 1985). When combined with a sensitive and selective luminescence chemical assay, it was not only discovered that cultured endothelial cells released NO (see below) in response to stimulation with endothelium-dependent vasodilators like bradykinin (Palmer *et al*. 1987; Moncada *et al*. 1991) but also with the bioassay running in sequence with the chemical assay, Palmer *et al*. (1987) were able to show critically that all the relaxing activity of EDRF released from these cells was acounted for by the amount of NO released.

The second aspect of EDRF highlights how serendipity often plays a key part in scientific discovery. In his 1981 review, Furchgott, in explaining how he discovered EDRF states:

In the course of one experiment in which rings rather than strips of aorta were being used, my technician accidentally added carbachol to a ring that was already contracted with NE (noradrenaline), and the ring partially relaxed.

Later, he added

Within a few weeks of our accidental finding, we had established that the lack of relaxing response to ACh in the helical strip was the result of unintentional rubbing of the intimal surface against foreign surfaces (including fingertips) during ordinary preparation.

Thus, the discovery of what has turned out to be one of the most important control mechanisms in the cardiovascular system was to a large extent serendipitous.

Chemical nature of EDRF

Furchgott's (1981) and many subsequent early studies indicated that EDRF was a small, labile factor possibly derived from arachidonic acid via a non-cyclooxygenase pathway (Angus and Cocks 1989) (Fig. 10.1). Most of these studies, however, often used poorly defined pharmacological tools to attempt to elucidate the pathway for EDRF production. Drugs such as quinacrine, hydroquinone, nordihydroguaruretic acid, ETYA, and metyrapone were all shown to block EDRF-mediated relaxation in various isolated blood vessels. For example, quinacrine

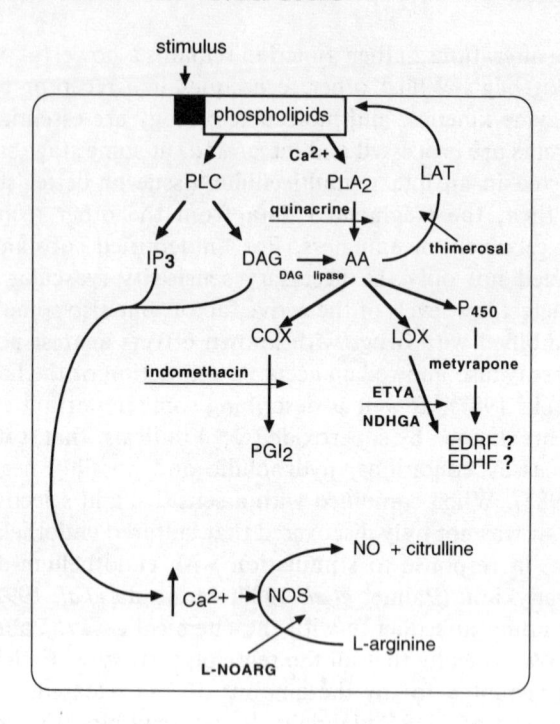

Fig. 10.1 Scheme of proposed and actual synthetic pathways for endothelium-derived relaxing factor (EDRF), endothelium-derived hyperpolarizing factor (EDHF), prostacyclin (PGI$_2$), and nitric oxide (NO) in vascular endothelial cells. Abbreviations; PLC, phospholipase C; PLA$_2$, phospholipase A$_2$; LAT, lysolecthicin acyltransferase; IP$_3$, inositol trisphosphate; DAG, diacylglycerol; AA, arachidonic acid; COX, cyclo-oxygenase; LOX, lipoxygenase; P$_{450}$, cytochrome P$_{450}$; NOS, nitric oxide synthase; N^G-nitro-L-arginine (L-NOARG). The intersecting arrows between synthetic steps represent block of that step by the indicated drug. Historically, EDRF was regarded as a LOX or P$_{450}$ product. As indicated by the question marks, EDRF (and EDHF) may still be such a product. For each factor (EDRF, EDHF, PGI$_2$ and NO) the cascade of events leading to their release is triggered by a specific stimulus (e.g. acetylcholine acting on a muscarinic receptor, an increase in shear stress)-induced increase in cell Ca^{2+}.

(mepacrine) was thought to block endothelial cell phospholipase A$_2$ activity and thus the release of arachidonic acid. Although EDRF was not a cyclo-oxygenase metabolite of arachidonic acid (e.g. prostacyclin), numerous studies indicated that other arachidonic acid metabolic pathways, particularly via lipoxygenases and mixed function monoxygenases like cytochrome P$_{450}$, could possibly be involved in the production of EDRF (for review see Angus and Cocks 1989). Most of these studies, however, did not take into consideration the important observation by Moncada *et al.* (1986) that some of the anti-EDRF drugs possibly blocked EDRF-mediated relaxations via generation of superoxide anion radicals (O$_2^-$). Whilst this property did not rule out an arachidonic acid metabolite as an EDRF, it certainly provided a key clue which aided the discovery of NO.

Regardless of the problems associated with the early pharmacology of EDRF, stimulation of endothelial cells with EDRF-releasing agents can theoretically increase cell arachidonic acid levels via two pathways (see Fig. 10.1). Crack and Cocks (1992) demonstrated that thimerosal, an inhibitor of acetyl CoA lysolecithin acyltransferase, an enzyme in endothelial cells responsible for re-incorporation of arachidonic acid into membrane phospholipids (Fig. 10.1), abolished the stimulated but not the basal release of EDRF in isolated ring segments of greyhound coronary artery. Thus, up to the discovery of NO, EDRF was generally regarded to be an oxygenated metabolite of arachidonic acid (see Angus and Cocks 1989).

Identification of the chemical nature of EDRF was made possible by the use of cultured endothelial cells (Cocks *et al.* 1985). Here, the amount of EDRF released from an endothelial cell source could be amplified many times by perfusing millions of cells growing on microcarrier beads in a small cell column. The amount of EDRF released from the cell column into the perfusate could then be detected by bioassay (i.e. relaxation of endothelium-denuded vascular smooth muscle preparations). Using this technique, properties such as the chemical half-life of EDRF (Angus and Cocks 1987), its degree of lipophilicity and charge (Cocks *et al.* 1985), its block by superoxide free radicals, and finally that all the relaxing activity of EDRF released by endothelial cells was NO (Palmer *et al.* 1987) were obtained.

NITRIC OXIDE (NO)

Even eight years after the discovery of NO, controversy still exists as to whether EDRF is simply NO or an NO-containing molecule (Feelisch *et al.* 1994), which in part may be due to the paucity of knowledge of NO chemistry in biological fluids . Therefore, since NO is such a reactive molecule and can exist as the free radical (NO•), as well as both the nitrosyl (NO$^+$) and nitroxyl (NO$^-$) ions in solution, it is difficult to determine if the NO produced in endothelial cells actually reaches its target cell (i.e, smooth muscle cells) as NO. Perhaps some of the tissue specialization in terms of the potency of endothelium-dependent dilator agonists and the degree of block of their relaxation responses by L-arginine analogues (see below) involves the chemical 'form' of NO at the level of the target cell. Thus, reaction between a hypothetical carrier or chaperone molecule for NO (i.e. RNO, see Fig. 10.2) effectively introduces another step in the already complicated cascade of steps from the stimulus to the relaxation response.

The enzyme that catalyses the synthesis of NO from the basic amino acid, L-arginine, NO synthase (NOS) (Moncada *et al.* 1991; Nathan 1992) exists in at least three distinct isoforms throughout a wide variety of tissues. These forms are referred to as the constitutive endothelial and brain NOSs (cNOS) and the inducible NOS (iNOS), and are coded for by separate genes. Each gene has been cloned and the enzymes' possess a number of intriguing and novel structural aspects related to their function such as activation by Ca^{2+} and the 'mini-electron

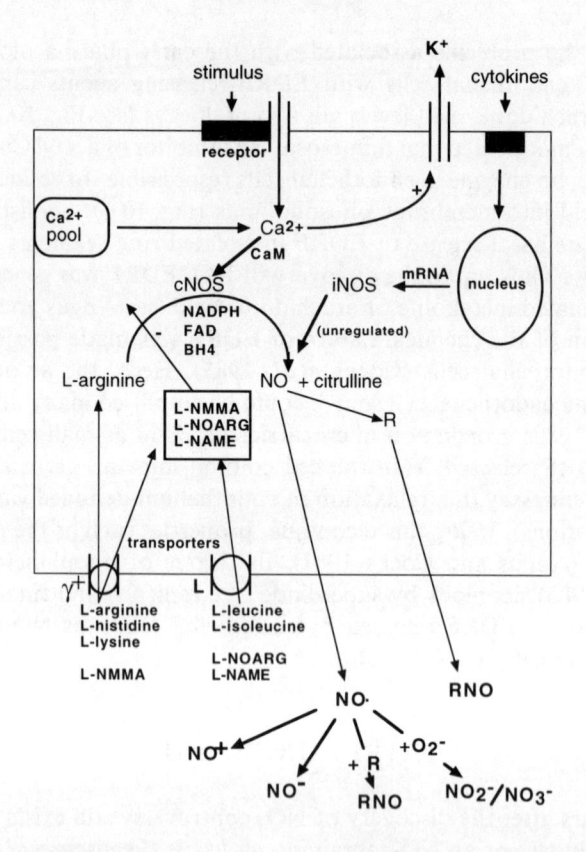

Fig. 10.2 Scheme depicting the regulatory mechanisms for the synthesis and release of nitric oxide (NO) from endothelial cells. The constitutive endothelial isoform of nitric oxide synthase (cNOS) is the major form found in these cells and (not depicted here) is located predominantly in the plasma membrane. Activity of cNOS is controlled by Ca^{2+}-activated calmodulin (CaM) binding and is dependent on cofactors such as NADPH, FAD, tetrahydrobiopterin (BH_4). The increase in cell Ca^{2+} (from both receptor operated channels and membrane bound intracellular pools) also activates plasma membrane K^+ channels which in turn results in endothelial cell membrane hyperpolarization. The substrate for NOS, L-arginine, is not rate limiting and whether the NO produced is released as NO or in combination with a specific carrier molecule (R) is unknown. Similarly, if NO is released from the cell as NO, it could then be picked up by a carrier molecule (R), converted to either the nitroxyl (NO_2^-) or nitrosyl (NO^+) ionic forms via redox reactions or inactivated to nitrite (NO_2^-) and nitrate (NO_3^-) ionic forms by superoxide free radicals (O_2^-). The amino acid transporters (γ^+ and L) also transport L-arginine analogue inhibitors of NOS (L-NNMA, L-NOARG, L-NAME) into the endothelial cell. The inducible isoform of NOS (iNOS), is regarded to be unregulated since it retains CaM tightly bound to the enzyme which is produced via cytokine-mediated increases in gene expression.

chain' involved in the complex five electron oxidation of one of the guanidino nitrogen atoms of L-arginine. Also, there is probably more heterogeneity within each enzyme isoform based on molecular weights, but any differences in terms of function have not been determined. This novel NOS/NO cell–cell signalling system appears to be implicated in such diverse biological processes as blood pressure control, haemostasis, memory, penile erection, peristalsis, and host defence. In terms of vascular control, both cNOS and iNOS appear to have important but different roles; cNOS as a physiological regulator of vascular tone and clotting, iNOS involved mostly in pathological conditions such as hypotension associated with sepsis and some forms of cardiomyopathy.

NO, or a closely related NO-containing compound like a nitrosothiol (but see Feelisch *et al.* 1994), is thought to be the main EDRF released from endothelial cells in response to stimuli which increase cell Ca^{2+} (see Fig. 10.3). A wide range of stimuli increase intracellular Ca^{2+}. These include activation of multiple surface receptors for agonists such as acetylcholine, substance P, bradykinin, noradrenaline, and 5-HT, and receptor-independent stimuli like calcium ionophores, and increases in shear stress on the cell surface, usually in response to increased laminar flow. Constitutive NOS, a Ca^{2+}-dependent membrane bound enzyme, then rapidly catalyses the conversion of L-arginine to NO plus citrulline. NO is then supposedly free to diffuse from the cell and activate guanylate cyclase in the underlying smooth muscle cell to initiate relaxation possibly via cGMP-dependent and protein kinase-mediated phosphorylation of a plasma membrane Ca^{2+} extrusion pump. Similarly, iNOS produces NO from L-arginine but is essentially regarded to be maximally regulated due to irreversible binding of calmodulin to the enzyme independent of changes in cell Ca^{2+}. This isoform, however, is regulated by transcription and translation of new protein, usually in response to growth factors and cytokines.

The physiology and pharmacology of NO have been greatly aided by the availability of potent and apparently selective inhibitors of NOS, the most commonly used being the substrate analogues of L-arginine. These compounds, modified chemically at one of the terminal guanidino nitrogens such as N^G-monomethyl-L-arginine (L-NMMA) and N^G-nitro-L-arginine (L-NOARG) are potent inhibitors of NOS, although their mechanism of block is unknown since the normal resonance of the free electron of the guanidino group is unaffected in these N^G-substituted arginine analogues. The analogues, however, are believed to bind to NOS at its active site but are not converted to NO and citrulline. Thus, these compounds act as substrate inhibitors of the enzyme. Their ability to prevent NO production in intact endothelial cells depends on a number of factors such as the kinetics of both uptake and binding of the L-arginine analogue to the enzyme, metabolism of the analogue within the endothelial cell, and the intracellular concentration of L-arginine. L-NMMA shares the same saturable amino acid uptake system in endothelial cells as L-arginine, the γ^+ basic amino acid transporter (Bogle *et al.* 1992; Schmidt *et al.* 1993) whereas L-NOARG is taken up into endothelial cells by another saturable amino acid transporter, the L-system, which also transports leucine and isoleucine into endothelial cells

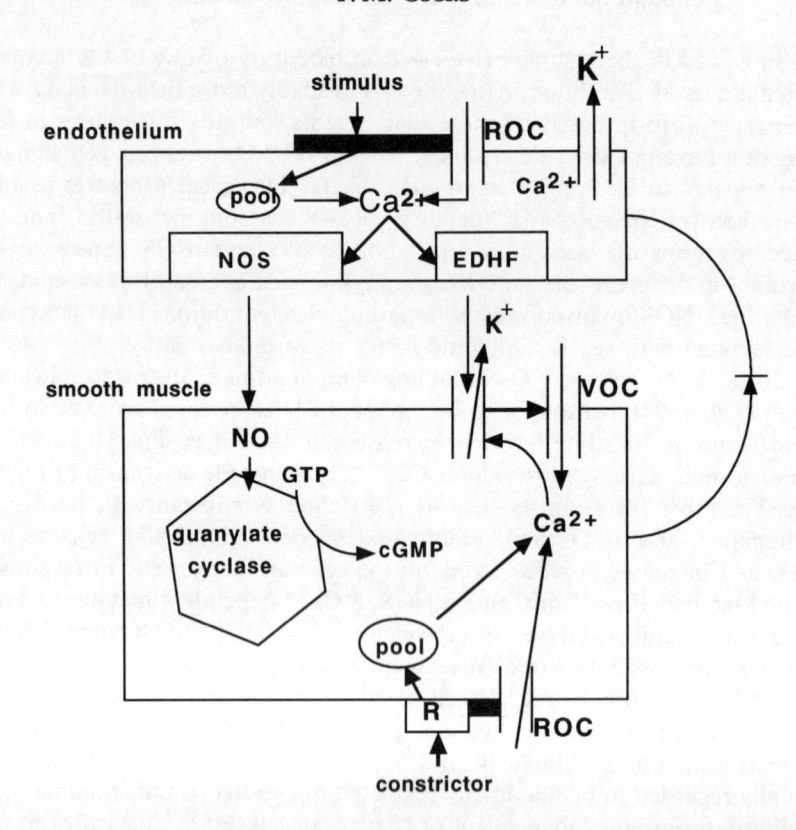

Fig. 10.3 Schema depicting possible roles of Ca^{2+}-activated K^+ channels in endothelium-dependent vascular relaxation responses. Increases in cellular Ca^{2+} (both from intracellular pools and entry via receptor operated Ca^{2+} channels; ROC) following appropriate stimulation activates both NOS and endothelial cell hyperpolarization. The latter response may act to reinforce Ca^{2+} entry but the hyperpolarizing current does not spread electrotonically to the smooth muscle cell (as it does in the opposite direction). This implies that endothelium-dependent smooth muscle hyperpolarization is mediated by release of EDHF, which activates Ca^{2+}-activated K^+ channels, closure of voltage operated Ca^{2+} channels (VOC) and thus relaxation.

(Schmidt *et al.* 1993). The kinetics of uptake for L-NMMA and L-NOARG differ considerably. Saturable uptake of L-NMMA into cultured endothelial cells occurs via high (K_m, 6 μM) and low (K_m, 0.8 mM) affinity sites, whereas that for L-NOARG only occurs via a low affinity site (K_m, 0.6 mM) (see Schmidt *et al.* 1993). Thus, the concentrations of each analogue attained within the endothelial cell will depend upon both the concentration used and the time of incubation. Nevertheless, even short incubation periods (30 min) with low concentrations of L-NOARG (10 μM), well below the K_m for uptake (600 μM), resulted in relatively low intracellular levels of L-NOARG yet still caused total block of both the increase in endothelial cell cGMP (Schmidt *et al.* 1993) and smooth muscle relaxation, in response to maximum stimulation of NOS with the calcium ionophore, A23187. Therefore, the capacity of the L-amino acid transporter to transport L-NOARG into endothelial cells appears greatly to exceed the intracellular concentrations of L-NOARG which abolish NOS activity.

Once the L-arginine analogues enter the endothelial cell, they compete with intracellular L-arginine for the active site of NOS. For L-NMMA this is readily reversible, but L-NOARG displays very slow kinetics of onset and offset of binding to NOS and may even covalently bind to the active site of the enzyme (Dwyer et al. 1991). Thus, whilst both L-NOARG and L-NMMA are competitive inhibitors of NOS, L-NOARG is a potent (K_i 1–10 μM) (Furfine et al. 1993), and effectively irreversible inhibitor due to its very slow rate of dissociation from the enzyme (Furfine et al. 1993), whilst L-NMMA is rapidly reversible. Finally, L-NMMA not L-NOARG is metabolized within endothelial cells (Hecker et al. 1990a,b), thus lowering the effective intraendothelial concentration of the analogue.

Therefore, the arginine analogue inhibitors of NOS are powerful tools for investigations of potential roles of NO in any particular biological system. Their acute use *in vivo* has been shown to cause a sustained and often large increase of blood pressure. If this reflects loss of endothelial cell-derived NO, then it is likely that the vasculature is in a permanent state of active dilatation from the endothelium (see above and Moncada et al. 1991). Some caution is required with this generalization, however, since

- other roles of the L-arginine analogues apart from inhibition of NOS should not be excluded (see also Cocks and Angus 1991)
- the role of NO in the regulation of tone in resistance vessels is increasingly controversial (see below)

The important issue to be addressed in terms of vascular control, however, is the effectiveness of the L-arginine analogue NOS inhibitors as inhibitors of endothelium-dependent relaxation.

INHIBITION OF ENDOTHELIUM-DEPENDENT RELAXATIONS BY L-ARGININE ANALOGUES

Many endothelium-dependent relaxation responses both *in vitro* and *in vivo* are only partially blocked or not blocked at all by these compounds even in millimolar concentrations, whilst similar responses in other vessels and the release of EDRF from cultured endothelial cells are completely inhibited. Examples of the two extremes of the heterogeneity of the effectiveness of L-arginine NOS inhibitors as inhibitors of endothelium-dependent relaxation responses in isolated artery preparations are the rat thoracic aorta where the response is effectively abolished by L-NOARG (Wu et al. 1993) or L-NAME (Cowan et al. 1993), and the rat small mesenteric artery, where it is largely unaffected by either compound (Garland and McPherson 1992; Wu et al. 1993; Waldron and Garland 1994).

There are at least two possible explanations for the heterogeneity of block of EDRF by potent L-arginine analogue inhibitors of NOS; either inhibition of NOS in endothelial cells *in situ* by the L-arginine analogues is incomplete or non-NO, endothelium-derived relaxing factors or mechanisms are present. The first explanation is that proposed by Martin *et al.* (1992), who theorized that differential block of endothelium-dependent relaxations by the L-arginine inhibitors of NOS was due to differences in the 'effector reserve' associated with any particular stimulus and tissue. Implicit in their argument is the assumption that the L-arginine analogues only partially block NOS and the degree of block of the resultant relaxation response depends on either the efficacy of the stimulating agonist or the efficiency of the smooth muscle's response to NO, both of which are incorporated in the effector reserve of the system. Martin *et al.* (1992) showed that relaxation responses to ACh in the rabbit isolated jugular vein were relatively resistant to block by L-NAME as compared to the near total block of similar responses in the rat thoracic aorta.

If the receptor reserve and therefore the effector reserve or efficacy of ACh in the jugular vein was reduced with phenoxybenzamine, then L-NAME markedly blocked the responses to ACh. Also, in jugular vein segments not treated with phenoxybenzamine, the relaxation responses to the partial muscarinic agonists pilocarpine and butyrylcholine were also markedly blocked by L-NAME. From these experiments, Martin *et al.* (1992) proposed that NO was the only factor involved in endothelium-dependent relaxation and that the differential block of the responses by L-arginine analogue inhibitors of NOS was due to differences in effector reserve, not different EDRFs.

A complication with the Martin *et al.* (1992) theory is that it is based entirely on the assumptions that NO is the only EDRF involved in endothelium-dependent relaxation and the L-arginine analogues therefore only partially inhibit NOS activity. Apart from the evidence that arginine analogues like L-NOARG and L-NAME are potent inhibitors of NOS (see above), three additional pieces of evidence strongly support the opposite conclusion, that the potent L-arginine analogues like L-NOARG and L-NAME in fact abolish NOS activity in endothelial cells *in situ*. First, in many isolated blood vessels, there is a ceiling for the maximum degree of block of endothelium-dependent relaxation obtainable by the L-arginine analogues. That is, the degree of block they produce is not improved by increasing either the concentration of the analogue or the time of its incubation with the tissue. Therefore, considering the kinetics for L-NOARG uptake and interaction with NOS (see above) this additional functional evidence indicates that NOS is effectively blocked.

The second piece of evidence in favour of NOS activity *in situ* being abolished by the irreversible L-arginine analogues like L-NOARG is that EDRF-mediated increases in cGMP, the recognized second messenger for NO (Moncada *et al.* 1991) are abolished by L-NOARG and L-NAME even though the accompanying relaxation responses are often largely unaffected (Cowan *et al.* 1993; Eckman *et al.* 1994; Holzmann *et al.* 1994). Finally, other inhibitors of endothelium-dependent relaxation such as LY 83583 (Mulsch *et al.* 1989) haemoglobin, and methylene blue (Angus and Cocks 1989) also abolish increases in cGMP in responses to increases in endothelial cell Ca^{2+} yet fail to block the relaxation response.

Therefore, the potency of certain L-arginine analogues (e.g. L-NNA and L-NAME) as inhibitors of NOS in endothelial cells and their ability to abolish increases in smooth muscle cGMP suggests that NO does not contribute to the functional response (i.e. relaxation) in the presence of such NOS inhibitors. L-NOARG- or L-NAME-resistant responses have been reported in arteries including the rat aorta (Cowan et al. 1993; Frew et al. 1993; Wu et al. 1993), guinea-pig coronary artery (Chen and Cheung 1992; Parkington et al. 1993; Eckman et al. 1994), pig coronary artery (Holzmann et al. 1994; Kilpatrick and Cocks 1994), rabbit carotid artery (Cowan et al. 1993; Najibi et al. 1994), and rat small mesenteric artery (Garland and McPherson 1992; Adeagbo and Triggle 1993; Wu et al. 1993; Hwa et al. 1994; Waldron and Garland 1994).

If the above conclusion that certain L-arginine analogue inhibitors of NOS abolish its activity in *in situ* cells, and thus the release of NO, is correct, then an alternative explanation is required for the resistance of endothelium-dependent relaxation to these inhibitors of NOS. The most likely is that other non-NO, endothelium-dependent vasodilator factors contribute to endothelium-dependent relaxation. Before the types of possible non-NO candidates are considered, it is important to mention that the two theories, i.e. NOS resistance to block by L-arginine analogues (Martin et al. 1992) and other factors (Kilpatrick and Cocks 1994) are not necessarily mutually exclusive. Most of the relaxation response resistant to NOS inhibition occurs over the higher concentration range of the stimulating agonist. Thus, maximum relaxation is depressed usually with only a small decrease in sensitivity. This characteristic pattern of non-surmountable block of endothelium-dependent relaxation by NOS inhibitors could be explained by either the release of two (or more) EDRFs or partial block of NOS with an irreversible competitive inhibitor (e.g. L-NOARG or L-NAME). In the former case, NO would be released over the lower concentration range of the stimulating agonist and the other non-NO factor over the higher concentration range. EDRF releasing agonists with low effector reserve (i.e. partial agonists at a particular receptor) would thus produce proportionally more NO than the other factor and as such, following inhibition of NOS, most if not all the relaxation response would be blocked. Conversely, agonists with high effector reserve would still be able to relax the tissue after NOS inhibition due to release of the non-NO factor.

The critical issue common to both theories is whether or not NOS activity is abolished by the L-arginine analogue inhibitors. If it is not, then the effector reserve theory of Martin et al. (1992) may be correct. If it is, however, Martin et al. (1992) effector reserve idea needs to be either modified to accommodate other EDRFs or rejected. The reported difference in sensitivity to block of ACh-mediated EDRF by L-NAME in different regions of the rat aorta (Cowan et al. 1993) provides a good example of this dilemma. Both sensitivity and maximum relaxation to ACh in the thoracic aorta are less than those in abdominal rings. Also, L-NAME nearly abolished the response in the thoracic aorta but only blocked that in the abdominal aorta by about 30%, although sensitivity was significantly reduced. At first, the pattern of responses appears to fit the effector reserve model of Martin *et al.* (1992). Cowan *et al.* (1993), however, showed:

- that the degree of block of endothelium-dependent relaxation was not increased by a tenfold higher concentration of L-NAME
- that the lower concentration of L-NAME abolished the smooth muscle cGMP response
- K^+ channel inhibitors like high extracellular K^+ and charybdotoxin blocked the L-NAME-resistant endothelium-dependent relaxation.

The last piece of evidence adds to the growing literature on hyperpolarization as a possible explanation for the resistance of endothelium-dependent relaxation to block by NOS inhibitors (see below).

ENDOTHELIUM-DEPENDENT HYPERPOLARIZATION (EDH) AND ITS CONTRIBUTION TO ENDOTHELIUM-DEPENDENT RELAXATION

Endothelium-dependent hyperpolarization factor (EDHF) is a hypothetical factor supposedly released simultaneously with EDRF from endothelial cells by endothelium-dependent vasodilators (Taylor and Weston 1988; Komori and Vanhoutte 1990; Bény and von der Weid 1991; Garland *et al.* 1995). Regardless of the controversy related to the existence of EDHF and the type of K^+ channels (large (maxi K^+), intermediate, and small conductance Ca^{2+}-activated, as well as ATP-sensitive (KATP) K^+ channels) involved in endothelium-dependent hyperpolarization, endothelial cells hyperpolarize in response to the same stimuli responsible for the release of EDRF (see Fig. 10.3). This, however, does not explain the ensuing hyperpolarization of the underlying smooth muscle, unless the cells are closely electrotonically coupled (Kuhberger *et al.* 1995). Bény and Paciccia (1994), however, found that a hyperpolarizing current initiated in smooth muscle cells could spread to the endothelium but not the reverse; i.e. from endothelial to smooth muscle cell. These authors concluded that the endothelial cell must release a factor to initiate smooth muscle hyperpolarization and that this factor was unlikely to be NO. NO is, however, able to activate Ca^{2+}-dependent K^+ channels as observed in patch-clamp experiments in cultured smooth muscle cells (Bolotina *et al.* 1994) but NO-induced hyperpolarizations are unlikely to be involved in endothelium-dependent relaxation of intact arteries (Garland and McPherson 1992).

The increase in K^+ conductance associated with hyperpolarization in endothelial cells may enhance entry of extracellular Ca^{2+} through receptor operated Ca^{2+} channels into endothelial cells and thus both promote and sustain activation of NOS and release of NO (Adams 1994). Alternatively, the y^+ basic amino acid transporter, which also transports L-NMMA into endothelial cells (Bogle *et al.* 1992; Schmidt *et al.* 1993) is activated by hyperpolarization (Kavanaugh 1993). Thus, endothelial cell hyperpolarization may be important *in vivo* to sustain or replenish levels of L-arginine. Regardless of the mechanism of endothelium-dependent hyperpolarization, numerous studies indicate that hyperpolarization or a K^+ channel-dependent mechanism may contribute to endothelium-dependent relaxation independently of NO (see Garland *et al.* 1995). In general, it has been accepted that this mechanism acts in parallel with NO to contribute to the final relaxation response. An important question is how does it contribute to the endothelium-dependent relaxation?

Many studies of endothelium-dependent relaxation in large arteries like the pig coronary artery indicated that a K^+ channel-dependent mechansim, not NO, was the main endothelium-dependent relaxation mechanism. Directly opposed to this suggestion, however, Kilpatrick and Cocks (1994) presented evidence in the same artery that NO was the dominant EDRF, with the K^+ channel-dependent mechanism acting as a 'backup' if NOS was blocked (Fig. 10.4). Two aspects of these apparently conflicting data are noteworthy. First, EDRF activity measured by bioassay relies on functional antagonism (by EDRF) of set levels of active contractions. It is usually necessary to contract isolated arteries since they possess little inherent active tone against which relaxation responses can be determined. The level of added active force required, however, is important. Too little and the assay tissue runs out of relaxation 'room' such that the lower part of the relaxation curve may be lost. Increases in cyclic GMP, however, would be expected to continue in a concentration-dependent manner. Too much contractile force would further functionally antagonize the relaxations, particulary to those agonists with either low efficacy at a particular receptor or ones which have less effector reserve. Again, changes in cyclic GMP would be expected to continue except in this case further increases in cyclic GMP would be unable to reduce further intracellular Ca^{2+} due to the higher constrictor drive. Therefore, it is important to set the contractions in isolated arterial preparations to an optimal level to measure relaxation responses. For EDRF releasing agents, this level is determined as that which a NO donor like SNP is able to cause potent and complete relaxation. Also, contractions between preparations should be normalized (usually to the tissue maximum, F_{max}) to allow for variations in smooth muscle mass. This is also important if the number of viable endothelial cells and thus the amount of EDRF released per unit stimuli remains constant between preparations. Therefore, careful experimental design is essential if potential roles for non-NO factors in endothelium-dependent relaxation are to be established.

At least three types of K^+ channel have been implicated in mediating non-NO endothelium-dependent vasorelaxation. Cowan *et al.* (1993) found that both charybdotoxin and glibenclamide, relatively selective inhibitors of large conductance Ca^{2+}-and ATP-sensitive K^+ channels respectively, blocked L-NAME resistant relaxations to ACh in the rabbit abdominal aorta but only glibenclamide blocked those in the rabbit carotid artery. Also, Hwa *et al.* (1994) reported that charydbotoxin but not glibenclamide partially blocked relaxations to ACh in the rat

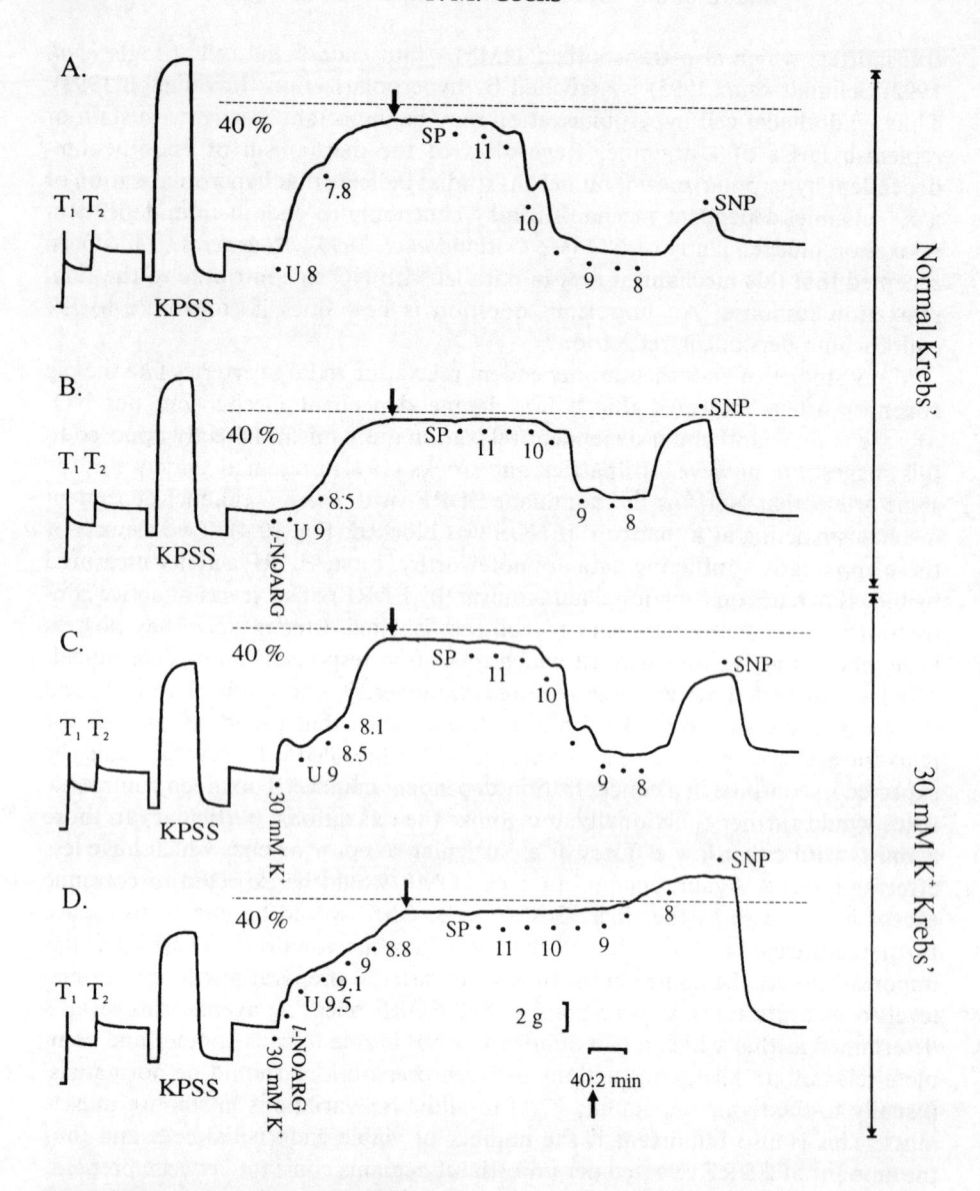

Fig. 10.4 Digitized traces of original chart recordings from four separate rings of pig, isolated coronary artery, showing the effect of L-NOARG (100 μM) on relaxation responses to cumulative half log concentrations of substance P (SP) in normal (A and B) and 30 mM K⁺ concentration (C and D) Krebs' solutions. In each case, the dotted horizontal line indicates 40% of the maximum contraction to KPSS, to which each tissue was approximately set by the addition of the thromboxane A_2 mimetic, U46619 (1–30 nM). Also note that the gain was reduced to obtain the initial KPSS contraction. T1 and T2 represent the initial passive stretches. The time calibration bar indicates 40, and 2 min before, and after the *arrow*, respectively. NIF = 0.3 μM nifedipine; U = U46619; SNP = 10 μM sodium nitroprusside; SP = substance P. Concentrations are expressed as −log[M].

mesenteric artery, a tissue in which a K$^+$ channel-dependent mechanism appeared to play a dominant role in endothelium-dependent relaxation. Apamin, an inhibitor of small conductance Ca^{2+}-activated K$^+$ channels, has also been claimed to block K$^+$ channel-mediated dilatation in the perfused rat mesenteric bed (Adeagbo and Triggle 1993), and Eckman *et al.* (1994) showed that the impure scorpion venom *Leiurus quinquestriatus habraeus* (SV), blocked non-NO-mediated relaxations in the guinea-pig isolated coronary artery whilst having no effect on the increase in cGMP. Also, the same authors claimed that SV, a reputed non-selective inhibitor of K$^+$ channels (Strong 1990), abolished the hyperpolarization to ACh in the guinea-pig coronary artery.

Whilst non-NO, endothelium-dependent relaxation of vascular smooth muscle may involve multiple types of K$^+$ channels (see Cowan *et al.* 1993), data available on different K$^+$ channel blockers are not convincing. A more reliable but non-selective method of inhibiting K$^+$ channel activity is to raise the concentration of extracellular K$^+$ (Garland *et al.* 1995). Chen and Suzuki (1989) showed that the amplitude of endothelium-dependent hyperpolarization to histamine and acetylcholine in rat pulmonary arteries linearly decreased with increasing concentration of extracellular K$^+$ and at 20–25 mM K$^+$ hyperpolarization was abolished. Therefore, whilst it will be important to identify the type(s) of K$^+$ channels involved in non-NO, endothelium-dependent relaxation of vascular smooth muscle, at present high extracellular K$^+$ remains the best method of determining, at least *in vitro*, how hyperpolarization may contribute to endothelium-dependent relaxation.

Apart from the apparent heterogeneity of K$^+$ channels mediating non-NO endothelium-dependent relaxations in blood vessels, tissue and species variation in the presence and contribution of K$^+$ channels to these responses need to be considered. Thus, all endothelium-dependent relaxation to ACh in the rat superior mesenteric artery is blocked by NOS inhibitors whereas that in rat small resistance mesenteric arteries is unaffected by the same inhibitors (Hwa *et al.* 1994). Although NO is the dominant EDRF in large arteries like the pig, dog, cow and human coronary arteries, a K$^+$ channel-dependent mechanism appears to act in 'reserve' or 'backup' if NO synthesis is inhibited (Kilpatrick and Cocks 1994). The reverse occurs in the rat small mesenteric artery. Here the K$^+$-dependent mechanism is the major EDRF with NO acting as backup or reserve. A projected trend is that as the arteries become smaller, the contribution of K$^+$ channels to endothelium-dependent relaxation becomes more important (Garland *et al.* 1995). What this means in terms of vascular function in both normal health and disease is unknown. It is tempting, however, to speculate that vascular resistance is controlled mainly by endothelium non-NO-dependent mechanisms which predominantly involve a novel K$^+$ channel opening compound (EDHF?). Given the range of different types of K$^+$ channels supposed to be present in vascular smooth muscle, perhaps the often reported failure to block non-NO relaxations with specific K$^+$ channel inhibitors (e.g. like charybdotoxin), is due to the hypothetical hyperpolarizing factor (EDHF) acting as a non-selective K$^+$ channel opener.

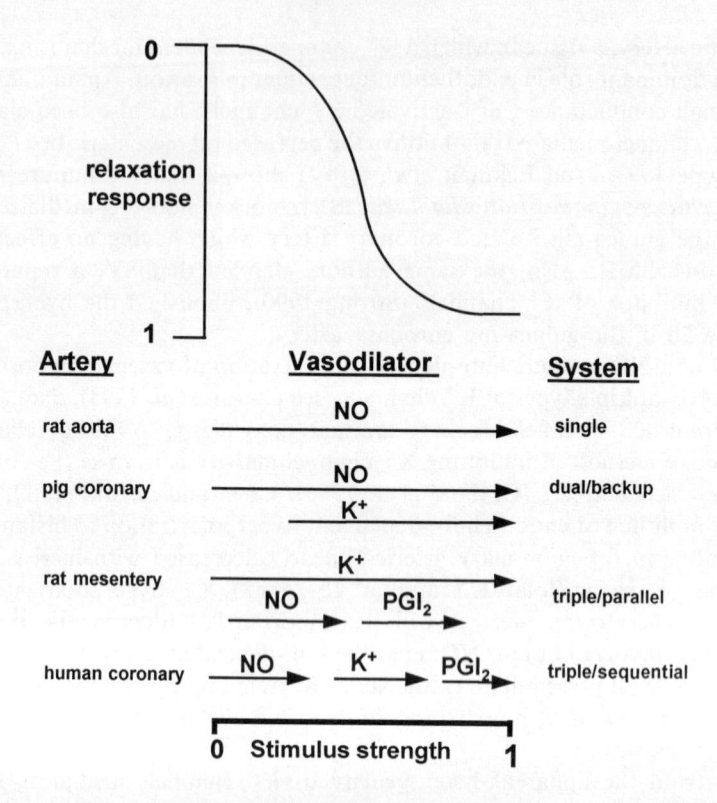

Fig. 10.5 Suggested schematic representation of examples of endothelium-dependent vasodilator systems in mammalian arteries. The arrows indicate the types of factors involved, their interactions, and the approximate range of stimulus strength over which they mediate relaxation.

CONCLUSION

Endothelium-dependent relaxation in blood vessels can be mediated by multiple factors or mechanisms, including NO, prostanoids, K^+ channels, and possibly other factors. Species and tissue specialization, however, appear to determine the type and degree of contribution of each factor or mechanism to the overall relaxation response (see Fig. 10.5). The challenge now is not only to characterize both the K^+ channel opener(s) and the different types of K^+ channels involved in endothelium-dependent relaxation, but also to show how their activity is integrated with other endothelium-dependent dilators like NO and PGI_2 throughout the vasculature.

REFERENCES

Adaegbo, A. S. and Triggle, C. R. (1993). Varying extracellular [K^+]: a functional approach to separating EDHF- and EDNO-related mechanisms in perfused rat mesenteric arterial bed. *J. Cardiovasc. Pharmacol.*, **21**, 423-9.

Adams, D. J. (1994). Ionic channels in vascular endothelial cells. *Trends Cardiovasc. Med.*, **4**, 18-26.

Angus, J. A. and Cocks, T. M. (1987). The half-life of endothelium-derived relaxing factor released from bovine aortic endothelial cell in culture. *J. Physiol.*, **388**, 71-81.

Angus, J. A. and Cocks, T. M. (1989). Endothelium-derived relaxing factor. *Pharmacol. Ther.*, **41**, 303-52.

Bény, J. L. and Paccica, C. (1994). Bidirectional electrical communication between smooth muscle and endothelial cells in the pig coronary artery. *Am. J. Pharmacol.*, **266**, H1465-72.

Bény, J. L. and von der Weid, P. Y. (1991). Hyperpolarising factors. *Coronary Artery Dis.*, **2**, 300-6.

Bogle, R. G., Moncada, S., Pearson, J. D., and Mann, G. E. (1992). Identification of inhibitors of nitric oxide synthase that do not interact with the endothelial cell L-arginine transporter. *Br. J. Pharmacol.*, **105**, 768-70.

Bolotina, V. M., Najibi, S., Palacino, J. J., Pagano, P. J., and Cohen, R. A. (1994). Nitric oxide directly activates calcium-dependent potassium channels in vascular smooth muscle. *Nature*, **368**, 850-53.

Chen, G. and Cheung, D. W. (1992). Characterisation of acetylcholine-induced membrane hyperpolarisation in endothelial cells. *Circ. Res.*, **70**, 257-63.

Chen, G. and Suzuki, H. (1989). Some electrical properties of the endothelium-dependent hyperpolarisation recorded from rat arterial smooth muscle cells, *J. Physiol.*, **410**, 91-106.

Cherry, P., Furchgott, R., and Zawadzki, J. (1982). The endothelium dependent relaxation of vascular smooth muscle by unsaturated fatty acids (Abstract). *Fed. Proc.*, **42**, 619.

Cocks, T. M. and Angus, J. A. (1983). Endothelium-dependent relaxation of coronary arteries by noradrenaline and serotonin. *Nature*, **305**, 627-30.

Cocks, T. M. and Angus, J. A. (1991). Evidence that contractions of isolated arteries by L-NMMA and NOLA are not due to inhibition of basal EDRF release. *J. Cardiovasc. Pharmacol.*, **17(Suppl. 3)**, S159-64.

Cocks, T. M., Angus, J. A., Campbell, J. H. and Campbell, G. R. (1985). Release and properties of endothelium-derived relaxing factor (EDRF) from endothelial cells in culture. *J. Cell Physiol.*, **123**, 315-20.

Cowan, C. L., Pasacino, J. J., Najibi, S., and Cohen, R. A. (1993). Potassium channel mediated relaxation to acetylcholine in rabbit arteries. *J. Pharmacol. Exp. Ther.*, **266**, 1482-9.

Crack, P. and Cocks, T. (1992). Thimerosal blocks stimulated but not basal release of endothelium-derived relaxing factor (EDRF) in dog isolated coronary artery. *Br. J Pharmacol.*, **107**, 566-72.

Dwyer, M. A., Bredt, D. S., and Snyder, S. H. (1991). Nitric oxide synthase: irreversible inhibitation by L-N^G-nitroarginine in brain *in vitro* and *in vivo*. *Biochem. Biophys. Res. Commun.*, **176**, 1136-41.

Eckman, D. M., Weinert, J. S., Buxton, I. L. O., and Keef, K. D. (1994). Cyclic GMP-independent relaxation and hyperpolarization with acetylcholine in guinea-pig coronary artery. *Br. J Pharmacol.*, **111**, 1053-60.

Feelisch, M., te Poel, M., Zamora, R., Deussen, A., and Moncada, S. (1994). Understanding the controversy over the identity of EDRF. *Nature*, **368**, 62-5.

Frew, J. D., Paisley, K., and Martin, W. (1993). Selective inhibition of basal but not agonist-stimulated activity of nitric oxide in rat aorta by N^G-monomethyl-L-arginine. *Br. J. Pharmacol.*, **110**, 1003-8.

Furchgott, R. F. (1981). The requirement for endothelial cells in the relaxation of arteries to acetylcholine and some other nitrovasodilators. *Trends Pharmacol. Sci.*, **2**, 173-6.

Furchgott, R. F. (1984). The role of the endothelium in the response of vascular smooth muscle to drugs. *Annu. Rev. Pharmacol. Toxicol.*, **24**, 175-97.

Furchgott, R. F. and Zawadzki, J. V. (1980). The obligatory role of endothelial cells in the relaxation of arterial smooth muscle by acetylcholine. *Nature*, **288**, 373-6.

Furfine, E. S., Harmon, M. F., Paith, J. E., and Garvey, E. P. (1993). Selective inhibition of constitutive nitric oxide synthase by L-N^G-nitroarginine. *Biochemistry*, **32**, 8512-17.

Garland, C. J. and McPherson, G. A. (1992). Evidence that nitric oxide does not mediate the hyperpolarisation and relaxation in the rat small mesenteric artery. *Br. J. Pharmacol.*, **2**, 429-35.

Garland, C. J., Plane, F., Kemp, B. K., and Cocks, T. M. (1995). Endothelium-dependent hyperpolarization: a role in the control of vascular tone. *Trends Pharmacol. Sci.*, **16**, 23-30.

Hecker, M., Mitchell, J., Harris, H. J., Katsura, M., Thiemermann, C., and Vane, J. R. (1990a). N^G-Monomethy-L-arginine but not N^G-nitro-L-arginine is metabolised by endothelial cells to L-citrulline. *Eur. J. Pharmacol.*, **183**, 648-9.

Hecker, M., Mitchell, J., Harris, H. J., Katsura, M., Thiermermann, C., and Vane, J. R. (1990b). Endothelial cells can metabolize N^G-monomethyl-L-arginine to L-citrulline and subsequently to L-arginine. *Bicheni. Biophys. Res. Commun.*, **167**, 1037-43.

Holzmann, S., Kukovetz, W. R., Windishhofer, W., Paschke, E., and Graier, W. F. (1994). Pharmacologic differentiation between endothelium-dependent relaxations sensitive and resistant to nitro-L-arginine in coronary arteries. *J. Cardiovasc. Pharmacol.*, **23**, 747-56.

Hwa, J. J., Ghiboudi, L., Williams, P., and Chatterjee, M. (1994). Comparison of acetylcholine-dependent relaxation in large and small arteries of rat mesenteric vascular bed. *Am. J. Physiol.*, **266**, H952-8.

Kavanaugh, M. P. (1993). Voltage dependence of facilitated arginine flux mediated by the system y^+ basic amino acid transporter. *Biochemistry*, **32**, 5781-5.

Kilpatrick, E. V. and Cocks, T. M. (1994). Evidence for differential roles of nitric-oxide (NO) and hyperpolarisation in endothelium-dependent relaxation of pig isolated coronary artery. *Br. J. Pharmacol.*, **112**, 557-65.

Komori, K. and Vanhoutte, P. M. (1990). Endothelium-derived hyperpolarising factor. *Blood Vessels*, **27**, 238-45.

Kuhberger, E., Grushner, K., Kukovetz, W. R., and Brunner, F. (1994). The role of myoendothelial cell contact in non-nitric oxide, non-prostanoid-mediated endothelium-dependent relaxation of porcine coronary artery. *Br. J. Pharmacol.*, **113**, 1289-94.

Martin, G. R., Bolofo, M. L., and Giles, H. (1992). Inhibition of endothelium-dependent vasorelaxation by arginine analogues: a pharmacological analysis of agonist and tissue dependence. *Br. J. Pharmacol.*, **105**, 643-52.

Moncada, S., Palmer, R. M. J., and Gryglewski, R. J. (1986). Mechansim of action of some inhibitors of endothelium-derived relaxing factor. *Proc. Natl Acad. Sci. USA*, **83**, 9164-8.

Moncada, S., Palmer, R. M. J., and Higgs, E. A. (1991). Nitric oxide: physiology, pathophysiology and pharmacology. *Pharmacol. Rev.*, **43**, 109-42.

Mulsch, A., Luckhoff, U. P., Busse, R., and Bassenge, E. (1989). LY83583 (6-anilino-5, 8-quinolinedione) blocks nitrovasodilator-induced cyclic GMP increases and inhibition of platelet activation. *Naunyn-Schmiedeberg's Arch. Pharmacol.*, **340**, 119-25.

Najibi, S., Cowan, C. L., Palacino, J. J., and Cohen, R. A. (1994). Enhanced role of potassium channels in relaxations to acetylcholine in hypercholesterolaemic rabbit carotid artery. *Heart Circ. Physiol.*, **351**, H2061-7.

Nathan, C. (1992). Nitric oxide as a secretory product of mammalian cells. *FASEB J.*, **6**, 3051-64.

Palmer, R. M. J., Ferrige, A. G., and Moncada, S. (1987). Nitric oxide release accounts for the biological activity of endothelium-derived relaxing factor. *Nature*, **327**, 524-6.

Parkington, H. C., Tonta, M. A., Tare, M., and Coleman, H. A. (1993). Stretch revealed three components in the hyperpolarisation of guinea-pig coronary artery in response to acetylcholine. *J. Physiol.*, **465**, 459-76.

Rusko, J., Tanzi, F., Van-Breeman, C., and Adams, D. J. (1992). Calcium-activated potassium channels in native endothelial cells from rabbit aorta: conductance; Ca^{2+} sensitivity and block. *J. Physiol.*, **455**, 601-21.

Schmidt, K., Klatt, P., and Mayer, B. (1993). Characterisation of endothelial cell amino acid transport systems involved in the actions of nitric oxide synthase inhibitors. *Mol. Pharmacol.*, **44**, 615-21.

Strong, P. N. (1990). Potassium channel toxins. *Pharmacol. Ther.*, **46**, 137-62.

Taylor, S. G. and Weston, A. H. (1988). Endothelium-derived hyperpolarising factor: a new endogenous inhibitor from the vascular endothelium. *Trends Pharmacol. Sci.*, **9**, 272-4.

Vane, J. R., Gryglewski, R. J., and Botting, R. M. (1987). The endothelial cell as a metabolic and endocrine organ. *Trends Pharmacol. Sci.*, **8**, 491-6.

Waldron, G. J. and Garland, C. J. (1994). Contribution of both nitric oxide and a change in membrane potential to acetylcholine-induced relaxation in the rat small mesenteric artery. *Br. J. Pharmacol.*, **112**, 831-6.

Wu, C. C., Chen, S. J., and Yen, M, H. (1993). Different responses to acetylcholine in the presence of nitric oxide inhibitor in rat aortae and mesenteric arteries. *Clin. Exp. Pharmacol. Physiol.*, **20**, 405-12.

11. Pharmacology of the cerebral circulation

P. A. T. Kelly and C. J. Garland

INTRODUCTION

It is now over a century since Roy and Sherrington (1890) proposed that cerebral blood flow is regulated to match closely the altered functional state of the brain. However, it is only relatively recently that experimental technology has advanced sufficiently to allow the concept of flow-metabolism coupling to be fully explored. Autoradiographic imaging techniques for the measurement of local cerebral blood flow (LCBF) with the tracer [^{14}C]iodoantipyrine (Sakurada *et al.* 1978), or local cerebral glucose utilization (LCMR$_{glu}$) with the glucose analogue [^{14}C]2-deoxyglucose (Sokoloff *et al.* 1977), have opened new avenues of investigation into the mechanisms controlling the perfusion of brain tissue. The similar levels of spatial resolution afforded by these two techniques have revealed that the phenomenon of flow-metabolism coupling in the brain can be highly localized (Kossut and Hand 1984). (Fig. 11.1). Moreover, the focal nature of many of the changes in the relationship between cerebral blood flow and metabolic demand elicited by experimental intervention has emphasized that the cerebrovascular bed is neither physiologically nor pharmacologically homogeneous (Graham *et al.* 1982; McBean *et al.* 1991; Kelly *et al.* 1993).

The precise mechanism by which vascular tone is coupled to regional neuronal metabolism is not known, but it is likely to be multifactorial, reflecting the concerted action of changes in the local ionic composition of the extracellular fluid (K^+, H^+, pCO_2, and pO_2) and changes in the concentration of chemical transmitters and neuromodulators released from the neurones of the brain. Superimposed upon these controlling processes is the influence of perivascular nerves, which appears to predominate in larger cerebral arteries, factors released from intimal endothelial cells, and the passive myogenic properties of cerebrovascular smooth muscle cells. The complex nature of the link between cerebral blood flow and metabolism, and the possible mediation of neurotransmitters, necessitates *in vitro* pharmacological studies, where the kinetics of agonist/receptor interactions can be examined under controlled, steady state conditions, and receptors can be classified without complications from changes in the local environment of the smooth muscle cells and the reflex activation of perivascular nerves (see Chapter 2). The use of isolated vascular smooth muscle preparations also enables studies of the cellular mechanisms which follow receptor activation, and assessment of the

Pharmacology of the cerebral circulation 253

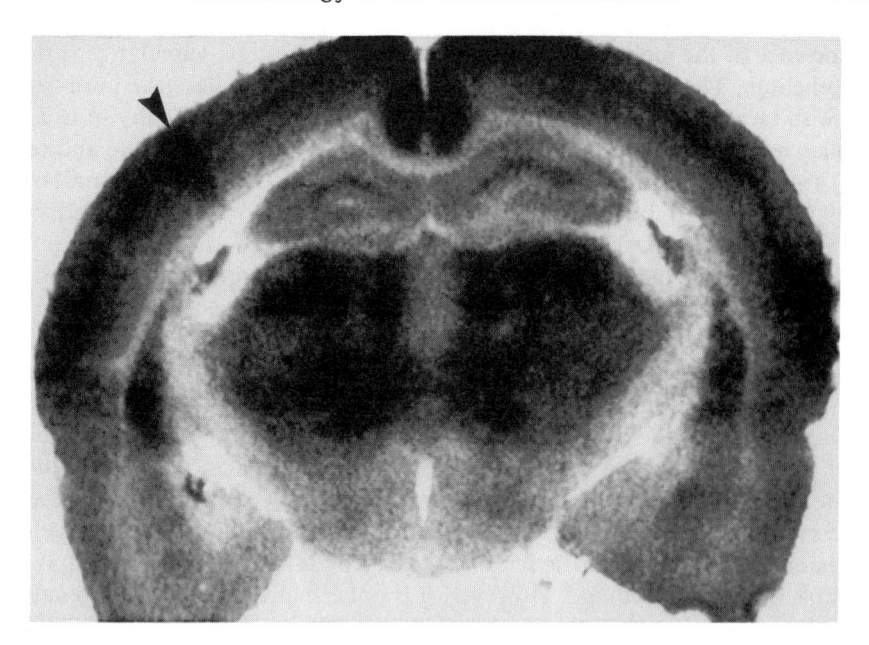

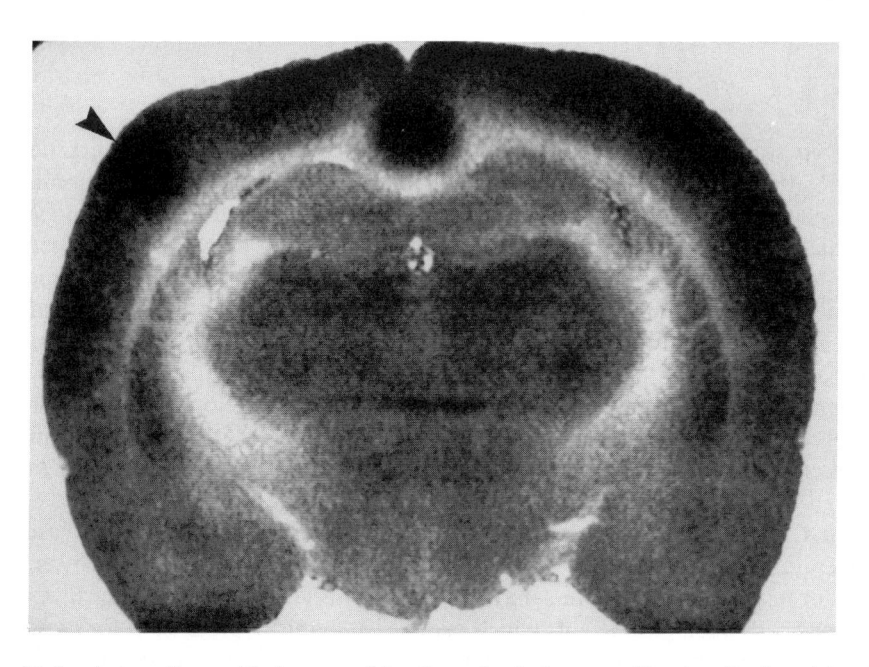

Fig. 11.1 Autoradiographic images of local cerebral glucose utilization (*top*) and local cerebral blood flow (*bottom*) derived from coronal sections of rat brain at the level of parietal cortex following unilateral stimulation of four adjacent vibissae. The column of increased grain density in the cortex contralateral to the stimulation (*arrows*) indicates that blood flow is coupled to the increased metabolic demands of cortical sensory processing.

importance of the modulatory influence which is exerted on vascular tone by the endothelium. The majority of *in vitro* pharmacological studies have been carried out with large cerebral arteries, the main reason being the difficulty in isolating smaller vessels in a viable form. Although the techniques for isolating and recording from small arteries have generally improved in recent years, studies with small arteries from the cerebrovascular bed are still somewhat limited and, apart from the work of Dacey and Duling (1984), restricted to pial arteries. The evidence available indicates variable smooth muscle membrane characteristics in different arterial branches (Hill *et al*. 1986; McPherson and Stork 1992), suggesting that the pharmacology of specific, large arteries such as the basilar artery, cannot be extrapolated to the cerebral circulation in general. However, studies with large cerebral arteries are of great importance in their own right, because these arteries provide a significant resistive element of between 25-50% of the total vascular resistance of the cerebral circulation under normal conditions (Baumbach and Heistad 1983). *In vitro* pharmacological studies are therefore necessary to complement *in vivo* experiments, allowing drug receptor and cellular mechanistic investigations under controlled conditions which are simply not possible in the intact animal. However, it is only finally in the intact animal that the physiological relevance of these mechanisms and their contribution to cerebrovascular disorders can be fully examined.

IN VIVO AND IN VITRO STUDIES

In vivo studies are hampered by the fact that most neurotransmitters/neuromodulators can modify cerebrovascular tone directly, as well as functioning as intraneuronal messengers, so they have tremendous potential to influence the intimate linkage that normally exists between synaptic activity, energy generation, and cerebral blood flow (Sokoloff 1977). Alterations in neuronal function elicited by neurotransmitters, which *in vivo* will effect changes in metabolic demand, will indirectly influence cerebral blood flow totally independently of vascular receptors, and sometimes in a manner diametrically opposed to that which would be predicted on the basis of a direct interaction with receptors on cerebral blood vessels (MacKenzie *et al*. 1976; Berntman *et al*. 1978; McCulloch *et al*. 1982). In addition, two further considerations are of importance in the design and interpretation of experiments in the intact animal.

First, the cerebrovascular bed is an integral part of the entire cardiovascular system of the body, so pharmacological interventions which alter cardiovascular and/or respiratory parameters may produce indirect effects upon cerebral vessels. Thus, pharmacological agents which produce systemic hypertension (or hypotension) will indirectly induce an autoregulatory vasoconstriction (or dilatation) in the cerebrovascular bed which must be considered (Kontos *et al*. 1978; MacKenzie *et al*. 1979), independent of direct local effects upon the cerebral vessels. Similarly, respiratory depression resulting in hypercapnia, or hyperventilation resulting in hypocapnia, can also induce profound cerebrovascular dilatation or constriction, respectively (Kuschinsky and Wahl 1978). In animals which are not artificially ventilated, considerable care must therefore be taken to ensure adequate monitoring of blood gas tensions.

Second, the range of drugs which might be useful in pharmacological investigations *in vivo* is limited by the presence of both the physical and enzymatic blood-brain barrier (Bradbury 1979). Although this problem has in many instances been overcome by the direct intracerebral application of agents, most notably in investigations of peptidergic systems (Klugman *et al.* 1980; Unterberg *et al.* 1983; Tuor *et al.* 1990*a,b*), this approach in itself can present problems arising from the local trauma of the intervention.

Another approach to the study of cerebrovascular pharmacology, which in effect combines some of the advantages of *in vitro* experiments with an *in vivo* environment, is provided by the pial window technique which has been applied in both cats and rats. The advantage of this method is that the blood vessels can be maintained in conditions which approach their normal physiological environment and with their normal intrinsic tone. Physiological parameters, such as arterial pCO_2 and blood pressure, can also easily be controlled. Whilst this approach is undoubtedly useful in the study of agonist/antagonist action, one is uncertain of the extent to which the larger pial vessels contribute to the total cerebrovascular resistance, and the interaction between responses and mechanisms responsible for the local regulation of cerebral blood flow. In addition, responses to the topical application of vasoactive agents to pial vessels may be modified by uptake into perivascular nerves, and thus induce different responses to those which follow intraluminal application, a route which is subject to both the diffusion-barrier properties of the endothelium and the possible release of dilator or constrictor agents from the endothelial cells themselves (Angus and Lew 1992).

By employing a variety of *in vitro* and *in vivo* techniques, the cerebrovascular pharmacology and physiology of a number of neurotransmitter systems has been characterized. Some types of perivascular innervation and their attendant smooth muscle receptors are also found in the peripheral circulation, but although the pharmacology may be similar, their physiological effects may differ. Others are unique to the cerebral circulation and include intrinsic GABAergic, serotonergic, and peptidergic nerves.

THE SYMPATHETIC NERVOUS SYSTEM

Although noradrenaline is a potent vasoconstrictor agent on vascular smooth muscle in peripheral blood vessels, cerebral arteries *in vitro* show a relative insensitivity to noradrenaline. *In vivo*, the effects of systemic noradrenaline injection are confounded by an effective blood-brain barrier to circulating catecholamines, and the metabolic effects of noradrenaline if this barrier is circumvented experimentally (Edvinsson and MacKenzie 1976). Cerebral blood vessels from a variety of species have been shown to be surrounded, to a greater or lesser extent, by a plexus of noradrenaline-containing or noradrenergic nerve fibres, derived in the main from the ipsilateral superior cervical ganglion (Edvinsson et al. 1972, 1976). Noradrenergic fibres form a perivascular plexus around large arteries arising from the carotid and vertebral arteries, and both the circle of Willis and its proximal branches. The density of innervation decreases and then disappears in pial vessels as they branch distally from the circle of Willis (Edvinsson et al. 1982). No role has yet been identified for this endogenous source of noradrenaline in the normal regulation of cerebrovascular tone.

Neither section nor stimulation of the cervical sympathetic nerves produces any significant change in cerebral blood flow under normal conditions (Harper et al. 1972), but sympathetic release of noradrenaline does fundamentally alter the cerebrovascular response to hypertension, protecting cerebral capillaries against acute and severe increases in blood pressure by a noradrenaline-induced constriction of the inflow and pial arteries. This effect is manifest in a shift in the autoregulatory curve, with the upper limit of autoregulation shifted to the right, i.e. towards higher pressure levels (Paulson et al. 1990). Noradrenergic nerve fibres have also been described in association with small penetrating blood vessels and capillaries (Swanson et al. 1977). These fibres apparently originate in the locus coeruleus, and their function is at present unknown. It has been suggested that they may play a role in the control of the permeability of the blood-brain barrier (Raichle et al. 1975).

The lack of a pronounced vasoconstrictor effect following sympathetic stimulation, which is indicated by *in vivo* data, is supported by *in vitro* studies. Transmural electrical stimulation of isolated segments of cerebral arteries, to activate the perivascular nerve fibres, only induces a very modest smooth muscle contraction compared to the capability of the tissue to contract in response to agonists. So for example, in isolated segments from either human or rabbit middle cerebral arteries, transmural stimulation induced a contraction of less than 10% of the total contractile capacity of these segments (Duckles 1979; Bevan et al. 1987; Duckworth et al. 1989). In addition, cerebrovascular smooth muscle is relatively insensitive to the constrictor action of exogenous noradrenaline, when compared to similar cells in peripheral arteries (Duckles and Bevan 1976; Harder et al. 1981; Garland 1989). The contraction to noradrenaline peaks at micromolar concentrations, before developing further with higher concentrations. The contraction, at least to the lower concentrations, appears to be mediated by α-adrenergic receptors (Harder et al. 1981; Garland 1989). The mechanism responsible for contraction in cerebral arteries is not clear, but involves a voltage-dependent contribution consequent to smooth muscle depolarization (Garland 1989; Plane and Garland 1992). Whether α-adrenergic receptors in cerebrovascular smooth muscle link to phospholipase C activation, as they do in peripheral vessels, is not known. If they do, noradrenaline-induced contraction may release internal calcium stores via IP_3 formation, and increase the myofilament calcium sensitivity by diacyglycerol-induced activation of protein kinases. Evidence has been presented to show that noradrenaline can cause contraction in cerebral arteries by the release of intracellular calcium, suggesting that voltage-independent mechanisms of this type are of importance (Aaronson 1993).

Smooth muscle contraction to neuronally released noradrenaline may also be modulated by cotransmitters such as ATP and NPY (see also Chapters 8 and 9), and possibly by the release of a constrictor agent(s) from the endothelium. Both ATP and NPY have been shown to contract cerebrovascular smooth muscle, although the size of this response appears to vary in different species (Karashima and Kuriyama 1981; Muramatsu et al. 1981; Fujiwara et al. 1982; Edvinsson et al. 1984a,b; Fallgren et al. 1990). The possibility also exists that NPY may synergize with noradrenaline to increase the constrictor response to this agent (Edvinsson et al. 1984a; Saville et al. 1990). The constrictor action of noradrenaline may also be increased indirectly, by a constrictor action in some species which is dependent on the endothelium (Usui et al. 1987).

Therefore, the main input from sympathetic nerves appears to be largely restricted to larger cerebral arteries, where nerve activation exerts an effect which is most relevant at the extremes of the autoregulatory range, when blood pressure is very high or very low. The lack of a functionally significant innervation to smaller pial arteries suggests a control by non-sympathetic mechanisms, and it has been suggested that the primary control of tone in these vessels is through alterations in myogenic tone in response to changes in blood pressure and flow (Bevan and Bevan 1993). Small arteries which penetrate into the brain parenchyma are ideally placed to respond rapidly to metabolites and neurotransmitters, and in so doing provide a very localized control of blood flow, closely matching the flow to cellular metabolism, obviating any requirement for a direct extrinsic neural control. A number of intrinsic sources for transmitters do, however, exist which may have a role to play in the modulation of cerebral blood flow.

CEREBROVASCULAR GABAERGIC SYSTEMS

Glutamic acid decarboxylase (GAD), the rate limiting enzyme in the synthesis of the inhibitory neurotransmitter GABA, and GABA transaminase (GABA-T), the principal enzyme involved with the degradation of GABA, have both been measured in large concentrations in cerebral vessels, but are not present in vessels from the peripheral circulation (Hamel et al. 1981; Krantis 1984). Pharmacological studies *in vitro* have demonstrated specific GABA binding (GABA$_A$) sites, and a positive correlation between binding affinity and potency of GABA agonists in eliciting dilatatory responses from preconstricted cerebral blood vessels. In contrast, GABA agonists have no action in vessels from the coronary, mesenteric, or hepatic vascular beds. These observations suggest that intrinsic cerebrovascular GABA systems may have an important role to play in the control of cerebral vasomotor activity (Edvinsson and Krause 1979; Krause et al. 1980).

In general, the *in vitro* characterization of cerebrovascular GABA receptors has been confirmed *in situ*. GABA, and the predominantly GABA$_A$ agonist muscimol elicited small but significant increases in pial diameter (dilatation) above threshold concentrations of 10^{-7} M in the microinjectate. The agonist effects could be blocked by the simultaneous injection of specific antagonists, while the absence of any effects of the antagonists alone suggested an absence of tonic GABA-induced dilatation (McCulloch *et al*. 1981).

Attempts to identify the effects which manipulating putative cerebrovascular GABA systems might have upon cerebral blood flow in intact experimental animals, have produced completely incompatible and diametrically opposite results. In these studies, where pharmacological agents are injected systemically, the use of GABA itself is precluded by the blood–brain barrier which, due probably to high vascular GABA-T enzymatic activity (Krantis 1984), is largely impermeable to GABA. The use of GABA antagonists in intact animals is precluded by their potent convulsive activity, so that the capacity for extensive pharmacological studies *in vivo* is very limited. However, the specific GABA$_A$ agonist muscimol, which has been used extensively in *in vitro* investigations, does cross the blood–brain barrier and has been used with some success in the intact animal (Baraldi *et al*. 1979).

Initial investigations in anaesthetized, artificially ventilated rats reported increases in cerebral blood flow, particularly in the cortex where increases of as much as 90% were reported following the systemic injection of muscimol (Edvinsson *et al*. 1980). These observations are completely in keeping with the known vasodilatory actions of the drug described *in vitro*. However, the results could not be reproduced in unanaesthetized animal preparations, where contrary to the proposed dilatatory properties of muscimol, local cerebral blood flow was significantly *reduced* throughout the brain (Kelly and McCulloch 1983). The reductions in cerebral blood flow in response to muscimol were identical in both magnitude and anatomical distribution to the reductions in metabolic demand measured in parallel groups of animals (Fig. 11.2).

A direct effect of muscimol upon the cerebral vessels in the intact animal cannot be totally discounted however. There is a tendency with increasing doses of muscimol for a slight resetting of the relationship between blood flow and glucose use (Fig. 11.2), suggesting that blood flow becomes progressively greater than would be predicted if flow remained tightly coupled to metabolism. Further evidence that there is an interaction between the opposing forces elicited by muscimol, comes from blood flow measurements immediately after the systemic injection of muscimol (Kelly *et al*. 1989) in which a clear negative correlation becomes evident between the intensity of the blood flow response and the density of vascular GABA$_A$ receptors (Napoleone *et al*. 1987). With increasing time delay between injection and the measurement of blood flow, the effect became progressively less pronounced, presumably as metabolic factors become more manifest. Although the significance of GABA-induced dilatation is not yet clear, it is tempting to speculate that the physiological role of cerebrovascular GABA may lie in its capacity to modulate the effects of vasoconstrictor stimuli (Shirakawa *et al*. 1989).

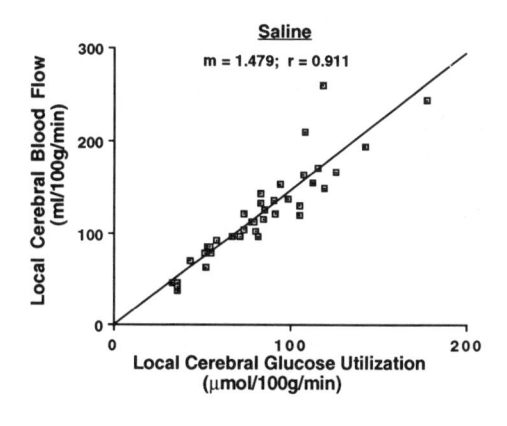

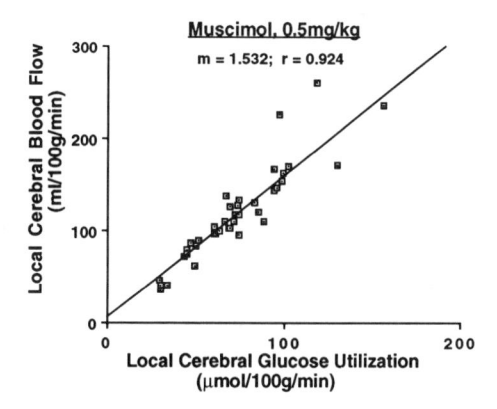

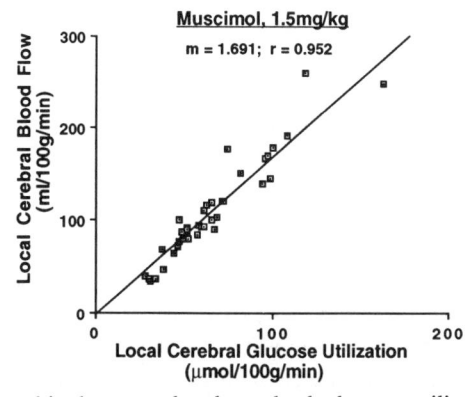

Fig. 11.2 The relationship between local cerebral glucose utilization and mean local cerebral blood flow in discrete regions of the conscious rat brain following intravenous injections of saline or the $GABA_A$ agonist, muscimol. The correlation coefficients (r) indicate that blood flow remains coupled to metabolic demand under all three conditions, but the progressive increase in the slope of the best fitting straight lines (m) suggests a slight resetting of the relationship, with global cerebral tissue perfusion in excess of metabolic demand with increasing doses of muscimol.

ENDOTHELIUM-DERIVED FACTORS

Endothelial cells can potentially exert a powerful influence on cerebrovascular smooth muscle by the release of dilator and constrictor factors (see also Chapter 10). Smooth muscle contraction which depends on the presence of an intact endothelial cell lining in cerebral arteries has been demonstrated in a number of species. Noradrenaline, 5-HT, arachidonic acid and even, in canine cerebral arteries acetylcholine have a contractile action, at least a component of which is endothelium-dependent (Shirahase et al. 1987; Usui et al. 1987; Seager et al. 1992). In addition, both tissue hypoxia and increases in transmural pressure stimulate endothelium-dependent contraction which has been shown to result from the release of a diffusible factor from endothelial cells (Rubanyi and Vanhoutte 1985; Harder 1987; Harder et al. 1989; Klaas and Wadsworth 1989). The factor which is responsible has not been identified, but at least in some cases it appears to be an arachidonic acid derivative. In addition, cerebrovascular endothelial cells can also release the potent constrictor peptide endothelin. The endothelin family of polypeptides has been identified as endothelium-derived constricting factors which can produce prolonged and potent cerebral artery constriction (Robinson and McCulloch 1990) which in the intact animal can reduce blood flow to ischaemic levels (Macrae et al. 1993). Although an endogenous release of endothelin has been described, it is almost invariably related to pathological conditions (Cintra et al. 1989; Rakugi et al. 1990; Suzuki et al. 1990). As yet no physiological role has been identified for this potent vasoconstrictor.

The principal dilator agent released by endothelial cells in response to a number of different vasoactive agents appears to be the simple diatomic molecule nitric oxide, derived from L-arginine by the action of the enzyme nitric oxide synthase (Chapter 10). The smooth muscle relaxation, which follows the release of NO is also associated with membrane hyperpolarization which appears to be largely independent of the action of NO, and may be due to the release of a separate factor, endothelium-derived hyperpolarizing factor-EDHF (Plane and Garland 1992). Although the experimental data are very limited, it appears that there could be a variation in the relative importance of NO and EDHF in different vascular beds, and possibly between separate branches of a specific bed. In isolated middle cerebral arteries from the rabbit and cat, the pharmacological agent ACh induces both smooth muscle relaxation and hyperpolarization, both of which are endothelium-dependent (Brayden and Wellman 1989; Brayden 1990). The hyperpolarization appears not to reflect an action of NO, as the increase in membrane potential and a component of relaxation persisted in the presence of methylene blue to inhibit guanylyl cyclase. In contrast, although ACh increased the membrane potential and relaxed smooth muscle in the rabbit basilar artery, the change in membrane potential appeared to have little influence on relaxation. The former response required higher concentrations of ACh (Fig. 11.3). Also, in contrast to the relaxation, it was both transient and desensitized rapidly. The relaxation was almost totally blocked in the presence of inhibitors for NO synthase, indicating a predominant role for NO, at least in response to ACh (Rand

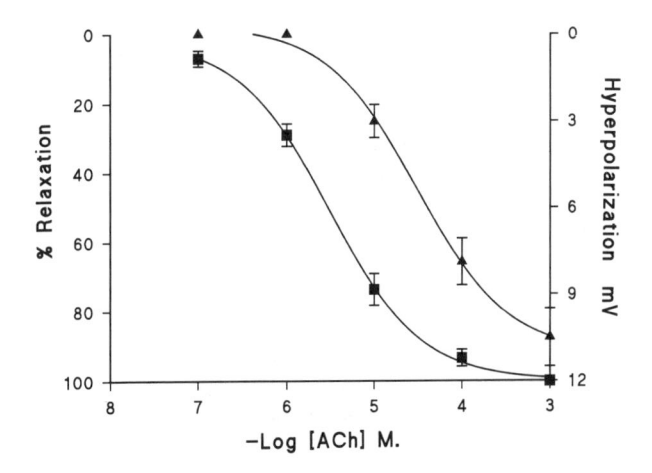

Fig. 11.3 Concentration–response curves for relaxation and repolarization to acetylcholine in rabbit basilar artery smooth muscle cells contracted and depolarized in the presence of noradrenaline. Points are the mean ± s.e. mean of at least five separate experiments. Hyperpolarization (■) relaxation (▲).

and Garland 1992). To what extent other, more physiologically relevant agonists induce relaxation through the release of NO and/or EDHF remains to be determined.

Although the inhibition of NO has been shown to result in the vasoconstriction of cerebral blood vessels *in vitro*, the conditions under which a similar action might occur in the intact animal are currently a matter of intense investigation. *In vivo*, NO synthase inhibitors and NO donors are currently the only pharmacological tools with which to manipulate endogenous NO activity, and in a number of studies marked decreases in cerebral blood flow have been described following administration of a variety of N^G-substituted arginine analogues, including N^G-nitro-L-arginine (NOLA) (Kovach *et al.* 1992; Wang *et al.* 1992; Dirnagl *et al.* 1993), N^G-monomethyl-L-arginine (Tanaka *et al.* 1991; Kozniewski *et al.* 1992), and N^G-nitro-L-arginine methyl ester (L-NAME), whether injected systemically (Goadsby *et al.* 1992; Northington *et al.* 1992; Prado *et al.* 1992; Iadecola *et al.* 1993; Pelligrino *et al.* 1993) or centrally (Kelly *et al.* 1992). There are however some inconsistencies. For example, no change in regional cerebral blood flow could be detected in anaesthetized dogs following inhibition of NO synthesis with L-NAME, despite clearly reduced flow in other organs of the body (Sonntag *et al.* 1992), and in both anaesthetized and conscious rats, neither L-NAME nor NOLA had any effect upon basal cerebral blood flow (Iadecola 1992; Wang *et al.* 1993). Data from anaesthetized cats adds a further level of complexity, showing a regional heterogeneity in the changes in cerebral blood flow to NOLA, with the cerebellum, pituitary, and medulla oblongata being markedly affected whilst cortical blood flow remained unchanged (Kovach *et al.* 1992).

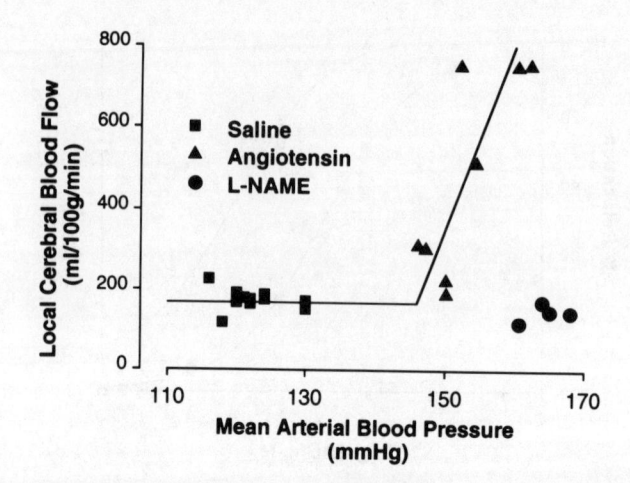

Fig. 11.4 The relationship between cortical blood flow and mean arterial blood pressure in conscious rats treated with saline, angiotensin II, or L-NAME. In rats treated with angiotensin II, blood flow was markedly increased when blood pressure exceeded approximately 150 mmHg. In contrast, there was no evidence of a breakdown in the autoregulation of blood flow in L-NAME treated rats, even when blood pressures were higher than those induced by angiotensin II.

These discrepancies cannot be ignored, but an explanation is not available. It is possible that there might be differences between species (dog, cat, and rats), between anaesthetic regimes during the measurement of cerebral blood flow (anaesthetized with halothane, chloralose/urethane, or pentobarbitone sodium, versus conscious), or between the methods used to measure blood flow (microspheres, laser Doppler, hydrogen clearance, intracarotid ^{133}Xe, quantitative iodoantipyrine autoradiography). To this list must also be added the possibility that the pharmacological profile of the arginine analogues may be subtly different. Using the same preparation (anaesthetized rat) the same authors found no change in basal blood flow with NOLA (Iadecola 1992) but a decreased flow following L-NAME (Iadecola et al. 1993).

Very recent studies have shown that despite inducing an increase in systemic blood pressure, higher than the upper limit of autoregulation, there is no evidence of the forced dilatation and increases in flow which follow when other hypertensive agents are used (Fig. 11.4) (Thomas et al. 1993). Moreover, injection of N^G-nitro-L-arginine methyl ester (L-NAME) directly into the brain of conscious rats, thus avoiding effects in the systemic circulation and maintaining normal homeostatic mechanisms, have confirmed that a decrease in local cerebral blood flow does follow the local inhibition of NO synthase (Kelly et al. 1992).

The growing evidence that NO synthase is also widely distributed in brain neurones (Bredt et al. 1990), where it is thought to act as an interneuronal messenger (Garthwaite et al. 1989), might suggest that manipulation of NO synthase may influence cerebral flood flow not only via direct effects on the vasculature, but also by altering underlying metabolic demand. It is worth noting in this respect that a uniquely vascular mechanism underlying NOS inhibitor-induced constriction has been identified, which occurs in the absence of any parallel changes in underlying metabolic demand (Goadsby et al. 1992; Kelly et al. 1994).

It has also been suggested that NO might function as a neurotransmitter in cerebral blood vessels, being released from perivascular nerve fibres. The evidence is based entirely on experiments conducted with isolated vessels. Smooth muscle relaxation follows transmural stimulation to activate perivascular nerves in isolated cerebral arteries from the dog and the monkey. Similar responses can be induced with exogenous nicotine which stimulates the nerve endings directly. These inhibitory responses were described as non-adrenergic and non-cholinergic (NANC), as they were not mediated by α or β-adrenergic receptors or muscarinic receptors. In addition, they were not mediated by purinoceptors, histamine receptors, peptidergic mechanisms, or the release of prostaglandins (Toda 1981, 1982; Okamura et al. 1989). However, the responses were not dependent on the presence of a functional endothelium, and were sensitive both to inhibitors of NO synthase and agents which block the action of NO on smooth muscle cells (Toda 1988; Toda et al. 1990; Toda and Okamura 1991). Support for the suggestion that NO releasing perivascular nerves specifically innervate cerebral blood vessels has come from immunohistochemical studies in the rat, where specific NO synthase activity was present in perivascular nerves as well as endothelial cells, but was absent from nerves supplying the aorta and coronary circulation (Bredt et al. 1990). Interestingly, the relaxation which followed the application of VIP or stimulation of perivascular nerves in isolated sheep cerebral arteries, with or without a functional endothelium, was greatly reduced by NO synthase inhibitors, while the effect of VIP was inhibited by either haemoglobin or methylene blue. This raises the possibility that nerve released VIP can cause smooth muscle relaxation via NO, possibly by an indirect release from perivascular nerves (Gaw et al. 1991).

5-HYDROXYTRYPTAMINE (5-HT)

Interest in the cerebrovascular actions of 5-HT stems mainly from the suggested involvement of this agent in a variety of cerebrovascular disorders. In addition to a possible involvement in stroke, 5-HT has been suggested to be involved in the generation of migraine headache and the responses of cerebral blood vessels to subarachnoid haemorrhage. Potential sources of 5-HT are blood platelets, with release occurring during activation and aggregation of these cells and access to the brain achieved via a compromised blood–brain barrier, and possibly specific cerebral perivascular nerves (Edvinsson et al. 1985). Receptors for 5-HT exist on cerebrovascular smooth muscle cells, and the predominant effect evoked by their activation is muscle contraction. Receptors which fall into the category 5-HT$_1$ and 5-HT$_2$ have been described in different species (see Chapter 5; Humphrey et al. 1993). In some cases, a heterogeneous population has been suggested, although the balance of evidence from most species favours the idea that the predominant receptor type is 5-HT$_1$, although which particular subtype is not clear. The ability of sumatriptan to constrict arteries in the human dura indicates that the functional subtype may be 5-HT$_{1D}$ (Humphrey and Feniuk 1991). Stimulation of this receptor on smooth muscle cells in large cerebral arteries has been suggested to form the basis of this agonists ability to reverse different types of migraine headache. In this scenario, intracranial vessels are distended during migraine headache. As a consequence, presynaptic trigeminal sensory nerve terminals are activated and release the dilator peptides, CGRP and substance P. These agents lead to a local inflammation of the blood vessel wall and pain perception via the trigeminal nerve. By constricting vascular smooth muscle cells in the cerebral vessels, sumatriptan reverses this process (Humphrey and Feniuk 1991). However, an alternative view has been presented by Moscowitz and co-workers (1992), who have suggested that the primary anti-migraine action of sumatriptan is due to a presynaptic effect, directly leading to a reduction in the release of neuropeptides from trigeminal nerve terminals. This effect is mediated by a receptor which closely resembles the vascular 5-HT$_{1D}$ receptor, and consequently inhibits plasma extravasation and this consequently blocks local blood vessel inflammation and thus alleviates migraine headache (Moskowitz 1992). Clinical data relating to the action of sumatriptan has recently been reviewed by Ferrai and Saxena (1993), who concluded that the balance of available evidence indicates a primary action of sumatriptan on the cerebrovasculature (Fig. 11.5).

The mechanism by which 5-HT contracts cerebrovascular smooth muscle has not been defined. 5-HT$_1$ receptor subtypes have recently been grouped in part on the basis of sequence homology and operational (pharmacological) similarities, and also on the basis of a common transduction mechanism (Humphrey et al. 1993). The activation of 5-HT$_1$ receptors leads to an inhibition of adenylyl cyclase. Whether this action can entirely account for the constrictor action of 5-HT on cerebral blood vessels is not known. Contraction in response to 5-HT is associated with smooth muscle depolarization in cerebral arteries (Harder and Waters 1983; Garland 1987), and voltage-dependent calcium channels do contribute to the contractile response (Worley et al. 1991; Clark and Garland 1993). However, the initiation of contraction appears to occur by voltage-independent mechanisms. In the rabbit basilar artery, 5-HT stimulates the production of membrane diacylglycerol, which is the endogenous activator of protein kinase C. The diacylglycerol appears to arise from membrane phospholipids other than phosphoinositide, and inhibitors of protein kinase C block the smooth muscle contraction (Clark and Garland 1991).

5-HT can also potentially modulate vascular tone by an indirect action exerted via the endothelium. A smooth muscle dilator effect exerted through an action on endothelial cell 5-HT$_1$ receptors has been reported in coronary arteries (Cocks and Angus 1983; Cohen and Vanhoutte 1983). A similar effect has not been reported for cerebral vessels, but conclusive experiments would require antagonism of the direct smooth muscle constrictor action of 5-HT, which is difficult in the absence of antagonists selective for the different 5-HT$_1$ receptor subtypes. A modest endothelium-dependent contractile effect of 5-HT has been reported

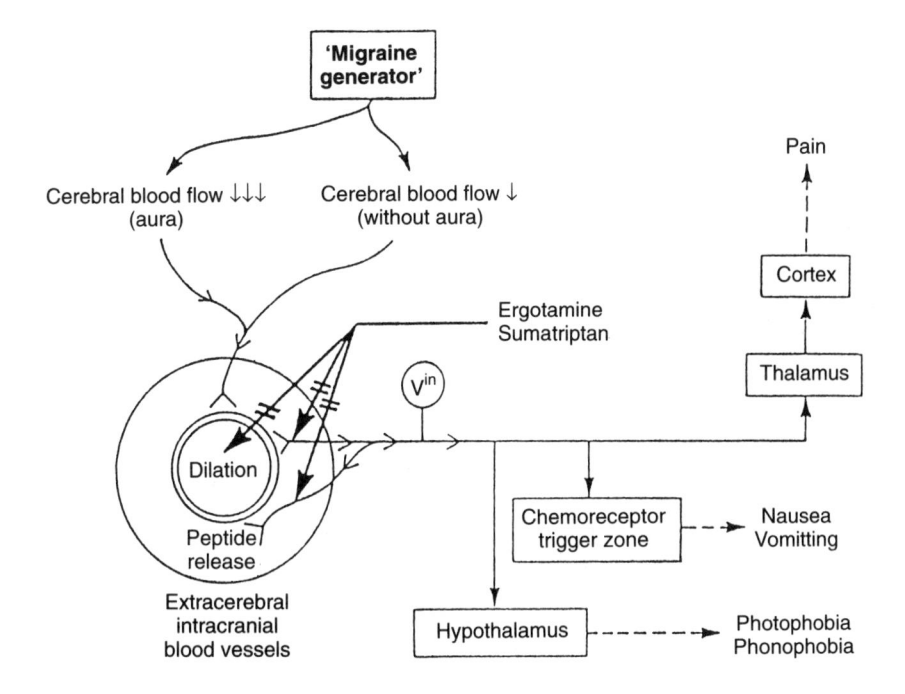

Fig. 11.5 Putative changes during migraine and sites of action of acutely acting antimigraine drugs (ergotamine and sumatriptan). Three phases of migraine can be distinguished: a 'generator' phase (mechanism unknown); a pre-headache phase where cerebral blood flow does (migraine with aura) or does not (migraine without aura) decrease below a critical value: and a headache phase with dilation of mainly extracerebral intracranial arteries and arteriovenous anastomoses, perhaps within the meningeal circulation and mediated by changes in the activity of raphé and/or locus coeruleus nuclei. This dilation would increase vascular pulsations, which, in turn, can stimulate perivascular sensory afferents of the Vth cranial nerve to cause the symptoms shown. In addition, neurogenic inflammation, via retrograde release of vasoactive neuropeptides and local ischaemia due to arteriovenous shunting may accentuate pain sensation. The ergot alkaloids and sumatriptan abort migraine attacks by potently constricting the dilated cephalic vessels and, possibly, also by inhibiting peptide release from perivascular nerve terminals, or neural transmission. Taken from Ferrai and Saxena (1993) with permission.

in rabbit cerebral arteries, which appears to be mediated by an arachidonic acid derivative, as the contraction was blocked in the presence of indomethacin (Seager *et al.* 1992). The localized nature of vascular responses to 5-HT, and its involvement in pathophysiological conditions, highlights the potential importance of any local modulating action exerted via the endothelium.

As with other neurotransmitter systems, the activity of 5-HT agonists or antagonists directed at cerebrovascular receptors may be confounded *in vivo* by the agents also binding to neuronal receptors and thereby altering underlying metabolic demand. In addition, the apparent innervation of cerebral vessels by serotonergic fibres arising from neurones in the midbrain raises a further complication.

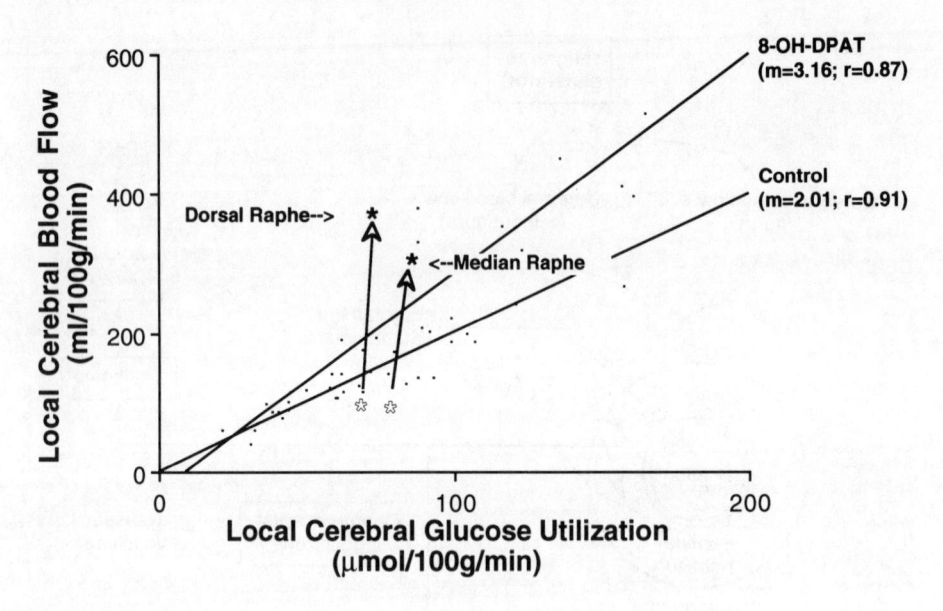

Fig. 11.6 The relationship between mean local cerebral glucose utilization and cerebral blood flow in discrete regions of the conscious rat brain measured in rat injected (IV) with either saline or the 5-HT$_{1A}$ agonist, 8-OH-DPAT. Treatment with 8-OH-DPAT produced both a global resetting of the flow-metabolism relationship, and a focal uncoupling which was manifest in both the dorsal and median raphe nuclei.

Thus binding of an agonist to 5-HT$_{1A}$ receptors on blood vessels might mediate vasoconstriction as *in vitro*, whilst the effects upon neuronal activity (Kelly *et al.* 1988), by increasing metabolic demand will induce dilatation. Inhibition of raphe neurones, via somatodendritic 5-HT receptors, may allow dilatation in the absence of any change in metabolic demand (by removing the constrictor effects of perivascular 5-HT release). This would require the presence of tonic input from 5-HT containing nerves. Available evidence does suggest that such a mechanism may well be functional *in vivo*. Systemic 8-OH-DPAT, a relatively selective 5-HT$_{1A}$ agonist, produces global increases in cerebral blood flow, increasing the flow-metabolism ratio by around 25% (McBean *et al.* 1991) (Fig. 11.6), whilst direct intracortical injection of 8-OH-DPAT, which avoids any interaction with somatodendritic raphé receptors, has no effect upon cerebral blood flow despite its presumed access to local vascular receptors (Kelly *et al.* 1987). Interestingly, the 5-HT$_{1B}$ agonist RU24969, increases blood flow locally when injected into the cortex, presumably once again by binding presynaptically to perivascular raphe terminals and inhibiting the release of 5-HT (Kelly *et al.* 1987). These pharmacological effects have been confirmed in animals treated with the specific serotonergic neurotoxin methylenedioxyamphetamine (MDA). Chronic exposure to MDA effects a severe depletion of serotonergic terminals, and although a minimal changes in metabolic demand results, cerebral blood flow is increased (McBean *et al.* 1990), an effect which becomes more marked under hypercapnic conditions

(Kelly et al. 1991). It has to be said however, that this result is in marked contrast to earlier work by Dahlgren et al. (1991) who were unable to detect any change in blood flow following intraventricular injections of 5,7-dihydroxytryptamine. The differences in these two studies serve to highlight a further source of confusion in the literature where opposite results are generated from experiments using conscious (Kelly et al. 1991) as opposed to anaesthetized animals (Dahlgren et al. 1981). It does seem that *in vivo* studies of cerebrovascular 5-HT systems are particularly prone to anaesthetic-induced artefact.

NEUROPEPTIDES

The observation of peptide-containing nerve fibres in association with cerebral blood vessels provided the initial stimulus for this important, and rapidly expanding area of cerebrovascular research. However, whilst the number of cerebrovascular peptidergic systems which have been identified has increased almost exponentially over the past ten years, the complexities of their anatomy and cellular physiology, together with limited pharmacological tools, have considerably hampered attempts to establish a clear role for these neuropeptides in cerebrovascular vasomotor control. Indeed for some peptides, most notably cholecystokinin and gastrin-releasing peptide, no vasoactive actions have been identified in cerebral vessels. To ascribe specific roles to specific peptide-releasing nerves *in vivo* is further complicated by the widespread co-existence of neuropeptides with other neurotransmitters. For example, in nerves arising from the superior cervical ganglia, neuropeptide Y (NPY) coexists with noradrenaline, trigeminal nerves contain substance P (SP), neurokinin A (NKA), and calcitonin gene-related peptide (CGRP), whilst the perivascular innervation from the sphenopalatine ganglion contains acetylcholine together with vasoactive intestinal polypeptide (VIP). These nerves also contain peptide histidine isoleucine (PHI) which is structurally related to VIP, is produced from the same precursor polypeptide (and is therefore part of the same gene product), and also has much the same biological profile, certainly in terms of its cerebrovascular effects (Edvinsson and McCulloch 1985; Tuor et al. 1990a). However, despite these difficulties, there are some areas in which real progress has been achieved.

The effects of NPY upon the cerebral circulation have been examined in intact rats where intracarotid injection of NPY produces reductions in cortical blood flow which are both profound (close to 100%) and prolonged (at least two hours) (Allen et al. 1984). It is not clear how a polypeptide such as NPY can circumvent the blood–brain barrier and gain access to cerebrovascular smooth muscle, and others have had some difficulty in reproducing these results (Tuor et al. 1985) or have been required to use very high concentrations of peptide (Suzuki et al. 1989). However, when the peptide is delivered directly to the abluminal side by direct intracerebral injection in conscious rats, localized, dose-dependent decreases in blood flow are measured (up to 45% at 200 pmol). This effect upon blood flow was found despite little or no change in local cerebral metabolism

(Tuor *et al.* 1990*b*), and it has been suggested that release of NPY from perivascular nerves *in vivo* might provide a direct vasoconstrictor stimulus of some importance under some pathophysiological conditions (Tuor *et al.* 1990*b*). Although there is evidence of a correlation between concentrations of NPY and the severity of vasospasm following subarachnoid haemorrhage, there is no evidence that absolute levels are any higher than in controls (Juul *et al.* 1991) and a causative link has yet to be established.

The role of neuropeptides in the trigeminal innervation of cerebral blood vessels has generated considerable interest over recent years, not least, as mentioned above, because of the possible role which this nociceptive pathway might subserve in the aetiology of migraine headache (Moskowitz 1984). In the periphery, sensory nerve fibres are capable of generating sustained vasodilatation and increased vascular permeability as a result of the action of SP release by antidromic stimulation (Lembeck and Holzer 1979), but in the cerebrovasculature there is no evidence that trigeminal release of SP alters vascular permeability. Capsaicin, which releases SP from cerebrovascular nerve terminals (Moskowitz *et al.* 1983), does not induce extravasation of neutral dye into the cerebral parenchyma (McCulloch and Reid 1986). Unilateral stimulation of the trigeminal nerve has been reported to increase cortical blood flow (Goadsby and Duckworth 1987), suggesting that in this respect at least there is analogy with peripheral vascular beds. However, the bilateral distribution of these changes in blood flow cannot be reconciled with the known unilateral distribution of trigeminal innervation and might therefore reflect a non-specific (possibly metabolic) effect of the stimulation.

Of all of the peptides so far identified in perivascular nerves, CGRP is the most potent in producing vasodilatation *in vitro* (McCulloch and Edvinsson 1987), but all of the peptides coexisting in the trigeminal nerve are dilatatory. Despite this potential to induce cerebrovascular dilatation, removal of the trigeminal nerve has no effect upon resting blood flow (McCulloch and Edvinsson 1987). However it has been the *in situ* investigation of pial vessels following lesions of the trigeminal nerve (McCulloch *et al.* 1986) which have done most to elucidate the role of trigemino-cerebrovascular peptide system in the control of cerebral blood flow. Lesion alone has no effect upon the magnitude of pial artery response to a variety of physiolgical and pharmacological constrictor stimuli, but the duration of these constrictor responses was substantially increased following trigeminal section. Taking the data from these studies together, it has been concluded that whilst peptide release from trigeminal nerve fibres has no influence upon the moment-to-moment control of cerebral blood flow, it may provide a neurogenic mechanism which is capable of responding to excessive vasoconstriction, providing a tempering vasodilatation which might serve to protect the brain from dangerously reduced blood flows.

REFERENCES

Aaronson, P. I. (1994). Intracellular calcium release in cerebral arteries. *Pharmacol. Ther.*, **64**, 493-507.
Allen, J. M., Schon, F., Todd, N., Yeats, J. C., Crockard, H. A., and Bloom, S. R. (1984). Presence of neuropeptide-Y in human circle of Willis and its possible role in cerebral vasospasm. *Lancet*, **2**, 550-2.
Angus, J. A. and Lew, M. J. (1992). Interpretation of the acetylcholine test of endothelial cell dysfunction in hypertension. *J. Hyperten.*, **10**, S179-86.
Baraldi, M., Grandison, L., and Guidotti, A. (1979). Distribution and metabolism of muscimol in the brain and other tissues of the rat. *Neuropharmacology*, **18**, 57-62.
Baumbach, G. L. and Heistad, D. D. (1983). Effects of sympathetic stimulation and changes in arterial pressure on segmental resistance of cerebral vessels in rabbits and cats. *Circ. Res.*, **52**, 527-33.
Berntman, L., Dahlgren, N., and Siesjö, B. K. (1978). Influence of intravenously administered catecholamines on cerebral oxygen consumption and blood flow in the rat. *Acta Physiol. Scand.*, **104**, 101-8.
Bevan, J. A. and Bevan, R. D. (1993). Is innervation a prime regulator of cerebral blood flow? *News Physiol. Sci.*, **8**, 149-53.
Bevan, J. A., Duckworth, J., Laher, I., Oriowo, M. A., McPherson, G. A., and Bevan, R. A. (1987). Sympathetic control of cerebral arteries: Specialization in receptor type, reserve, affinity and distribution. *FASEB J.*, **1**, 193-8.
Bradbury, M. (1979). *The concept of a blood-brain barrier.* John Wiley, Chichester.
Brayden, J. E. (1990). Membrane hyperpolarization is a mechanism of endothelium-dependent cerebral vasodilation. *Am. J. Physiol.*, **259**, H668-73.
Brayden, J. E. and Wellman, G. C. (1989). Endothelium-dependent dilation of feline cerebral arteries: role of membrane potential and cyclic nucleotides. *J. Cereb. Blood Flow Metab.*, **9**, 256-63.
Bredt, D. S., Hwang, P. M., and Snyder, S. H. (1990). Localization of nitric oxide synthase indicating a neural role for nitric oxide. *Nature*, **347**, 768-70.
Cintra, A., Fuxe, K., Anggard, E., Tinner, B., Staines, W., and Agnati, L. F. (1989). Increased endothelin-like immunoreactivity in ibotenic acid-lesioned hippocampal formation of the rat brain. *Acta Physiol. Scand.*, **137**, 557-8.
Clark, A. H. and Garland, C. J. (1991). 5-Hydroxytryptamine-stimulated accumulation of 1,2-diacylglycerol in the rabbit basilar artery: a role for protein kinase C in smooth muscle contraction. *Br. J. Pharmacol.*, **102**, 415-21.
Clark, A. H. and Garland, C. J. (1993). Ca^{2+} channel antagonists and inhibition of protein kinase C each block contraction but not depolarizationn to 5-hydroxytryptamine in the rabbit basilar artery. *Eur. J. Pharmacol.*, **235**, 113-16.
Cocks, T. M. and Angus, J. A. (1983). Endothelium-dependent relaxation of coronary arteries by noradrenaline and serotonin. *Nature*, **305**, 627-30.
Cohen, R. A. and Vanhoutte, P. M. (1983). 5-Hydroxytryptamine can mediate endothelium-dependent relaxation of coronary arteries. *Am. J. Physiol.*, **245**, H1077-80.
Dacey, R. G. and Duling, B. R. (1984). Effect of norepinephrine on penetrating arterioles of rat cerebral cortex. *Am. J. Physiol.*, **246**, H380-5.
Dahlgren, N., Lindvall, O., Nobin, A., and Stenevi, U. (1981). Cerebral circulatory response to hypercapnia: Effects of lesions of central dopaminergic and serotonergic neuron systems. *Brain Res.*, **230**, 221-33.
Dirnagl, U., Lindauer, U., and Villringer, A. (1993). Role of nitric oxide in the coupling of cerebral blood flow to neuronal activation. *Neurosci. Lett.*, **149**, 43-6.

Duckles, S. P. (1979). Neurogenic dilator and constrictor responses of pial arteries *in vitro*. *Circ. Res.*, **44**, 482-90.

Duckles, S. P. and Bevan, J. A. (1976). Pharmacological characterization of adrenergic receptors of a rabbit cerebral artery *in vitro*. *J. Pharmacol. Exp. Ther.*, **197**, 371-8.

Duckworth, J. W., Wellman, G. C., Walters, C. L., and Bevan J. A. (1989). Aminergic histofluorescence and contractile responses to transmural electrical field stimulation and norepinephrine of human cerebral arteries otained promptly after death. *Circ. Res.*, **65**, 316-24.

Edvinsson, L. and Krause, D. N. (1979). Pharmacological characterization of GABA receptors mediating vasodilatation of cerebral vessels *in vitro*. *Brain Res.*, **173**, 89-97.

Edvinsson, L. and McCulloch, J. (1985). Distribution and vasomotor effects of peptide HI (PHI) in feline cerebral blood vessels *in vitro* and *in situ*. *Reg. Peptides*, **10**, 345-56.

Edvinsson, L. and MacKenzie, E. T. (1976). Amine mechanisms in the cerebral circulation. *Pharmacol. Rev.*, **2**, 275-348.

Edvinsson, L., Owman, C., Rosengren, E., and West, K. A. (1972). Concentration of noradrenaline in pial vessels, choroid plexus, and iris during two weeks after sympathetic ganglionectomy or decentralization. *Acta Physiol. Scand.*, **85**, 201-6.

Edvinsson, L., Owman, C., and Sjöberg, N.-O. (1976). Autonomic nerves, mast cells, and amine receptors in human brain vessels. A histochemical and pharmacological study. *Brain Res.*, **115**, 377-93.

Edvinsson, L., Larsson, B., and Skärby, T. (1980). Effects of the GABA agonist muscimol on regional cerebral blood flow in the rat. *Brain Res.*, **185**, 445-58.

Edvinsson, L., McCulloch, J., and Uddman, R. (1982). Feline cerebral veins and arteries: comparison of autonomic innervation and vasomotor responses. *J. Physiol.*, **325**, 161-73.

Edvinsson, L., Ekblad, E., Hakanson, R., and Wahlestedt, C. (1984*a*). Neuropetide Y potentiates the effect of various vasoconstrictor agents on rabbit blood vessels. *Br. J. Pharmacol.*, **83**, 519-25.

Edvinsson, L., Emson, P., McCulloch, J., Tatemoto, K., and Uddman, R. (1984*b*). Neuropeptide Y: immunocytochemical localization to and effect upon feline pial arteries and veins *in vitro* and *in situ*. *Acta Physiol. Scand.*, **122**, 155-163.

Edvinsson, L., Deguerce, A., Duverger, D., MacKenzie, E. T., and Scatton, B. (1985). Central serotonergic nerves project to the pial vessels of the brain. *Nature*, **306**, 55-7.

Fallgren, B., Arlock, P., Jansen, I., and Edvinsson, L. (1990). Neuropeptide Y in cerebrovascular function: comparison of membrane potential changes and vasomotor responses evoked by NPY and other vasoconstrictors in the guinea-pig basilar artery. *Neurosci. Lett.*, **114**, 117-22.

Ferrai, M. D. and Saxena, P. R. (1993). Clinical and experimental effects of sumatriptan in humans. *Trends Pharmacol. Sci.*, **14**, 129-33.

Fujiwara, S., Itoh, T., and Suzuki, H. (1982). Membrane properties and excitatory neuromuscular transmission in the smooth muscle of dog cerebral arteries. *Br. J. Pharmacol.*, **77**, 197-208.

Garland, C. J. (1987). The role of membrane depolarization in the contractile response of the rabbit basilar artery to 5-hydroxytryptamine. *J. Physiol.*, **392**, 333-48.

Garland, C. J. (1989). Influence of the endothelium and α-adrenoreceptor antagonists on responses to noradrenaline in the rabbit basilar artery. *J. Physiol.*, **418**, 205-17.

Garthwaite, J., Garthwaite, G., Palmer, R. M. J., and Moncada, S. (1989). NMDA receptor activation induces nitric oxide synthesis from arginine in rat brain slices. *Eur. J. Pharmacol.*, **172**, 413-16.

Gaw, A. J., Aberdeen, J., Humphrey, P. P. A., Wadsworth, R. M., and Burnstock, G. (1991). Relaxation of sheep cerebral arteries by vasoactive intestinal polypeptide and

neurogenic stimulation: inhibition by L-N^G-monomethyl arginine in endothelium-denuded vessels. *Br. J. Pharmacol.*, **102**, 567–72.
Goadsby, P. J. and Duckworth, J. W. (1987). The effect of stimulation of the trigeminal ganglion on regional cerebral blood flow in the cat. *Am. J. Physiol.*, **253**, R270–4.
Goadsby, P. J., Kaube, H., and Hoskin, K. L. (1992). Nitric oxide synthesis couples cerebral blood flow and metabolism. *Brain Res.*, **595**, 167–70.
Graham, D. I., Grome, J. J., Kelly, P. A. T., MacKenzie, E. T., McCulloch, J., Reis, D. J., *et al.* (1982). Cerebral circulatory effects of fulminating neurogenic hypertension. In *Cerebral blood flow: effects of nerves and neurotransmitters* (ed. D. D. Heistad and M. L. Marcus), pp. 493–502. Elsevier, New York.
Hamel, E., Krause, D. N., and Roberts, E. (1981). Specific cerebrovascular localization of glutamate decarboxylase activity. *Brain Res.*, **223**, 199–204.
Harder, D. R. (1987). Pressure-induced myogenic activation of cat cerebral arteries is dependent on intact endothelium. *Circ. Res.*, **60**, 102–7.
Harder, D. R. and Waters, A. (1983). Electromechanical coupling in feline basilar artery in response to serotonin. *Eur. J. Pharmacol.*, **93**, 95–100.
Harder, D. R., Abel, P. W., and Hermsmeyer, K. (1981). Membrane electrical mechanism of basilar artery constriction and pial artery dilation by norepinephrine. *Circ. Res.*, **49**, 1237–42.
Harder, D. R., Sanchez-Ferrer, C. F., Kauser, K., Stekiel, W. J., and Rubanyi, G. M. (1989). Pressure releases a transferable endothelial contractile factor in cat cerebral arteries. *Circ. Res.*, **65**, 193–98.
Harper, A. M., Deshmukh, V. D., Rowan, J. O., and Jennett, W. B. (1972). The influence of sympathetic nervous activity on cerebral blood flow. *Arch. Neurol.*, **27**, 1–6.
Hill, C. E., Hirst, G. D. S., Silverberg, G. D., and Van Helden, D. F. (1986). Sympathetic inervation and excitability of arterioles originating from the rat middle cerebral artery. *J. Physiol.*, **371**, 305–16.
Humphrey, P. P. A. and Feniuk, W. (1991). Mode of action of the anti-migraine drug sumatriptan. *Trends Pharmacol. Sci.*, **12**, 444–6.
Humphrey, P. P. A., Hartig, P., and Hoyer, D. (1993). A proposed new nomenclature for 5-HT receptors. *Trends Pharmacol. Sci.*, **14**, 233–6.
Iadecola, C. (1992). Does nitric oxide mediate the increase in cerebral blood flow elicited by hypercapnia? *Proc. Natl. Acad. Sci. USA*, **89**, 3913–16.
Iadecola, C., Zhang, F., and Xu, X. (1993). Role of nitric oxide synthase-containing vascular nerves in cerebrovasodilation elicited from cerebellum. *Am. J. Physiol.*, **264**, R738–46.
Juul, R., Edvinsson, L., Fredriksen, T. A., Ekman, R., Brubakk, A. O., and Gisvold, S. E. (1991). Changes in the levels of neuropeptide Y-LI in the external jugular vein in connection with vasoconstriction following subarachnoid hemorrhage in man. Involvement of sympathetic neuropeptid Y in cerebral vasospasm. *Acta Neurochi.*, **107**, 75–81.
Karashima, T. and Kuriyama, H. (1981). Electrical properties of smooth muscle cell membrane and neuromuscular transmission in the guinea-pig basilar artery. *Br. J. Pharmacol.*, **74**, 495–504.
Kelly, P. A. T. and McCulloch, J. (1983). The effects of the GABA agonist muscimol upon the relationship between local cerebral blood flow and glucose utilization. *Brain Res.*, **258**, 338–42.
Kelly, P. A. T., Davis, C. J., and Goodwin, G. M. (1987). Differential effects of selective 5-HT$_1$ agonists upon local cerebral glucose utilization and flow-metabolism coupling. *J. Cereb. Blood Flow Metab.*, **7(Suppl. 1)**, 269.

Kelly, P. A. T., Davis, C. J., and Goodwin, G. M. (1988). Differential pattern of local cerebral glucose utilization in response to 5-hydroxytryptamine$_1$ agonist. *Neuroscience*, **25**, 907–15.

Kelly, P. A. T., Faulkner, A. J., and Burrow, A. P. (1989). The effects of the GABA agonist muscimol upon blood flow in different vascular territories of the rat cortex. *J. Cereb. Blood Flow Metab.*, **9**, 754–8.

Kelly, P. A. T., McBean, D. E., and Sharkey, J. (1991). The effect of central 5-hydroxytryptaminergic lesions on the cerebrovascular response to hypercapnia. *Br. J. Pharmacol.*, **104**, 367P.

Kelly, P. A. T., Ritchie, I. M., Wright, A. K., and Arbuthnott, G. W. (1992). Oligaemia induced by direct injection of N^G-nitro-L-arginine methyl ester into the rat striatum. *Br. J. Pharmacol.*, **107**, 398P.

Kelly, P. A. T., Sharkey, J., Philip, R., and Ritchie, I. M. (1993). Acute cocaine alters cerebrovascular autoregulation in the rat neocortex. *Brain Res. Bull.*, **31**, 581–5.

Kelly, P. A. T., Thomas, C. L., Ritchie, I. M., and Arbuthnott, G. W. (1994). Cerebrovascular autoregulation in response to hypertension induced by N^G-nitro-L-arginine methyl ester. *Neuroscience*, **59**, 13–20.

Klaas, M. and Wadsworth, R. (1989). Contraction followed by relaxation in response to hypoxia in the sheep isolated middle cerebral artery. *Eur. J. Pharmacol.*, **168**, 187–92.

Klugman, K. P., Lembeck, F., Markowitz, S., Mitchell, G., and Rosendorff, C. (1980). Substance-P increases hypothalamic blood flow via an indirect adrenergic-cholinergic interaction. *Br. J. Pharmacol.*, **71**, 623–9.

Kontos, H. A., Wei, E. P., Navari, R. M., Levasseur, J. E., Rossenblum, W. I., and Patterson, J. L. (1978). Responses of cerebral arteries and arterioles to acute hypotension and hypertension. *Am. J. Physiol.*, **234**, H371–83.

Kossut, M. and Hand, P. (1984). The development of the vibrissal column: A 2-deoxyglucose study in the rat. *Neurosci. Lett.*, **46**, 1–6.

Kovách, A. G. B., Szabó, C., Benyó, Z., Csáki, C., Greenberg, J. H., and Reivich, M. (1992). Effects of N^G-nitro-L-arginine and L-arginine on cerebral blood flow in the cat. *J. Physiol.*, **449**, 183–96.

Kozniewski, E., Oseka, M., and Stys, T. (1992). Effects of endothelium-derived nitric oxide on cerebral circulation during normoxia and hypoxia in the rat. *J. Cereb. Blood Flow Metab.*, **12**, 311–17.

Krantis, A. (1984). The involvement of GABA-transaminase in the blood–brain barrier to radiolabelled GABA. *Acta Neuropathol.*, **64**, 61–7.

Krause, D. N., Wong, E., Degener, P., and Roberts, E. (1980). GABA receptors in bovine cerebral blood vessels: binding studies with [^{3}H]muscimol. *Brain Res.*, **185**, 51–7.

Kuschinsky, W. and Wahl, M. (1978). Local chemical and neurogenic regulation of cerebral vascular resistance. *Physiol. Rev.*, **58**, 656–89.

Lembeck, F. and Holzer, P. (1979). Substance P as neurogenic mediator of antidromic vasodilatation and neurogenic plasma extravasation. *Naunyn-Schmeideberg's Arch. Pharmacol.*, **310**, 106–8.

McBean, D. E., Sharkey, J., Ritchie, I. M., and Kelly, P. A. T. (1990). Evidence for a possible role for serotonergic systems in the control of cerebral blood flow. *Brain Res.*, **537**, 307–10.

McBean, D. E., Sharkey, J., Ritchie, I. M., and Kelly, P. A. T. (1991). Cerebrovascular and metabolic consequences of 5-HT$_{1A}$ receptor activation. *Brain Res.*, **555**, 159–63.

McCulloch, J. and Edvinsson, L. (1987). Calcitonin gene-related peptide and the trigeminal innervation of the cerebral circulation. In *Peptidergic mechanisms in the cerebral circulation* (ed. L. Edvinsson and J. McCulloch), pp. 132–51. VPH Verlagsgesellschaft, Weinheim.

McCulloch, J. and Reid, J. (1986). The effect of capsaicin on blood-brain barrier permeability in the rat. *J. Physiol.*, **374**, 208.

McCulloch, J., Kelly, P. A. T., and Grome, J. J. (1981). GABAergic influences upon cerebral metabolism and perfusion. In *Cerebral microcirculation and metabolism* (ed. J. Cervos-Navarro and E. Firtschka), pp. 189-93. Raven Press, New York.

McCulloch, J., Kelly, P. A. T., and Ford, I. (1982). Effect of apomorphine on the relationship between local cerebral glucose utilization and local cerebral blood flow (with an appendix on its statistical analysis). *J. Cereb. Blood Flow Metab.*, **2**, 487-99.

McCulloch, J., Uddman, R., Kingman, T. A., and Edvinsson, L. (1986). Calcitonin gene-related peptide: functional role in cerebrovascular regulation. *Proc. Natl. Acad. Sci. USA*, **83**, 5731-5.

MacKenzie, E. T., McCulloch, J., O'Keane, M., Packard, J. D., and Harper, A. M. (1976). Cerebral circulation and norepinephrine: Relevance of the blood-brain barrier. *Am. J. Physiol.*, **231**, H483-8.

MacKenzie, E. T., Strangaard, S., Graham, D. I., Jones, J. V., Harper, A. M., and Farrar, J. K. (1979). Effects of acutely induced hypertension in cats on pial arteriolar caliber, local cerebral blood flow, and the blood-brain barrier. *Circ. Res.*, **39**, 33-41.

McPherson, G. A. and Stork, A. P. (1992). The resistance of some rat cerebral arteries to the vasorelaxant effect of cromakalim and other K^+-channel openers. *Br. J. Pharmacol.*, **105**, 51-58.

Macrae, I. M., Robinson, M. J., Graham, D. I., Reid, J. L., and McCulloch, J. (1993). Endothelin-1-induced reductions in cerebral blood flow: Dose dependency, time course, and neuropathological consequences. *J. Cereb. Blood Flow Metab.*, **13**, 276-84.

Moskowitz, M. A. (1984). The neurobiology of vascular head pain. *Ann. Neurol.*, **16**, 157-68.

Moscowitz, M. A. (1992). Neurogenic versus vascular mechanisms of sumatriptan and ergot alkaloids in migraine. *Trends Pharmacol. Sci.*, **13**, 307-11.

Moskowitz, M. A., Brody, M., and Liu-Chen, L.-Y. (1983). *In vitro* release of immunoreactive substance P from putative afferent nerve endings in bovine pia arachnoid. *Neuroscience*, **9**, 809-14.

Muramatsu, I., Fujiwara, M., Miura, A., and Sakakibara, Y. (1981). Possible involvement of adenine nucleotides in sympathetic neuroeffector mechanism of dog basilar artery. *J. Pharmacol. Exp. Ther.*, **216**, 401-9.

Napoleone, P., Erdo, S., and Amenta, F. (1987). Autoradiographic localization of the $GABA_A$ receptor agonist [^{3}H] muscimol in rat cerebral vessels. *Brain Res.*, **423**, 109-15.

Northington, F. J., Matherne, G. P., and Berne, R. M. (1992). Competitive inhibition of nitric oxide synthase prevents the cortical hyperaemia associated with peripheral nerve stimulation. *Proc. Natl. Acad. Sci. USA*, **89**, 6649-52.

Okamura, R., Inoue, S., and Toda, N. (1989). Action of atrial natriuretic peptide (ANP) on dog cerebral arteries: evidence that neurogenic relaxation is not mediated by release of ATP. *Br. J. Pharmacol.*, **97**, 1258-64.

Paulson, O. B., Strandgaard, S., and Edvinsson, L. (1990). Cerebral autoregulation. *Cerebrovas. Brain Metab. Rev.*, **2**, 161-92.

Pelligrino, D. A., Koenig, H. M., and Albrecht, R. F. (1993). Nitric oxide synthesis and regional cerebral blood flow responses to hypercapnia and hypoxia in the rat. *J. Cereb. Blood Flow Metab.*, **13**, 80-7.

Plane, F. and Garland, C. J. (1992). Electrophysiology of cerebral vessels. *Pharmacol. Ther.*, **56**, 341-58.

Prado, R., Watson, M. D., Kuluz, J., and Dietrich, W. D. (1992). Endothelium-derived nitric oxide synthase inhibition. Effects on cerebral blood flow, pial artery diameter, and vascular morphology in rats. *Stroke*, **23**, 1118–24.

Raichle, M. E., Hartman, B. K., Eichling, J. O., and Sharpe, L. G. (1975). Central noradrenergic regulation of cerebral blood flow and vascular permeability. *Proc. Natl. Acad. Sci. USA*, **72**, 3726–30.

Rakugi, H., Tabuchi, Y., and Nakamani, M. (1990). Evidence for endothelin-1 release from resistance vessels of rats in response to hypoxia. *Biochem. Biophys. Res. Commun.*, **169**, 973–7.

Rand, V. E. and Garland, C. J. (1992). Endothelium-dependent relaxation to acetylcholine in the rabbit basilar artery: importance of membrane hyperpolarization. *Br. J. Pharmacol.*, **106**, 143–50.

Robinson, M. J. and McCulloch, J. (1990). Contractile responses to endothelin in feline cortical vessels *in situ*. *J. Cereb. Blood Flow Metab.*, **10**, 285–9.

Roy, C. S. and Sherrington, C. S. (1890). On the regulation of the blood supply of the brain. *J. Physiol.*, **11**, 85–108.

Rubanyi, G. M. and Vanhoutte, P. M. (1985). Hypoxia releases a vasoconstrictor substance from a canine vascular endothelium. *J. Physiol.*, **364**, 45–56.

Sakurada, O., Kennedy, C., Jehle, J., Brown, J. D., Carbin, G. L., and Sokoloff, L. (1978). Measurement of cerebral blood flow with iodo-[^{14}C]-antipyrine. *Am. J. Physiol.*, **234**, H59–66.

Seville, V. L., Maynard, K. I., and Burnstock, G. (1990). Neuropeptide Y potentiates purinergic as well as adrenergic responses of the rabbit ear artery. *Eur. J. Pharmacol.*, **176**, 117–25.

Seager, J. M., Clark, A. H., and Garland, C. J. (1992). Endothelium-dependent contractile responses to 5-hydroxytryptamine in the rabbit basilar artery. *Br. J. Pharmacol.*, **105**, 424–8.

Shirahase, H., Fujiwara, M., Usui, H., and Kurahashi, K. (1987). A possible role of thromboxane A_2 in endothelium in maintaining resting tone and producing contractile response to acetylcholine and arachidonic acid in canine cerebral arteries. *Blood Vessels*, **24**, 117–19.

Shirakawa, J., Hosoda, K., Taniyama, K., Matsumoto, S., and Tanaka, C. (1989). γ-Aminobutyric acid-A receptor-mediated suppression of 5-hydroxytryptamine-induced guinea pig basilar artery smooth muscle contractility. *Blood Vessels*, **26**, 129–36.

Sokoloff, L. (1977). Relationship between physiological function and energy metabolism in the central nervous system. *J. Neurochem.*, **29**, 13–26.

Sokoloff, L., Reivich, M., Kennedy, C., Des Rosiers, M. H., Patlak, C. S., Pettigrew, K. D., *et al.* (1977). The [^{14}C]-deoxyglucose method for the measurement of local cerebral glucose utilization: theory, procedure, and normal values in the conscious and anaesthetized albino rat. *J. Neurochem.*, **28**, 897–916.

Sonntag, M., Deussen, A., and Schrader, J. (1992). Role of nitric oxide in local blood flow control in the anaesthetized dog. *Pflugers Arch.*, **420**, 194–9.

Suzuki, Y., Sato, S., Ikegaki, I., Okada, T., Shibuya, M., Sugita, K., *et al.* (1989). Effects of neuropeptide Y and calcitonin gene-related peptide on local cerebral blood flow in rat striatum. *J. Cereb. Blood Flow Metab.*, **9**, 268–70.

Suzuki, H., Sato, S., Suzuki, Y., Takekoshi, K., Ishihara, N., and Shimoda, S. (1990). Increased endothelin concentration in CSF from patients with subarachnoid hemorrhage. *Acta Neurol. Scand.*, **81**, 553–4.

Swanson, L. W., Connelly, M. A., and Hartmen, B. K. (1977). Ultrastructural evidence for central monoamine innervation of blood vessels in the paraventricular nucleus of the hypothalamus. *Brain Res.*, **136**, 166–73.

Tanaka, K., Gotoh, F., Gomi, S., Takashima, S., Mihara., T., Shirai, T., *et al.* (1991).

Inhibition of nitric oxide synthesis induces a significant reduction in local cerebral blood flow in the rat. *Neurosci. Lett.*, **127**, 129–32.

Thomas, C. L., Kelly, P. A. T., Ritchie, I. M., Sharkey, J., and Arbuthnott, G. W. (1993). Cerebrovascular autoregulation to hypertension induced by inhibition of nitric oxide synthesis. *Br. J. Pharmacol.*, **108**, 129P.

Toda, N. (1981). Non-adrenergic, non-cholinergic innervation in monkey and human cerebral arteries. *Br. J. Pharmacol.*, **72**, 281–3.

Toda, N. (1982). Relaxant responses to transmural stimulation and nicotine of dog and monkey cerebral arteries. *Am. J. Physiol.*, **243**, H145–53.

Toda, N. (1988). Hemosylate inhibits cerebral artery relaxation. *J. Cereb. Blood Flow Metab.*, **8**, 46–53.

Toda, N. and Okamura, T. (1990). Possible role of nitric oxide in transmitting information from vasodilator nerve to cerebroarterial muscle. *Biochem. Biophys. Res. Commun.*, **170**, 308–13.

Toda, N. and Okamura, T. (1991). Role of nitric oxide in neurally induced cerebroarterial relaxation. *J. Pharmacol. Exp. Ther.*, **258**, 1027–32.

Toda, N., Minami, Y., and Okamura, T. (1990). Inhibitory effects of L-N^G-nitro arginine on the synthesis of EDRF and the cerebroarterial response to vasodilator nerve stimulation. *Life Sci.*, **47**, 345–51.

Tuor, U. I., Edvinssion, L., and McCulloch, J. (1985). Neuropeptide Y and cerebral blood flow. *Lancet*, **1**, 1271.

Tuor, U., Edvinsson, L., Kelly, P. A. T., and McCulloch, J. (1990a). Local cerebral blood flow following the intrastriatal administration of vasoactive intestinal polypeptide or peptide histidine isoleucine in the rat. *Reg. Peptides*, **28**, 255–64.

Tuor, U., Kelly, P. A. T., Edvinsson, L., and McCulloch, J. (1990b). Neuropeptide Y and the cerebral circulation. *J. Cereb. Blood Flow Metab.*, **10**, 591–601.

Unterberg, A., Baethmann, A., and Hack, U. (1983). Cerebral blood flow and metabolism during bradykinin exposure. In *Cerebral blood flow metabolism and epilepsy* (ed. M. Baldy-Moulinier, D. H. Ingvar, and B. D. Meldrum), pp. 174–9. John Libbey, London.

Usui, H., Kurahashi, K., Shirahase, H., Fukui, K., and Fujiwara, M. (1987). Endothelium-dependent vasoconstriction in response to noradrenaline in the canine cerebral artery. *Jap. J. Pharmacol.*, **44**, 228–31.

Wang, Q., Paulson, O. B., and Lassen, N. A. (1992). Effects of nitric oxide blockade by N^G-nitro-L-arginine on cerebral blood flow response to changes in carbon dioxide tension. *J. Cereb. Blood Flow Metab.*, **12**, 591–601.

Wang, Q., Kjaer, T., Jørgensen, M. B., Paulson, O. B., Lassen, N. A., Diemer, N. H., *et al.* (1993). Nitric oxide does not act as a mediator coupling cerebral blood flow to neural activity following somatosensory stimuli in rats. *Neurol. Res.*, **15**, 33–6.

Worley, J. F., Quayle, J. M., Standen, N. B., and Nelson, M. T. (1991). Regulation of single calcium channels in cerebral arteries by voltage, serotonin and dihydropyridines. *Am. J. Physiol.*, **261**, H1951–60.

12. Pharmacology of human isolated large and small coronary arteries

J. A. Angus and T. M. Cocks

INTRODUCTION

Human epicardial conduit and small 'resistance' coronary arteries, like many other blood vessels, possess a broad spectrum of receptors on the smooth muscle cells which when activated by endogenous and exogenous ligands, mediate either vasoconstriction or vasodilatation. In addition indirect vasodilatation or vasoconstriction can be caused by substances released by receptor activation on the endothelium. For conduit vessels, changes in contractility are not usually important under normal physiological conditions because maximum changes in lumen diameter are generally not sufficient to affect vascular resistance and blood flow. This may change, however, in pathological conditions associated with coronary artery disease (CAD). First, progressive structural changes within the vessel wall associated with CAD, including intimal proliferation and accumulation of lipid, would narrow the lumen diameter (lumen encroachment) so that small contractions of the wall (fall in diameter) could alter blood flow as the lesion becomes flow limiting. Secondly, the change in wall composition may alter the reactivity of the smooth muscle cells in relation to loss of factors from endothelium, inflammatory cell invasion, hypertrophy, or change in phenotype of smooth muscle cells and even altered innervation. Thirdly, changes in reactivity may also result from disease related alterations in receptor populations and signal transduction mechanisms in either smooth muscle or endothelial cells. Finally, a reduction in vessel elasticity through calcification for example may allow the same degree of muscle shortening to a standard contractile stimulus to lead to a reduced vasoconstriction. Thus, under certain circumstances both structural and pharmacological changes in epicardial coronary arteries may enable them to cause an exaggerated contraction or even 'spasm' to reduce blood flow to zero. Clinically, such 'spasm' manifests itself as variant (Prinzmetal's) angina and is readily relieved by vasodilators (Maseri and Chierchia 1982).

Unlike large arteries, reactivity in human small coronary arteries less than 250 μm in internal diameter under normal conditions are critically involved in control of resistance and flow. These vessels are surprisingly devoid of structural changes associated with atherosclerosis as seen in conduit arteries of patients with CAD. As in large arteries adrenergic innervation, circulating humoral factors together with constrictor and dilator factors released from the endothelium are important determinants of small artery diameter and thus blood flow to the coronary bed. The pharmacological properties of these vessels is beginning to emerge as access to tissue is improved and technology is refined. Reactivity of coronary collateral arteries which become of major importance following an infarct and in some instances are critical for survival, is largely unknown.

The first half of this chapter will review current data on the *in vitro* findings of the effect of a range of vasoactive substances on human large coronary arteries. Particular attention will be given to spontaneous or phasic contractions, the role of nitric oxide in the relaxation to a range of agents, and importantly the question of synergy of two constrictor agents. In the second half, data will be presented on the electrophysiology and contractility of human isolated right atrial coronary resistance vessels in response to acetylcholine, noradrenaline, and 5-hydroxytryptamine.

LARGE CORONARY ARTERIES

Structure

Large coronary arteries from humans have structural adaptations which make them relatively unique from other species. This is particularly true for the intimal layer, i.e. that region from the luminal surface of the endothelium to the luminal margin of the media (Stary *et al.* 1992). Most large human coronary arteries possess either diffuse or eccentric adaptive intimal thickenings, made up mostly of endothelial and synthetic state smooth muscle cells as well as macrophages (Fig. 12.1). Also, extracellular matrix consisting of proteoglycans, collagens, elastin, laminin, and fibronectin makes up a major part of the intimal thickening of normal coronary arteries. The role of this 'adaptive' thickening is unclear. There may be an evolutionary advantage if the vessel can rapidly adapt to changes in pulsatile pressure, shear stress, and flow rate, particularly in response to altered demand downstream in the coronary bed. Interest in these 'normal' intimal lesions is their predisposition to becoming atherogenic and how this transition will alter the artery's reactivity to vasoactive substances. Before this is considered, however, it is necessary to describe how to optimally determine reactivity in human isolated coronary arteries.

Reactivity

In vitro reactivity describes the potency and efficacy of vasoactive substances in isolated blood vessels. This information can help to predict mechanism *in vivo* but cannot be used explicitly to determine action *in vivo* because of the greater complexity of the integrated environment in intact vascular beds (see Chapter 4). For example, progressive coronary atherosclerosis is associated with gradual accumulation of lipid and calcification of the intima and eventually results in luminal encroachment. *In vivo*, this is associated with the gradual loss of endothelium-

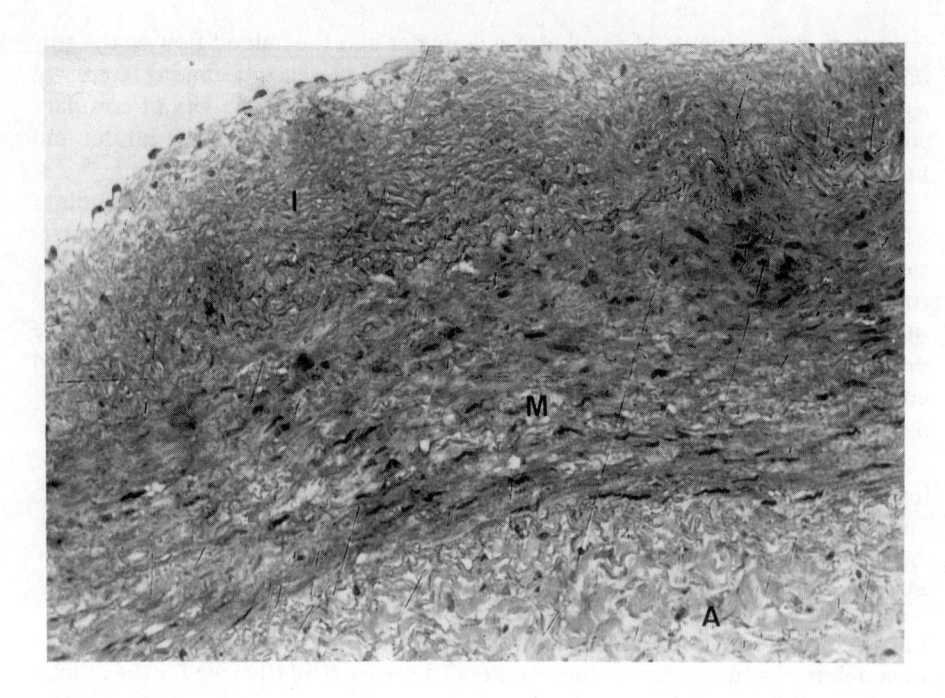

Fig. 12.1 High power magnification (×20) of a cross-section of a ring of human distal right coronary artery. Note the presence of an intima (I). M, media; A, adventitia.

dependent vasodilator capacity. Yet, from *in vitro* reactivity studies, loss of endothelium-dependent relaxation responses in isolated coronary arteries appears to be affected only in the advanced stages of the disease. Thus, atherosclerosis *per se* may not reduce endothelial cells' capacity to manufacture dilator factors like NO and PGI_2, but rather it is the changing thickness, and cellular and chemical nature of the intima which affects the transition of these factors from the endothelium to the underlying smooth muscle cells.

When arteries are removed from the body and set-up in organ-baths, they are also removed from the majority of endogenous factors which may affect their contractility. These include circulating hormones, nerves, and other factors such as cytokines and growth factors released from many different, interacting cell types (Ross 1993). Furthermore, the arteries are usually incubated in artificial salt solutions with very high pO_2 levels (> 400 mmHg). Under these conditions, the vessels are then stretched to set optimum levels of passive force if measuring isometric contraction. This passive force is either normalized to the pressure the vessels would be subjected to *in vivo* or is the optimum point for active force development of the particular vessel's passive length–tension curve (Angus *et al.* 1986).

Spontaneous and constrictor-induced phasic activity

Human epicardial coronary arteries *in vitro* usually exhibit spontaneous contractile activity when arranged as ring segments on wires under isometric conditions. This activity consists of contractions of variable amplitudes, lasting between 30 sec and 10 min at variable frequencies of approximately two to six per hour (Cocks *et al.* 1993; Stork and Cocks 1994*a*). Spontaneous contractions often occur either immediately the vessels are set-up in Krebs' solution at 37 °C triggered by the passive stretch procedure and/or by stimulation with contractile agents — (see below and Fig. 12.2). Either situation can make it difficult to set the arteries at optimal levels of stretch. Another characteristic of some spontaneous contractions is that upon reaching and holding a maximum level of active force, they relax rapidly to levels of force below the initial starting level if any active force was present at the start. Active force then slowly increases back towards the original level at which point another contraction is triggered. Thus, there appears to be a type of 'slow wave' of **tonic** contractile activity in some human isolated coronary arteries which modulates spontaneous **phasic** contractile activity. These phasic contractions appear to depend on entry of extracellular Ca^{2+} through L-type voltage operated Ca^{2+} channels (VOCCs; Golenhofen 1978; Ross *et al.* 1980; Stork and Cocks 1994*a*) which is interesting since other vasodilators, which lower any inherent active force, like glyceryl trinitrate and cromakalim block spontaneous but not constrictor-induced phasic activity (Stork and Cocks 1994*a*). Also, either removal of the endothelium or block of nitric oxide synthase (NOS) has no effect on either spontaneous or agonist-induced phasic activity. These findings suggest that the availability and open-state probability of VOCCs, underlie the major determinant of phasic activity *in vitro*. This conclusion is supported by data shown in Fig. 12.2 where increasing concentration of U46619 over the EC_{10} to EC_{70} range resulted in a concentration-dependent increase in the amplitude of phasic contractions. It is clear that with the agonist-induced phasic activity abolished by nifedipine, the remaining tonic contraction curve to U46619 lies virtually on top of the lower plateau phasic contraction curve (Fig. 12.3). The same pattern of phasic and tonic contractions were also observed for endothelin-1 and 5-HT (Fig. 12.3) (Stork and Cocks 1994*a*). Thus, in human isolated coronary arteries, phasic contractions due to entry of extracellular Ca^{2+} through L-type VOCCs are additive with any tonic component of the same stimulus due to non-VOCC-mediated increases of intracellular Ca^{2+}. This in turn implies that phasic activity is able to markedly augment contractions to vasoconstrictors over physiologically relevant concentration ranges. If the same occurs *in vivo* then the resultant amplification of constrictor responses to physiologically/pathologically important stimuli like noradrenaline, 5-HT, endothelin, and thromboxane A_2 could, given appropriate conditions (e.g. lumen encroachment), cause an exaggerated contraction or 'spasm'. Furthermore, apparent amplification of contractions to one vasoconstrictor by another via second messenger interactions needs careful consideration when determining the overall reactivity profiles of vasoconstrictors in human coronary arteries.

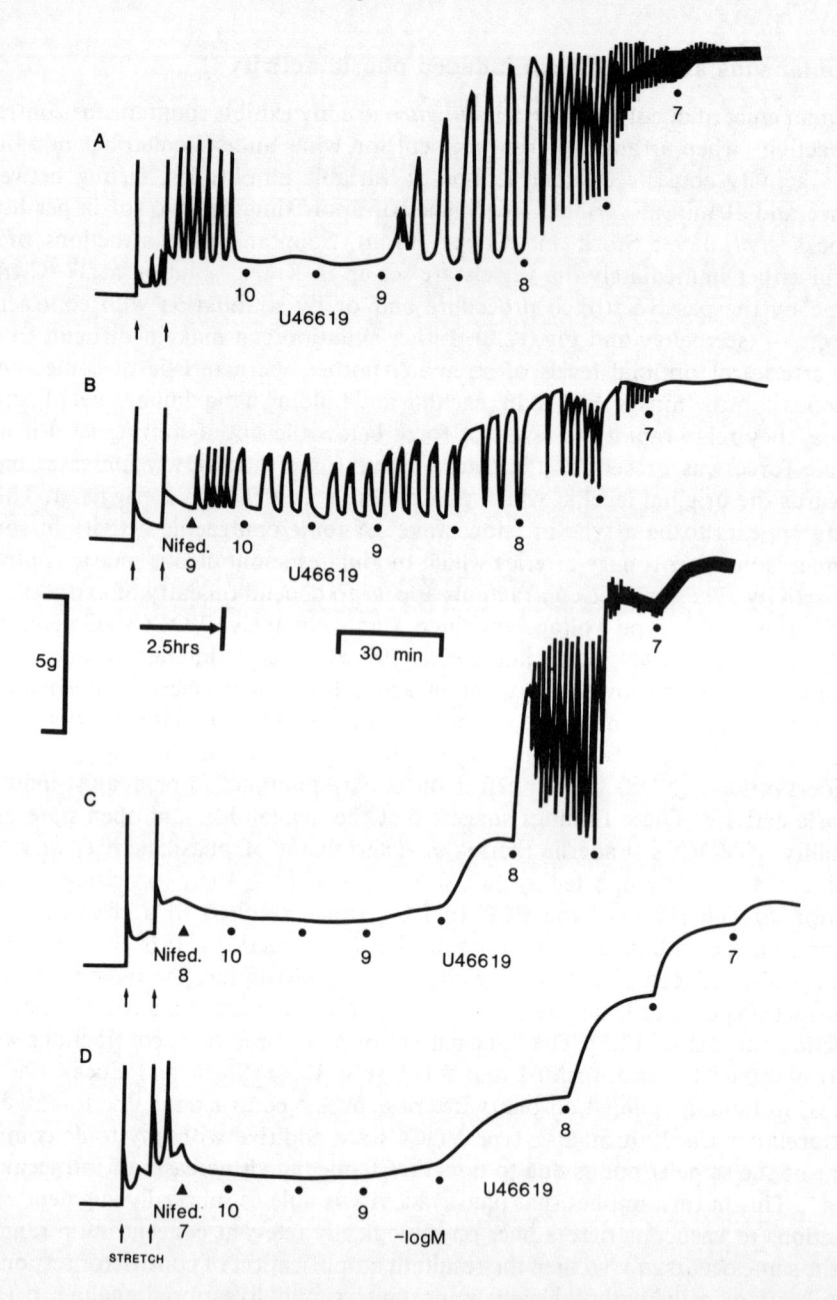

Fig. 12.2 Effect of increasing concentrations of nifedipine (Nifed.) on phasic activity and the concentration–contraction responses to U46619 in human coronary artery (all concentrations in −log M). Nifedipine concentrations are (A) control, (B) 9, (C) 8, and (D) 7. Traces are of chart recordings from four consecutive rings of a circumflex coronary artery from a 42-year-old male. The recordings are representative of four separate experiments. (Reproduced from Stork and Cocks 1994a with permission.)

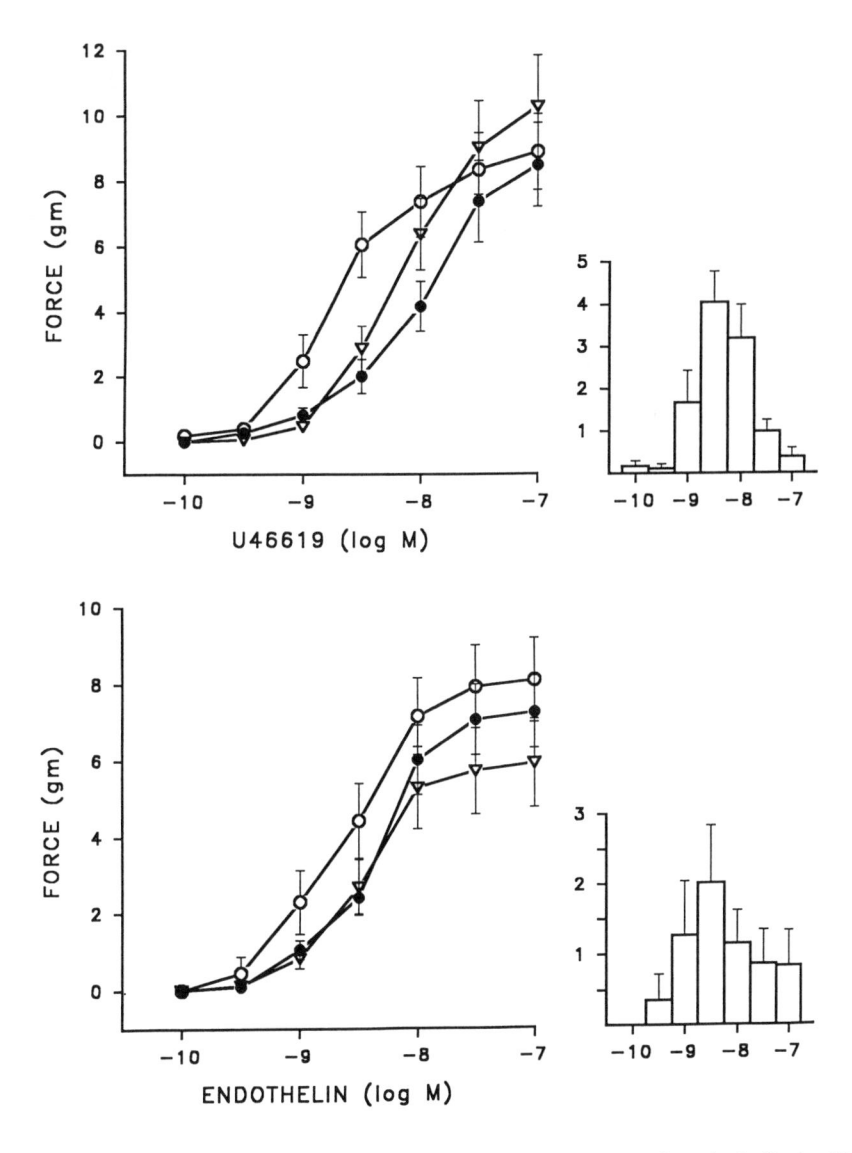

Fig. 12.3 Response of human coronary artery to U46619 and endothelin-1. Mean cumulative concentration–response curves (line graphs) and the mean range of phasic contractions for each concentration (histograms) were determined for (A) U46619 ($n = 10$) and (B) endothelin-1 in control [upper (○) and lower (●) levels of phasic contraction] and nifedipine treated (0.1 μM, ▽) arterial rings. (Reproduced from Stork and Cocks 1994a with permission.)

Human large coronary arteries at least *in vitro*, appear to have pacemaker-type electrical activity which has the potential to critically modify vascular reactivity. For example, if focal loss or damage to the endothelium occurs due to localized thrombosis or mechanical damage and if endothelial cell factors like NO help maintain coronary arterial tone below the threshold for activation of spontaneous contractions, then even partial loss of this inhibitory influence may tip the segment into the threshold range for spontaneous contractions. As such, stimulation with contractile agents like 5-HT (released from the aggregating platelets) could result in spasm whereas normally the same stimulus may only cause small tonic contractions.

Vasoconstrictor substances

5-hydroxytryptamine (5-HT)

5-HT mediates contraction of human large coronary artery *in vitro* via both 5-HT$_2$ and 5-HT$_1$-like receptors, the latter resembling cloned 5-HT$_{1D\beta}$ receptors (Kaumann *et al.* 1993, 1994). There has been considerable controversy, however, as to the fractional contribution of each receptor subtype to the response to 5-HT, mainly as a result of the development of a selective 5-HT$_1$-like agonist, sumatriptan (Bradley *et al.* 1986; Van Heuven-Nolsen 1988) for the treatment of migraine (Perrin *et al.* 1989; Humphrey *et al.* 1990; Ferrari *et al.* 1991). Thus regardless of sumatriptan's anti-migraine mechanism of action in the brain (Moskowitz 1992), sumatriptan was reported to be a poor contractile agonist in coronary arteries due to few 5-HT$_1$-like receptors and since 5-HT-induced contractions were mostly blocked by the 5-HT$_2$-selective receptor antagonist, ketanserin (Connor *et al.* 1989).

In vitro

Human large coronary arteries *in vitro* display a wide degree of interpatient variability with respect to the proportion of 5-HT contractions mediated by 5-HT$_1$ receptors (Kaumann *et al.* 1994). Such variability is, however, expected given the variability in age, sex, disease status, and medication histories of the heart transplant patients from where the coronary arteries are normally taken (Kaumann *et al.* 1994). Nevertheless, Kaumann *et al.* (1994) showed that sumatriptan can be a full agonist at 5-HT$_1$ receptors in human coronary arteries and Cocks *et al.* (1993) demonstrated that contractions to 5-HT in similar arteries were likely to be mediated equally by 5-HT$_2$ and 5-HT$_1$ receptors (see below). These receptors are considered to be on the smooth muscle cells but in porcine and canine coronary arteries endothelial cells express functional 5-HT$_1$ receptors which mediate endothelium-dependent relaxation (Cocks and Angus 1983). However, there are no reports of similar endothelial receptors in human coronary arteries. Regardless of whether 5-HT releases endothelium-derived vasodilators (e.g. nitric oxide, see Chapter 10), however, the integrity of the endothelium as a diffusion barrier is an important determinant of reactivity to 5-HT in large coronary arteries *in vivo* (see Chapter 2).

The importance of human coronary artery 5-HT receptors is related to circumstances under which they are likely to be activated or blocked by either endogenous ligands or exogenous drugs. Nearly all the 5-HT in plasma is stored in dense-cored platelet granules. Therefore, activation of coronary smooth muscle 5-HT receptors by the endogenous ligand (5-HT) depends upon release of platelet stores, predominantly during aggregation. Thromboxane A_2 is also a potent vasoconstrictor released from platelets and although it is important to assess the reactivity to each of these platelet-derived vasoconstrictors individually, it is equally important to assess how they interact at the level of the smooth muscle cells. For human large coronary artery reactivity, ketanserin should have little effect on artery calibre unless aggregation of platelets occurs and then it would be expected to be beneficial, i.e. block of contraction due to activation of 5-HT_2 receptors. For 5-HT receptor-agonists like methysergide and sumatriptan, in migraine therapy however, any coronary constrictor effects *in vivo* will depend not only upon relative proportions of 5-HT_2 and 5-HT_1 receptors present in any particular segment of artery but importantly on the geometry of the wall if coronary artery disease is present (see above).

In vivo studies in man, show that both the coronary arterial bed and large epicardial arteries normally dilate in response to intracoronary injection of 5-HT (Golino and Maseri 1994). The type and location of the 5-HT receptors mediating both responses is unclear, although ketanserin fails to antagonize either suggesting they are not mediated via 5-HT_2 receptors. The increase in lumen diameter in the larger conduit arteries in response to 5-HT, however, is probably unrelated to activity of dilator 5-HT receptors, but a result of flow-induced release of endothelium-dependent vasoactive factors. The mechanisms of the dilator response to 5-HT in the smaller vessels, however, is likely to be a direct effect of 5-HT_1 receptor activation either on the endothelium or smooth muscle (Angus 1989 and below).

In patients with angiographic evidence of mild atherosclerosis the response to intracoronary 5-HT is reversed compared with that in normal subjects. Now there is both a decrease in large artery diameter and a reduction in coronary flow. There are mixed reports as to the effect of ketanserin on these responses (Golino *et al.* 1991; McFadden *et al.* 1992) which may be explained by Kaumann *et al.* (1994) finding that variable fractional contributions of 5-HT_1 and 5-HT_2 receptors to contractions to 5-HT in human isolated coronary arteries. However, the change with atherogenesis of dilatation to constriction in both large and presumably small coronary arteries suggests a generalized impairment of endothelial cell-mediated vasodilator function (see below) and/or an increase in *in vivo* constrictor reactivity to 5-HT in large arteries. Also, loss of endothelium-derived vasodilator tone in large arteries with mild atheroma could be due to either the indirect effect of reduced flow or a direct effect of the disease on the large artery endothelial cells. Thus, the 'primary' response of coronary arteries to 5-HT *in vivo* (see below) may be attenuated normally by tonic release of vasodilators (i.e. NO) from the endothelium.

Adrenoceptor agonists

Contractions of large coronary arteries to noradrenaline (and adrenaline) are mediated by both α_1- and α_2-adrenoceptors, since they are attenuated by phentolamine as well as the α_1- and α_2-selective antagonists, prazosin and yohimbine respectively. Furthermore the α_1- and α_2-selective agonists, phenylephrine and clonidine respectively cause similar contractions in isolated arteries (Toda 1986; Isikawa *et al.* 1991). The relative magnitudes of these α-adrenoceptor-mediated contractions are, however, extremely poor compared to either maximum contraction with KCl or 5-HT. As such the physiological relevance of α-adrenoceptors on smooth muscle of large coronary arteries in man is unclear. By contrast, β-adrenoceptor-mediated relaxation in similar arteries is greater in absolute magnitude than α-adrenoceptor-mediated contractions (Ginsburg *et al.* 1980) and the use of non-selective β-antagonists is usually required to see contractions to adrenoceptor agonists in this tissue. The subtype of β-adrenoceptor mediating these responses is likely to be β_1 since isoprenaline-mediated relaxation is antagonized by the relatively β_1-selective antagonist, atenolol (Berkenboom *et al.* 1987) and metoprolol (Toda and Okamura 1990) but not by the β_2-selective antagonist zinterol (Ginsburg 1984). There may be some functional β_2-adrenoceptors in human large coronary arteries since terbutaline, a β_2-adrenoceptor selective agonist has been shown to generate a small relaxation (Toda and Okamurai 1990). β_1-Adrenoceptors have been localized autoradiographically to the medial layer in human coronary arteries whilst β_2-adrenoceptors seem to be located only on the intima and adventitia (Amenta *et al.* 1991). This suggests that β_2-adrenoceptors are located on endothelial cells although there is no functional evidence that their activation mediates or inhibits the release of endothelium-derived vasoactive factors. As also mentioned above, however, the barrier effects of the intimal layer in large coronary arteries will have important effects of the *in vivo* reactivity to circulating catecholamines. The role of sympathetic nerves in controlling vascular tone in human large coronary arteries is largely unexplored.

Human isolated coronary arteries contract to other naturally occurring compounds including histamine, neuropeptide Y, thromboxane A_2, and endothelin-1. Compounds which cause relaxation include calcitonin gene-related peptide (cGRP), adenosine, ATP, prostacyclin (PGI$_2$), and many endothelium-dependent substances which release NO or other factors (see below).

Interactions between vasoconstrictor agents

5-Hydroxytryptamine (5-HT) and thromboxane A_2 (TXA$_2$)

The interactions between vasoconstrictor agents to be discussed here are not unique to 5-HT and TXA$_2$ nor to the human coronary artery. But such interactions may be the key to vasospasm and variant angina. Our example should highlight the need for caution when attempting to compare the relative contractile effectiveness in *in vitro* studies of different agents acting through the same or different mechanism. The example chosen may be clinically relevant since thromboxane A_2 and 5-HT are released from aggregating platelets and intracoronary thrombus formation has been shown to result in focal vasoconstriction in patients with coronary artery disease (Zeiher et al. 1991b).

Human isolated large coronary arteries are, like most isolated arteries, devoid of intrinsic and *in vivo* circulating factors which in combination interact to mediate what is termed arterial vascular 'tone'. In the isolated arteries, tone was raised with a thromboxane A_2 mimetic U46619 before applying an increasing concentration of 5-HT or sumatripan. In vessels in which active force was raised above the resting initial level with U46619, contraction curves to each constrictor agent were increased in potency and efficacy compared with the curves constructed in the absence of U46619 (Fig. 12.4). Similar results were shown for methysergide and ergometrine in the presence of U46619 (Cocks et al. 1993).

Thus, at least *in vitro*, the reactivity of the human coronary artery is critically dependent on active force. This tone can markedly alter the 'effector reserve' for any particular agent. Two important conclusions can be made about the contractions to 5-HT in this tissue. First, sumatriptan is a full agonist at 5-HT_1-like receptors (Kaumann et al. 1993, 1994), and secondly the fractional contribution of 5-HT_1-like receptors to contractions to 5-HT is on average 50% (Cocks et al. 1993) but can be as high as 100% in certain patients (Kaumann et al. 1994). These facts need to be carefully considered for newly developed 5-HT_1-like agonists particularly since 5-HT has been shown to induce ketanserin-resistant spasm at the sites of stenoses in instances of advanced atherosclerosis and vasospastic disease (McFadden et al. 1991, 1992).

Therefore, inherent active force as well as receptor populations are crucial determinants of reactivity to vasoconstrictor agents with differing efficacy in human coronary artery *in vitro*.

Endothelium-dependent vasodilators

Use of nifedipine

As discussed above, quantitative relaxation in human isolated coronary arteries could only be achieved if the phasic contractions were absent. We have again employed nifedipine to readily abolish all constrictor agonist-induced phasic activity without affecting the tonic response to the precontraction stimulus. Fortunately, nifedipine has no effect on endothelium-dependent relaxation in dog large arteries (Schoeffter and Miller 1986; Angus and Cocks 1989; Mugge et al. 1991). This is also true for human large coronary arteries where nifedipine has no effect on relaxations to both substance P and bradykinin, two endothelium-dependent dilator agents (Fig. 12.5).

Functional antagonism

Functional antagonism underscores dilator capacity of a test agent in human isolated coronary arteries. Stork and Cocks (1994b) reported that contractions

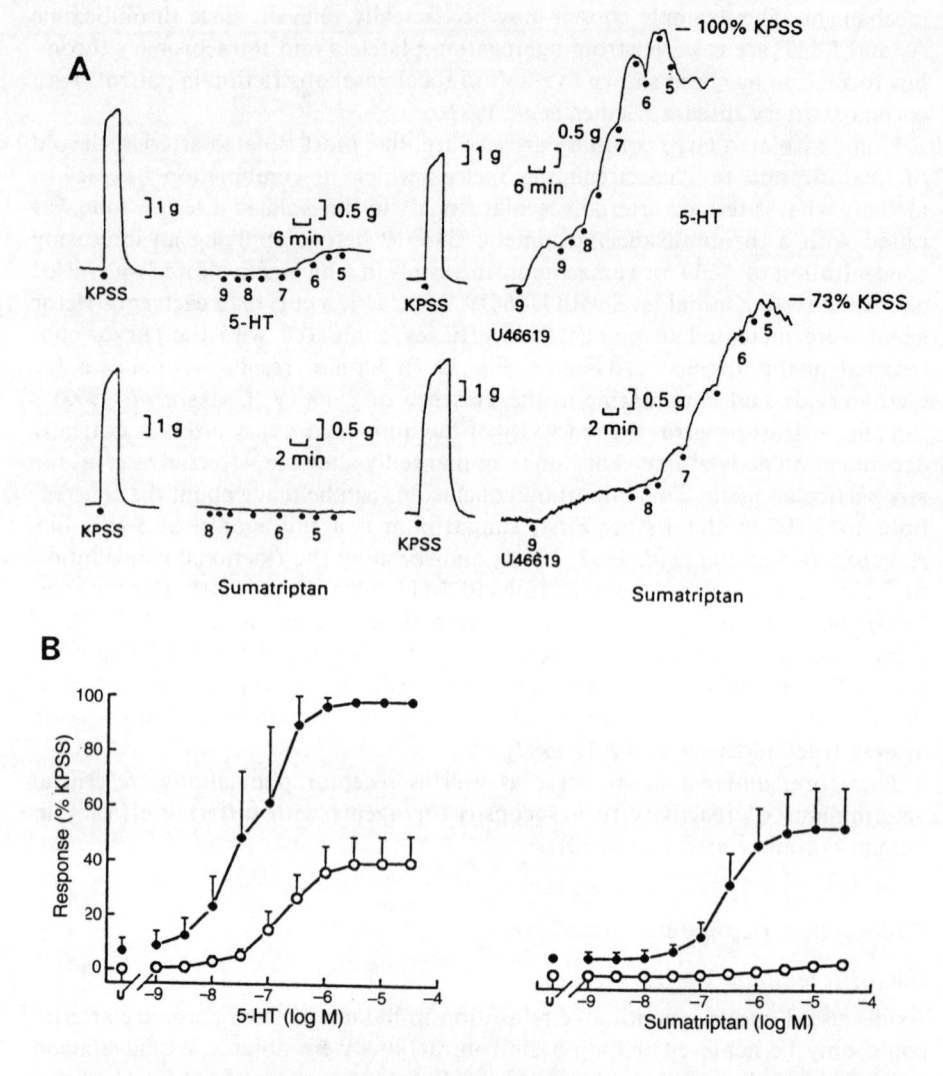

Fig. 12.4 Traces of original traces (A) and group data (B) showing the effect of precontraction with the thromboxane A_2 mimetic, U46619 (1 nM) on contractions to 5-HT and sumatriptan in isolated rings of human epicardial coronary artery. Contractions are expressed as percentages of the maximum contraction to 124 mM K^+ Krebs' solution (KPSS). (Reproduced from Cocks *et al.* 1993 with permission.)

above approximately 40% of tissue maximum resulted in progressive functional antagonism of both endothelium-dependent and independent relaxing agents. To compare the effect of drugs on relaxation responses, it is therefore important to set each tissue at similar levels of active force in the presence of nifedipine to prevent phasic contraction. It is our experience to obtain an estimation of each tissue's maximum contraction to a standard contracting agent, for example maximum depolarization with isotonic KCl (K^+ 124 mM). Relaxation can be compared

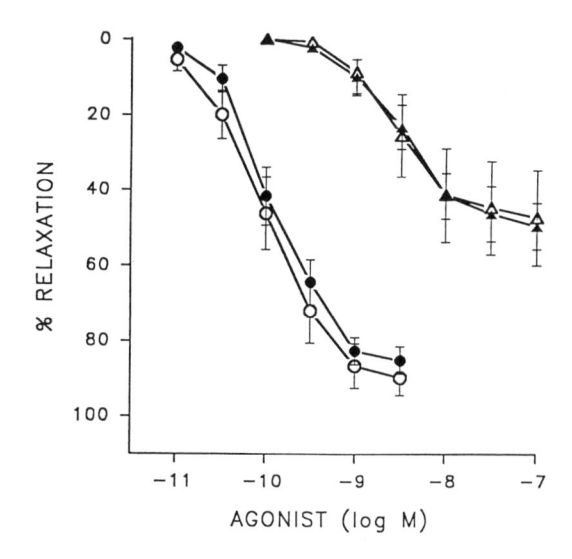

Fig. 12.5 Lack of effect of nifedipine (0.1 μM) on relaxation responses to substance P (circles) and bradykinin (triangles) in human coronary artery. Relaxation curves were obtained in rings precontracted with U46619 (1-3 nM) in the absence (open symbols) and presence (closed symbols). (Reproduced for Stork and Cocks 1994*b* with permission.)

from standardized levels of initial active force achieved by adjusting the concentration of the constrictor agents of choice (e.g. U46619). Relaxation responses to the test agent are then normalized as percentages of the maximum relaxation to sodium nitroprusside.

When optimal conditions are used (nifedipine, U46619 precontraction) endothelium-dependent relaxations to substance P, bradykinin, histamine, and the calcium ionophore A23187 and ionomycin are relatively insensitive to the L-arginine analogue inhibitors of NO synthase ^GN-nitro-L-arginine (L-NNA) also Chapter 10 (Fig. 12.6). This relatively poor degree of inhibition of endothelium-dependent relaxation by L-NNA is surprising, particularly for bradykinin since if the responses were due to NO then the submaximal relaxation should have been abolished by the NO synthase inhibitors (see Martin *et al.* 1992). The fact that L-NNA was only partially effective implies that other factors like prostnoids and a K^+ channel-dependent hyperpolarizing mechanism may be involved in endothelium-dependent relaxation in large coronary arteries (see Chapter 10).

It is important here to again stress that human coronary arteries are not usually taken from healthy individuals, but rather from patients either in end stage heart disease or from unused donor hearts. Although age, sex, and disease can be often matched, there is little control for drug histories in the case of explant hearts or of the effects of cardioplegia and trauma associated with preparing 'normal' donor hearts.

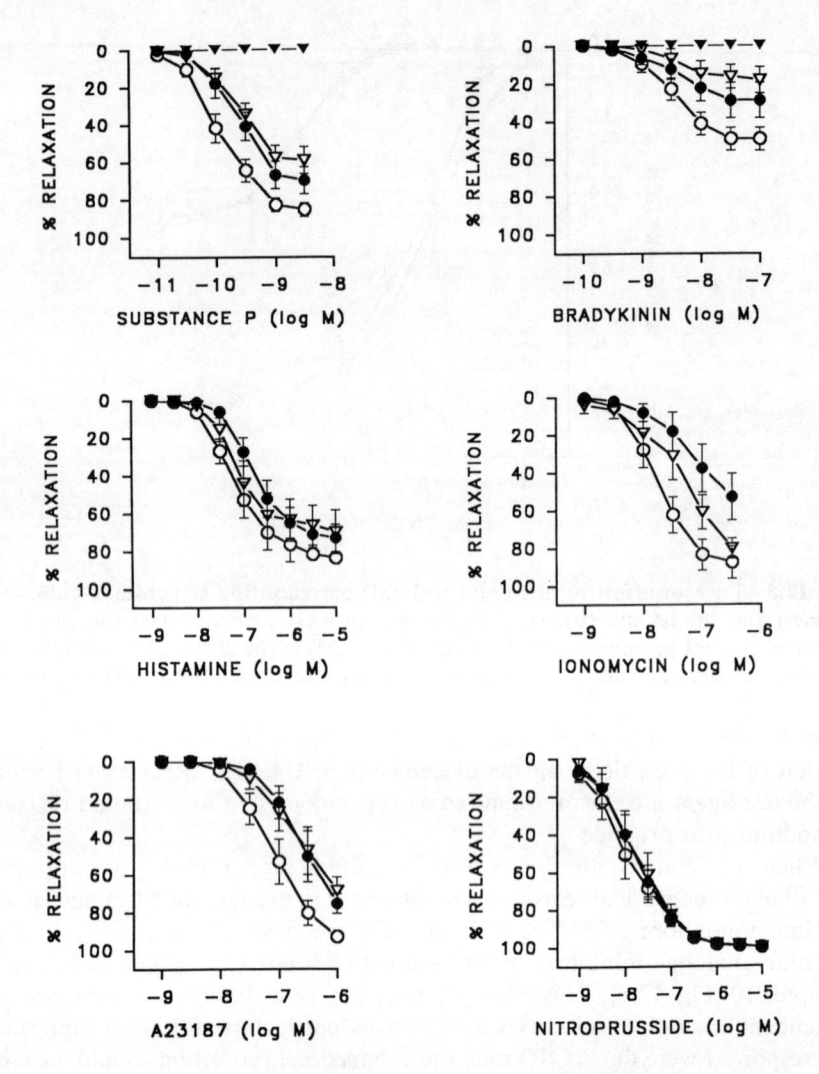

Fig. 12.6 Mean cumulative concentration–relaxation curves for EDRF-releasing agents in human coronary artery. Arterial rings were (○) control, (●) L-NNA (0.1 mM), (▽) L-NMMA (0.1 mM), and (▼) endothelium denuded. Agents examined were substance P, bradykinin, histamine, A23187, ionomycin A23187, and the endothelium-independent dilator sodium nitroprusside. (Reproduced form Stork and Cocks 1994*b* with permission.)

Acetylcholine and coronary atherosclerosis

Atherosclerosis is a progressive disease in large coronary arteries (Davies and Woolf 1993; Ross 1993). Its clinical effects, manifest as coronary artery disease (CAD) and myocardial ischaemia however, are usually only observed in mid to late age groups when the disease is well advanced. For men in these groups, CAD remains the major cause of death whereas for women CAD is more prevalent

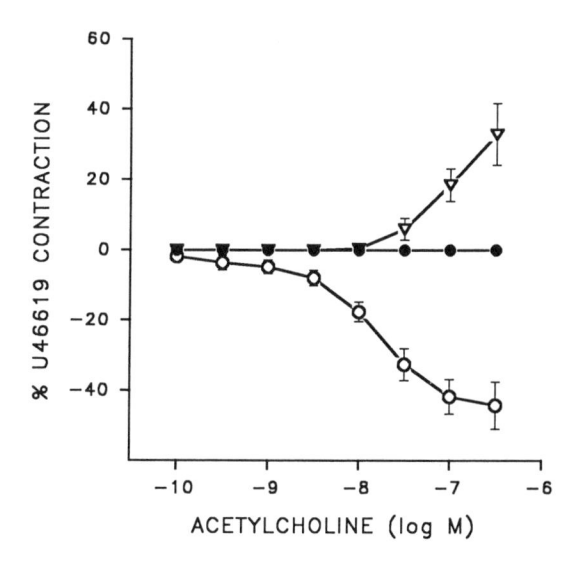

Fig. 12.7 Acetylcholine responses in U46619 precontracted rings of human epicardial coronary artery rings isolated from 15 patients. Acetylcholine caused relaxation (○; $n = 31$ rings), no response (●; $n = 31$ rings), or contraction (△; $n = 38$ rings).

following menopause. Since early CAD is thought to be associated with loss of NO-mediated vasodilatation, the presence of multiple endothelium-dependent relaxation systems and knowledge of their cellular mechardsm(s) of action, may have an important therapeutic potential.

In our hands acetylcholine relaxes only about 30% of human isolated large coronary arteries (Fig. 12.7). In normal human subjects, however, without angiographic evidence of coronary atherosclerosis, intracoronary infusions of acetylcholine causes dilatation of both the bed as measured by increases in flow and increases in diameter of large conduit vessels (Ludmer *et al.* 1986; Vita *et al.* 1990; Zeiher *et al.* 1991*a*). The apparent difficulty with detecting relaxations to acetylcholine *in vitro* may be due to:

(a) The presence of muscarinic receptors on both endothelial and smooth muscle cells which mediate endothelium-dependent relaxation and direct contraction respectively.
(b) The large ratio of smooth muscle to endothelial cells in such large arteries.
(c) The exposure of all surfaces of the artery to acetylcholine *in vitro* but only the intima *in vivo*.

Autoradiographic evidence suggests that M_1 and M_2 receptors are present on the smooth muscle of human large coronary arteries and probably mediate contraction. M_1 receptors are also found primarily in the media and also in the adventitia whilst M_2 receptors are mainly present on the adventitia (Amenta *et al.* 1992).

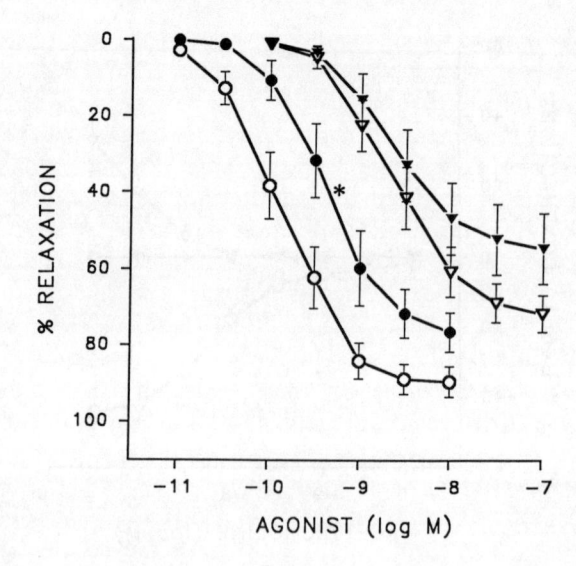

Fig. 12.8 Substance P (circles) and bradykinin (triangles) responses in human coronary artery rings sequential to rings which relaxed (open symbols) or failed to relax (closed symbols) to acetylcholine. * indicates significantly different ($p > 0.05$) pEC_{50} for vessels which did not relax to ACh compared to those that did relax.

The response to acetylcholine in human large coronary arteries either *in vitro* or *in vivo* is a 'balance' or net effect between the two opposing effects, direct contraction and indirect, endothelium-dependent relaxation. Fig. 12.7 illustrates this balancing effect for acetylcholine in human isolated coronary arteries which either relaxed, gave no response, or contracted. Sensitivity but not maximum response to the more efficient endothelium-dependent relaxing agent, substance P, was also reduced in segments of artery adjacent to those which failed to relax to acetylcholine (Fig. 12.8). It has been argued therefore, acetylcholine, not substance P (Kushwaha *et al.* 1991) is a highly sensitive test for coronary artery endothelial vasodilator dysfunction. However, an increase in muscarinic receptors on smooth muscle cells could lead to the same finding without there being any change in the endothelium-dependent dilator signal. It is not established, however, how this is related to coronary vasospasm, particularly since other potential endothelial dilator factors are able to compensate remarkably well for loss of NO-mediated relaxation (see Chapter 10).

HUMAN SMALL CORONARY ARTERIES

Introduction

The view that pharmacology of isolated large arteries mirrors that of resistance arteries in a particular vascular bed is now rejected with the emerging information coming from the development of the Mulvany-Halpern (1977) small vessel myograph. To be able to mount small arteries of 100–200 μm i.d., and measure isometric force in controlled *in vitro* organ chamber conditions with simultaneous intracellular recordings of membrane potential has given much insight into the regional differences among vascular beds within species and between species. Underlying any use of short segments of large conduit coronary arteries or resistance arteries is the caution that the information is still only a snapshot of a selected part of the entire bed. For example how representative is a 2 mm long artery 150 μm i.d. of the remaining arteriolar resistance vessels at the precapillary level? Moreover, for studying the human coronary bed, cardiac surgery can provide the tip of the right atrial appendage from where vessels of 100–300 μm i.d. can be obtained. But are these small arteries representative of the reactivity of similarly sized arteries from left atrium or ventricular tissue? In addition, the clinical condition of the coronary circulation needs to be considered when attempting to ascribe 'normal' reactivity to segments harvested from atrial appendages taken before cross-clamping at bypass surgery versus explant hearts in failure, from cardiomyopathy or ischaemia, or from 'normal' unused donor hearts but subject to perfusion with cardioplegia. Having recognized these difficulties, the following is a summary of the techniques and results we have obtained in human right atrial small coronary arteries in response to a variety of pharmacological stimuli.

Technique of vessel isolation and mounting

The tip of the right atrial appendage (0.5–1 cm long) was removed from 30 patients (40–75 years) during routine heart–lung bypass surgery for the placement of the venous drain and immediately placed in ice-cold physiological saline solution (PSS) saturated with 5% CO_2 in O_2 (Angus *et al.* 1988). For comparison, buttock skin biopsies were taken under local anaesthesia from eight patients with untreated essential hypertension or from eight normotensive volunteers (Angus *et al.* 1991*a*). Small arteries (2 mm long) were dissected from the atrial appendage and skin biopsy and suspended on 40 μm diameter stainless steel wires in a modified Mulvany–Halpern double myograph (Mulvany and Halpern 1977). The myograph was heated to 37 ± 0.1 °C and the vessels subjected to a normalized passive stretch procedure (Angus *et al.* 1988).

Acetylcholine

The majority of arteries had negligible active force after mounting and normalizing for passive stretch. In a sample of 24 human small coronary arteries the internal diameter was 169 ± 8 μm (mean ± s.e.m.) at a passive stretch equivalent to a transmural pressure of 100 mmHg. At the first stable intracellular impalement the resting E_m was −62 ± 3 mV. Acetylcholine, applied as a bolus 'upstream' from the artery caused a rapid depolarization to as high as −20 mV followed by a rapid repolarization to near resting E_m before a further cycle of depolarization-repolarization was repeated. In most arteries (> 60%) the bolus caused 4–12 oscillations of E_m accompanied by a contraction. Careful examination of the force record showed that every time the E_m depolarized there was a small, sharp rise in force similar to a 'staircase' phenomenon (Fig. 12.9). Note that if the oscillation of E_m stopped, the contraction was maintained even though the E_m was near pre-stimulation levels. These oscillations in E_m should not be confused with the oscillatory-phasic **contractions** observed in human large coronary arteries. In the large arteries the contractions are of very slow frequency (one every 5-20 min) compared with the regular 0.5 Hz observed on E_m in the small arteries. Differentiation of the E_m showed that the first depolarization gave the highest $+dV/dt$ which tendered to wane to a steady peak after four or five depolarizations (Angus et al. 1991a).

In later experiments we have used an infusion protocol which generally caused a sustained oscillation in E_m at a frequency of 0.5 Hz (0.54 ± 0.8 Hz $n = 11$ arteries) with sustained contraction (Fig. 12.10). The infusion of substance P (30 nM) in the presence of acetylcholine rapidly repolarized the artery and reduced the force presumably as NO was released from the endothelium (Fig. 12.10). If substance P was infused prior to infusing acetylcholine, there was only a single depolarization and repolarization and no contraction. Clearly then, the human right atrial small coronary artery set-up in the myograph has acetylcholine receptors on smooth muscle cells to cause depolarization and contraction and probably a paucity of receptors on the endothelium. Cumulative concentration-contraction curves to acetylcholine had an EC_{50} of 6.52 ± 0.15 ($-\log$ M, $n = 10$). This is in contrast to human buttock skin arteries of (100-400 μm i.d.) where acetylcholine only hyperpolarized and relaxed U46619 (a stable thromboxane mimetic) precontracted vessels in the classical fashion with an EC_{50} of 7.27 ± 0.2 ($-\log$ M $n = 5$). In dog small coronary arteries precontracted with K^+, acetylcholine relaxed while rabbit coronary vessels relaxed before contracting at higher concentrations. Under the same K^+ contracted conditions, acetylcholine further contracted human atrial small coronary arteries (Angus et al. 1991b). In an anecdotal experiment, a human ventricular coronary artery (417 μm i.d.) contracted only briefly to acetylcholine (1 μM). In an experiment with a larger coronary artery (783 μm i.d.) from human left ventricle taken from an explant heart acetylcholine (1-10 μM) caused a poorly sustained contraction of only 11% of the maximum contraction to K^+ depolarization (K^+ 124 mM). Acetylcholine depolarized the vessel from -50 mV to -45 mV transiently with no oscillation in E_m. Other experiments from human *left* atrial coronary arteries of 367 ± 41 μm i.d. relaxed to acetylcholine with an EC_{50} of 7.22 ± 0.06 ($n = 16$) in endothelin-1 precontracted arteries (A. Stork and T. M. Cocks unpublished observations). No electrophysiological measurements were made. Taken together these observations highlight the variation in acetylcholine responses in human isolated small coronary arteries from different regions. Therefore careful studies are needed to be made of the size, location, and conditions of the vasculature before drawing firm conclusions. One consistent finding of all these studies has been the maximum relaxation to substance P indicating the integrity of the endothelium and its ability to release EDRF/NO. Morphological examination of atrial arteries removed

Pharmacology of human isolated coronary arteries

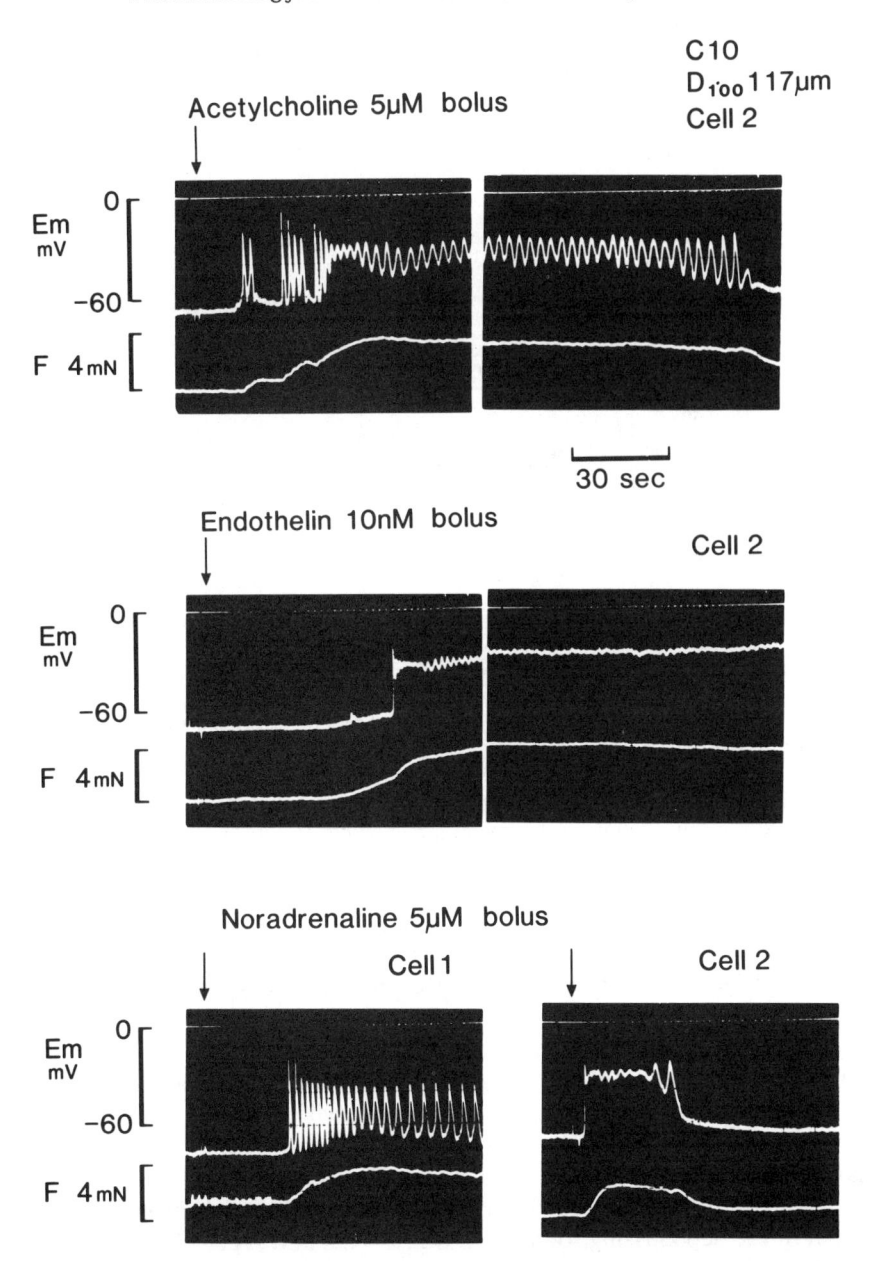

Fig. 12.9 Polaroid photographs of the membrane potential (E_m) and isometric force (mN) taken from the same human small atrial coronary artery (117 μm i.d.) and cell impalement. Drugs were applied as a bolus to the myograph chamber (7 ml) which was being perfused with drug-free solution at 5 ml/min. Note the similar oscillatory behaviour of E_m for both acetylcholine and noradrenaline and the prolonged depolarization and contraction to endothelin-1. (Reproduced from Angus *et al*. 1991a with permission.)

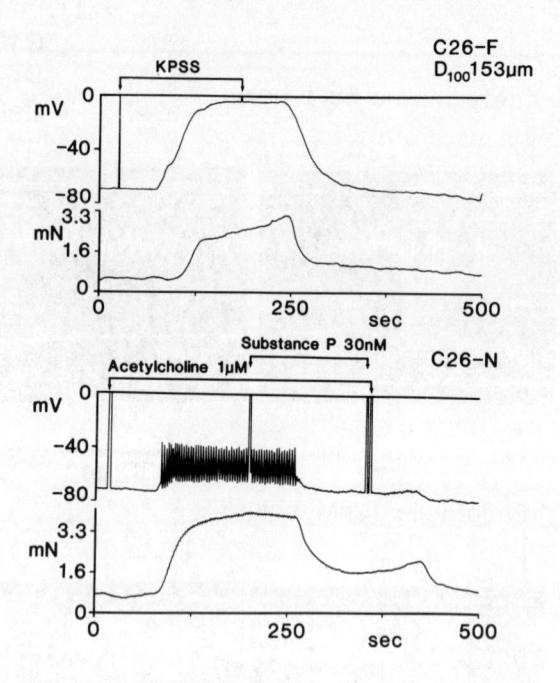

Fig. 12.10 Simultaneous records of membrane potential (mV, top traces) and active force (mN, bottom traces) recorded from the same human small coronary artery (153 μm diameter) in response to K$^+$ (124 mM, KPSS, *top*) and acetylcholine, with substance P (*bottom*). The bar indicates the infusion period. There was a 60 s delay between the pump switching and the drug change in the myograph chamber (Reproduced from Angus *et al.* 1993 with permission.)

from the myograph revealed that endothelial cells were present except where the wires had made contact with the intima. The average small coronary artery diameter was 156 ± 8.3 μm (n = 30) (circumference = 490 μm) with an intimal wire contact of circumference 126 μm. Thus the maximum loss of endothelium from the wires would be theoretically 26%.

To date we have noted that the pig small atrial coronary artery behaves similarly to the large coronary artery in that species whereby acetylcholine steadily depolarizes and contracts the artery but did not cause the unique oscillatory behaviour in E_m seen in human right atrial small arteries (Angus *et al.* 1991*a*).

To highlight the peculiar behaviour of the human right atrial coronary arteries, infusion of the depolarizing solution KPSS (K$^+$ 124 mM replacing Na$^+$) steadily raised E_m to near zero and contracted the artery. Contrast these traces with the E_m and force responses to acetylcholine in the same artery (153 μM) (Fig. 12.10).

The mechanism of the acetylcholine response

In the human small coronary arteries, the oscillation of E_m and contraction in response to acetylcholine (1–10 μM) were apparently mediated by muscarinic receptors since atropine (0.1 μM) completely prevented these responses. More specifically, the receptors are consistent with an M_2-subtype classification since 4-DAMP (4-diphenylcetoxy-N-methyl piperidine methiodide, 0.01 μM) shifted the acetylcholine contraction concentration–contraction curve in parallel by 52-fold giving an estimated pK_B of 9.7, a similar value to that reported for contraction in the pig large coronary artery (Van Charldorp and Van Zwieten 1989). Methocratamine up to 1 μM and pirenzipine (0.03 μM) did not alter the contraction responses to acetylcholine.

The E_m and force responses to acetylcholine were unaffected by tetrodotoxin (0.1 μM) or by the N-type calcium channel antagonist ω-conotoxin GVIA (1 nM). Two chemically distinct L-type calcium channel antagonists diltiazem (1 μM) and felodipine (0.1 μM) (2 h contact) had no significant effect on the level of depolarization or on the oscillation of the E_m in response to acetylcholine or noradrenaline. However, the peak contractions to these agents were reduced by 30% and 60% respectively. Presumably, this reduction reflected the component of the force response due to voltage-dependent calcium channels recruited by acetylcholine-induced E_m oscillations. In pilot studies, felodipine (0.1 μM) reduced the contraction induced by 124 mM K^+ by 96.3 ± 1.3% ($n = 4$) in rat mesenteric resistance vessels, evidence that this concentration of felodipine was effective at the voltage-dependent, L-type calcium channels.

In ion substitution experiments, lowering Ca^{2+} in PSS (from 2.5 to 0 mM) slowly depolarized the coronary resistance arteries and in some arteries transiently lowered the resting force. Acetylcholine then induced further slow depolarization without any oscillation in E_m. The contraction was weak and short-lived. After the acetylcholine was removed from the muscle chamber, the artery remained depolarized until Ca^{2+} was restored to 2.5 mM, presumably because Ca^{2+}-activated K^+ conductance required for repolarization was inactivated. The slow depolarization in low Ca^{2+} solution was prevented by the removal of external sodium (completely replaced by N-methyl-D-glucamine, a solution (zero Na) that did not alter the resting E_m or force). Acetylcholine still caused depolarization and E_m oscillation in this zero Na^+ solution when the calcium concentration was normal (2.5 mM) (Fig. 12.11, left). Given that KSS depolarization (K^+ 124 mM) takes less than five minutes to reach equilibrium (see Fig. 12.10) we used a five minute exposure to zero Na before challenging with acetylcholine and then returning to PSS. Exposure to zero Na containing Ca^{2+} (2.5 mM) for five minutes slightly reduced the contractile response and the peak depolarization but did not abolish the oscillation in E_m ($n = 3$) (Fig. 12.11, frame C45-E). When Ca^{2+} was lowered to 1.0 mM the oscillation in E_m was abolished and only a small depolarization occurred with little contraction (Fig. 12.11, right). When Ca^{2+} 2.5 mM in PSS was reapplied, the force and oscillatory E_m responses to acetylcholine were restored.

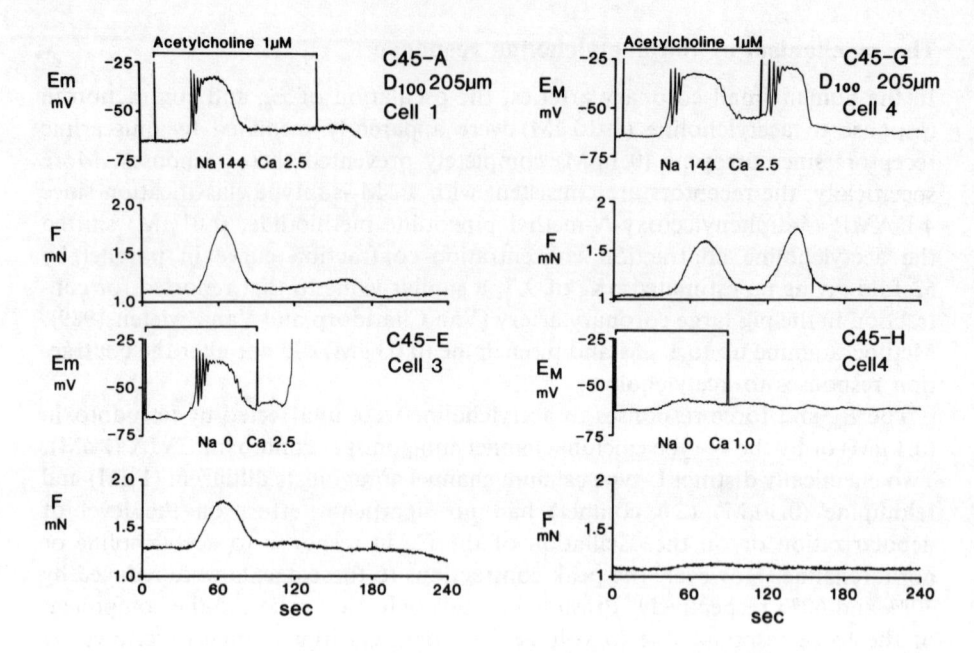

Fig. 12.11 Computer regenerated paired traces of membrane potential (E_m) and force (F) in the same human atrial coronary artery (205 μm i.d.). *Left*: traces C45-E, lowering extracellular Na$^+$ to zero was achieved by replacing NaCl with *N*-methyl-D-glucamine (NMDG) and buffering with HCl. (The 25 mM NaHCO$_3$ was replaced with 5 mM KHCO$_3$ and 20 mM NMDG.) Vigorous aeration with 5% CO$_2$ in O$_2$ generated NHDG$^+$ and HCO$_3^-$ in solution. This O Na$^+$, Ca^{2+} 2.5 mM solution (trace C45-E) for 5 min equilibration only slightly affected the response to acetylcholine. Trace C45-G is another control response to acetylcholine in PSS. Lowering the extracellular Ca^{2+} to 1.0 mM in O Na$^+$ for 5 min (trace C45-H) now almost abolished both the E_m and F response to acetylcholine.

Further evidence that acetylcholine was probably causing calcium-induced calcium release (CCR) was the finding that ryanodine (10 μM) for 20 min exposure prevented the E_m oscillation and contraction to acetylcholine (1 μM) but the responses were restored 90 min after removal of ryanodine (Angus *et al.* 1992). In addition, the intracellular Ca^{2+} chelating agent BAPTA-AM 20 μM for 30 min also prevented the oscillation in E_m and contraction to acetylcholine 1–10 μM (Fig. 12.12). In separate experiments this concentration of BAPTA depressed the concentration–contraction curve to acetylcholine but had very little effect on the peak contraction to KPSS (Fig. 12.13) indicating the relatively specific effect on intracellular Ca^{2+} rather than Ca^{2+} entry via the voltage operated calcium channel.

These studies show that the human right atrial resistance artery responds more like cardiac myocytes than vascular smooth muscle cells because of the importance of calcium-induced calcium release presumably from sarcoplasmic reticulum (SR) (Fig. 12.14). The trigger for this SR calcium release probably comes from the

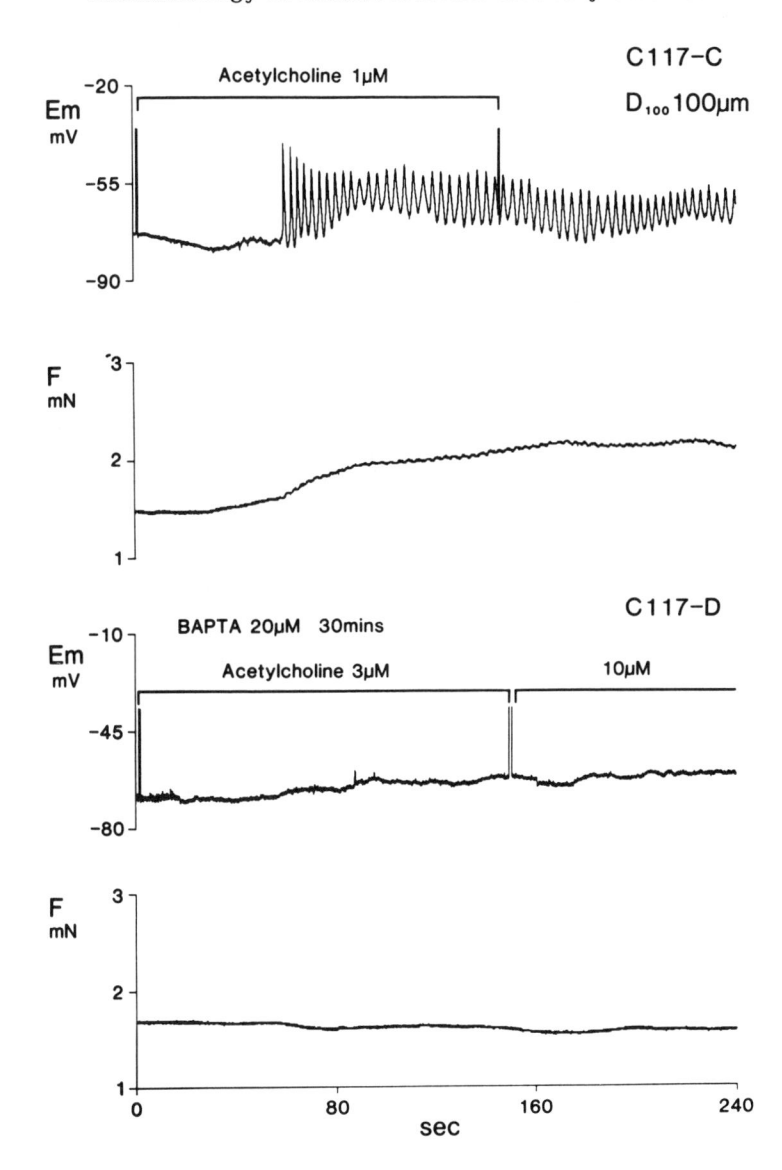

Fig. 12.12 Computer regenerated records of membrane potential (E_m) and isometric force (F) response to a acetylcholine infusion in a human right atrial coronary artery (100 μm i.d.). BAPTA-AM (20 μM) pre-treatment (30 min) prevented the oscillation in E_m and contraction to 3 and 10 μM acetylcholine. Note there was a 60 s delay from pump onset/offset of the acetylcholine entry/exit from the chamber.

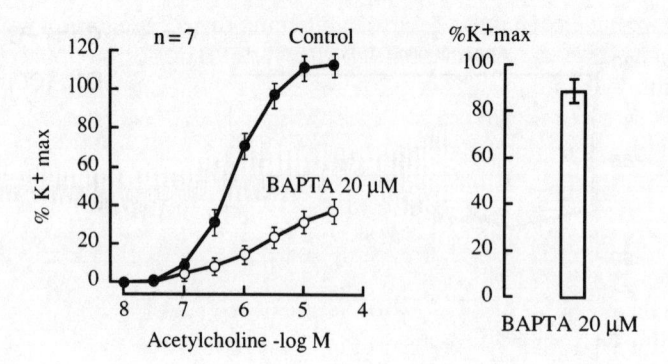

Fig. 12.13 Average concentration–contraction curves for acetylcholine in human atrial small coronary vessels in the absence (solid symbol) and presence of BAPTA-AM (20 μM, 30 min exposure). Right: bar graph shows the contraction to K^+ 124 mM in the presence of BAPTA-AM (20 μM) compared with the contraction to K^+ 124 mM (100%) in the absence of BAPTA-AM.

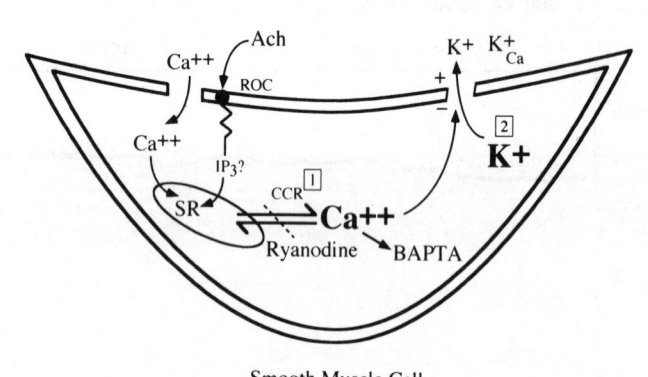

Fig. 12.14 Schematic diagram of the possible sites of action of acetylcholine, ryanodine, and BAPTA-AM in smooth muscle cells of human right atrial coronary microvessels. Terms are: Ach, acetylcholine; ROC, receptor operated channel; IP_3, inositol triphosphate; SR, sarcoplasmic reticulum; CCR, calcium-induced calcium release; K^+_{Ca}, calcium-activated potassium channel. Oscillation in E_m may be caused by $[Ca^{2+}]_i$ rising through CCR and falling through repolarization via the opening of K^+_{Ca} channels. BAPTA-AM is [1,2-bis(*o*-aminophenoxy)-ethane-*N*, *N*, *N'*, *N'*-tetraacetic acid tetra acetoxymethyl)-ester].

acetylcholine receptor activating second messenger systems such as IP_3 as occurs in aortic vascular smooth muscle (Ehrlich and Watras 1988). Whether the IP_3 concentration fluctuates is debatable but a sharp rise in $[Ca^{2+}]_i$ would rapidly open the Ca^{2+}-activated K^+-selective channels. The increase in K^+ conductance (g_K) would rapidly repolarize the cell. These processes may explain the regular oscillation in the E_m in response to acetylcholine and the failure of K^+ depolarization to cause a similar phenomenon.

To date we have been unsuccessful in blocking the E_m oscillation with K^+ channel blockers such as glibenclamide, charybdotoxin, or apamin. Tetraethylamomonium (TEA) has anticholinoceptor activity at a concentration > 0.1 mM and is therefore not useful (Angus and Broughton unpublished).

The lack of a sustained E_m oscillation and contraction in the presence of continued acetylcholine infusion in some arteries (as in Fig. 12.10) could be due to the additional action of acetylcholine on the endothelial cells. Here release of EDRF (nitric oxide) could rapidly repolarize the smooth muscle by opening the calcium-activated K^+ channel or by sequestering $[Ca]_i$ into intracellular stores or out of the cell through its well known action on cGMP (Taylor and Weston 1988). Acetylcholine only transiently hyperpolarizes isolated endothelial cells and raises $[Ca]_i$ in an oscillatory manner (Busse et al. 1988). This could explain the variable functional antagonism observed between the smooth muscle direct effects and the indirect release of EDRF by acetylcholine. Additional EDRF release by substance P shows that the actions of acetylcholine on the smooth muscle can be terminated or almost prevented by appropriately timed infusions of substance P. Presumably, the muscarinic receptors on the endothelial cells in both skin and coronary arteries release EDRF. But in pig and human coronary arteries, there appears to be a large population of muscarinic (M_2) receptors on the smooth muscle cells. Why the contraction response associated with E_m oscillation is confined to the human atrial resistance vessel is not clear from these experiments. However, we cannot exclude an age-dependent effect on endothelial cells or smooth muscle cell dysfunction.

These observations indicate that the human isolated small coronary arteries are unusually excited by receptor stimulation and emphasize the importance of EDRF in functionally antagonizing membrane depolarization and contraction. Whether endogenous acetylcholine is ever presented to small coronary arteries in sufficient concentration to affect vessel calibre is unknown. But both choline acetyltransferase and substance P have been localized in rat coronary endothelial cells (Milner et al. 1989) and a possible role for the parasympathetic nervous system in exercise-induced coronary artery spasm has been reported (Yasue et al. 1986).

5-Hydroxytryptamine

Given that 5-HT and the 5-HT_1-like receptor agonist, sumatriptan, contracted the human large coronary artery especially in the presence of additional active tone from U46619, we tested how the small coronary arteries responded to this receptor stimulation. A group of 18 arteries, one per patient were divided retrospectively into those that responded (R) to a high concentration of 5-HT (10 μM) or those that failed to contract — the non responders (NR). To assess the vessels' contractile viability, responses to KPSS (K^+ 124 mM) and acetylcholine (10 μM) were also tested.

Only seven arteries (39%) contracted to 5-HT and the maximum contraction was only 43 ± 14% of the depolarized contraction to KPSS compared with 82 ± 20% in the R and 78 ± 9% in the NR for acetylcholine. Thus 5-HT was a poor constrictor of the atrial small arteries with an EC_{50} of 6.7 ± 0.2 ($-\log M$ ± s.e.m.). Of 11

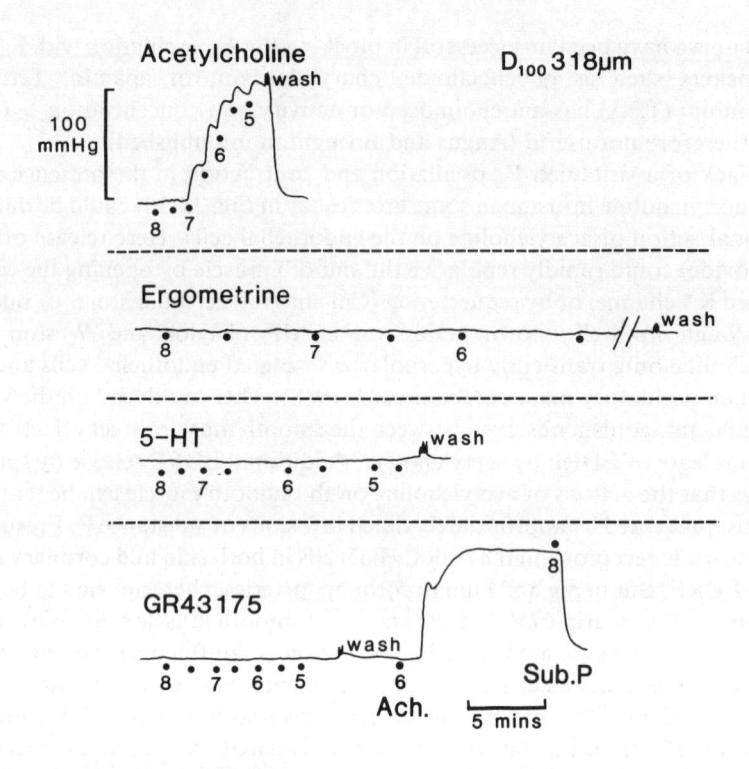

Fig. 12.15 Chart record of force changes in a human small coronary artery (318 μm diameter) in response to acetylcholine, ergometrine, 5-HT, and sumatriptan (GR43175). Endothelium was mainly intact given the relaxation to substance P. Concentrations are −log M at 0.5 units steps. Force change is in active pressure units (ΔP = Δtension/radius). (Reproduced from Angus et al. 1993 by permission.)

arteries tested, only one artery contracted to sumatriptan (0.01–1 μM) to 12% of KPSS. Similarly, ergometrine (1–1000 nM) was without effect in seven arteries tested where 5-HT (10 μM) contracted three vessels of this group (Fig. 12.15). To test the possible synergy of sumatriptan with other constrictor agents, five arteries were exposed to acetylcholine (0.3 μM) which caused a steady contraction of 9 ± 2% of KPSS (range 6–17%). In the presence of this contraction, sumatriptan 3 μM raised the force to 16 ± 4% in three out of five arteries (range 6–31% of KPSS). In two arteries of 760 and 435 μm i.d. taken from the ventricle of an explant heart, neither sumatriptan nor 5-HT (from 0.01–30 μM) caused any contraction. In an atrial artery (351 μm) and a vessel from the ventricle (783 μm) precontracted with endothelin 10 nM to about 65% of KPSS, 5-HT 10 μM failed to further contract these vessels.

Thus, the majority of human small coronary arteries (> 60%) failed to contract to 5-HT. But where contraction occurred the maximum effect was similar to the contraction in large arteries, i.e. 40–50% of KPSS. A predominant relaxation to 5-HT is unlikely since the 5-HT$_4$-receptor agonist BMIU8 0.01–30 μM was without effect in K$^+$ (25-35 μM) contracted atrial arteries (Angus *et al.* 1993). We could find little evidence of synergy between sumatriptan and acetylcholine but because the thromboxane mimetic U46619 failed to contract the small vessels, we could not test the sumatriptan — U46619 interaction that was observed in large coronary arteries (see above).

These studies suggest that there is relatively little role for 5-HT and 5-HT$_1$-like receptor activity in the small arteries. Therefore selective agonists such as sumatriptan may have little affect on coronary resistance if these results from isolated tissue assays can be extrapolated to the more general intact coronary vasculature.

Adrenoceptors

There is little information on the adrenoceptors located on human coronary microvessels. We found that relatively high doses of noradrenaline ($> 1 \mu$M) caused rapid depolarization and contraction of right atrial arteries (Fig. 12.1). The record shows a similar oscillation of E_m and contraction to noradrenaline as for acetylcholine, for the first exposure at least. In separate cumulative/concentration response curves, noradrenaline caused a weak contraction of 23 ± 3% of KPSS, ($n = 5$) at 10 μM. However, 10 min after exposure to propranolol (1 μM) noradrenaline was about tenfold more potent as the contraction was raised to 55% ± 10% of KPSS at 10 μM. These contractions and E_m depolarization to noradrenaline were completely prevented by the prior exposure to prazosin (0.1 μM). In contrast to the oscillatory E_m response to noradrenaline in human coronary arteries, the human buttock skin vessels only contracted with a slowly developing depolarization.

Thus, the atrial small coronary vessels appear to be endowed with β-adrenoceptors and α_1-adrenoceptors. These experiments offer an explanation for a rise in coronary blood flow resistance in the setting of β-adrenoceptor blockade.

Future work

These studies in human atrial small coronary arteries have highlighted a most unusual oscillatory membrane potential behaviour especially in response to acetylcholine. What relevance this activity has to normal or abnormal coronary resistance is unknown. If the phenomenon was caused by the artificial experimental environment it would be expected that similar arteries from other species would also display this phenomenon. The apparent role for calcium-induced calcium release in the phenomenon points to potential targets for therapeutic intervention.

Future work should be directed to exploring the pharmacology of as many different parts of the human coronary bed as possible including the endocardial vessels subjected to hypoxia. At experiment, rigorous attention must be given to tissue procurement, vessel dissection, and mounting in the myograph if we are to define reactivity of the resistance bed, isolated from myocardial cell influences, in normal, aged, and/or diseased vessels. This area of human vascular pharmacology has been neglected for too long. We now have the tools to explore the important role of the coronary vasculature under varied clinical conditions. In the end, clinical observation of what **does** occur in the intact coronary circulation must consider the information of what **can** occur in isolated segments of a range of vessels albeit under the artificial, controlled environment of the myograph or organ chamber.

ACKNOWLEDGEMENTS

We thank Ms Fanoula Penou for help with preparing the manuscript and Mr Peter Coles and Mr Mark Ross-Smith for the illustrations. This work was supported by the National Health and Medical Research Council (NHMRC), National Heart Foundation (NHF), and Glaxo Australia Pty Ltd.

REFERENCES

Amenta, F., Coppola, L., Gallo, P., Ferrante, F., Forlani, A., Momopoli, A., et al. (1991). Autoradiographic localization of β-adenergic receptors in human large coronary arteries. Circ. Res., 68, 1591-9.

Amenta, F., De Michele, M., Strocchi, P., Ferrante, F., and Gallo, P. (1992). Muscarinic cholinergic receptors in the human right coronary artery: a receptor binding and autoradiographic study. Naunyn-Schmiedeberg's Arch. Pharmacol., 345, 251-4.

Angus, (1989). 5-HT receptors in the coronary circulation. Trends Pharmacol. Sci., 10, 89-90.

Angus, J. A. and Cocks, T. M. (1989). Endothelium-derived relaxing factor. Pharmacol. Ther., 41, 303-51.

Angus, J. A., Cocks, T. M., and Satoh, K. (1986). α-Adrenoceptors and endothelium-dependent relaxation in canine large ateries. Br. J. Pharmacol., 88, 767-77.

Angus, J. A., Broughton, A., and Mulvany, M. J. (1988). Role of α-adrenoceptors in constrictor responses of rat, guinea pig and rabbit small arteries to neural activation. J. Physiol., 403, 495-570.

Angus, J. A., Broughton, A., and McPherson, G. A. (1991a). Membrane potential and contractility responses to acetylcholine and other vasoconstrictor stimuli in human small coronary arteries. In Resistance arteries, structure and function (ed. M. J. Mulvany, C. Aalkjaer, A. M. Heagerty, N. C. B. Nyborg, and S. Strandgaard), pp. 254-60. Elsevier Science.

Angus, J. A., Cocks, T. M., McPherson, G. A., and Broughton, A. (1991b). The acetylcholine paradox — a contrictor of human small coronary arteries even in the presence of endothelium. Clin. Exp. Pharmacol. Physiol., 18, 33-6.

Angus, J. A., Broughton, A., and Ross-Smith, M. (1992). Mechanism of acetylcholine-induced contraction of human small coronary arteries. Clin. Exp. Pharmacol. Physiol., Suppl. 21, 2 (Abstract).

Angus, J. A., Cocks, T. M., and Ross-Smith, M. (1993). Pharmacological analysis of 5-HT receptors in human small coronary arteries. In Serotonin (ed. P. M. Vanhoutte, P.R. Saxena, R. Paoletti, N. Brunello, and A.S. Jackson), pp. 297-305. Klumer Academic Publishers, Netherlands.

Berkenboom, G., Fontaine, J., Desmet, J.-M., and Degre, S. (1987). Comparison of beta adrenergic antagonists with different ancillary properties on isolated canine and human coronary arteries. *Cardiovasc. Res.*, **21**, 299–304.

Bradley, P. B., Engel, G., Feniuk, W., Fozard, J. R., Humphrey, P. P. A., Middlemiss, D. N., *et al.* (1986) Proposals for the classification and nomenclature of functional receptors for 5-hydroxytryptamine. *Neuropharmacology*, **25**, 563–76.

Busse, R., Fichtner, H., Luckoff, A., and Kohlhardt, M. (1988). Hyperpolarisation and increased free calcium in acetylcholine-stimulated endothelial cells. *Am. J. Physiol.*, **255**, H965–9.

Cocks, T. M., and Angus, J. A. (1983). Endothelium-dependent relaxation of coronary arteries by noradrenaline and serotonin. *Nature*, **305**, 627–30.

Cocks, T. M., Kemp, B. K., Pruneau, D., and Angus, J. A. (1993). Comparison of contractile responses to 5-hydroxytryptamine and sumatriptan in human isolated coronary artery: synergy with the thromboxane A_2-receptor agonist, U46619. *Br. J. Pharmacol.*, **110**, 360–8.

Connor, H. E., Feniuk, W., and Humphrey, P. P. A. (1989). 5-hydroxytryptamine contracts human coronary arteries predominantly via 5-HT$_2$ receptor activation. *Eur. J. Pharmacol.*, **161**, 91–4.

Davies, M. J. and Woolf, N. (1993). Atherosclerosis: what is it and why does it occur? *Br. Heart J.*, **69**, S3–11.

Ehrich, B. E. and Watras, J. (1988). Inositol 1, 4, 5-trisphosphate activates a channel from smooth muscle sarcoplasmic reticulum. *Nature*, **336**, 583–6.

Ferrari, M. D., Melamed, E., Gawel, M. J., Nappi, G., Luben, V., Tranchant, C., *et al.* (1991). Treatment of migraine attacks with sumatriptan. *N. Eng. J. Med.*, **325**, 316–21.

Ginsburg, R. C. (1984). Myogenic tone of the isolated human epicardial artery: regulatory controls. *Acta Med. Scand.*, **694**, 29–37.

Ginsburg, R., Bristow, M. R., Harrison, D. C., and Stinson, E. B. (1980). Studies with isolated human coronary arteries: some general observations, potential mediators of spasm, role of calcium antagonists. *Chest*, **78**, 180–6.

Golenhofen, K. (1978). Activation mechanisms in smooth muscle of human coronary arteries and their selective inhibition. *Naunyn-Schmiedeburg's Arch. Pharmacol.*, **302**, R36.

Golino, P. and Maseri, A. (1994). Serotonin receptors in human coronary arteries. *Circulation*, **90**, 1573–5.

Golino, P., Piscione, F., Willerson, J. T., Cappelli-Bigazzi, M., Focaccio, A., Villari, B., *et al.* (1991). Divergent effects of serotonin on coronary artery dimensions and blood flow in patients with coronary atherosclerosis and control patients. *N. Eng. J. Med.*, **324**, 641–8.

Humphrey, P. P. A., Apperley, E., Feniuk, W., and Perren, M. J. (1990). A rational approach to identifying a fundamentally new drug for the treatment of migraine. In *Cardiovascular pharmacology of 5-hydroxytryptamine* (ed. P. R. Saxena, D. I. Wallis, W. Wouters, and P. Bevan), pp. 417–31, Kluwer Academic Publishers, Dordrecht.

Ishikawa, Y., Umemura, S., Uchino, K., Shindou, T., Yasuda, G., Minamisawa, K., *et al.* (1991). Identification of an alpha$_2$ adrenoceptor in human coronary arteries by radioligand binding assay. *Life Sci.*, **48**, 2513–18.

Kaumann, A. J., Parsons, A. A., and Brown, A. M. (1993). Human arterial constrictor serotonin receptors. *Cardiovasc. Res.*, **27**, 2094–103.

Kaumann, A. J., Frenken, M., Posival, H., and Brown, A. M. (1994). Variable participation of 5-HT$_1$-like receptors and 5-HT$_2$ receptors in serotonin-induced contraction of human isolated coronary arteries.: 5-HT$_1$-like receptors resemble cloned 5-HT$_{1D\beta}$ receptors. *Circulation*, **90**, 1141–53.

Kushwaha, S. S., Crossman, D. C., Bustami, M., Davies, G. J., Mitchell, A. G., Maseri,

A., et al. (1991). Substance P for evaluation of coronary endothelial function after cardiac transplantation. *J. Am. Coll. Cardiol.*, **17**, 1537-44.

Ludmer, P. L., Selwyn, A. P., Shook, T. L., Wayne, R. P., Mudge, G. H., Alexander, R. W., et al. (1986). Paradoxical vasoconstriction induced by acetylcholine in atherosclerotic coronary arteries. *N. Engl. J. Med.*, **315**, 1046-51.

McFadden, E. P., Clarke, J. G., Davies, G. J., Kaski, J. C., Haider, A. W., and Maseri, A. (1991). Effect of intracoronary serotonin on coronary vessels in patients with stable angina and patients with variant angina. *N. Engl. J. Med.*, **324**, 648-54.

McFadden, E. P., Bauters, C., Lablanche, J. M., Leroy, F., Clarke, J. G., Henry, M., et al. (1992) Effect of ketanserin on proximal and distal coronary constrictor responses to intracoronary infusion of serotonin in patients with stable angina, patients with variant angina and control patients. *Circulation*, **86**, 187-95.

Martin, G. R., Bolofo, M. L., and Giles, H. (1992). Inhibition of endothelium-dependent vasorelaxation by arginine analogues: a pharmacological analysis of agonist and tissue dependence. *Br. J. Pharmacol.*, **105**, 643-52.

Maseri, A. and Chierchia, S. (1982). Coronary artery spasm: demonstration, definition, diagnosis, and consequences. *Prog. Cardiovasc. Dis.*, **25**, 169-92.

Milner, P., Ralevic, V., Hopwoud, A. M., Feher, E., Lincoln, J., Kirkpatrick, K. A., et al. (1989). Ulstrastructural localisation of substance P and choline acetyltransferase in endothelial cells of rat coronary artery and release of substance P and acetylcholine during hypoxia. *Experentia*, **45**, 121-5.

Moskowitz, M. A. (1992). Neurogenic versus vascular mechanisms of sumatriptan and ergot alkaloids in migraine. *Trends Pharmacol. Sci.*, **13**, 307-11.

Mügge, A., Peterson, T., and Harrison, D. G. (1991). Release of nitrogen oxides from cultured bovine aortic endothelial cells is not impaired by calcium channel antagonists. *Circulation*, **83**, 1404-9.

Mulvany, M. J. and Halpern, W. (1977). Contractile properties of small arterial resistance vessels in spontaneously hypertensive and normotensive rats. *Circ. Res.*, **41**, 19-26.

Perrin, V. L., Farkkila, M., Goasguen, J., Doenicke, A., Brand, J., and Tfelt-Hansen, P. (1989). Overview of initial clinical studies with intravenous and oral GR43175 in acute migraine. *Cephalagia*, **9**, 63-72.

Ross, R. (1993). The pathogenesis of atherosclerosis: a perspective for the 1990s. *Nature*, **362**, 801-9.

Ross, G., Stinson, E., Schroeder, J., and Ginsburg, R. (1980). Spontaneous phasic activity of isolated human coronary arteries. *Cardiovasc. Res.*, **14**, 613-18.

Schoeffter, P. and Miller, R. C. (1986). Role of sodium-calcium exchange and effects of calcium entry blockers on endothelial-mediated responses in rat isolated aorta. *Mol. Pharmacol.*, **30**, 53-7.

Stary, H. C., Blankenhorn, D. H., Chandler, A. B., Glagov, S., Insull, W., Richardson, M., et al. (1992). A definition of the intima of human arteries and of its atherosclerosis-prone regions: a report from the Committee on Vascular Lesions of the Council on Arteriosclerosis, American Heart Association. *Circulation*, **85**, 391-405.

Stork, A. P. and Cocks, T. M. (1994a). Pharmacological reactivity of human epicardial coronary arteries: phasic and tonic responses to vasoconstrictor drugs differentiated by nifedipine. *Br. J. Pharmacol.*, **113**, 1093-8.

Stork, A. P. and Cocks, T. M. (1994b). Pharmacological reactivity of human epicardial coronary arteries: characterization of relaxation responses to endothelium-dependent relaxing factor. *Br. J. Pharmacol.*, **113**, 1099-104.

Taylor, S. G. and Weston, A. H. (1988). Endothelium derived hyperpolarising factor — a new endogenous inhibitor from the vascular endothelium. *Trends Pharmacol. Sci.*, **9**, 212-74.

Toda, N. (1986). α-Adrenoceptor subtypes and diltiazem actions in isolated human coronary arteries. *Am. J. Physiol.*, **250**, H718-24.
Toda, N. and Okamura, T. (1990). Beta adrenoceptor subtype in isolated human, monkey and dog epicardial coronary arteries. *J. Pharmacol. Exp. Ther.*, **253**, 518-24.
Van Charldorp, K. J. and Van Zwieten, P. A. (1989). Comparison of the muscarinic receptors in the coronary artery, cerebral artery and atrium of the pig. *Naunyn-Schmiedeberg's Arch. Pharmacol.*, **339(4)**, 403-8.
Van Heuven-Nolsen, D. (1988). 5-HT receptor subtype-specific drugs and the cardiovascular system. *Trends Parmacol. Sci.*, **9**, 423-5.
Vita, J. A., Treasure, C. B., Nagel, E. G., Mclenachan, J. M., Fish, R. D., Yeung, A. C., et al. (1990). Coronary vasomotor response to acetylcholine relates to risk factors for coronary artery disease. *Circulation*, **81**, 491-7.
Yasue, H., Horio, Y., Nakamura, N., Fujii, H., Imoto, N., Sonoda, M. D., Kugiyama, K., Obata, K., Morikami, Y., and Kimura, T. (1986). Induction of coronary artery spasm by acetylcholine in patients with variant angina — possible role of parasympathetic nervous system in the pathogenesis of coronary artery spasm. *Circulation*, **74**, 955-63.
Zeiher, A. M., Drexler, H., Wollschläger, H., and Just, H. (1991a). Modulation of coronary vasomotor tone in humans: progressive endothelial dysfunction with different early stages of coronary atherosclerosis. *Circulation*, **83**, 391-401.
Zeiher, A. M., Drexler, H., Wollschläger, H., and Just, H. (1991b). Endothelial dysfunction of the coronary microvasculature is associated with impaired coronary blood flow regulation in patients with early atherosclerosis. *Circulation*, **83**, 1984-92.

13. Pharmacology of the renal circulation

David P. Brooks and Richard M. Edwards

INTRODUCTION

The function of the kidney has intrigued scientists from the time of Aristotle (384 to 322 BC), who provided one of the early descriptions of renal anatomy (Fine 1987; Eknoyan 1989), through the experiments of Galen (130 to 200 AD), who described the formation of urine, and the research of the 19th century physiologists, William Bowman and Carl Ludwig, who made significant advances toward our understanding of glomerular filtration and renal blood flow (Fine 1987; Thurau et al. 1987). Considerable work is still being conducted in order to better our understanding of the dominant role of the kidney in the regulation of both blood pressure and the internal millieu. Much work remains to be performed for us to comprehend fully the processes and mechanisms involved in both renal function and dysfunction. This chapter is intended to provide some general information on one particular aspect of kidney function, the renal circulation. We describe some of the different methods used to study the renal circulation (Table 13.1) and provide a synopsis of some factors which affect blood flow through the kidney (Table 13.2). Where appropriate, we also provide information on the pathophysiological role these factors may have in renal disease.

Methods for studying renal circulation and renal vascular smooth muscle pharmacology

Measurement of total renal blood flow

Total blood flow to the kidneys constitutes 25% of the cardiac output and thus in a 70 kg human represents over 1 litre/min. Renal blood flow, however, can vary considerably and ranges from a low of 12% to a high of 30% of cardiac output; thus measurement of renal blood flow is of great importance. Historically, a number of methods for measuring total renal blood flow have been utilized (Knox and Spielman 1983), however, two have predominated. The renal clearance method that provides an estimate of renal plasma flow and direct measurement of renal blood flow using a variety of flow transducers and meters.

1. Clearance as a measure of renal plasma flow. The renal clearance of any substance by definition is the volume of plasma completely cleared of that substance

Pharmacology of the renal circulation

Table 13.1 Methods for study of renal blood flow and microvascular reactivity

Measurement of total renal blood flow
- Electromagnetic flow probes
- Pulsed Doppler flow probes
- PAH clearance
- Inert gas washout (^{133}Xe, ^{85}Kr)
- Radioactive or coloured microspheres
- Phase-contrast cinemagnetic imaging

Measurement of intrarenal vascular reactivity
- Micropuncture
- Isolated arterioles
- Hydronephrotic kidney — intravital microscopy
- Isolated perfused juxtamedullary nephron
- Vascular casts

Table 13.2 Location and function of receptors in the renal microcirculation

	Preglomerular	Postglomerular
Noradrenaline	$+(\alpha_1)$	$+(\alpha_1)$
Dopamine	$-(DA_1)$	$-(DA_1)$
Acetylcholine	$-(m)$	$-(m)$
Serotonin	$+(5\text{-}HT_1)$	0
	$-(5\text{-}HT_2)$	
Angiotensin II	$+(AT_1)$	$+(AT_1)$
Vasopressin	0	$+(V_1)$
Bradykinin	0	$-$
Atrial natriuretic factor	$-$	0
Endothelin	$+$	$+$
Adenosine	$+(A_1)$	$-(A_2)$
PGI$_2$	$-$	$-$
PGE$_2$	$-$	0

$+$, vasoconstriction; $-$, vasodilatation; 0, no response. Receptor subtype where known is shown in parentheses.

per unit/time. Thus, the clearance of the compound that is freely filterable and removed completely from the remaining plasma by tubular secretion will represent renal plasma flow. An example of such a substance is *para*-aminohippuric acid (PAH) whose clearance averages in excess of 90% of the plasma load to the kidney. Thus, measurement of PAH clearance provides a good estimate of renal plasma flow (the clearance of inulin or polyfructosan which are only filtered, but not secreted or reabsorbed, represent a good measure of glomerular filtration rate). Clearance of PAH is measured by infusing it at a constant rate, collecting urine samples over a fixed period (~30 min) and assaying PAH in both the urine and plasma using a colorimetric assay (Smith *et al.* 1945). The amount of PAH excreted (U_{PAH} × urine flow rate) divided by the plasma concentration provides a measure of renal plasma flow. A more accurate measure of total renal plasma flow can be determined by measuring the concentration of PAH in renal venous plasma and determining plasma flow using the Fick principle. Both these methods require accurate collection of urine and thus indwelling bladder catheters, a measurable flow rate and irrigation of the bladder. Methods have been described to obviate the need for urine collection and these depend upon measuring the rate of disappearance from the circulation of markers such as PAH following an IV injection. These methods, however, do require serial blood samples and are unsuitable for repeated measurements within a short period of time. A simplified method for the measurement of renal plasma flow (and glomerular filtration rate) involves measuring the renal clearance of PAH (or inulin for GFR) by assaying the infusion rate rather than excretion rate of marker (Earle and Berliner 1946). Given that the marker is not metabolized and solely excreted in the urine, one can assume that, at equilibrium, the amount of marker infused intravenously per unit/time is equal to the amount excreted. Thus, with an accurate measurement of the pump rate and the concentration of PAH in both the infusate and plasma, the clearance of PAH (and thus effective renal plasma flow) at equilibrium is calculated as the infusion rate (mg/min) divided by the plasma concentration (mg/ml). This method relies on ensuring that following initiation of the PAH infusion and when renal blood flow has changed, enough time is allowed to reach steady state conditions and a new equilibrium.

2. Direct measurement of renal blood flow. A more direct measurement of renal blood flow can be achieved using a variety of flow probes and meters. These methods usually rely on placing either an electromagnetic or pulsed Doppler flow probe around the renal artery. Both methods can be used acutely or chronically. The latter type in particular has been successfully miniaturized for use in small animals such as rats and can be chronically implanted for long-term studies. The Doppler flow system measures the Doppler shift in the frequency of ultrasound reflected from moving red blood cells, a variable which is proportional to the velocity of the reflecting cells (Haywood *et al.* 1981). Larger versions of ultrasonic flow probes have been developed and have been used successfully in chronic dog studies. The flow probe connectors can either be exteriorized with a skin button or excised from a subcutaneous pocket under local anaesthesia on the day of the experiment (Brooks *et al.* 1990*b*).

More recently, non-invasive techniques have been used clinically to measure normal renal blood flow. One example is measurement of renal blood flow using phase-contrast cinemagnetic resonance imaging (Sommer *et al.* 1992).

Measurement of the renal microcirculation

As in other vascular beds, renal blood flow is critically dependent on the contractile state of small intrarenal resistance vessels. In the kidney, the major sites of vascular resistance are the afferent arteriole, which carries blood to the glomerulus, and the efferent arteriole, which exits the glomerulus and gives rise to the peritubular capillaries. Micropuncture measurements have revealed that ~60% of total renal vascular resistance is located proximal to the glomerulus, mainly in the afferent arteriole, whereas the efferent arteriole accounts for ~30% of the total resistance. By virtue of their pre- and postglomerular location, the afferent and efferent arterioles are strategically positioned to regulate glomerular capillary pressure and hence, glomerular filtration rate and overall renal function. Unfortunately, these important segments of the renal microvasculature are not accessible for direct study in the intact kidney. Therefore, the vascular reactivities of the glomerular arterioles have, until recently, been inferred from studies using conventional micropuncture and clearance techniques which are often difficult to interpret because of the accompanying changes in systemic haemodynamics and the complex interaction between the nervous system and extra- and intrarenal vasoactive hormonal systems. However, over the past decade, a number of new techniques have been developed that allow the direct study of the physiology and pharmacology of the renal microvasculature *in situ* and *in vitro*. We will describe four innovative techniques that span the spectrum from the study of single glomerular arterioles *in vitro* to the *in situ* observation of arterioles in the whole kidney. These techniques include the isolated arteriole method, the split hydronephrotic kidney model, the blood perfused juxtamedullary nephron preparation, and fluorescence videomicroscopy of the medullary microcirculation.

Isolated arterioles The isolated arteriole technique permits the direct *in vitro* assessment of vascular reactivity of the glomerular arterioles under controlled conditions free from any systemic influences (Edwards 1983). In this technique single afferent or efferent arterioles are dissected free-hand from the renal cortex and are transferred to a temperature controlled bath mounted on the stage of an inverted microscope. One end of the arteriole is cannulated with micropipettes similar to those used in the isolated perfused tubule method (Burg *et al.* 1966). The other end of the arteriole is occluded with another micropipette and intraluminal pressure is set at a physiological value. Alternatively, the arteriole can be freely perfused (Weihprecht *et al.* 1991). The image of the arteriole is displayed on a video monitor and changes in lumen diameter in response to addition of compounds to the bathing medium are measured directly. Arterioles having lumen diameters on the order of 10–20 μm can routinely be studied with this technique (Edwards 1983). The rate limiting step in this procedure is the dissection of the arterioles. The rabbit renal microvasculature has been the most extensively studied with this technique (Edwards 1988; Ito *et al.* 1991) because of the amenability of the rabbit kidney to dissection. However, both rat (Yuan *et al.* 1990) and dog arterioles (Ohishi *et al.* 1988) have also been studied with the technique. Isolated renal arterioles appear to lack functional nerve terminals as demonstrated by the failure of tyramine to evoke contraction and do not develop spontaneous tone consistently (Edwards 1983), however, they are responsive to a number of vasoactive agents (see below) and are exquisitely sensitive to peptides such as angiotensin II (Edwards 1983; Yuan *et al.* 1990) and endothelin (Edwards *et al.* 1990; Lanese *et al.* 1992).

Split hydronephrotic kidney The split hydronephrotic kidney preparation allows the application of epi- and transillumination microscopic techniques to study the glomerular arterioles as well as the circulation in single glomerular loops during perfusion with systemic blood (Steinhausen *et al.* 1983). In this model, rats first undergo unilateral ureteral ligation. During the development of hydronephrosis, the tubular system atrophies, leaving the vascular system intact. After 6-8 weeks, the rat is anaesthetized and the ligated kidney is transsected with a cautery knife. One-half of the kidney is immobilized and placed in a tissue bath while still connected to the systemic circulation. Virtually the entire intrarenal microcirculation can be viewed using intravital microscopy. Changes in diameter of the various segments of the renal microvasculature can be increased following systemic and/or local application of drugs. This technique has been used exclusively in the rat and has yielded valuable information on the reactivity of various segments of the renal microvasculature to a number of vasoactive agents (Steinhausen *et al.* 1983; Loutzenhiser *et al.* 1990).

Blood perfused juxtamedullary nephron This technique takes advantage of a unique population of nephrons present on the inside cortical surface of the rat kidney that lies in direct opposition to the pelvic cavity (Casellas and Navar 1984). In this technique, the kidney is cannulated *in situ* and removed from the abdominal cavity. The kidney is bisected longitudinally and the papilla reflected to expose the pelvic mucosa. The mucosa is then peeled off to reveal the underlying vasculature. Addition of fluorescence in isothiocyanate–bovine serum albumin to the blood perfusing the kidney helps to visualize the microvasculature by video microscopy (Carmines *et al.* 1986). This technique permits the measurement of lumen diameter of the various segments of the renal microvasculature and in addition, the hydrostatic pressure profile along the vascular tone can be measured with micropipettes using a servonuiling apparatus (Casellas and Navar 1984). This preparation is responsive to a number of vasoactive agents and has the additional advantage of permitting the study of glomerular and tubular dynamics concomitant with vascular measurements (Casellas and Navar 1984).

Videomicroscopy of the medullary microcirculation The renal medulla derives its blood flow from juxtamedullary afferent arterioles that branch into descending vasa recta which terminate in capillary plexuses. Blood from the inner medulla returns to the arcuate vein via the ascending vasa recta (Zimmerhackl *et al.* 1985). Direct observation of the medullary microcirculation by microscopic techniques has been performed primarily in the rat. With this technique the papilla is exposed by severing the ureter and placing the kidney in a small holder. Video microscopy combined with fluorescence epillamination facilitates the measurement of vasa recta diameters (Zimmerhackl *et al.* 1985). Fluorescence isothyiocyamate labelled red blood cells can be used to measure red cell velocity. Velocity measurements combined with diameter measurements can be used to calculate vasa recta blood flow (Navar *et al.* 1986). These and similar techniques have been used primarily to study the influence of vasopressin (Zimmerhackl *et al.* 1985; Kiberd *et al.* 1987*a*) and prostaglandin (Lemley *et al.* 1984) on inner medullary blood flow.

Factors affecting the renal circulation

α-Adrenoceptors

Morphological and histochemical studies have demonstrated that the kidney has a dense sympathetic innervation (Barajas 1978) which, together with the renin-angiotensin system, is probably the most important system involved in the acute regulation of renal blood flow. Adrenergic nerve fibres and terminals are associated with all the major blood vessels of the kidney, including the interlobular arteries and the afferent and efferent arterioles (Barajas 1978). Radioligand binding studies have revealed the existence of α_1, α_2, β, and β_2 receptors in the kidney (McPherson and Summers 1983; Summers and Kuhar 1983; Summers 1984), however, there appears to be a substantial species difference with regard to the number, proportion, and intrarenal distribution of the various receptor subtypes (Summers 1984).

Stimulation of α-adrenoceptors in the kidney either by renal nerve stimulation (Kon and Ichikawa, 1983) or by infusion of α-adrenoceptor agonists (Myers *et al.* 1975) results in a decrease in renal blood flow, an increase in renal vascular resistance, and a decrease in the glomerular ultrafiltration coefficient. The renal vascular effects of α-adrenoceptor stimulation appear to be mediated predominantly, if not exclusively by activation of α_1-adrenoceptors (DiBona 1982; Summers 1984), however, under some circumstances, a small α_2-adrenoceptor-mediated vasoconstriction can be observed in some species (Hesse and Johns 1984). Direct study of rabbit glomerular arterioles *in vitro* has shown that noradrenaline and the α_1-selective agonist, phenylephrine, contract both the afferent and efferent arterioles (Edwards and Trizna 1988). The selective α_2-adrenoceptor agonist, B-HT 933, had no effect on the arterioles. Furthermore, the contractile effects of noradrenaline were antagonized by the selective α_1-adrenoceptor antagonist, prazosin, but not by raulwoscine, a selective α_2-receptor antagonist. α_1-Adrenoceptor-mediated contraction of both the afferent and efferent arterioles may explain the near constancy of glomerular filtration rate, despite a reduction of renal blood flow that occurs following α-adrenergic stimulation *in vivo* (DiBona 1982).

Although postsynaptic α_2-adrenoceptors are present in the kidney, they do not appear to participate in an important way to the regulation of renal blood flow. Rather, they appear to inhibit hormone-induced activation of adenylate cyclase at the tubular (Edwards and Gellai 1988) and glomerular level (Umemura *et al.* 1986) and also inhibit renin release (Pettinger *et al.* 1976). Significant species differences exist in some of these responses (Brooks *et al.* 1991*b*,*c*; Edwards *et al.* 1992*b*).

β-Adrenoceptors

Activation of renal vascular β-adrenoceptors results in vasodilatation and a decrease in renal vascular resistance (Insel and Snavely 1981). However, α-adrenoceptors appear to greatly outnumber β-adrenoceptors, and β-adrenoceptor-mediated vasodilatation occurs to a lesser degree in the kidney than in other vascular beds (Insel and Snavely 1981). β-Adrenoceptors can, however, indirectly influence renal haemodynamics by their role in the release of renin from the juxtaglomerular apparatus. Stimulation of renal nerves under conditions that do not affect renal perfusion pressure, renal blood flow, or glomerular filtration rate results in renin release (Osborn *et al.* 1981). Renal β-adrenoceptors can also be stimulated by infusions of dopamine (see below).

Cholinergic receptors

Muscarinic cholinergic receptors have been identified in the renal vasculature (Edwards 1985*b*), glomeruli (Torres *et al.* 1978; Edwards *et al.* 1992*b*), and certain tubule segments (Snyder *et al.* 1991). Acetylcholine increases renal blood flow *in vivo* (Baylis *et al.* 1976) and causes both afferent and efferent relaxation *in vitro* (Edwards *et al.* 1985*b*). The physiological relevance of these receptors, however, is not clear since the existence of a distinct cholinergic innervation of the kidney is controversial (DiBona 1982).

Dopamine

Dopamine receptors of both the DA_1 and DA_2 subtypes have been identified in the kidney (Felder *et al.* 1984*a,b*). At low concentrations, dopamine stimulates both DA_1 and DA_2 receptors in the kidney (Goldberg 1972; Goldberg *et al.* 1978) and thus, at low infusion rates (0.5–2 µg/kg·min in humans) dopamine leads to renal vasodilatation and a natriuresis. These responses likely involve both vascular and proximal tubular dopamine receptors. At higher concentrations, dopamine activates systemic and renal β-adrenoceptors and thus, infusion rates of 2–4 µg/kg·min increase cardiac output. At higher infusion rates (>4 µg/kg ·min), dopamine activates alpha adrenoceptors and overrides the initial vasodilatation and causes alpha adrenoceptor-mediated vasoconstriction. Modification of the phenethylamine structure of dopamine produced a series of compounds, one of which, fenoldopam, produces selective activation of dopamine DA_1 receptors (Nichols *et al.* 1990). *In vitro* fenoldopam, like dopamine, relaxes afferent and efferent arterioles in both the rat (Steinhausen *et al.* 1986) and rabbit (Edwards 1985*b*, 1986). *In vivo*, stimulation of dopamine DA_1 receptors with fenoldopam (Brooks *et al.* 1990*d*; Nichols *et al.* 1992) or a fenoldopam prodrug (Brooks *et al.* 1990*b*) results in a significant increase in renal blood flow. Low dose dopamine is used clinically in cases of oliguric acute renal failure (Parker *et al.* 1981) and higher doses can help maintain blood pressure without compromising renal blood flow. Pre-clinical studies have demonstrated that stimulation of renal dopamine receptors with fenoldopam or a fenoldopam prodrug is beneficial in both amphotericin B (Brooks *et al.* 1991d; Nichols *et al.* 1992) and cyclosporine A (Brooks *et al.* 1990c) nephrotoxicity.

Histamine

Both H_1 and H_2 histamine receptors have been identified in the renal vasculature (Banks *et al.* 1978; Ichikawa and Brenner 1979) and glomerulus (Torres *et al.* 1978). Infusion of histamine increases renal blood flow with little change in glomerular filtration rate (Ichikawa and Brenner 1979). Histamine also decreases the glomerular ultrafiltration coefficient (Ichikawa and Brenner 1979) and stimulates cAMP formation in the glomerulus via the H_2 receptor (Torres *et al.* 1978), supporting a role for a direct glomerular action of histamine.

5-Hydroxytryptamine (5-HT)

The renal vascular effects of 5-HT are complex and often contradictory. 5-HT has been shown to both vasoconstrict and to vasodilate renal vessels (Charlton *et al.* 1984; Blackshear *et al.* 1986,1991; Wright and Angus 1987; Verbeuren *et al.* 1991). Whether these conflicting results are due to species differences or the presence of multiple 5-HT receptor subtypes remains to be determined. In the rat, 5-HT and 5-HT agonists decrease renal blood flow in conscious (Janssen *et al.* 1989; Zink *et al.* 1990) and anaesthetized preparations (Ding *et al.* 1989) as well as in the isolated perfused kidney (Charlton *et al.* 1984; Janssen and van Nueten 1986). This vasoconstrictor action of 5-HT appears to be due to activation of $5-HT_2$ receptors (Alper 1990; Lameire *et al.* 1990; Zink *et al.* 1990). Similar $5-HT_2$-induced decreases in renal blood flow have been observed in the rabbit (Ikeda *et al.* 1987; Wright and Angus 1987), although 5-HT-mediated contraction of isolated rabbit renal arteries appears to be due to stimulation of $5-HT_1$ receptors (Tadipatri *et al.* 1991). Intrarenal administration of 5-HT to anaesthetized dogs transiently decreased the increased renal blood flow (Blackshear *et al.* 1986; Shoji *et al.* 1989; Takahashi *et al.* 1991). In one study (Blackshear *et al.* 1986) it was concluded that the 5-HT-mediated decrease in dog renal blood flow was due to $5-HT_2$ receptors, while the increase in renal blood flow was attributed to $5-HT_1$-like receptors. The opposite conclusions were reached in another study (Shoji *et al.* 1989). Erdlich *et al.* (1993) have conducted a detailed study of the effects of 5-HT on the microvasculature of the hydronephrotic rat kidney. They observed that 5-HT contracted the large intrarenal arteries such as the arcuate artery but caused vasodilatation of the interlobular and afferent arterioles. The $5-HT_2$ receptor antagonist, ritanserin, given alone, dilated all preglomerular vessels, suggesting the presence of endogenous 5-HT tone. Ritanserin also blocked all the vascular effects of 5-HT. Finally, pre-treatment of the kidney with indomethacin inhibited the vasoconstriction of the large intrarenal vessels but had no effect on the vasodilatation observed in the small preglomerular vessels. They interpreted their results as showing that 5-HT contracts large intrarenal vessels via a $5-HT_2$ receptor and that this action of 5-HT is modulated by the prostaglandin system. Although no direct data were given, they inferred that the

5-HT-induced vasodilatation of the small preglomerular vessels was due to activation of 5-HT$_1$ receptors.

Angiotensin

Angiotensin II in its capacity as a regulator of cardiovascular function has a number of direct and indirect actions on the kidney. Indeed, the primary role of the kidney in determining long-term blood pressure involves angiotensin II receptors. Recently, the synthesis of highly selective nonpeptide angiotensin II receptor antagonists and the expression cloning of the angiotensin receptor have demonstrated the existence of at least two angiotensin II receptor subtypes, designated as AT$_1$ and AT$_2$. Autoradiography and ligand binding studies have shown that the kidney has a mixture of both receptor subtypes. The AT$_1$ receptor is coupled via G proteins to traditional signal transduction mechanisms such as stimulation of phospholipase C, Ca^{2+} mobilization, and inhibition of adenylate cyclase. The AT$_2$ receptor does not appear to be coupled to G proteins, and the signal transduction pathway(s) associated with this receptor is not known but may involve cGMP. In the kidney, as in the periphery, all of the major physiological actions of angiotensin II appear to be mediated by activation of the AT$_1$ receptor. Infusion of angiotensin II in a number of species elicits a dose-dependent decrease in renal blood flow with smaller and more variable effects on glomerular filtration rate (Navar and Rosivall 1984). Since filtration fraction increases, it has been proposed that angiotensin II preferentially increases efferent arteriolar resistance (Hall *et al.* 1977). This notion is supported by *in vitro* studies in which isolated rabbit afferent arterioles failed to respond to angiotensin II, whereas efferent arterioles were highly sensitive to the vasoconstrictor effects of angiotensin II (Edwards 1983). Morphometric analysis of vascular casts of rabbit renal arterioles also indicate a greater effect of angiotensin II on efferent arteriolar resistance (Denton *et al.* 1992). The idea of angiotensin II having greater vasoconstrictor activity in the efferent arteriole is controversial and has been challenged (Carmines *et al.* 1986), and recent studies have indicated that if rabbit arterioles are dissected with glomeruli attached, they are capable of responding to angiotensin II; however, the vasoconstrictor response to angiotensin II is largely eliminated by removal of the glomerulus and the distal portion of the afferent arteriole (Weihprecht *et al.* 1991). These studies may explain why under certain conditions, angiotensin II may also increase preglomerular resistance (Navar and Rosivall 1984). Thus, when angiotensin II is infused during inhibition of prostaglandin synthesis, the vasoconstrictor effect of angiotensin II, especially on preglomerular resistance vessels, is most pronounced (Baylis and Brenner 1978). Therefore, the alteration of renal haemodynamics observed with angiotensin II may depend in part on the status of other intrarenal hormone systems. Angiotensin II plays an important role in controlling renal function and particularly glomerular filtration (Hall *et al.* 1977; Brooks *et al.* 1992*a*), however, it also is an important factor in hypertension, congestive heart failure and possibly chronic renal failure. Angiotensin converting enzyme inhibitors as well as the newly discovered nonpeptide angiotensin II antagonists (Timmermans et al. 1991, Brooks et al. 1992b) are potent antihypertensive agents.

Vasopressin

Under normal physiological conditions, the kidney appears to be relatively insensitive to the vasoconstrictor action of vasopressin. This may be due to vasopressin-induced intrarenal formation of vasodilatory prostaglandins which attenuate the vasoconstrictor action of the peptide (Yared et al. 1985). Cyclo-oxygenase inhibition unmasks the renal vascular effects of vasopressin and vasopressin antagonists (Cooper and Malik 1984; Yared et al. 1985). In vitro studies in the rabbit have shown that vasopressin elicits a concentration-dependent contraction of efferent but not afferent arterioles (Edwards et al. 1989). This effect of vasopressin was blocked by V_1 but not V_2 receptor antagonists. Physiological concentrations of vasopressin have been shown to reduce inner medullary blood flow without altering renal blood flow or glomerular filtration rate (Zimmerhackl et al. 1985; Kiberd et al. 1987b). There appears to be both a non-vascular V_2 component as well as a vascular V_1 component to the observed vasopressin-induced decrease in medullary blood flow. V_2 receptors indirectly decrease medullary flow as a consequence of a reduction in capillary intake of reabsorbed fluid from the collecting ducts (Kiberd et al. 1987b), however, V_1 receptor antagonists attenuate vasopressin-induced decreases in medullary blood flow (Zimmerhackl et al. 1985), suggesting a direct vascular effect of vasopressin in this portion of the renal microvasculature. There is little evidence that vasopressin-induced effects on the renal vasculature have any pathophysiological role (Brooks et al. 1990e).

Bradykinin

Bradykinin is a potent renal vasodilator, increasing renal blood flow without altering glomerular filtration rate (Baylis et al. 1976). All the components of the kallikrein-kinin system are present in the kidney (Orstavik and Inagami 1982) and it is likely that bradykinin acts in a paracrine or autocrine manner in the kidney. This is supported by the observation showing that bradykinin receptor antagonists reduce renal blood flow under conditions known to activate the renal kallikrein-kinin system (Beierwaltes et al. 1988). Both the B_1 and B_2 bradykinin receptor subtypes appear to be involved in the vasodilatation produced by bradykinin (Regoli and Barabe 1980). In addition to a direct action on the renal microvasculature, bradykinin is a potent stimulus of renal prostaglandin synthesis (Flamenbaum et al. 1979) which appears to be mediated by the B_2 receptor (Regoli and Barabe 1980). Increased vasodilatory prostaglandin synthesis may, in part, account for some of the vascular and non-vascular effects of bradykinin in the kidney (Nasjletti and Malik 1981).

Bradykinin appears to influence medullary blood flow since bradykinin receptor blockade reduces papillary blood flow, while inhibition of bradykinin degradation increases papillary blood flow (Roman et al. 1988). There is little information on the sites of action of bradykinin in the renal microcirculation. In the rabbit, bradykinin was shown to relax only efferent arterioles (Edwards 1985b), while in the rat split hydronephrotic kidney model, bradykinin appears to relax both afferent and efferent arterioles (Carmines and Fleming 1990).

Atrial natriuretic peptide

Autoradiography has localized receptors for atrial natriuretic peptide (ANP) in the glomerulus and most of the renal microvasculature including the inner medullary circulation (Chai *et al.* 1986; Healy and Fanestil 1986). While it appears that the natriuretic and diuretic actions of ANP are not totally dependent on the haemodynamic effects of the peptide, ANP has been shown to exert direct effects on the renal vasculature. ANP increases medullary blood flow with little change in outer cortical blood flow or whole kidney blood flow (Kiberd *et al.* 1987; Takezawa *et al.* 1987) and may contribute to the natriuretic and diuretic actions of the peptide. Micropuncture studies have shown that ANP increases single nephron glomerular filtration rate without significantly altering glomerular plasma flow (Carmines and Fleming 1990), suggesting a preglomerular vasodilatation coupled with postglomerular vasoconstriction. Direct microvascular studies have shown that ANP relaxes afferent arterioles from dogs (Ohishi *et al.* 1988) but not rabbits (Edwards and Weidley 1987). Preglomerular vasodilatory responses to ANP have also been observed in the rat *in vitro* juxtamedullary preparation (Veldkamp *et al.* 1988) and in the rat split hydronephrotic kidney model (Marin-Gerz 1986). In this latter preparation, ANP was also observed to cause efferent arteriolar vasoconstriction but only at peptide concentrations 1000 times that needed to cause preglomerular vasodilatation. Thus, it appears that the major vascular action of ANP in the kidney is localized to the preglomerular microvasculature.

Endothelin

Endothelin (ET) is a potent renal vasoconstrictor. Intravenous administration of ET causes a long lasting increase in systemic arterial pressure and profound decreases in renal blood flow and glomerular filtration rate (Goetz *et al.* 1988; King *et al.* 1989). Micropuncture studies in the rat have shown that ET increases both preglomerular and postglomerular resistance (Badr *et al.* 1989; King *et al.* 1989; Kon *et al.* 1989). Studies designed to assess directly the renal microvascular effects of ET have yielded results in agreement with the micropuncture studies. Thus, in rabbit (Edwards *et al.* 1990) and rat (Yuan *et al.* 1990), ET-1 causes concentration-dependent contraction of both afferent and efferent arterioles *in vitro*. Similarly, in the rat hydronephrotic kidney (Loutzenhiser *et al.* 1990), ET-1 contracted both afferent and efferent arterioles. Interestingly, in both the rat (Loutzenhiser *et al.* 1990) and rabbit (Edwards *et al.* 1990), the contractile effects of ET-1 could be attenuated by Ca^{2+} channel antagonists in the afferent but not the efferent arteriole. These results suggest that Ca^{2+} entry through voltage-gated channels play an important role in ET-induced contraction of afferent arterioles but that Ca^{2+} from other sources, presumably intracellular stores, is required to support ET-induced contraction of efferent arterioles.

Binding studies have demonstrated that both ET_A and ET_B receptor subtypes are present in the kidney, although their relative distribution within the kidney and between species may vary. In canine cortical, medullary and papillary membranes, the ratio of ET_A to ET_B receptor subtypes is 20:80, 40:60, and 50:50, respectively (Brooks et al. 1994). In the rat kidney cortex there appears to be a higher proportion of ET_A receptors than in the dog (Nambi et al. 1992). There may also be species differences in ET receptor subtype function. Thus, ET-1-mediated vasoconstriction in the dog is mediated by the ET_A subtype (Brooks et al. 1994), whereas in the rat it appears to be mediated by ET_B receptors (Cristol et al. 1993; Pollock and Opgenforth 1993). In the rat, activation of ET_B receptors also increases glomerular cGMP via an L-arginine-dependent pathway (Edwards et al. 1992a). In addition to being a potent constrictor of the renal vasculature, endothelin may have tubular and mesangial cell proliferative effects which could be important in certain renal diseases. Evidence is growing that endothelin production, metabolism, and receptor number may be altered in such diseases as chronic renal failure (Brooks et al. 1991a), cyclosporine nephrotoxicity (Nambi et al. 1990; Brooks et al. 1991e), and acute renal failure (Nambi et al. 1993).

Adenosine

Adenosine, which in most organs is a vasorelaxant, is a potent renal vasoconstrictor. When injected directly into the renal artery, adenosine causes a dramatic fall in renal blood flow, however, if administered as a continuous infusion, adenosine will have a biphasic effect, causing an initial vasoconstriction and subsequent modest increase in blood flow (Spielman and Thompson 1982; Spielman and Arend 1991). In addition to decreasing renal blood flow, adenosine will cause a fall in glomerular filtration rate, a response associated with increased preglomerular and decreased postglomerular resistances. Adenosine has effects on renin release, tubular salt, and water reabsorption and appears to be an important mediator of the tubuloglomerular feedback mechanism. Adenosine receptors have been classified into two subtypes. The A1 (high affinity) subtype, which inhibits adenyl cyclase, and the A2 (low affinity) subtype, which stimulates adenyl cyclase. The kidney contains both A1 and A2 receptor subtypes but unlike other organs, both receptor subtypes may exist on the same cell (Spielman and Arend 1991). Adenosine-induced vasoconstriction has been reported to be mediated by the A1 receptor subtype and the vasodilatation by the low affinity A2 subtype (Murray and Churchill 1985; Rossi et al. 1988).

EDRF

Production of nitric oxide from L-arginine in renal endothelial cells plays an important role in the renal circulation. The vascular smooth muscle, juxtaglomerular apparatus, mesangium, and renal tubular cells respond to EDRF. In animals, EDRF-induced renal vasodilatation appears to be an important component of acetylcholine and bradykinin-induced increases in renal blood flow. In isolated renal arteries and arterioles EDRF is a potent vasodilator and mediates the relaxation induced by a number of agents including acetylcholine (Lüscher and Bock 1991; Romero *et al.* 1992). Inhibition of nitric oxide synthase with agents such as L-NMMA or L-NAME leads to decreased renal blood flow and increased renal vascular resistance, indicating an important role for EDRF in renal function. Chronic inhibition of nitric oxide synthase causes hypertension and renal failure (Baylis *et al.* 1992).

Amino acids

It has been known for many years that infusion of amino acids or indeed ingestion of a protein meal increases renal blood flow and glomerular filtration rate (Premen 1988). The hyperaemia induced by high protein meal is thought to be due to a subsequent elevation of plasma amino acid concentration, especially glycine. It is not clear what the mediators of amino acid-induced renal hyperfiltration are, however, evidence suggests that glucoregulatory hormones, prostaglandins, endothelium-derived relaxing factor, dopamine, and/or the renin-angiotensin system may be involved (Premen 1988; Wang and Brooks 1992*b*). It has been suggested that inhibition of the tubuloglomerular feedback mechanism may also be involved in amino acid-induced hyperaemia and hyperfiltration (Premen 1988). Consistent with this hypothesis is the observation that pharmacological inactivation of the TDF mechanism with a dopamine DA_1 receptor agonist (Wang *et al.* 1992) or inhibition of adenosine A-1 receptors (Wang and Brooks 1992*b*), or the renin-angiotensin system (Wang and Brooks 1992*a*) inhibit amino acid-induced hyperfiltration and not hyperaemia. Reduction in amino acid-induced changes in the renal vasculature by reducing dietary protein intake has been proposed as a treatment for chronic renal failure (Mitch 1991).

Eicosanoids

Many studies have established that arachidonic acid metabolites, mainly PGE_2 and PGI_2, are potent renal vasodilators and participate in the control of renal blood flow (Walker and Fröhlich 1987). Under normal conditions, prostaglandins do not appear to contribute in a major way in the control of renal blood flow. However, in pathological states, or when vasoconstrictor tone is increased as a consequence of increased sympathetic drive to the kidney or increased formation of AII, prostaglandin synthesis is enhanced. The prostaglandins thus formed attenuate the action of the vasoconstrictors and serve to maintain renal blood flow. Evidence in support of this view are the findings that vasoconstrictors such as AII stimulate prostaglandin synthesis in renal arterioles (Chaudhari and Kirschenbaum 1988; Hura and Kunau 1988), and that cyclo-oxygenase inhibitors enhance the renal vasoconstrictor effects of noradrenaline and AII (Baylis and Brenner 1978). Furthermore, direct application of arachidonic acid on noradrenaline contracted renal arterioles *in vitro* results in a rapid relaxation that is blocked by meclofenamate (Edwards 1985*a*). Both PGE_2 and PGI_2 relax afferent and efferent arterioles contracted with noradrenaline or AII (Edwards 1985*a*). In addition, direct observation of the inner medullary microcirculation revealed a significant reduction in red blood cell velocity following indomethacin of meclofenamate (Lemley et al. 1984). Inhibition of cyclo-oxygenase can be detrimental to renal failure (DiBona 1986), however, administration of the PGE_2 analogue, misoprostal, improves renal function in renal transplant recipients treated with cyclosporine (Moran et al. 1990).

Other arachidonic acid metabolites with renal effects include the thromboxanes, leukotrienes, and lipoxins. Thromboxane A_2 is formed from cyclic endoperoxide by thromboxane A_2 synthase, both in the periphery by platelets and by renal tissue, and is a potent renal vasoconstrictor and contracts mesangial cells (Lote and Haylor 1989). There is little evidence for a physiological role for thromboxane in renal function, however, measurement of increased thromboxane production and the use of thromboxane synthase inhibitors and receptor antagonists have indicated that thromboxane may play a role in the pathophysiology of a number of renal diseases, including renal uretral obstruction (Morrison et al. 1977; Klotman et al. 1986), cyclosporine nephrotoxicity (Benigni et al. 1988; Spurney et al. 1990), renal transplant rejection (Perico et al. 1992), and ablation-induced chronic renal failure (Purkerson et al. 1985). It should be noted, however, that the role of thromboxane in chronic renal failure is controversial (Brooks et al. 1990a).

Leukotrienes have significant indirect and direct effects on the renal vasculature. Given systemically, LTC_4 causes a reduction in renal blood flow which is in part due to a reduction in cardiac output (Badr et al. 1984). It also reduces plasma volume and results in haemoconcentration (Badr et al. 1984). In the perfused kidney both LTC_4 and D_4 result in potent vasoconstriction (Rosenthal and Pace-Asciak 1983), and micropuncture studies have indicated that leukotrienes result in a significant increase in efferent arteriolar resistance, with an associated fall in glomerular plasma flow, and an increase in glomerular capillary hydraulic pressure (Badr et al. 1987). As with the thromboxanes, increased production and use of receptor antagonists and synthesis inhibitors have provided evidence for the importance of leukotrienes in renal disease, particularly ureteral obstruction-induced hydronephrosis (Albrightson et al. 1987) and lupus nephritis (Spurney et al. 1991).

Finally, it has been shown recently that lipoxins which are lipoxygenase products involved in glomerular inflammation have significant effects on the renal vasculature. Thus, lipoxin A causes a cyclo-oxygenase-dependent increase in renal blood flow and GFR, while lipoxin B4 and 7-cys-11-trans lipoxan A4 decreases both renal blood flow and GFR. The decrease in renal blood flow and GFR induced by 7-cys-11-trans lipoxan A4 may be mediated by LTD_4 (Katoh et al. 1992).

ACKNOWLEDGEMENT

The authors are grateful to Sue Tirri for preparing this manuscript.

REFERENCES

Albrightson, C. R., Evers, A. S., Griffin, A. C., and Needleman, P. (1987). Effect of endogenously produced leukotrienes and thromboxane on renal vascular resistance in rabbit hydronephrosis. *Circ. Res.*, **61**, 514–22.

Alper, R. H. (1990). Hemodynamic and renin responses to (±)-DOI, a selective 5-HT$_2$ receptor agonist in conscious rats. *Eur. J. Pharmacol.*, **175**, 323–32.

Badr, K. F., Baylis, C., Pfeffer, J. M., Pfeffer, M. A., Soberman, R. J., Lewis, R. A., et al. (1984). Renal and systemic hemodynamic responses to intravenous infusion of leukotriene C$_4$ in the rat. *Cir. Res.*, **54**, 492–9.

Badr, K. F., Brenner, B. M., and Ichikawa, I. (1987). Effects of leukotriene D$_4$ on glomerular dynamics in the rat. *Am. J. Physiol.*, **253**, F239–43.

Badr, K. F., Murray, J. J., Breyer, M. D., Takahashi, K., Inagami, T., and Harris, R. C. (1989). Mesangial cell, glomerular and renal vascular responses to endothelin in the rat kidney. *J. Clin. Invest.*, **83**, 336–42.

Banks, R. O., Fondacaro, J. D., Schwaiger, M. M., and Jacobson, E. D. (1978). Renal histamine H$_1$ and H$_2$ receptors: characterization and functional significance. *Am. J. Physiol.*, **235**, F570–5.

Barajas, L. (1978). Innervation of the renal cortex. *Fed. Proc.*, **37**, 1192–201.

Baylis, C. and Brenner, B. M. (1978). Modulation by prostaglandin synthesis inhibitors of the action of exogenous angiotensin II on glomerular ultrafiltration in the rat. *Circ. Res.*, **43**, 889–98.

Baylis, C., Deen, W. M., Myers, B. D., and Brenner, B. M. (1976). Effects of some vasodilator drugs on transcapillary fluid exchange in renal cortex. *Am. J. Physiol.*, **230**, 1148–58.

Baylis, C., Mitruka, B., and Deng, A. (1992). Chronic blockade of nitric oxide synthesis in the rat produces systemic hypertension and glomerular damage. *J. Clin. Invest.*, **90**, 278–81.

Beierwaltes, W. H., Carretero, O. A., and Scicli, A. G. (1988). Renal hemodynamics in response to a kinin analogue antagonist. *Am. J. Physiol.*, **255**, F408–14.

Benigni, A., Chiabrando, C., Piccinelli, A., Perico, N., Gavinelli, M., Furci, L., et al. (1988). Increased urinary excretion of thromboxane B$_2$ and 2,3-dinor-TxB$_2$ in cyclosporin A nephrotoxicity. *Kidney Int.*, **34**, 164–74.

Blackshear, J. L., Orlandi, C., and Hollenberg, N. K. (1986). Serotonin and the renal blood supply: Role of prostaglandins and the 5-HT$_2$ receptor. *Kidney Int.*, **30**, 304–10.

Blackshear, J. L., Orlandi, C., and Hollenberg, N. K. (1991). Constrictive effect of serotonin on visible renal arteries: A pharmacoangiographic study in anesthetized dogs. *J. Cardiovasc. Pharmacol.*, **17**, 68–73.

Brooks, D. P., Contino, L. C., Trizna, W., Edwards, R. M., Ohlstein, E. H., and Solleveld, H. A. (1990*a*). Effect of enalapril or the thromboxane receptor antagonist, daltroban, in rats with subtotal renal ablation. *J. Pharmacol. Exp. Ther.*, **253**, 119–23.

Brooks, D. P., DePalma, P. D., Cyronak, M. J., Bryant, M. A., Karpinski, K., Mico, B., et al. (1990*b*). Identification of fenoldopam prodrugs with prolonged renal vasodilator activity. *J. Pharmacol. Exp. Ther.*, **254**, 1084–9.

Brooks, D. P., Drutz, D. J., and Ruffolo, R. R., Jr. (1990*c*). Prevention and complete reversal of cyclosporine A-induced renal vasoconstriction and nephrotoxicity in the rat by fenoldopam. *J. Pharmacol. Exp. Ther.*, **254**, 375–9.

Brooks, D. P., Goldstein, R., Koster, P. F., DePalma, P. D., DiCristo, M., Karpinski, K., et al. (1990*d*). Effect of fenoldopam in dogs with spontaneous renal insufficiency. *Eur. J. Pharmacol.*, **184**, 195–9.

Brooks, D. P., Solleveld, H. A., and Contino, L. C. (1990*e*). Vasopressin and the pathogenesis of chronic renal failure. *Br. J. Pharmacol.*, **100**, 79–82.

Brooks, D. P., Contino, L. C., Storer, B., and Ohlstein, E. H. (1991a). Increased endothelin excretion in rats with renal failure induced by partial nephrectomy. *Br. J. Pharmacol.*, **104**, 987-9.

Brooks, D. P., Edwards, R. M., DePalma, P. D., Fredrickson, T. A., Hieble, J. P., and Gellai, M. (1991b). The water diuretic effect of the alpha-2 adrenoceptor agonist, AGN 190851, is species-dependent. *J. Pharmacol. Exp. Ther.*, **259**, 1277-82.

Brooks, D. P., Gellai, M., DePalma, P. D., and Edwards, R. M. (1991c). Modulation of vasopressin antidiuretic action by α_2-adrenoceptors is species specific. *Am. J. Physiol.*, **261**, F1242-6.

Brooks, D. P., Mitchell, M. P., Short, B. G., Ruffolo, R. R., Jr., and Nichols, A. J. (1991d). Attenuation of amphotericin B nephrotoxicity in the dog by the fenoldopam prodrug, SK&F R105058. *J. Pharmacol. Exp. Ther.*, **257**, 1243-7.

Brooks, D. P., Ohlstein, E. H., Contino, L. C., Storer, B., Pullen, M., Caltabiano, M., et al. (1991e). Effect of nifedipine on cyclosporine A-induced nephrotoxicity, urinary endothelin excretion and renal endothelin receptor number. *Eur. J. Pharmacol.*, **194**, 115-17.

Brooks, D. P., DePalma, P. D., and Ruffolo, R. R. Jr. (1992a). Effect of captopril and the nonpeptide angiotensin II antagonists, SK&F 108566 and EXP3174, on renal function in dogs with a renal artery stenosis. *J. Pharmacol. Exp. Ther.*, **263**, 422-7.

Brooks, D. P., Fredrickson, T. A., Weinstock, J., Ruffolo, R. R., Jr., Edwards, R. M., and Gellai, M. (1992b). Antihypertensive activity of the non-peptide angiotensin II receptor antagonist, SK&F 108566, in rats and dogs. *Arch. Pharmacol.*, **345**, 673-8.

Brooks, D. P., DePalma, P. D., Pullen, M., and Nambi, P. (1994). Characterization of canine renal endothelin receptor subtypes and their function. *J. Pharmacol. Exp. Ther.*, **268**, 1091-7.

Burg, M., Grantham, J., Abramow, M., and Orloff, J. (1966). Preparation and study of fragments of single rabbit nephrons. *Am. J. Physiol.*, **210**, 1296-8.

Carmines, P. K. and Fleming, J. T. (1990). Control of the renal microvasculature by vasoactive peptides. *FASEB J.*, **4**, 3300-9.

Carmines, P. K., Morrison, T. K., and Navar, L. G. (1986). Angiotensin II effects on microvascular diameters of *in vitro* blood perfused juxtamedullary nephrons. *Am. J. Physiol.*, **251**, F610-18.

Casellas, D. and Navar, L. G. (1984). *In vitro* perfusion of juxtamedullary nephrons in rats. *Am. J. Physiol.*, **246**, F349-58.

Chai, S. Y., Sexton, P. M., Allen, A. M., Figor, R., and Mendelsohn, F. A. 0. (1986). *In vitro* autoradiographic localization of ANP receptors in rat kidney and adrenal gland. *Am. J. Physiol.*, **250**, F753-7.

Charlton, K. G., Johnson, T. D., and Clarke, D. E. (1984). Vasoconstrictor and noradrenaline potentiating action of 5-hydroxykynuramine in the isolated perfused rat kidney: Involvement of serotonin receptors and alpha$_1$-adrenoceptors. *Naunyn Schmiedebergs Arch. Pharmacol.*, **328**, 154-9.

Chaudhari, A. and Kirschenbaum, M. A. (1988). A rapid method for isolating rabbit renal microvessels. *Am. J. Physiol.*, **254**, F291-6.

Cooper, C. L. and Malik, K. U. (1984). Mechanism of action of vasopressin on prostaglandin synthesis and vascular function in the isolated rat kidney: effect of calcium antagonists and calmodulin inhibitors. *J. Pharmacol. Exp. Ther.*, **229**, 139-47.

Cristol, J.-P., Warner, T. D., Thiemermann, C., and Vane, J. R. (1993). Mediation via different receptors of the vasoconstrictor effects of endothelins and sarafotoxins in the systemic circulation and renal vasculature of the anaesthetized rat. *Br. J. Pharmacol.*, **108**, 776-9.

Denton, K. M., Fennessy, P. A., Alcorn, D., and Anderson, W. P. (1992). Morphometric analysis of the actions of angiotensin II on renal arterioles and glomeruli. *Am. J. Physiol.*, **262**, F367-72.

DiBona, G. F. (1982). The function of the renal nerves. *Rev. Physiol. Biochem. Pharmacol.*, **94**, 75-181.

DiBona, G. F. (1986). Prostaglandins and nonsteroidal anti-inflammatory drugs. Effects on renal hemodynamics. *Am. J. Med.*, **80(Suppl. 1A)**, 12-21.

Ding, X. R., Stier, C. T., and Itskovitz, H. D. (1989). Serotonin and 5-hydroxytryptophan on blood pressure and renal blood flow in anesthetized rats. *Am. J. Med. Sci.*, **297**, 290-3.

Earle, D. P. and Berliner, R. W. (1946). A simplified clinical procedure for measurement of glomerular filtration rate and renal plasma flow. *Proc. Soc. Exp. Biol.* **62**, 262-4.

Edwards, R. M. (1983). Segmental effects of noradrenaline and angiotensin II on isolated renal microvessels. *Am. J. Physiol.*, **244** F526-34.

Edwards, R. M. (1985a). Effects of prostaglandins on vasoconstrictor action in isolated renal arterioles. *Am. J. Physiol.*, **248**, F779-84.

Edwards, R. M. (1985b). Responses of isolated renal arterioles to acetylcholine, dopamine and bradykinin. *Am. J. Physiol.*, **248**, F183-9.

Edwards, R. M. (1986). Comparison of the effects of fenoldopam, SK&F R-87516 and dopamine on renal arterioles *in vitro*. *Eur. J. Pharmacol.*, **126**, 167-70.

Edwards, R. M. (1988). Direct assessment of glomerular arteriole activity. *News Physiol. Sci.*, **3**, 216-19.

Edwards, R. M. and Gellai, M. (1988). Inhibition of vasopressin-stimulated cyclic AMP accumulation by alpha-2 adrenoceptor agonists in isolated papillary collecting ducts. *J. Pharmacol. Exp. Ther.*, **244**, 526-30.

Edwards, R. M. and Trizna, W. (1988). Characterization of α-adrenoceptors on isolated rabbit renal arterioles. *Am. J. Physiol.*, **254**, F178-F83.

Edwards, R. M. and Weidley, E. F. (1987). Lack of effect of atriopeptin II on rabbit glomerular arterioles *in vitro*. *Am. J. Physiol.*, **252**, F317-21.

Edwards, R. M., Trizna, W., and Kinter, L. B. (1989). Renal microvascular effects of vasopressin and vasopressin antagonists. *Am. J. Physiol.*, **256**, F274-8.

Edwards, R. M., Trizna, W., and Ohlstein, E. H. (1990). Renal microvascular effects of endothelin. *Am. J. Physiol.*, **259**, F217-21.

Edwards, R. M., Pullen, M., and Nambi, P. (1992a). Activation of endothelin ET_B receptors increases glomerular cGMP via an L-arginine dependent pathway. *Am. J. Physiol.*, **263**, F1020-5.

Edwards, R. M., Stack, E. J., Gellai, M., and Brooks, D. P. (1992b). Inhibition of vasopressin-sensitive cAMP accumulation by α_2-adrenoceptor agonists in collecting tubules is species dependent. *Pharmacology*, **44**, 26-32.

Eknoyan, G. (1989). The origins of nephrology — Galen, the founding father of experimental renal physiology. *Am. J. Nephrol.*, **9**, 66-82.

Erdlich, K., Kühn, R., and Steinhausen, M. (1993). Visualization of serotonin effects on renal vessels of rats. *Kidney Int.*, **43**, 314-23.

Felder, R. A., Blecher, M., Calcagno, P. L., and Jose, P. A. (1984a). Dopamine receptors in the proximal tubule of the rabbit. *Am. J. Physiol.*, **247**, F499-505.

Felder, R. A., Blecher, M., Eisner, G. M., and Jose, P. A. (1984b). Cortical tubular and glomerular dopamine receptors in rat kidney. *Am. J. Physiol.*, **246**, F557-68.

Fine, L. G. (1987). Evolution of renal physiology from earliest times to William Bowman. In *Renal physiology: people and ideas* (ed. C. W. Gottschalk, R. W. Berkner, and G. H. Giebish), pp. 1-30. Am. Physiol. Soc., Bethesda, MD.

Flamenbaum, W., Gagnon, J., and Ramwell, P. (1979). Bradykinin-induced renal hemodynamic alterations: renin and prostaglandin relationships. *Am. J. Physiol.*, **237**, F433-40.

Goetz, K. L., Wang, B. C., Madwed, J. B., Zhu, J. L., and Leadley, R. J. Jr. (1988). Cardiovascular, renal and endocrine responses to intravenous endothelin in conscious dogs. *Am. J. Physiol.*, **255**, R1064-8.

Goldberg, L. (1972). Cardiovascular and renal actions of dopamine potential clinical applications. *Pharmacol. Rev.*, **24**, 1-29.

Goldberg, L., Volkman, P. H., and Kohli, J. D. (1978). A comparison of the vascular dopamine receptor with other dopamine receptors. *Annu. Rev. Pharmacol. Toxicol.*, **18**, 57-79.

Hall, J. E., Guyton, A. C., Jackson, T. E., Coleman, T. G., Lohmeier, T. E., and Trippodo, N.C. (1977). Control of glomerular filtration rate by renin-angiotensin system. *Am. J. Physiol.*, **233**, F366-72.

Haywood, J. R., Shaffer, R. A., Fastenow, C., Fink, G. D., and Brody, M. J. (1981). Regional blood flow measurement with pulsed Doppler flow meter in conscious rat. *Am. J. Physiol.*, **241**, H273-8.

Healy, D. P. and Fanestil, D. D. (1986). Localization of atrial natriuretic peptide binding sites within the rat kidney. *Am. J. Physiol.*, **250**, F573-8.

Hesse, I. F. A. and Johns, E. J. (1984). An *in vivo* study of the adrenoceptor subtypes on the renal vasculature of the anesthetized rabbit. *J. Auton. Pharmacol.*, **4**, 145-52.

Hura, C. E. and Kunau, R. T. (1988). Angiotensin II-stimulated prostaglandin production by canine renal afferent arterioles. *Am. J. Physiol.*, **254**, F734-8.

Ichikawa, I. and Brenner, B. M. (1979). Mechanism of action of histamine and histamine antagonists on the glomerular microcirculation. *Circ. Res.*, **45**, 737-45.

Ikeda, K., Takata, M., Tomoda, F., Mikawa, M., Iida, H., and Sasayama, S. (1987). Differences in vasodilating action between ketanserin, a 5-HT$_2$-serotonergic receptor antagonist, and terazosin, an alpha$_1$-adrenoceptor antagonist, in anesthetized rabbits. *J. Cardiovasc. Pharmacol.*, **10(Suppl. 3)**, S69-72.

Insel, P. A. and Snavely, M. D. (1981). Catecholamines and the kidney: receptors and renal function. *Annu. Rev. Physiol.*, **43**, 625-36.

Ito, S., Johnson, C. S., and Carretero, O. A. (1991). Modulation of angiotensin II-induced vasoconstriction by endothelium-derived relaxing factor in the isolated microperfused rabbit afferent arteriole. *J. Clin. Invest.*, **87**, 1651-63.

Janssen, W. J. and van Nueten, J. M. (1986). The direct and amplifying effects serotonin are increased with age in the isolated perfused kidney of Wistar and spontaneously hypertensive rats. *Naunyn Schmiedebergs Arch. Pharmacol.*, **334**, 327-32.

Janssen, B. J. A., van Essen, H., Struyker-Doudier, H. A. J., and Smits, J. F. M. (1989). Hemodynamic effects of activation of renal and mesenteric sensory nerves in rats. *Am. J. Physiol.*, **257**, R29-36.

Katoh, T., Takahashi, K., DeBoer, D. K., Serhan, C. N., and Badr, K. F. (1992). Renal hemodynamic actions of lipoxins in rats: a comparative physiological study. *Am. J. Physiol.*, **263**, F436-42.

Kiberd, B. A., Larson, T. S., Robertson, C. R., and Jamison, R. L. (1987*a*). Effect of atrial natriuretic peptide on vasa recta blood flow in the rat. *Am. J. Physiol.*, **252**, F1112-17.

Kiberd, B., Robertson, C. R., Larson, T., and Jamison, R. L. (1987*b*). Effect of V$_2$-receptor-mediated changes on inner medullary blood flow induced by AVP. *Am. J. Physiol.*, **253**, F576-81.

King, A. J., Brenner, B. M., and Anderson, S. (1989). Endothelin: a potent renal and systemic vasoconstrictor peptide. *Am. J. Physiol.*, **256**, F1051-8.

Klotman, P. E., Smith, S. R., Volpp, B. D., Coffman, T. M., and Yarger, W. E. (1986). Thromboxane synthetase inhibition improves function of hydronephrotic rat kidney. *Am. J. Physiol.*, **250**, F282-7.

Knox, F. G. and Spielman, W. S. (1983). Renal circulation. In *The handbook of physiology: the cardiovascular system*, (ed. F. Abboud and J. T. Shepherd), pp. 183-218. American Physiological Society, Bethesda, MD.

Kon, V. and Ichikawa, I. (1983). Effect on loci for renal nerve control of cortical microcirculation. *Am. J. Physiol.*, **245**, F545-53.

Kon, V., Yoshioka, T., Fogo, A., and Ichikawa, I. (1989). Glomerular actions of endothelin in vivo. *J. Clin. Invest.*, **83**, 1762-7.

Lameire, N. H., Matthys, E., Kesteloot, D., and Waterloos, M. A. (1990). Effect of a serotonin blocking agent on renal hemodynamics in the normal rat. *Kidney Int.*, **38**, 823-9.

Lanese, D. M., Yuan, B. H., McMurtry, I. F., and Conger, J. D. (1992). Comparative sensitivities of isolated rat renal arterioles to endothelin. *Am. J. Physiol.*, **263**, F894-9.

Lemley, K., Schmitt, J. L., Holligen, C., Dunn, M. J., Robertson, C. R., and Jamison, R. L. (1984). Prostaglandin synthesis inhibitors and vasa recta velocities in the rat. *Am. J. Physiol.*, **247**, F562-7.

Lote, A. J. and Haylor, J. (1989). Eicosanoids in renal function. *Prostag. Leuk. Essen. Fatty Acids*, **36**, 203-17.

Loutzenhiser, R., Epstein, M., Hayashi, K., and Horton, C. (1990). Direct visualization of effects of endothelin on the renal microvasculature. *Am. J. Physiol.*, **258**, F61-8.

Lüscher, T. F. and Bock, H. A. (1991). The endothelial L-arginine/nitric oxide pathway and the renal circulation. *Klin. Wochenschr.*, **69**, 603-9.

McPherson, G. A. and Summers, R. J. (1983). Evidence from binding studies for α_2-adrenoceptors directly associated with glomeruli from rat kidney. *Eur. J. Pharmacol.*, **90**, 333-41.

Marin-Gerz, M., Fleming, J. T., and Steinhausen, M. (1986). Atrial natriuretic peptide causes preglomerular vasodilatation and post-glomerular vasoconstriction in rat kidney. *Nature*, **324**, 473-41.

Mitch, W. E. (1991). Dietary protein restriction in patients with chronic renal failure. *Kidney Int.*, **40**, 326-41.

Moran, M., Mozes, M. F., Maddux, M. S., Veremis, S., Bartkus, C., Ketel, B., et al. (1990). Prevention of acute graft rejection by the prostaglandin E_1 analogue misoprostol in renal-transplant recipients treated with cyclosporine and prednisone. *N. Engl. J. Med.*, **322**, 1183-8.

Morrison, A. R., Nishikawa, K., and Needleman, P. (1977). Unmasking of thromboxane A_2 synthesis by ureteral obstruction in the rabbit kidney. *Nature*, **267**, 259-60.

Murray, R. D. and Churchill, P. C. (1985). The concentration-dependency of the renal vascular and renin secretory responses to adenosine receptor agonists. *J. Pharmacol. Exp. Ther.*, **232**, 189-93.

Myers, B. D., Deen, W. M., and Brenner, B. M. (1975). Effects of noradrenaline and angiotensin II on the determinants of glomerular ultrafiltration and proximal tubule fluid reabsorption in the rat. *Circ. Res.*, **37**, 101-10.

Nambi, P., Pullen, M., Contino, L. C., and Brooks, D. P. (1990). Upregulation of renal endothelin receptors in rats with cyclosporine A-induced nephrotoxicity. *Eur. J. Pharmacol.*, **187**, 113-16.

Nambi, P., Wu, H.-L., Pullen, M., Aiyar, N., Bryan, H., and Elliott, J. (1992). Identification of endothelin receptor subtypes in rat kidney cortex using subtype-selective ligands. *Mol. Pharmacol.*, **42**, 336-9.

Nambi, P., Pullen, M., Jugus, M., and Gellai, M. (1993). Rat kidney endothelin receptors in ischemia-induced acute renal failure. *J. Pharmacol. Exp. Ther.*, **264**, 345-8.

Nasjletti, A. and Malik, K. U. (1981), Renal kinin-prostaglandin relationship-implications for renal function. *Kidney Int.*, **19**, 860-8.

Navar, L. G. and Rosivall, L. (1984). Contribution of the renin-angiotensin system to the control of intrarenal hemodynamics. *Kidney Int.*, **25**, 857-68.

Navar, L. G., Gilmore, J. P., Joyner, W. L., Steinhausen, M., Edwards, R. M., Casellas, D., et al. (1986). Direct assessment of renal microcirculatory dynamics. *Fed. Proc.*, **45**, 2851-61.

Nichols, A. J., Ruffolo, R. R. Jr., and Brooks, D. P. (1990). The pharmacology of fenoldopam. *Am. J. Hypertens.*, **3**, 1165-95.

Nichols, A. J., Koster, P. F., Brooks, D. P., and Ruffolo, R. R. Jr. (1992). Effect of fenoldopam on the acute and subacute nephrotoxicity produced by amphotericin B in the dog. *J. Pharmacol. Exp. Ther.*, **260**, 269-74.

Ohishi, K., Hishida, A., and Honda, N. (1988). Direct vasodilatory action of atrial natriuretic factor on canine glomerular afferent arterioles. *Am. J. Physiol.*, **255**, F415-20.

Orstavik, T. B. and Inagami, T. (1982). The localization of kallikrein in the rat kidney and its anatomical relationship to renin. *J. Histochem-Cytochem.*, **39**, 385-90.

Osborn, J. L., DiBona, G. F., and Thames, M. D. (1981). Beta-1 receptor mediation of renin secretion elicited by low frequency renal nerve stimulation. *J. Pharmacol. Exp. Ther.*, **216**, 265-9.

Parker, S., Carlon, G. C., Isaacs, M., Howland, W. S., and Kehn, R. C. (1981). Dopamine administration in oliguria and oliguric renal failure. *Crit. Care Med.*, **9**, 630-2.

Perico, N., Rossini, M., Imberti, O., Malanchini, B., Comejo, R. P., Gaspari, F., et al. (1992). Thromboxane receptor blockade attenuates chronic cyclosporine nephrotoxicity and improves survival in rats with renal isograft. *J. Am. Soc. Nephrol.*, **2**, 1398-404.

Pettinger, W. A., Keeton, T. K., and Campbell, W. B. (1976). Evidence for a renal α-adrenergic receptor inhibiting renin release. *Circ. Res.*, **38**, 338-46.

Pollock, D. M. and Opgenorth, T. J. (1993). Evidence for endothelin-induced renal vasoconstriction independent of ET_A receptor activation. *Am. J. Physiol.*, **264**, R222-6.

Premen, A. J. (1988). Potential mechanisms mediating postprandial renal hyperemia and hyperfiltration. *FASEB J.*, **2**, 131-7.

Purkerson, M. L., Joist, J. H., Yates, J., Valdes, A., Morrison, A., and Klahr, S. (1985). Inhibition of thromboxane synthesis ameliorates the progressive kidney disease of rats with subtotal renal ablation. *Proc. Natl. Acad. Sci. USA*, **82**, 193-7.

Regoli, D. and Barabe, J. (1980). Pharmacology of bradykinin and related kinins. *Pharmacol. Rev.*, **32**, 1-46.

Roman, R. J., Kaldunski, M. L., Scicli, A. G., and Carretero, O. A. (1988). Influence of kinins and angiotensin II on the regulation of papillary blood flow. *Am. J. Physiol.*, **255**, F690-8.

Romero, J. C., Lahera, V., Salom, M. G., and Biondi, M. L. (1992). Role of the endothelium-dependent relaxing factor nitric oxide on renal function. *J. Am. Soc. Nephrol.*, **2**, 1371-87.

Rosenthal, A. and Pace-Asciak, C. R. (1983). Potent vasoconstriction of the isolated perfused rat kidney by leukotrienes C_4 and D_4. *Can. J. Physiol. Pharmacol.*, **61**, 325-8.

Rossi, N. F., Churchill, P. C., and Amore, B. (1988). Mechanism of adenosine receptor induced renal vasoconstriction in the rat. *Am. J. Physiol.*, **255**, H885-90.

Shoji, T., Tamaki, T., Fukui, K., Iwao, H., and Abe, Y. (1989). Renal hemodynamic responses to 5-hydroxytryptamine (5-HT): Involvement of the 5-HT receptor subtypes in the canine kidney. *Eur. J. Pharmacol.*, **171**, 219-8.

Smith, H. W., Findelstein, N., Aliminosa, L., Crawford, B., and Graber, M. (1945). The renal clearances of substituted hippuric acid derivatives and other aromatic acids in dogs and man. *J. Clin. Invest.*, **42**, 388-404.

Snyder, H. M., Fredin, D. M., and Breyer, M. D. (1991). Muscarinic receptor activation inhibits AVP-induced water flow in rabbit cortical collecting ducts. *Am. J. Physiol.*, **260**, F929-36.

Sommer, G., Noorbehesht, B., Pelc, N., Jamison, R., Pinevich, A. J., Newton, L., *et al.* (1992). Normal renal blood flow measurement using phase-contrast cine magnetic resonance imaging. *Inv. Rad.*, **27**, 465-70.

Spielman, W. S. and Arend, L. J. (1991). Adenosine receptors and signaling in the kidney. *Hypertension*, **17**, 117-30.

Spielman, W. S. and Thompson, C. I. (1982). A proposed role for adenosine in the regulation of renal hemodynamics and renin release. *Am. J. Physiol.*, **242**, F423-35.

Spurney, R. F., Mavros, S. D., Collins, D., Ruiz, P., Klotman, P. E., and Coffman, T. (1990). Thromboxane receptor blockade improves cyclosporine nephrotoxicity in rats. *Prostaglandins*, **39**, 135-46.

Spurney, R. F., Ruiz, P., Pisetsky, D. S., and Coffman, T. M. (1991). Enhanced renal leukotriene production in murine lupus: role of lipoxygenase metabolites. *Kidney Int.*, **39**, 95-102.

Steinhausen, M., Snoei, H., Parekh, N., Baker, R., and Johnson, P. C. (1983). Hydronephrosis: a new method to visualize vas afferens, efferens and glomerular network. *Kidney Int.*, **23**, 794-806.

Steinhausen, M., Weis, S., Fleming, J., Dussel, R., and Parekh, N. (1986). Responses of *in vivo* renal microvessels to dopamine. *Kidney Int.*, **30**, 361-70.

Summers, R. J. (1984). Renal α-adrenoceptors. *Fed. Proc.*, **43**, 2917-22.

Summers, R. J. and Kuhar, M. J. (1983). Autoradiographic localization of β-adrenoceptors in rat kidney. *Eur. J. Pharmacol.*, **91**, 305-10.

Tadipatri, S., Van Heuven-Nolsen, D., Feniuk, W., and Saxena, P. R. (1991). Analysis of the 5-HT receptors mediating contractions in the rabbit isolated renal artery. *Br. J. Pharmacol.*, **104**, 887-94.

Takahashi, T., Hisa, H., and Satoh, S. (1991). Serotonin-induced renin release in the dog kidney. *Eur. J. Pharmacol.*, **193**, 315-20.

Takezawa, K., Cowley, A. W., Jr., Skelton, M., and Roman, R. J. (1987). Atriopeptin III alters renal medullary hemodynamics and the pressure-diuresis response in rats. *Am. J. Physiol.*, **252**, F992-1002.

Thurau, K., Davis, J. M., and Häberle, D. A. (1987). Renal blood flow and dynamics of glomerular filtration. Evolution of a concept from Carl Ludwig to the present day. In *Renal physiology: people and ideas* (ed. C. W. Gottschalk, R. W. Berkner, and G. H. Giebish), pp. 31-62, Am. Physiol. Soc., Bethesda, MD.

Timmermans, P. B. M. W. M., Wong, P. C., Chiu, A. T., and Herblin, W. F. (1991). Nonpeptide angiotensin II receptor antagonists. *Trends Pharm. Sci.*, **12**, 55-61.

Torres, V. E., Northrup, T. E., Edwards, R. M., Shah, S. V. and Dousa, T. P. (1978). Modulation of cyclic nucleotides in isolated rat glomeruli. *J. Clin Invest.*, **62**, 1334-43.

Umemura, S., Smyth, D. D., and Pettinger, W. A. (1986). α-Adrenoceptor stimulation and cellular cAMP levels in microdissected rat glomeruli. *Am. J. Physiol.*, **250**, F103-8.

Veldkamp, P. J., Carmines, P. K., Inscho, E. W., and Navar, L. G. (1988). Direct evaluation of the microvascular actions of ANP in juxtamedullary nephrons. *Am. J. Physiol.*, **254**, F440-4.

Verbeuren, T. J., Mennecier, P. and Laubie, M. (1991). 5-hydroxytryptamine-induced vasodilatation in the isolated perfused rat kidney: Are endothelial 5-HT$_{1A}$ receptors involved? *Eur. J. Pharmacol.*, **201**, 17-27.

Walker, L. A. and Frölich, J. C. (1987). Renal prostaglandins and leukotrienes. *Rev. Physiol. Biochem. Pharmacol.*, **107**, 1-72.

Wang, Y.-X. and Brooks, D. P. (1992*a*). Renin-angiotensin system inhibition reduces glycine-induced glomerular hyperfiltration in conscious rats. *J. Pharmacol. Exp. Ther.*, **261**, 95-100.

Wang, Y.-X. and Brooks, D. P. (1992*b*). The role of adenosine in glycine-induced glomerular hyperfiltration in rats. *J. Pharmacol. Exp. Ther.*, **263**, 1188-94.

Wang, Y.-X., Gellai, M. and Brooks, D. P. (1992). Dopamine DA_1 receptor agonist, fenoldopam, reverses glycine-induced hyperfiltration in rats. *Am. J. Physiol.*, **262**, F1055-60.

Weihprecht, H., Lorenz, J. N., Briggs, J. P., and Schnermann, J. (1991). Vasoconstrictor effect of angiotensin and vasopressin in isolated rabbit afferent arterioles. *Am. J. Physiol.*, **261**, F273-F282.

Wright, C. E. and Angus, J. A. (1987). Diverse vascular responses to serotonin in the conscious rabbit: Effects of serotonin antagonists on renal artery spasm. *J. Cardiovasc. Pharmacol.*, **10**, 415-23.

Yared, A., Kon, V., and Ichikawa, I. (1985). Mechanism of preservation of glomerular perfusion and filtration during acute extracellular fluid volume depletion: importance of intrarenal vasopressin-prostaglandin interaction for protecting kidneys from contraction action of vasopressin. *J. Clin. Invest.*, **75**, 1477-87.

Yuan, B. H., Robinette, J. B., and Conger, J. D. (1990). Effect of angiotensin II and noradrenaline on isolated rat afferent and efferent arterioles. *Am. J. Physiol.*, **258**, F741-F750.

Zimmerhackl, B., Robertson, C.R., and Jamison, R. L. (1985). The microcirculation of the renal medulla. *Circ. Res.*, **57**, 657-67.

Zink, M. H., Pergola, P. E., Doane, J. F., Sved, A. F., and Alper, R. H. (1990). Quipazine increases renin release by a peripheral hemodynamic mechanism. *J. Cardiovasc. Pharmacol.*, **15**, 1-9.

14. Atherosclerosis

Xiao-Jun Du and Anthony M. Dart

INTRODUCTION

It has now become clear that the physiological and pharmacological behaviour of vascular smooth muscle, particularly in the coronary circulation, is abnormal throughout the evolution of atherosclerosis (Vanhoutte and Shimokawa 1989; Bassenge and Heusch 1990). This chapter will review these pathophysiological alterations and the consequently modified (or even paradoxical) pharmacological characteristics of coronary vasculature.

CORONARY RISK FACTORS AND ABNORMAL CORONARY VASOACTIVITY

The well documented coronary risk factors include hyperlipidaemia, hypertension, cigarette smoking, diabetes, age, and family history. Several recent studies have demonstrated an association between these risk factors and a high prevalence of abnormal vasomotor responses. Hypertension, cigarette smoking, and diabetes are accompanied by endothelial dysfunction and an increased incidence of coronary vasospasm. In the presence of multiple risk factors even angiographically normal coronary arteries show abnormal responses (vasoconstriction) to acetylcholine (ACh, Fig. 14.1) (Vita *et al.* 1990). Whilst multiple risk factor status impairs endothelium-dependent vasorelaxation, responses to endothelium-independent relaxants are maintained.

Abnormalities in coronary vasoactivity and responses to a range of vasoactive agents have become particularly apparent in human and animals with hypercholesterolaemia *prior to* any evident morphological changes in vascular wall and endothelial cells (Zeiher *et al.* 1991*a*). In various species hypercholesterolaemia attenuates endothelium-dependent vasorelaxation or even induces vasoconstrictor response to agents such as ACh whilst vasoconstrictor responses are themselves substantially enhanced (Bassenge and Heusch 1990). These vascular abnormalities are likely the direct effect of elevated lipids because similar dysfunction occurs in arteries from normal animals when exposed to oxidized low density lipoprotein (LDL) in the medium (Galle *et al.* 1990; Jacobs *et al.* 1990).

The mechanisms involved in this impaired vasomotor control by elevated lipids are probably multifactorial. Hypercholesterolaemia is accompanied by increased circulating endothelin-1 (ET-1) level (Lüscher *et al.* 1992), indicating an enhanced

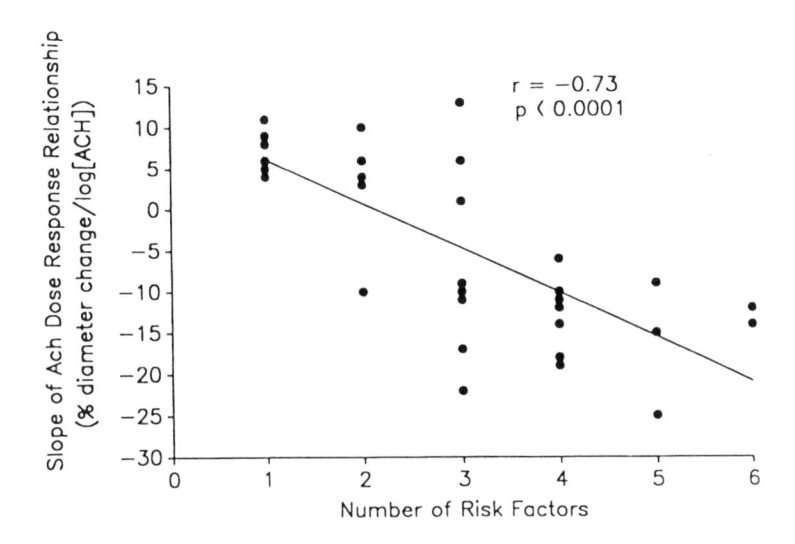

Fig. 14.1 Plot of the relation between the vasomotor response to acetylcholine and the number of coronary risk factors. The acetylcholine response is expressed as the slope of the dose–response relations (% change in coronary diameter/log [acetylcholine]), where a positive slope reflects dilation and a negative slope reflects constriction. By univariate analysis, a significant negative correlation occurred between the acetylcholine response and the number of coronary risk factors. Adopted with permission from Vita *et al.* (1990).

synthesis and/or release of ET-1 from the vascular wall or decreased breakdown. A cytotoxic effect of oxidized LDL on endothelial cells has been demonstrated (Hennig and Chow 1988). LDL may itself become pharmacologically active following cell-mediated oxidation in the vessel wall. Thus in precontracted rabbit aorta strips vasodilator responses to ACh are well maintained after incubation with native LDL, but lost after incubation with oxidized LDL despite preserved vasodilator response to nitroglycerin (Kugiyama *et al.* 1990; Mangin *et al.* 1993). In contrast to the adverse effects of LDL, and interestingly in view of the epidemiologically demonstrated *inverse* relation between high density lipoprotein (HDL) levels and coronary artery disease, preliminary studies indicate a protection by HDL of endothelium function. Subjects with a normal vasodilator response to ACh have significantly higher HDL levels than those with an abnormal (vasoconstrictive) response (Kuhn *et al.* 1991).

ATHEROSCLEROTIC DAMAGE AND VASCULAR DYSFUNCTION

Clinical and experimental studies on atherosclerotic coronary arteries have demonstrated an abnormal vasoconstriction in response to various pharmacological agents which induce vasodilation in non-atherosclerotic arteries. Intracoronary injection of ACh or 5-HT in man induces a dose-dependent vasoconstrictor response in segments with atherosclerotic damage but the vasodilator response to nitroglycerin is intact (Bassenge and Heusch 1990; Golino *et al.* 1991; Zeiher *et al.* 1991*a*). This selective loss of endothelium-dependent relaxation in atherosclerotic arteries can be reversed by intracoronary injection of L-arginine or by treatment with 5-HT receptor antagonists indicating a dual mechanism of reduced formation/activity of endothelium-derived relaxing factor (EDRF) and direct vasoconstriction mediated by 5-HT receptors. An impairment of endothelial-dependent vasodilatation has been demonstrated in hypercholesterolaemia-induced atherosclerosis in various species. Both *in vivo* and cell culture experiments have indicated that EDRF release is stimulated by high shear stress and this flow-dependent vasodilatation is also impaired in atherosclerotic coronary arteries in man (Nabel *et al.* 1990). Impaired endothelium-dependent vasodilatation in resistance arteries has recently been demonstrated in angina patients with angiographically normal large conduit coronary arteries (Zeiher *et al.* 1991*a*; Egashira *et al.* 1993). The documented abnormalities in coronary vasomotion and response to mechanical and pharmacological interventions, which occur in both resistance and conduit arteries, constitute an important aspect for the pathogenesis of variant angina pectoris and acute myocardial ischaemia in subjects with coronary atherosclerosis. Clinical approaches to identifying subjects with predominantly vasospastic angina and ischaemia are also based on enhanced vasoconstrictive activity. Such patients are particularly benefited by vasodilator anti-anginal therapy.

Impairment of endothelium-dependent relaxation in atherosclerotic vessels could be due to depressed EDRF release and/or limited EDRF diffusion due to intimal thickening (Bassenge and Heusch 1990; Chester *et al.* 1990). Peroxidized lipoproteins present in atheromatous lesions may scavenge EDRF (Haberland *et al.* 1988). A reduced sensitivity of underlying smooth muscle seems unlikely since responses to L-arginine and exogenous nitric oxide are well maintained. G_i protein mediates endothelium-dependent vasodilator responses to certain agonists (5-HT, α_2- adrenergic agonists, and thrombin), and recent evidence has implicated a loss of G_i protein function in atherosclerotic coronary arteries (Shimokawa *et al.* 1991).

Increased production and activity of endogenous vasoconstrictors also contributes to enhanced vasoconstriction in atherosclerotic coronary vessels. Coronary sinus blood obtained from patients with atheromatous coronary disease exhibits vasoconstrictor activity (Rubanyi *et al.* 1987). Several recent studies have reported an increase in tissue and circulating levels of ET-1 in patients with atherosclerosis, indicating an augmented production and local release (Lerman *et al.* 1991). Besides its direct vasoconstrictive activity, ET-1 potentiates adrenergic vasoconstriction even at subpressor doses (Yang *et al.* 1990). Both ET-1-mediated vasoconstriction and its synergistic potentiation of adrenergic vasoconstriction can be attenuated by calcium antagonists, indicating a role of enhanced calcium influx in ET-1-dependent vasoconstriction. In addition, there may be an enhanced production and release of other endothelium-derived constricting factors (EDCFs) in atherosclerotic arteries, superoxide anion and prostaglandin H_2 (Vanhoutte and Shimokawa 1989). Several studies have demonstrated that regression of atherosclerotic lesions and correction of hypercholesterolaemia is associated with a recovery of endothelium-dependent relaxation and a reduction in the hypercontractile response of atherosclerotic vessels (Heistad et al. 1987).

Intact endothelium inhibits smooth muscle cell proliferation both by releasing inhibitory factors such as heparin and by preventing release of growth promoting factors from activated platelets. Thus, in addition to functional vasomotor effects endothelial dysfunction may promote the development of morphological stenoses.

CORONARY VASCULAR DYSFUNCTION IN ACUTE MYOCARDIAL ISCHAEMIA

Although previous studies on ischaemia/reperfusion injury of the heart concentrated on the myocardium *per se*, endothelial damage is an important component of ischaemic damage and may play a central role in reperfusion injury (Hearse et al. 1993).

Several studies in dogs have demonstrated that vasorelaxation is impaired following reperfusion after 60 min ischaemia. Although morphological changes, including microcirculatory blockage by neutrophils and platelets, are already evident substantial evidence indicates an impairment of endothelium-dependent relaxation and an augmented response to vasoconstrictor agents (Mehta et al. 1989a; Kim et al. 1992; Sobey et al. 1992). Investigation of the time course in canine hearts has shown that short (15 min) periods of combined ischaemia and reperfusion impair responses to ACh, which are reversed after 90 min of reperfusion. Extension of the duration of ischaemia to 20-30 min results in almost complete loss of endothelium-dependent relaxation to ACh and bradykinin when tested after 20 min reperfusion (Fig. 14.2). Morphological damage of endothelium also occurs when ischaemia extends to 20-30 min and causes a sustained impairment with functional changes similar to those seen with vascular denudation (Kim et al. 1992). Studies have also shown that coronary resistance vessels are more vulnerable than large conduit vessels to ischaemia-reperfusion injury on endothelium-dependent function (Hearse et al. 1993).

Reduced production and release of EDRF is an important mechanism for these altered responses (Kim et al. 1992; Ma et al. 1993). It is well documented that reperfusion or reoxygenation induces a massive formation of oxygen-derived free radicals, which can scavenge nitric oxide. Treatment with superoxide dismutase or other agents to inhibit free radical formation is protective against subsequent endothelial injury (Mehta et al. 1989b, Tsao and Lefer 1990). Ischaemia/reperfusion may also be associated with an enhanced formation and activity of vasoconstrictive substances. Production of ET-1 by coronary arteries is enhanced by hypoxia and a number of other factors that exist during ischaemia/reperfusion (Lüscher et al. 1992). Vascular sensitivity to EDCFs may be increased in arteries with

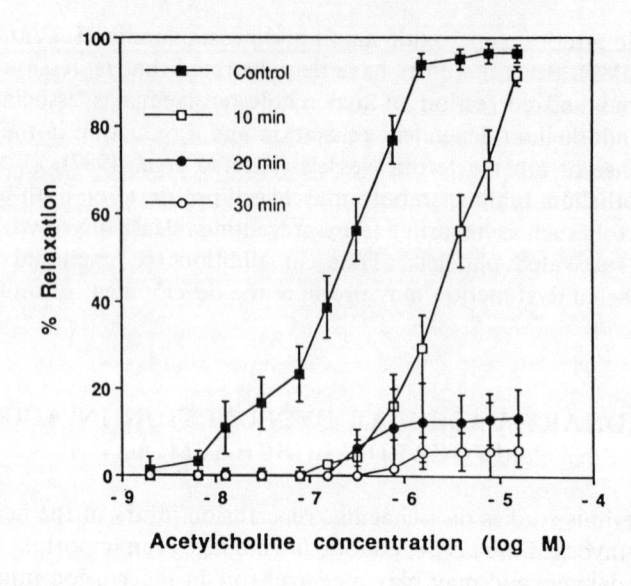

Fig. 14.2 Relaxation response to acetylcholine of canine coronary arterial rings precontracted with KCl. Relaxation to maximal concentrations (15 μmol/litre) in rings pre-exposed to 10 min of ischaemia–reperfusion was similar to control, but responses to submaximal concentrations were blunted, resulting in a rightward shift of the response curve. As ischaemic duration extended to 20 and 30 min, relaxation to acetylcholine was almost abolished, indicating severe impairment of endothelium-dependent vasodilation in ischaemically injured rings. Data are expressed as mean ± s.e.m. Adopted with permission from Kim *et al.* (1992).

ischaemia and hypoxia (Lüscher *et al.* 1992). An additional explanation for potentiated vasoconstriction is an enhanced calcium influx into smooth muscle cells, perhaps together with an impaired intracellular handling of calcium. This view is supported by evidence that calcium blockers are effective in preventing ischaemia/reperfusion-induced vascular dysfunction (Mehta *et al.* 1989*a*; Sobey *et al.* 1992). Propranolol is also effective although the mechanism is not clear (Sobey *et al.* 1992).

AUTONOMIC NEUROTRANSMISSION IN ATHEROSCLEROTIC CORONARY VESSELS AND IN MYOCARDIAL ISCHAEMIA

Adrenergic mechanisms in atherosclerotic coronary arteries

Accumulating evidence suggests an important role for sympathoadrenergic mechanisms in the regulation of coronary vasoactivity throughout the progession of coronary artery disease from the pre-atherosclerotic stage to myocardial infarction.

In *in vivo* dog hearts, a normal vasodilator response to α-adrenergic agonists can be changed into vasoconstriction after inhibition of nitric oxide synthetase, indicating that endothelium-dependent relaxation competes with α-adrenergic vasoconstriction (Jones *et al.* 1993). Several clinical studies have observed a marked focal vasospasm in atherosclerotic coronary arteries in response to exercise or cold pressor test while normal vessels respond with vasodilation (Gage *et al.* 1986; Nabel *et al.* 1988; Zeiher *et al.* 1991*a*). Such an abnormal vasoconstriction by sympathetic activation can be reversed by nitroglycerin or by calcium antagonists. In normal segments of coronary arteries vasorelaxation to a stressor test is mediated by β-adrenergic relaxation, increased EDRF release due to increased pressure and coronary flow (shear stress), and an enhanced adenosine production in response to β- and $α_2$-adrenergic stimulation. The paradoxical vasoconstriction in diseased arteries appears to be mediated by α-adrenoceptors as it can be attenuated by α-antagonists. However, several other factors may be also involved. First, the local concentration of noradrenaline (NA) may be high in atherosclerotic arteries due to exaggerated sympathetic activation in coronary patients during dynamic exercise (McCance and Forfar 1989). Secondly, uptake of NA released by endothelium contributes to NA clearance and suppression of postsynaptic effects (Tesfamariam *et al.* 1987). It is possible that such effect is attenuated in atherosclerotic arteries leading to enhanced vasoconstriction. Thirdly, vasoconstrictors such as ET-1, neuropeptide Y, and 5-HT may potentiate α-adrenergic vasoconstrictor activity (Bassenge and Heusch 1990; Yang *et al.* 1990). Finally, neurotransmitter(s) which mediate the vasoconstriction by sympathetic stimulation may be altered in atherosclerotic arteries. Cohen *et al.* (1987) have reported that the tissue content of NA was reduced by 40% but 5-HT increased by 17-fold in canine coronary arteries 24 hours after endothelium injury by balloon expansion. The authors proposed that endothelium injury promotes local adhesion and activation of platelets followed by release of 5-HT, which were taken up by local adrenergic nerves and released upon nerve activation to induce vasoconstriction.

Cholinergic mechanism in atherosclerotic coronary arteries

In normal coronary arteries, the predominant response to exogenous ACh given from the luminal (endothelial) site is relaxation, whilst in atherosclerotic or denuded coronary arteries the predominant response is constriction. However it is unclear if vagally released ACh, acting from the non-endothelial (advential) surface, behaves similarly and results from vagal stimulation are inconsistent (Kalsner 1989). Further studies are required to examine vasomotor regulation by endogenous ACh in pathological conditions such as endothelial damage, anoxia, and ischaemia. However, hypersensitivity of vascular smooth muscles to ACh, with or without an endothelial dysfunction, may contribute to the pathogenesis of focal vasospasm.

Sympathoadrenergic mechanism in acute myocardial ischaemia

Although acute myocardial ischaemia is accompanied by a systemic sympathetic activation with elevated circulating catecholamines the major source of an enhanced adrenergic stimulation to the ischaemic myocardium comes from locally released NA (Schömig 1990; Dart and Du 1993). NA release in response to nerve fibre activation, and its modulation by a range of drugs, is profoundly influenced by myocardial ischaemia. Whilst blockade of presynaptic adenosine receptors normally has little effect on NA release their blockade during ischaemia results in a marked increase of release. This difference is attributed to the normally low levels of extracellular adenosine becoming greatly increased during ischaemia to levels sufficient to exert a presynaptic inhibition. In contrast, the usually potent presynaptic inhibition of NA release by vagal nerve stimulation or by administration of muscarinic receptor agonists fails shortly after the induction of ischaemia (Dart and Du 1993). In normoxic preparations increase in K^+ concentration to 15–20 mM suppresses exocytotic NA release whilst further increase above 20 mM induces NA release by depolaring nerve varicosities. In perfused hearts exposed to energy depleted conditions to simulate ischaemia, a significant NA overflow can be induced by K^+ at 10 mM, and the quantities of NA overflow evoked by various concentrations of K^+ (10–40 mM) are substantially higher than that with the corresponding concentrations during normoxic perfusion due to attenuated neuronal reuptake and an enhanced exocytosis (Dart and Du 1993). Propranolol and lignocaine, when tested in normally perfused conditions, show no effect on NA release at doses up to 10 μM, but produce a potent inhibition on NA release in ischaemic conditions even at 0.1 μM. This inhibitory effect is due to a synergism between ischaemic environment (mainly raised extracellular K^+) and the Na^+ channel blocking activity of both agents, leading to an impairment of neuronal conduction (Dart and Du 1993). Later in ischaemia massive NA release is mediated by the neuronal Uptake$_1$ carrier acting in the reverse of its normal transporting direction driven by increased intraneuronal Na^+ and NA (Schömig 1990). Inhibition of Uptake$_1$ normally potentiates overflow of NA released by nerve activation, but paradoxically and markedly suppresses spontaneous NA release in hearts with ischaemia or with energy depletion (Dart and Du 1993). Although these observations have been made in perfused whole hearts it is likely that similar changes occur in the coronary vasculature.

Postsynaptic β- and α-adrenergic pathways are also profoundly altered during myocardial ischaemia. Although β-adrenergic stimulation induces vasodilation in normal hearts, activation of arterial β-receptors in the ischaemic heart results in an unfavourable redistribution of coronary blood flow from subendocardium, usually the most severely ischaemic, to the less ischaemic subepicardium (Heusch 1990).

Experimental studies have also shown a substantially increased density of α_1-adrenoceptors in the myocardium shortly after ischaemia or hypoxia as a result of receptor externalization. Increased α-adrenoceptors in the ischaemic myocardium maintain functional coupling with the intracellular system as indicated by the increased breakdown of inositol phosphates and by the arrhythmogenic property of α_1-adrenergic stimulation. In vascular smooth muscle there is an enhanced formation of phosphoinositides by α_1-adrenergic stimulation during ischaemia and reperfusion. Other factors including thrombin, histamine, ET-1, TXA_2, bradykinin, and intracellularly accumulated calcium following ischaemia and reperfusion, could also enhance, via the activation of phospholipase C, the formation of inositol 1,4,5-triphosphate (IP_3) and diacylglycerol (DAG) leading to increased intracellular calcium and vasoconstriction (Otani et al. 1988; Marsden et al. 1989; Schrör 1990; Berridge 1993). Intracellular accumulation of lysophosphatidylcholine, which occurs in ischaemia, potentiates the DAG-dependent activation of protein kinase C (Nishizuka 1992).

Clinical and experimental studies have provided evidence for an important role of α-adrenergic vasoconstriction in myocardial ischaemia. In non-ischaemic conditions, α-adrenergic stimulation induces a direct vasoconstriction in large arteries and indirect metabolic relaxation in small resistance arterioles. Coronary hypoperfusion may exhaust this indirect vasodilator reserve in response to α-stimulation, thereby leading to an enhanced vasoconstriction (Heusch 1990). Such a poststenotic α-adrenergic vasoconstriction and the resulting ischaemia during sympathetic activation can be attenuated or prevented by α-antagonists.

Although it has been widely accepted that α-adrenergic vasoconstriction is deleterious in acute myocardial ischaemia, several studies in dogs have demonstrated a beneficial effect of α-adrenergic vasoconstriction during coronary hypoperfusion. In the presence of critical coronary restriction, sympathetic activation (in the presence of β-blockade) or α-agonists reduce the existing transmural gradient by redistributing blood flow to the most ischaemic subendocardium (Chilian and Ackell 1988; Kitakaze et al. 1990). This is due to a more pronounced α-adrenergic vasoconstriction in subepicardial coronary arteries and an enhanced adenosine release from ischaemic myocardium by α-stimulation. This α-adrenergic anti-steal mechanism may also play a role in subacute or chronic myocardial infarction when an area of myocardium is supported by collateral circulation. As collateral vessels have no functional α-adrenoceptors, α-adrenergic stimulation would be expected to divert blood flow through the collateral circulation (Harrison et al. 1990; Heusch 1990).

Transmural infarction induces a sympathetic denervated area apical to the infarct zone with a resultant catecholamine supersensitivity of the denervated myocardium but it is unknown if these changes also occur in the vasculature.

PHARMACOLOGICAL FEATURES OF COLLATERAL VESSELS

Following acute myocardial infarction or a period of critical coronary stenosis, collateral circulation develops to provide blood supply to potentially ischaemic myocardium. These collateral vessels, whether studied at immature or mature stages, show certain pharmacological features which differ from native coronary arteries (Harrison et al. 1990). Although endothelial morphology appears normal, endothelial relaxation has been found to be abnormal in some but not all studies. Endothelium-independent relaxation was well maintained according to all studies. Studies with aspirin have suggested that canine collateral vessels are particulary sensitive to the vasodilatory influence of endogenous PGI_2 (Altman et al. 1993). Clinical studies have indicated that dihydropyridine calcium antagonists may reduce the collateral flow via a steal mechanism (Egstrup and Andersen 1993).

Mature collateral vessels have little, if any, functional α-receptors. In contrast, β_1- and β_2-adrenergic vasoactivity is preserved which is in agreement with findings from ligand binding studies (Harrison et al. 1990). Such an alteration in adrenergic vasomotor regulation seems beneficial in protecting the potentially ischaemic myocardium during condition of cardiac sympathetic activation. Mature collateral vessels retain vasoconstrictor responses to 5-HT, vasopressin, and TXA_2.

PLATELET ACTIVATION, THROMBOSIS, AND CORONARY VASOCONSTRICTION

There is now strong evidence that in most patients, acute coronary events are the consequence of platelet aggregation and thrombus formation at segments of coronary arteries with atherosclerotic stenosis, ulceration, and endothelial injury.

During the onset of unstable angina, there is an increased intracoronary production of TXA_2, 5-HT, prostaglandins (PGH_2 and PGE_2), and platelet-derived growth factor, indicating platelet activation (Hirsh et al. 1981; van van den Berg et al. 1989; Ogawa et al. 1992). In arteries with severe endothelial injury, vasoconstrictor response to these platelet-released substances is extremely pronounced because of impairment of EDRF release in response to stimuli by these substances, together with an enhanced release of EDCFs (Vanhoutte and Shimokawa 1989). On the other hand, there is a paradoxical and exaggerated vasoconstriction to platelet-released substances in atherosclerotic vessels with associated endothelial injury (Golino et al. 1989; Kaul et al. 1991).

Recently agents have been developed which inhibit synthesis and activity of the vasoconstrictive substances released upon platelet activation allowing investigation of the role of these substances during acute coronary syndromes. In the canine heart, a severe coronary artery stenosis together with endothelial injury causes cyclic coronary flow reduction due to thrombus formation and embolism, a model simulating clinical unstable and variant angina. Using this model and the newly developed agents, an important role of TXA_2 and 5-HT in mediating such cyclic coronary flow reduction and vasospasm has been demonstrated. Golino et al. (1989) have observed a marked vasospasm at the site of platelet aggregation and this focal vasospasm can be prevented by the blockade of TXA_2 or 5-HT receptors. This experimental finding has been supported by a recent clinical study by Zeiher et al. (1991b). They observed that in patients receiving coronary angioplasty, those who developed intracoronary thrombus during angioplasty had an evident vasoconstriction distal to the expanded segment leading to 27% reduction in coronary luminal area. Other recent studies have shown that coronary vasoconstriction to various vasoconstrictors is sustantially augmented by activated platelet or TXA$_2$ (Martin *et al.* 1992; Weyrich *et al.* 1992). In human coronary arteries, activation of TXA$_2$ receptors markedly potentiates vasoconstriction mediated by 5-HT$_1$ receptors present in regions distal to atherosclerotic lesion (Chester *et al.* 1993). These observations strongly indicate that platelet aggregation and thrombus formation is associated with coronary artery spasm, either at the site of (proximal) or downstream to (distal) the site of thrombosis, which is mediated by platelet-released vasoconstrictors. Thus, at least in some cases, this combination of mechanical and dynamic coronary restriction may form a viscous cycle leading to a more complete coronary occlusion and the onset of acute myocardial infarction.

REFERENCES

Altman, J. D., Dulas, D., Pavek, T., and Bache, R. J. (1993). Effect of aspirin on coronary collateral blood flow. *Circulation*, **87**, 583–9.

Bassenge, E. and Heusch, G. (1990). Endothelial and neuro-humoral control of coronary blood flow in health and disease. *Rev. Physiol. Biochem. Pharmacol.*, **116**, 77–165.

Berridge, M. J. (1993). Inositol trisphosphate and calcium signalling. *Nature*, **361**, 315–25.

Chester, A. H., O'Neil, G. S., Moncada, S., Tadjkarimi, S., and Yacoub, M. H. (1990). Low basal and stimulated release of nitric oxide in atherosclerotic epicardial coronary arteries. *Lancet*, **336**, 897–900.

Chester, A. H., Allen, S. P., Tadjkarimi, S., and Yacoub, M. H. (1993). Interaction between thromboxane A$_2$ and 5-hydroxytryptamine receptor subtypes in human coronary arteries. *Circulation*, **87**, 874–80.

Chilian, W. M. and Ackell, P. (1988). Transmural differences in sympathetic coronary constriction during exercise in the presence of coronary stenosis. *Circ. Res.*, **62**, 216–25.

Cohen, R. A., Zitnay, K. M., and Weisbrod, R. M. (1987). Accumulation of 5-hydroxytryptamine leads to dysfunction of adrenergic nerves in canine coronary artery following intimal damage *in vivo*. *Circ. Res.*, **61**, 829–33.

Dart, A. M. and Du, X.-J. (1993). Unexpected drug effects on autonomic function during myocardial ischaemia. *Cardiovasc. Res.*, **27**, 906–14.

Egashira, K., Inou, T., Hirooka, Y., Yamada, A., Urabe, Y., and Takeshita, A. (1993). Evidence of impaired endothelium-dependent coronary vasodilatation in patients with angina pectoris and normal coronary angiograms. *N. Eng. J. Med.*, **328**, 1659–64.

Egstrup, K. and Andersen, P. E. Jr. (1993). Transient myocardial ischaemia during nifedipine therapy in stable angina pectoris, and its relation to coronary collateral flow and comparison with metoprolol. *Am. J. Cardiol.*, **71**, 177–83.

Gage, J. E., Hess, O. M., Murakami, T., Ritter, M., Grimm, J., and Krayenbuehl, H. P. (1986). Vasoconstriction of stenotic coronary arteries during dynamic exercise in patients with classic angina pectoris: reversibility by nitroglycerin. *Circulation*, **73**, 865–76.

Galle, J., Bassenge, E., and Busse, R. (1990). Oxidized low density lipoproteins potentiate vasoconstrictions to various agonists by direct interaction with vascular smooth muscle. *Circ. Res.*, **66**, 1287–93.

Golino, P., Ashton, J. H., Buja, L. M., Rosolowsky, M., Taylor, A. L., McNatt, J., et al. (1989). Local platelet activation causes vasoconstriction of large epicardial canine coronary arteries in vivo. *Circulation*, **79**, 154–66.

Golino, P., Piscione, F., Willerson, J. T., Cappelli-Bigazzi, M., Focaccio, A., Villari, B., et al. (1991). Divergent effects of serotonin on coronary-artery dimensions and blood flow in patients with coronary atherosclerosis, and control patients. *N. Eng. J. Med.*, **324**, 641–8.

Haberland, M. E., Fong, D., and Cheng, L. (1988). Malondialdehyde-altered protein occurs in atheroma of Watanabe heritable hyperlipidemic rabbits. *Science*, **241**, 215–18.

Harrison, D. G., Sellke, F. W., and Quillen, J. E. (1990). Neurohumoral regulation of coronary collateral vasomotor tone. *Basic Res. Cardiol.*, **85 (suppl 1)**, 121–9.

Hearse, D. J., Maxwell, L., Saldanha, C., and Gavin, J. B. (1993). The myocardial vasculature during ischemia and reperfusion: a target for injury and protection. *J. Mol. Cell. Cardiol.*, **25**, 759–800.

Heistad, D. D., Mark, A. L., Marcus, M. L., Piegors, D. J., and Amstrong, M. L. (1987). Dietary treatment of atherosclerosis abolishes hyperresponsiveness to serotonin: implications for vasospasm. *Circ. Res.*, **61**, 346–51.

Hennig, B. and Chow, C. K. (1988). Lipid peroxidation and endothelial cell injury: Implications in atherosclerosis. *Free Radical Biol. Med.*, **4**, 99–106.

Heusch, G. (1990). α-adrenergic mechanisms in myocardial ischemia. *Circulation*, **81**, 1–13.

Hirsh, P. D., Hillis, L. D., Campbell, W. B., Firth, B. G., and Willerson, J. T. (1981). Release of postaglandins and thromboxane into the coronary circulation in patients with ischemic heart disease. *N. Eng. J. Med.*, **304**, 685–91.

Jacobs, M., Plane, F., and Bruckdorfer, K. R. (1990). Native and oxidized low-density lipoproteins have different inhibitory effects on endothelium-derived relaxing factor in the rabbit aorta. *Br. J. Pharmacol.*, **100**, 21–6.

Jones, C. J. H., DeFily, D. V., Patterson, J. L., and Chilian, W. M. (1993). Endothelium-dependent relaxation competes with α_1- and α_2-adrenergic constriction in the canine epicardial coronary microcirculation. *Circulation*, **87**, 1264–74.

Kalsner, S. (1989). Cholinergic constriction in the general circulation and its role in coronary artery spasm. *Circ. Res.*, **65**, 237–57.

Kaul, S., Heistad, D. D., Mügge, A., Armstrong, M. L., Piegors, D. J., and Lopez, J. A. G. (1991). Vascular responses to platelet activation in normal and atherosclerotic primates in vivo. *Arterioscler. Thromb.*, **11**, 1745–51.

Kim, Y. D., Fomsgaard, J. S., Heim, K. F., Ramwell, P. W., Thomas, G., Kagan, E., et al. (1992). Brief ischemia-reperfusion induces stunning of endothelium in canine coronary artery. *Circulation*, **85**, 1473–82.

Kitakaze, M., Hori, M., Gotoh, K., Sato, H., Iwakura, K., Kitabatake, A., et al. (1990). Vascular reactivity during the progression of atherosclerotic plaque. *Circ. Res.*, **66**, 1112–26.

Kuhn, F. E., Mohler, E. R., Satler, L. F., Reagan, K., Lu, D. Y., and Rackley, C. E. (1991). Effects of high-density lipoprotein on acetylcholine-induced coronary vasoreactivity. *Am. J. Cardiol.*, **68**, 1425–30.

Kugiyama, K., Kerns, S. A., Morrisett, J. D., Roberts, R., and Henry, P. D. (1990). Impairment of endothelium-dependent arterial relaxation by lysolecithin in modified low-density lipoproteins. *Nature*, **344**, 160–2.

Lerman, A., Edwards, B. S., Hallett, J. W., Heublein, D. M., Sandberg, S. M., and Burnett, J. C. Jr. (1991). Circulating and tissue endothelin immunoreactivity in advanced atherosclerosis. *N. Eng. J. Med.*, **325**, 997–1001.

Lüscher, T. F., Boulanger, C. M., Dohi, Y., and Yang, Z. (1992). Endothelium-derived contracting factors. *Hypertension*, **19**, 117-30.

McCance, A. J. and Forfar, J. C. (1989). Selective enhancement of the cardiac sympathetic response to exercise by anginal chest pain in humans. *Circulation*, **80**, 1642-51.

Ma, X., Weyrich, A. S., Lefer, D. J., and Lefer, A. M. (1993). Diminished basal nitric oxide release after myocardial ischemia and reperfusion promotes neutrophil adherence to coronary endothelium. *Circ. Res.*, **72**, 403-12.

Mangin, E. L., Kugiyama, K., Nguy, J. H, Kerns, S. A., and Henry, P. D. (1993). Effects of lysolipids and oxidatively modified low density lipoprotein on endothelium-dependent relaxation of rabbit aorta. *Circ. Res.*, **72**, 161-6.

Marsden, P. A., Danthuluri, N. R., Brenner, B. M., Ballermann, B. J., and Brock, T. A. (1989). Endothelin action on vascular smooth muscle involves inositol triphosphate and calcium mobilization. *Biochem. Biophys. Res. Commun.*, **158**, 86-93.

Martin, S. E., Kuvin, J. T., Offenbacher, S., Odle, B. M., and Patterson, R. E. (1992). Neuropeptide Y and coronary vasoconstriction: role of thromboxane A_2. *Am. J. Physiol.*, **263**, H1045-53.

Mehta, J. L., Nichols, W. W., Donnelly, W. H., Lawson, D. L., and Saldeen, T. G. P. (1989*a*). Impaired canine coronary vasodilator response to acetylcholine and bradykinin after occlusion-reperfusion. *Circ. Res.*, **64**, 43-54.

Mehta, J. L., Lawson, D. L., and Nichols, W. W. (1989*b*). Attenuated coronary relaxation after reperfusion: effects of superoxide dismutase and TxA_2 inhibitor U 63557A. *Am. J. Physiol.*, **257**, H1240-6.

Nabel, E. G., Ganz, P., Gordon, J. B., Alexander, R. W., and Selwyn, A. P. (1988). Dilation of normal and constriction of atherosclerotic coronary arteries caused by the cold pressor test. *Circulation*, **77**, 43-52.

Nabel, E. G., Selwyn, A. P., and Ganz, P. (1990). Large coronary arteries in humans are responsive to changing blood flow: An endothelium-dependent mechanism that fails in patients with atherosclerosis. *J. Am. Coll. Cardiol.*, **16**, 349-56.

Nishizuka, Y. (1992). Intracellular signaling by hydrolysis of phospholipids and activation of protein kinase C. *Science*, **258**, 607-14.

Ogawa, H., Yasue, H., Misumi, I., Masuda, T., Okumura, K., Bannai, S., *et al.* (1992). Plasma platelet-derived growth factor levels in coronary circulation in unstable angina pectoris. *Am. J. Cardiol.*, **69**, 453-6.

Otani, H., Prasad, M. R., Engelman, R. M., Otani, H., Cordis, G. A., and Das, D. K. (1988). Enhanced phosphodiesteratic breakdown and turnover of phosphoinositides during reperfusion of ischemic rat heart. *Circ. Res.*, **63**, 930-6.

Rubanyi, G. M., Frye, R. L., Holmes, D. R. Jr., and Vanhoutte, P. M. (1987). Vasoconstrictor activity of coronary sinus plasma from patients with coronary artery disease. *J. Am. Coll. Cardiol.*, **9**, 1243-9.

Schömig, A. (1990). Catecholamines in myocardial ischemia: Systemic and cardiac release. *Circulation*, **82 (suppl II)**, 13-22.

Schrör, K. (1990). Thromboxan A_2 and platelets as mediators of coronary arterial vasoconstriction in myocardial ischemia. *Eur. Heart J.*, **11 (suppl B)**, 27-34.

Shimokawa, H., Flavahan, N. A., and Vanhoutte, P. M. (1991). Loss of endothelial pertussis toxin-sensitive G protein function in atherosclerotic porcine coronary arteries. *Circulation*, **83**, 652-60.

Sobey, C. G., Dalipram, R. A., Dusting, G. J., and Woodman, O. L. (1992). Impaired endothelium-dependent relaxation of dog coronary arteries after myocardial ischaemia and reperfusion: prevention by amlodipine, propranolol and allopurinol. *Br. J. Pharmacol.*, **105**, 557-62.

Tesfamariam, B., Weisbrod, R. M., and Cohen, R. A. (1987). Endothelium inhibits responses of rabbit carotid artery to adrenergic nerve stimulation. *Am. J. Physiol.*, **253**, H792–8.

Tsao, P. S. and Lefer, A. M. (1990). Time course and mechanism of endothelial dysfunction in isolated ischemic- and hypoxic-perfused rat hearts. *Am. J. Physiol.*, **259**, H1660–6.

van den Berg, E. K., Schmitz, J. M., Benedict, C. R., Malloy, C. R., Willerson, J. T., and Dehmer, G. J. (1989). Transcardiac serotonin concentration is increased in selected patients with limiting angina and complex coronary lesion morphology. *Circulation*, **79**, 116–24.

Vanhoutte, P. M. and Shimokawa, H. (1989). Endothelium-derived relaxing factor and coronary vasospasm. *Circulation*, **80**, 1–9.

Vita, J. A., Treasure, C. B., Nabel, E. G., McLenachan, J. M., Fish, R. D., Yeung, A. C., *et al.* (1990). Coronary vasomotor response to acetylcholine relates to risk factors for coronary artery disease. *Circulation*, **81**, 491–7.

Weyrich, A. S., Solis, G. A., Li, K. S., Tulenko, T. N., and Santamore, W. P. (1992). Platelet amplification of vasospasm. *Am. J. Physiol.*, **263**, H349–58.

Yang, Z., Richard, V., von Segesser, L., Bauer, E., Stulz, P., Turina, M., *et al.* (1990). Threshold concentrations of endothelin-1 potentiate contractions to norepinephrine and serotonin in human arteries. *Circulation*, **82**, 188–95.

Zeiher, A. M., Drexler, H., Wollschlager, H., and Just, H. (1991a). Modulation of coronary vasomotor tone in humans. Progressive endothelial dysfunction with different early stages of coronary atherosclerosis. *Circulation*, **83**, 391–401.

Zeiher, A. A., Schächinger, V., Weitzel, S. H., Wollschläger, H., and Just, H. (1991b). Intracoronary thrombus formation causes focal vasoconstriction of epicardial arteries in patients with coronary artery disease. *Circulation*, **83**, 1519–25.

15. Vessel wall injury and growth: pharmacological considerations in atherosclerosis and collateral artery function

Norman K. Hollenberg

INTRODUCTION

Atherosclerosis is the leading cause of morbidity and mortality in societies that enjoy a typical western life-style. Until recently, the pathogenesis of ischaemia secondary to atherosclerotic disease was considered largely to reflect the progression of a fixed, organic process. If a functional element was thought to complicate the process, that consideration largely involved the acute and dramatic mechanical effects of local thrombosis. Growing recognition during the past two decades that the interaction of platelets with the vessel wall, part of the thrombotic process, could result in a sequence that is far more complex and interesting than the mere creation of a mechanical haemostatic plug, through the release of a host of agents which can influence vascular function has brought atherosclerosis as a subject of investigation to a much wider range of investigators. The more recent recognition of the interaction between the intima and vascular smooth muscle contractile state and growth, and that intimal function could be altered very early in the atherosclerotic process, served to expand that interest further. Arteries relax in response to some vasodilators only if the endothelium is present, as reviewed in detail in earlier chapters. The obligatory role for vasodilatation of a diffusible factor from endothelium termed 'EDRF' for endothelial-dependent relaxing factor, now identified as nitric oxide or a related nitroso-thiol has been demonstrated for many agents, including acetylcholine, bradykinin, substance P, ATP, other adenine nucleotides — and especially important for this essay — the vasodilator action of 5-HT. Other vasodilator agents, however, such as nitrates, papaverine, isoproterenol, and prostaglandins do not require endothelium. This chapter will focus on pharmacological considerations relevant to the processes defined above in the atherosclerotic wall, and in the collateral arteries that grow in response to the vascular occlusion that so often occurs with atherosclerosis. A bias will be evident in the selection of material for this discussion, reflecting the author's opinion that platelet:vessel wall interactions are especially important. Given necessary editorial limitations on space, and the broad scope of this chapter, it will be necessary to omit or limit discussion of a number of relevant subjects. No attention will be given, for example, to pharmacological factors that can influence lipid metabolism and deposition, or what has been learned of the contribution of growth factors to pathogenesis. Therapeutics, including the fascinating possible contribution of calcium channel blocking agents to delaying the process will also be given minimal attention.

CHOLESTEROL, ATHEROSCLEROSIS, AND VASCULAR REACTIVITY

Hypercholesterolaemia can clearly influence vascular responses. Rosendorff *et al.* (1981) rendered dogs hypercholesterolaemic by cholesterol feeding for 26 to 32 days, too short a time for atherosclerosis to develop, and showed enhanced coronary vascular resistance in response to noradrenaline. No explanation was offered on the possible mechanism. Wright and Angus (1986) documented a reduction in the vasodilator response to acetylcholine in rabbits made hypercholesterolaemic by means of a four week high cholesterol diet, suggesting that altered endothelial function could be a contributor. Vasodilator responses of the limb resistance vessels to 5-HT, however, were unchanged by this regimen. No attempt was made to assess the large artery response in either study.

Prompted by evidence that epicardial coronary artery spasm participates in the pathophysiology of ischaemic heart disease, and that some patients show a potentiated coronary vascular response to the vasoconstrictor actions of the ergot alkaloid ergonovine, Henry and Yokoyama (1980) examined the responses of the rabbit aorta after about ten weeks on a high cholesterol diet, a sufficient time to increase substantially not only serum cholesterol but also the cholesterol content of the vascular tissue. They documented supersensitivity of the isolated arterial strips to ergonovine, and to 5-HT, but not to noradrenaline. Supersensitivity expressed itself in a reduced 5-HT dose required to induce a threshold response, and an increase in the maximum response. They speculated that the functional changes in the atherosclerotic arteries were unlikely to be attributable to alterations in their structure, since responses to alpha receptor agonists were unaltered. Moreover, a structural change was unlikely to alter the threshold concentration of 5-HT required to induce a response.

Yokoyama *et al.* (1983) went on to document supersensitivity to ergonovine and to 5-HT not only in the aorta, but also in the coronary arteries of 8-12 month-old rabbits of the Watanabe strain, that develop hyperlipidaemia and atherosclerosis as a result of a genetic abnormality. Again, the supersensitivity was specific, as responses to phenylephrine were not altered. This study suggested regional arterial differences that are still unexplained: neither the carotid nor the femoral artery in this strain of rabbit showed a potentiated response to 5-HT or ergonovine. Regional vascular differences in endothelial function still require study, as they might provide clues on the crucial factors linking the atherosclerotic process and the attendant functional alterations.

Among the possible mechanisms responsible for loss of endothelial-dependent vasodilatation in these models, suggestions included a decrease in EDRF production or its release, or production of an abnormal EDRF. Minor et al. (1990) confirmed a dramatic impairment in the vasodilator activity of EDRF released from the aorta of rabbits fed a high cholesterol diet, but made an unanticipated observation. They measured the release of nitrogen oxides by a chemiluminescence method and found that release of these agents from the diet-induced atherosclerotic vessels was not decreased. Moreover, their production was increased in response to acetylcholine, so that impairment in synthesis or signal transduction was not responsible for impaired vasodilator activity. Mugge et al. (1991) went on to test the hypothesis that the factor responsible for endothelial dysfunction in this model, at least in part, involves rapid inactivation of the EDRF by superoxide radicals. They reasoned that the response reflected an imbalance between intrinsic superoxide dismutase activity, and the generation of superoxide radicals in atherosclerotic arteries. They found that treatment of cholesterol fed rabbits with polyethylene-glycolated superoxide dismutase increased vascular superoxide dismutase in normal and cholesterol fed rabbits and improved endothelium-dependent relaxation. Thus, the dysfunction of endothelium which leads to impaired endothelial-dependent relaxation reflects not an abnormality in synthesis or release, but rather an abnormality in local EDRF metabolism. Whether these observations in cholesterol fed rabbits apply to other models of vascular injury in which abnormalities in endothelial-dependent relaxation have been documented is not yet know.

The first observation of potentiated responses to 5-HT occurred in atherosclerotic vessels *in vivo* was made by Heistad et al. (1984) in hypercholesterolaemic and atherosclerotic monkeys treated for three to five years with an atherogenic diet. They studied the hindlimb, perfused at constant flow, so that changes in perfusion pressure indicated changes in vascular resistance, and segmental pressure and resistance could be assessed. The pressure gradient from the iliac to the dorsal pedal artery was employed to assess the response of the large artery segment. 5-HT decreased total hindlimb vascular resistance in normal and hypercholesterolaemic monkeys, but increased total vascular limb vascular resistance in the atherosclerotic monkeys. The constrictor response of large arteries to 5-HT in the atherosclerotic monkeys was increased a remarkable tenfold, and was largely responsible for the increase in total vascular resistance. Vasoconstrictor responses to noradrenaline were more complex, since they were increased in hypercholesterolaemic monkeys prior to the development of atherosclerosis, confirming Rosendorff et al. (1981), but were normal when atherosclerosis had supervened. Moreover, the enhanced response to noradrenaline was confined to the arteriolar level: large artery responses to noradrenaline were unaltered by either hypercholesterolaemia or atherosclerosis. Ketanserin reduced the vasoconstrictor responses to 5-HT in the atherosclerotic monkeys and the dose of ketanserin employed did not influence the response to nonadrenaline, suggesting that the enhanced large artery response to 5-HT reflected an action on the 5-HT$_2$ receptor, and that the influence of ketanserin did not reflect alpha adrenergic blockade.

These observations in animal models found strong support in recent studies in patients with coronary atherosclerosis. Golino *et al.* (1991) and McFadden *et al.* (1991) reported that infusion of 5-HT directly to the coronary artery in humans caused dilatation of coronary arteries that were free of atherosclerosis, but consistent, dose-related constriction of arteries with atherosclerosis and stable angina pectoris. This response was prevented or reversed by ketanserin (Golino *et al.* 1991; McFadden *et al.* 1992). In patients with vasospasm and atypical angina pectoris, the vasoconstrictor response to 5-HT was especially striking, with disappearance of the arterial lumen at 5-HT concentrations that caused only moderate constriction of adjacent arterial segments (McFadden *et al.* 1991, 1992). Ketanserin did not prevent the response in atypical angina (McFadden *et al.* 1992). Of interest is the fact that aspirin was employed as pre-treatment in all of these studies. Thus, it is clear that these conclusions apply to combined blockade. Whether the failure of ketanserin to reverse 5-HT-induced responses in variant angina reflects the presence of a different 5-HT receptor is not yet known.

VASCULAR INJURY, PLATELETS, AND PLATELET PRODUCTS

Even minimal injury to the endothelium results in platelet aggregation at the site of injury (Ashford 1968). Any break in the continuity of the vessel wall is met with an instant response from platelets, which contact the zone of injury and release a host of vasoactive factors. Although the molecular mechanisms responsible for platelet attachment to subendothelial tissues or abnormal endothelium are not known, recent research into the determinants of cell adhesion has identified a number of endothelial receptors, which are candidates to serve as an adhesive anchor (Ware and Heistad 1993). Especially intriguing is PECAM-1, a platelet: endothelial cell adhesion molecule which is found not only on endothelial cells, but is also abundant on platelets and neutrophils (Albelda *et al.* 1991). Although the specific ligand has not been identified, this receptor belongs to a family of endothelial receptors that are related to immunoglobulins, and which have cellular integrins and selectins as their ligands (Ware and Heistad 1993).

Only recently have we come to recognize from *in vitro* studies the potential interactions among the vasoactive agents that bathe the vessel wall during the platelet release action and we know far less of their actions and interactions *in vivo*, where the static fluids of the tissue bath are replaced by the dynamics of flowing blood. Isolated vessels often demonstrate a striking contraction, in response to aggregating platelets and their products (DeClerck and Van Newten 1982; Cohen *et al.* 1983*a,b*; Lindblad *et al.* 1984). The platelet release reaction releases a host of candidates with the ability to induce vascular smooth muscle contraction, which raises important questions about the responsible mediators. Pharmacological antagonists have provided an index of the relative contribution to the *in vitro* response of various mediators released by platelets. In the case of human digital arteries, studies with ketanserin suggested that 5-HT was responsible for about 50% of the response (Moulds *et al.* 1984), in the case of the rat caudal artery, about 60% of the response was 5-HT mediated (DeClerck and Van Newton 1982). In canine pulmonary arteries, by contrast, 5-HT accounted for virtually all of the response (McGoon and Vanhoutte 1984), reflecting the insensitivity of this vascular bed to thromboxane A_2. A constrictor response to aggregating platelets in each system assessed to date seems to have been accounted for by 5-HT and thromboxane, but dilator responses may be accounted for by other platelet factors, such as adenine nucleotides (Houston *et al.* 1985).

5-HT, thromboxane A_2, and thromboxane mimetics induce contraction of the rat caudal artery (DeClerck and Van Neuten 1982), the canine and porcine coronary artery (Ellis *et al.* 1976; Mullane *et al.* 1982; Cohen *et al.* 1983*a,b*), and human digital arteries (Moulds *et al.* 1984; Young *et al.* 1986). In all three systems, 5-HT not only induced a contractile response directly, but also potentiated thromboxane-induced contractions. Of equal interest, a thromboxane mimetic amplified responses to 5-HT, which raised the intriguing possibility that their mutual amplification plays a role in the vasospasm that may accompany the platelet release reaction (DeClerck and Van Neuten 1982; Mullane *et al.* 1982). This possibility was evaluated in greatest detail in the isolated digital artery obtained from humans post-mortem (Young *et al.* 1986) where the response of the arteries to aggregating platelets was substantially larger than the sum of the anticipated contractile response to the quantity of thromboxane A_2 and 5-HT released. A thromboxane mimetic enhanced substantially the responses to 5-HT. 5-HT appeared to amplify the responses to thromboxane rather less. As the response was abolished by a combination of ketanserin and thromboxane synthetase inhibitors, amplification of the response rather than the presence of additional mediators accounted for the enhanced response.

DeClerck *et al.* (1986) independently extended these observations to the platelet, and to events *in vivo*. They found that the combination of ketanserin and a thromboxane antagonist induced significantly more pronounced inhibition in the extent of the irreversible platelet aggregation that is elicited by ADP, than when the individual blockers were used alone. The possibility of synergism in the interaction between 5-HT and thromboxane in this process — combined release of which is a primary event in the interaction of platelets with a damaged vessel wall — led them to explore the interaction *in vivo*. The employed tail bleeding time in rats as an *in vivo* model of the platelet: vessel wall interaction. The simultaneous administration of both classes of antagonist resulted in a much more marked prolongation of bleeding time than when either agent was employed alone. Similar considerations apply to vascular smooth muscle responses to platelet activation in animals (Hollenberg *et al.* 1988) and in humans (Janicek *et al.* 1990, 1992). These are considered in detail below.

There are quantitatively important regional differences, perhaps species related (Somlyo and Somlyo 1970), in vascular responsiveness to 5-HT and thromboxane A_2. For example, the canine pulmonary artery shows little or no response to thromboxane A_2, whereas 5-HT induces a striking response (McGoonand Vanhoutte 1984). The coronary artery and the basilar artery of the dog, on the other hand, are sensitive to both thromboxane A_2 and to 5-HT (Ellis *et al.* 1976;

Van Neuten and Vanhoutte 1981; Mullane et al. 1982; Muller-Schweinitzer and Engel 1983) with possible implications for the pathogenesis of heart attack and stroke.

COLLATERAL REACTIVITY

A growing body of evidence indicates that collateral vessels and their responsiveness are complex: collateral arteries are not passive conduits, but rather a reactive system. Intrinsic vascular tone, reversible by vasodilators, is evident in the collateral blood supply to the limb of the dog (Thulesius 1962; Coffman 1966). There are a series of striking parallels to the questions raised by the atherosclerosis story, including the features of endothelial function, responsiveness to platelet products, and their implications for vascular tone and reactivity.

Acute occlusion of the terminal aorta in the cat resulted in substantially more ischaemia of the spinal cord and limb when the occlusion involved thrombus, leading to speculation that thrombus might release vasoactive factors that further reduced blood flow, through an action on the collateral arterial supply (Imhoff 1962). An alternative to release by the thrombus of vasoactive factors was embolization or extension beyond its initial size, to occlude collateral vessels mechanically. Schaub et al. (1976) showed that neither extension of the thrombus nor embolism, could not account for the more substantial impact of thrombus on hindlimb perfusion in the cat. They next evaluated 5-HT as a logical candidate (Schaub et al. 1977). Limb blood flow fell strikingly in response to 5-HT three days after aortic ligation. Both the 5-HT antagonist, cinanserin, or depletion of platelet 5-HT stores with reserpine, sustained collateral circulation to the limb. A reduction in platelet count induced by an antiserum directed against platelets, on the other hand, was not effective in restoring a limb circulation, despite a striking fall in platelet count. A remarkably small number of activated platelets, it appears are required to induce collateral arterial spasm.

Their observations were rapidly confirmed and extended. 5-HT induced striking ischaemia in the rat limb from five days to eight weeks after femoral artery ligation (Verheyen et al. 1984). Ketanserin, the $5-HT_2$ receptor antagonist, prevented that response, and blunted the blood flow reduction and tissue damage induced by acute thrombotic obstruction of the aorta in the cat (Nevelsteen et al. 1984). An action of thromboxane A_2 released by platelets was thought unlikely, as ketanserin appeared to be fully effective, and ketanserin does not inhibit the production, the release or the actions of thromboxane A_2.

The application of quantitative arteriography to pharmacology provided important insights into these processes (Orlandi et al. 1986). In the normal dog, 5-HT induced the anticipated, dose-related reduction in large artery calibre: limb blood flow increased. The reduction in large artery calibre was prevented or reversed by ketanserin, but not the blood flow increase (Blackshear et al. 1985). The larger was the normal artery, the larger the absolute and relative reduction in arterial lumen induced by 5-HT (Blackshear et al. 1985).

Collateral arteries were strikingly more sensitive to 5-HT than were normal intact arteries (Orlandi *et al.* 1986), and that enhanced response was also reversed by ketanserin. The increase in sensitivity expressed itself as a 10- to 30-fold reduction in the threshold 5-HT dose required to induce vasoconstriction in the profunda femoris and the medial and lateral circumflex remoral arteries, the major stem vessels giving rise to the collateral tree. The slope relating 5-HT dose to the degree of vasoconstriction, moreover, became much steeper. Calf blood flow, assessed with radioxenon, fell with 5-HT infusion in the collateral-dependent limb, and rose, as anticipated, in the normal limb. Responses of the collateral arterial supply to noradrenaline were not potentiated and prazosin did not influence the response to 5-HT. Taken in all, these data indicated that growing collateral arterial vessels display a specific increase in sensitivity to 5-HT via the $5\text{-}HT_2$ receptor, and that the potentiated response was sufficient to limit blood flow.

The isolated, perfused hind quarters of rats studied from five days to two months after vascular occlusion, showed a striking increase in sensitivity of the collateral bed to 5-HT, but not for noradrenaline, or a thromboxane A_2 mimetic, or angiotensin II (Verheyen *et al.* 1987). The increase in sensitivity was clearly 5-HT-specific. The fact that the responses to the thromboxane mimetic were not potentiated suggests that the 5-HT–thromboxane A_2 interaction *in vivo*, described below, may reflect 5-HT-induced amplification of the response to thromboxane A_2, as described earlier *in vitro* (DeClerck and Van Newten 1982; McGoon and Vanhoutte 1984; Moulds *et al.* 1984).

The duration of the supersensitivity of collateral vessels to 5-HT is prolonged. Studies, performed three days after femoral artery occlusion revealed an enhanced response (Nevelsteen *et al.* 1984; Verheyen *et al.* 1984). The longest study reported suggested that collateral vessel supersensitivity in the limb continues for at least eight weeks in the rat (Verheyen *et al.* 1984). Our studies (unpublished data) suggest that supersensitivity to 5-HT of limb collateral vessels in the rabbit continues for at least eight months after femoral artery occlusion, and supersensitivity of epicardial coronary collateral arteries to 5-HT in the dog was sustained for at least one year.

Does 5-HT released from platelets account for the entire collateral arterial response when thrombus complicates vascular occlusion? Helenski *et al.* (1980) suggested that thromboxane A_2 might play a role, but others disagreed (Nevelsteen *et al.* 1984). When platelet activation was induced *in vivo* by endothelial injury above the origin of the limb collateral arteries in the rabbit, spasm of the collateral vessels occurred routinely (Hollenberg *et al.* 1988). Ketanserin in doses too low to influence the response to noradrenaline (30 μg/kg) partially reversed the spasm. Thromboxane synthetase inhibition or a thromboxane antagonist also induced a partial reversal, somewhat less in degree than that induced by ketanserin. When the two classes of agent were combined, a striking reversal of spasm occurred, substantially greater than when either was employed alone. The efficacy of combined blockade for collateral function has been confirmed for humans with advanced atherosclerosis (Janicek *et al.* 1992).

The mechanism of the supersensitivity of collateral arterial arteries to 5-HT is as yet unclear. One possibility has involved the vasodilator influence of the endothelium (Cohen et al. 1983a,b). Endothelial cells of rapidly growing collateral arteries show marked changes, including hyperplasia demonstrated by radioautography with tritiated thymidine (Ilich et al. 1979; Odori et al. 1983). Multiple studies have suggested that dividing endothelial cells, and their daughter cells for some time after division, lose their ability to release the relaxant factor (Weldinger et al. 1990, 1991). Thus, one might anticipate, in view of the burst of endothelial proliferation during early collateral growth, that dysfunction of the daughter endothelial cells, leaving an unopposed constrictor response to 5-HT, could account for the apparent supersensitivity.

Knowledge of endothelial function in growing collaterals is limited. The acute opening of preformed collateral arteries after sudden arterial occlusion in the rabbit ear was reversed by an arginine analogue (L-NAME), the influence of which, in turn, was reversed by an excess of L-arginine (Randall and Griffith 1992). Thus, the acute vascular response appears to be endothelial-dependent, perhaps reflecting an influence of the rise in intimal shear stress (Cooke et al. 1990; Buga et al. 1991) in the collaterals consequent to increased flow velocity that must accompany the sharp rise in the pressure gradient. This study assessed only the first 100 minutes after acute occlusion, and endothelial hyperplasia requires at least 24 hours to become evident (Ilich et al. 1979, Odari et al. 1983). In studies performed three to six months after gradual coronary artery occlusion in the dog, the blood flow increase induced by acetylcholine carried by collateral arteries suggested that endothelial-dependent vasodilator mechanisms were intact (Altman et al. 1993). A number of studies of major epicardial collateral arteries in a similar model studied over a similar interval revealed intact acetylcholine-induced relaxation (Sellke et al. 1990; Angus et al. 1991; Flynn et al. 1991), although Sellke reported an impairment of acetylcholine-induced relaxation of coronary microvessels 100 to 200 microns in diameter in the collateral-dependent zone. This observation led Altman et al. (1993) to conclude that the crucial action of acetylcholine to induce a rise in blood flow was at the large collateral artery level. A similar conclusion was achieved independently based on similar considerations in the limb blood supply (Paskins-Hurlburt and Hollenberg 1992).

Unfortunately, there are no reported studies on endothelial function in growing collateral arteries in the crucial interval between 100 minutes and 3 months — as reviewed above. Our unreported, and still preliminary, studies in the rat and rabbit indicate that endothelial-dependent relaxation of limb collateral arteries is certainly intact, and probably enhanced during this interval. Thus, loss of endothelial-dependent relaxation, leaving an unopposed constrictor response, cannot account for collateral arterial supersensitivity to 5-HT. More intriguing — at least to the author — is another question. Why do replicating endothelial daughter cells after vascular injury lose this function (Weidinger et al. 1990, 1991) whereas replicating endothelial daughter cells in growing collateral arteries retain, or even enhance this function? Perhaps earlier explanations for this speciflc loss of function were too facile?

There are no species-related exceptions: exquisite sensitivity of the limb collateral arterial tree to 5-HT has been documented in the cat (Nevelsteen *et al.* 1984), the rat (Verheyen *et al.* 1984), the dog (Orlandi *et al.* 1986), and the rabbit (Hollenberg *et al.* 1988). Ketanserin dilated limb collaterals in over 50% of human patients with advanced atherosclerosis (Janicek *et al.* 1990). The combination of ketanserin and aspirin was more effective than ketanserin alone (Janicek *et al.* 1992). The unpredictable, but occasionally striking improvement in symptoms of intermittent claudication and limb perfusion in the patient with peripheral vascular disease treated with ketanserin (DeCree *et al.* 1983) may reflect these findings: Patients differ in the degree to which limb ischaemia reflects an influence of activated platelets and release of vasoactive factors acting on the collateral-dependent limb. The fact that the combination of ketanserin superimposed on aspirin produced a more predictable and striking collateral response on angiography (Janicek *et al.* 1992) is consistent with earlier studies in animals and has obvious therapeutic implications.

VASCULAR GROWTH REGULATION AND INJURY

Vascular embryogenesis remains as mysterious today as it was when Thoma performed his classical studies on the chick embryo and chorioallantoic membrane over 100 years ago. As little is known about the determinants of vascular growth during childhood. Perhaps it is not surprising, then, that so little is known of the determinants of hyperplasia and hypertrophy in response to vascular injury in the adult. Recent reviews on the determinants of vascular hyperplasia and hypertrophy have focused on the surprising finding that agents that act as vasoconstrictors and vasodilators in the short run are also candidates to serve as determinants of cardiovascular growth. In general, endogenous vasoconstrictors act as growth promoters and endogenous vasodilators act as growth inhibitors (Jackson and Schwartz 1992; Dzau 1993). An important caveat is that virtually all of the information has come from *in vitro* studies. There are a host of other known growth factors that have the capacity to influence growth of vascular elements, and have been incorporated into schemata design to explore atherosclerosis and collateral arterial formation (Jackson and Schwartz 1992; Schaper *et al.* 1992; Dzau 1993). Among the candidates that have received substantial emphasis in this essay is nitric oxide, which was shown to inhibit mitogenesis and proliferation of vascular smooth muscle cells, albeit only in a tissue culture system (Garg and Hassid 1989). Another relevant agent is PDGF, the platelet-derived growth factor that is released along with 5-HT and thromboxane A_2 during the platelet release reaction. Many would implicate PDGF in the vascular response to injury (Ross 1986; Jackson and Schwartz 1992).

Substantial credibility for these speculations was provided by the earlier studies of Langille and O'Donnell (1986). They exploited the long-recognized influence of chronic blood flow changes on arterial diameter to assess the contribution of endothelium to that vascular response. In the common carotid artery of rabbits, partial ligation to induce a 70% reduction in blood flow rate was associated with a 21% fall in the diameter of the artery within two weeks. This reduction in diameter reflected an organic change, which was abolished when the endothelium was removed from the vessel either by mechanical means, with a balloon catheter, or by local administration of Triton-X-100. They speculated on the possibility that loss of endothelial vasoactive factor release provided the link, which has found strong support from subsequent studies. Lessons learned from collateral blood vessel formation, a convenient method for provoking blood vessel growth in otherwise stable adult animals, might provide insights into not only embryogenesis, but also into the pathogenesis of atherosclerosis. We are as unlikely to understand atherosclerosis in the absence of these insights as we are to understand cancer without deep knowledge of normal growth processes.

THERAPEUTIC IMPLICATIONS

Although attempts to exploit the emerging concepts reviewed in this chapter for treatment are in their infancy, some of the implications are already evident (Luscher 1993; Ware and Heistad 1993). Attempts to reduce serum cholesterol with drugs and diet, for example, probably involved more than the local, mechanical effects of lipid deposition. To the extent that oxidized low density lipoproteins could contribute to the impairment of endothelium-dependent arterial relaxation in atherosclerosis, reduction in serum cholesterol and the action of omega-3 fatty acids in fish oil may have an additional action (Kugiyama *et al.* 1990; Simon *et al.* 1990; Tanner *et al.* 1991). Certainly in animal models, dietary treatment of atherosclerosis can restore endothelium-dependent relaxation (Harrison *et al.* 1987). Oestrogen replacement might share a similar mechanism (Williams *et al.* 1990). Whether the acute improvement in endothelium-dependent vasodilatation induced by administration of arginine (Girerd *et al.* 1990; Drexler *et al.* 1991) can be translated into a chronic, sustained response remains to be determined. Endothelial dysfunction has also been ameliorated by treatment with antioxidant agents in the atherosclerosis induced by cholesterol feeding in rabbits (Mugge *et al.* 1991).

There are other examples. Attempts to preserve endothelial capacity to release prostacyclin while inhibiting platelet synthesis of thromboxane A_2 have been the goal of low dose aspirin treatment (Pedersen and Fitz Gerald 1984). Diabetes, hypertension, and other risk factors clearly contribute to the impairment of endothelial function not only in animal models, but also in patients with atherosclerotic disease (Luscher 1993; Ware and Heistad 1993). In animal models, antihypertensive therapy appears to improve endothelial function (Luscher *et al.* 1987).

What does the future hold? Certainly, attempts are ongoing to influence the binding of platelets and other formed elements of the blood to endothelium, to limit destruction of nitric oxide, to enhance local nitric oxide production through several strategies, and to limit the influence of platelet-derived 5-HT and thromboxane A_2 on blood vessels. It seems likely that many of these treatments directed at the atherosclerotic vessel wall will also have a salutary influence on collateral arterial function. Given the number of variables involved, the number of potential targets for the strategies that are emerging, and the pace of current research, the design of therapeutic trials to assess their efficacy should prove to be an interesting challenge.

REFERENCES

Albelda, S. M., Muller, W. A., Buck, C. A., and Newman, P. J. (1991). Molecular and cellular properties of PECAM-1 (endoCAM/CD3): a novel vascular cell-cell adhesion molecule. *J. Cell. Biol.*, **114**, 1059-68.

Altman, J., Dulas, D., Pavek, T., Laxson, D. D., Homans, D. C., and Bache, R. J. (1993). Endothelial function in well-developed canine coronary collateral vessels. *Am. J. Physiol.*, **264**, H567-72.

Angus, J. A., Ward, J. E., Somlich, J. J., and McPherson, G. A. (1991). Reactivity of canine isolated epicardial collateral coronary arteries. *Circ. Res.*, **69**, 1340-52.

Ashford, T. (1968). Platelet aggregation at sites of minimal endothelial injury. *Am. J. Pathol.*, **53**, 599-607.

Blackshear, J. L., Orlandi, C., Garnic, J. D., and Hollenberg, N. K. (1985). Differential large and small vessel responses to serotonin in the dog hind limb *in vivo*: Role of the 5HT-2 receptor. *J. Cardiovasc. Pharmacol.*, **7**, 45-9.

Brazenor, R. M. and Angus, J. A. (1981). Ergometrine contracts isolated canine coronary arteries by a serotonergic mechanism: no role for alpha adrenoceptors. *J. Pharmacol. Exp. Ther.*, **218**, 530-6.

Brum, J. M., Sufan, Q., Lane, G. and Bove, A. A., (1984). Increased vasoconstrictor activity of proximal coronary arteries with endothelial damage in intact dogs. *Circulation*, **70**, 1066-73.

Buga, G. M., Gold, M. E., Fukuto, J. M., and Ignarro, L. J. (1991). Shear stress-induced release of nitric oxide from endothelial cells grown on beads. *Hypertension*, **17**, 187-93.

Cocks, T. M. and Angus, J. A. (1993). Endothelium-dependent relaxation of coronary arteries by noradrenaline and serotonin. *Nature*, **305**, 627-30.

Coffman, J. D. (1966). Peripheral collateral blood flow and vascular reactivity in the dog. *J. Clin. Invest.*, **45**, 923-31.

Cohen, R. A., Shepherd, J. T., and Vanhoutte, P. M. (1983*a*). 5-Hydroxytryptamine can mediate endothelium-dependent relaxation of coronary arteries. *Am. J. Physiol.*, **245**, H1077-80.

Cohen, R. A., Shepherd, J. T., and Vanhoutte, P. M. (1983*b*). Inhibitory role of the endothelium in the response of isolated coronary arteries to platelets. *Science*, **22**, 273-4.

Cooke, J. P., Stamler, J., Andon, N., Davies, P. F., McKinley, G., and Loscalzo, J. (1990). Flow stimulates endothelial cells to release a nitrovasodilator that is potentiated by reduced thiol. *Am. J. Physiol.*, **259**, 28, H804-12.

Cowan, D. F., Hollenberg, N. K., Connelly, C. M., Williams, D. H., and Abrams, H. L. (1978). Increased collateral arterial and venous endothelial cell turnover after renal artery stenosis in the dog. *Invest. Radiol.*, **13**, 143-9.

Creager, M. A., Cooke, J. P., Mendelsohn, M. E., Gallagher, S. J., Coleman, S. M., Loscalzo, J., *et al.* (1990). Impaired vasodilation of forearm resistance vessels in hypercholesterolemic humans. *J. Clin. Invest.*, **86**, 228-34.

DeClerck, F. and Van Neuten, J. M. (1982). Platelet-mediated vascular contractions: Inhibition of the serotonergic component by ketanserin. *Thromb. Res.*, **32**, 765-71.

DeClerck, F., Xhonneux, B., Van Gorp, L. J., and Beetens, P. A. J. (1986). S₂-Serotonergic receptor inhibition (ketanserin), combined with thromboxane A₂/prostaglandin endoperoxide receptor blockade (BM 13.177): Enhanced anti-platelet effect. *Thromb. Hemost.*, **56**, 236.

DeCree, J., Leempoels, J., Geukens, H., and Verhaegen, H. (1983). Placebo controlled double blind trial of ketanserin in the treatment of intermittent claudication. *Lancet*, **ii**, 775-9.

Drexler, H., Zeiher, A. M., Meinzer, K., and Just, H. (1991). Correction of endothelial dysfunction in coronary microcirculation of hypercholesterolemic patients by L-arginine. *Lancet*, **338**, 1546-50.

Dzau, V. (1993). The role of the mechanical and humoral factors in growth regulation of vascular smooth muscle and cardiac myocytes. *Curr. Opin. Nephrol. Hypertens.*, **2**, 27-32.

Egashira, K., Inou, T., Hirooka, Y., Yamada, A., Maruoka, Y., Kai, H., *et al.* (1993). Impaired coronary blood flow response to acetylcholine in patients with coronary risk factors and proximal atherosclerotic lesions. *J. Clin. Invest.*, **91**, 29-37.

Ellis, E. F., Oelz, O., Roberts, L. J., Payne, N. A., Sweetman, B. J., Niess, A. S., *et al.* (1976). Coronary arterial smooth muscle contraction by a substance released from platelets: Evidence that it is thromboxane A₂. *Science*, **193**, 1135-7.

Flynn, N. M., Kenny, D., Pelc, L. R., Warltier, D. C., Bosnjak, Z. J., and Kampine, J. P. (1991). Endothelium-dependent vasodilation of canine coronary collateral vessels. *Am. J. Physiol.*, **261**, H1797-801.

Folts, J. D., Crowell, E. B., and Rowe, G. G. (1976). Platelet aggregation in partially obstructed vessels and its elimination with aspirin. *Circulation*, **54**, 365-70.

Freeman, P. C., Mitchell, G. G., Heistad, D. D., Armstrong, M. L., and Harrison, D. G. L. (1996). Atherosclerosis impairs endothelium-dependent vascular relaxation to acetylcholine and thrombin in primates. *Circ. Res.*, **58**, 783-9.

Garg, U. C., and Hassid, A. (1989). Nitric oxide-generating vasodilators and 8-Bromo-cyclic guanosine monophosphate inhibit mitogenesis and proliferation of cultured rat vascular smooth muscle cells. *J. Clin. Invest.*, **83**, 1774-7.

Girerd, X. J., Hirsch, A. T., Cooke, J. P., Dzau, V. J., and Creager, M. A. (1990). L-Arginine jugments endothelium-dependent vasodilation in cholesterol-fed rabbits. *Circ. Res.*, **67**, 1301-8.

Golino, P., Piscione, F., Willerson, J. T., Cappelli-Bigazzi, M., Focaccio, A., Villari, B., *et al.* (1991). Divergent effects of serotonin on coronary artery dimensions and blood flow in patients with coronary atherosclerosis and control patients. *N. Engl. J. Med.*, **324**, 641-8.

Harrison, D. G., Armstrong, M., Freiman, P. C., and Heistad, D. D. (1987). Restoration of endothelium-dependent relaxation by dietary treatment of atherosclerosis. *J. Clin. Invest.*, **80**, 1808-11.

Heistad, D. D., Armstrong, M. L., Marcus, M. L., Piegor, D. J., and Mark, A. L. (1984). Augmented responses to vasoconstrictor stimuli in hypercholesterolemic and atherosclerotic monkeys. *Circ. Res.*, **54**, 711-18.

Helenski, C., Schaub, R. G., and Roberts, R. (1980). Improvement of collateral circulation after aortic thrombosis with indomethacin therapy. *Thromb. Haemostas.*, **44**, 69-71.

Henry, P. D. and Yokoyama, M. (1980). Supersensitivity of atherosclerotic rabbit aorta to ergonovine. Mediation by a serotonergic mechanism. *J. Clin. Invest.*, **66**, 306-13.

Hollenberg, N. K. (1993). Collateral arterial growth and reactivity: Lessons from the limb and renal blood supply. In *Collateral circulation* (ed. W. Schaper and J. Schaper), pp. 1-15. Kluwer Academic Publishers, Germany.

Hollenberg, N. K. and Odori, T. (1987). Centripetal spread of arterial collateral endothelial cell hyperplasia after renal artery stenosis in the rat. *Circ. Res.*, **60**, 398-401.

Hollenberg, N. K., Monteiro, K., and Sandor, T. (1988). Endothelial injury provokes collateral arterial spasm: Role of thromboxane and serotonin. *J. Pharmacol. Exp. Ther.*, **244**, 1164-8.

Houston, D. S., Shepherd, J. T., and Vanhoutte, P. M. (1985). Adenine nucleotides, serotonin, and endothelium-dependent relaxations to platelets. *Am. J. Physiol.*, **17**, H389-95.

Ilich, N., Hollenberg, N. K., Williams, D. H., and Abrams, H. L. (1979). Time course of increased collateral arterial and venous endothelial cell turnover after renal artery stenosis in the rat. *Circ. Res.*, **45**, 579-82.

Imhoff, R. K. (1962). Production of aortic occlusion resembling acute aortic embolisni syndrome in cats. *Nature*, **192**, 979-80.

Jackson, C. L. and Schwartz, S. M. (1992). Pharmacology of smooth muscle cell reproduction. *Hypertension*, **20**, 713-36.

Janicek, M., Grassi, C. J., Meyerovitz, M., Callahan, M. B., Sandor, T., Whittemore, A., et al. (1990). Atherosclerosis, peripheral arterial disease and the vascular response to ketanserin. *Invest. Radiol.*, **25**, 495-503.

Janicek, M. J., Meyerovitz, M., Harrington, D. P., and Hollenberg, N. K. (1992). Arterial response to ketanserin and aspirin in patients with advanced peripheral atherosclerosis. *Invest. Radiol.*, **27**, 415-21.

Kugiyama, K., Kerns, S. A., Morrisett, J. D., Roberts, R., and Henry, P. D. (1990). Impairment of endothelium-dependent arterial relaxation by lysolecithin in modified low-density lipoproteins. *Nature*, **344**, 160-2.

Langille, B. L. and O'Donnell, F. (1986). Reductions in arterial diameter produced by chronic decreases in blood flow are endothelium-dependent. *Science*, **231**, 405-7.

Liebow, A. A. (1963). Situations which lead to changes in vascular patterns. In (ed. *Handbook of physiology* and W. F. Hamilton and P. Dow), Vol. II, pp. 125-76. Circ., Am. Physiological Soc., NY.

Lindbland, L. E., Shepherd, J. T., and Vanhoutte, P. M. (1984). Cooling augments platelet-induced contraction of peropheral arteries of the dog. *Proc. Soc. Exp. Biol. Med.*, **176**, 119-22.

Ludmer, P. L., Selwyn, A. P., Shook, T. L., Wayne, R. R., Mudge, G. H., Alexander, R. W., et al. (1986). Paradoxical vasoconstriction induced by acetylcholine in atherosclerotic coronary arteries. *N. Engl. J. Med.*, **315**, 1046-51.

Luscher, T. F. (1993). Possibilities and perspectives of pharmacotherapy for endothelial protection. *Curr. Opin. Nephrol. Hypertens.*, **2**, 129-36.

Luscher, T. F., Vanhoutte, P. M., and Raij, L. (1987). Antihypertensive therapy normalizes endothelium-dependent relaxations in salt-induced hypertension of the rat. *Hypertension*, **9**, 193-7.

McFadden, E. P., Clarke, J. G., Davies, G. J., Kaski, J. C., Haider, A. W., and Maseri, A. (1991). Effect of intracoronary serotonin on coronary vessels in patients with stable angina and patients with variant angina. *N. Engl. J. Med.*, **324**, 648-54.

McFadden, E. P., Bouters, C., Lablanche, J. M., Leroy, F., Clarke, J. G., Henry, M., et al. (1992). Effect of ketanserin on proximal and distal coronary constrictor responses to intracoronary infusion of serotonin in patients with stable angina, patients with variant angina, and control patients. *Circulation*, **86**, 187-95.

McGoon, M. D. and Vanhoutte, P. M. (1984). Aggregating platelets contract isolated canine pulmonary arteries by releasing 5-hydroxtryptamine. *J. Clin. Invest.*, **74**, 828-33.

Maseri, A., Chierchia, S., and Davies, G. (1986). Pathophysiology of coronary occlusion in acute infarction. *Platelets Vasc. Occlusion*, **73**, 233-9.

Minor, R. L., Jr., Myers, P. R., Guerra, R. Jr., Bates, J. N., and Harrison, D.G. (1990). Diet-induced atherosclerosis increases the release of nitrogen oxides from rabbit aorta. *J. Clin. Invest.*, **86**, 109–16.

Morikawa, E., Huang, Z., and Moskowitz, M. A. (1992). L-Arginine decreases infarct size caused by middle cerebral arterial occlusion in SHR. *Am. J. Physiol.*, **263**, H1632–5.

Moulds, R. F. W., Iwanov, V., and Medcalf, R. L. (1984). The effects of platelet-derived contractile agents on human digital arteries. *Clin. Sci.*, **66**, 443–51.

Mugge, A., Elwell, J. H., Peterson, T. E., Hofmeher, T. G., Heistad, D. D., and Harrison, D. G. (1991). Chronic treatment with polyethylene-glycolated superoxide dismutase partially restores endothelium-dependent vascular relaxations in cholesterol fed rabbits. *Circ. Res.*, **69**, 1293–300.

Mullane, K. M., Bradley, G., and Moncada, S. (1982). The interactions of platelet-derived mediators on isolated canine coronary arteries. *Eur. J. Pharmacol.*, **84**, 115–18.

Muller-Schweinitzer, E., and Engel, G. (1983). Evidence for mediation by 5HT-2 receptors of 5-hydroxytryptamine-induced contraction of canine basilar artery. *Naunyn Schmiedebergs Arch. Pharmacol.*, **324**, 287–92.

Nevelsteen, A., DeClerck, F., Loots, W., and De Gryse, A. (1984). Restoration of post-thrombotic peripheral collateral circulation in the cat by ketanserin, a selective 5HT$_2$-receptor antagonist. *Arch. Int. Pharmacodyn. Ther.*, **270**, 268–79.

Oates, J. A., Hawiger, J., and Ross, R. (1985). Interaction of platelets with the vessel wall. Am. Physiol. Soc. Bethesda.

Odori, T., Paskins-Hurlburt, A., and Hollenberg, N. K. (1983). Increase in collateral arterial endothelial cell proliferation induced by captopril after renal artery stenosis in the rat. *Hypertension*, **5**, 307–11.

Orlandi, C., Blackshear, J. L., and Hollenberg, N. K. (1986). Specific increase in sensitivity to serotonin of the canine hind-limb collateral arterial tree via the 5-hydroxytryptamine-2 receptor. *Microvasc. Res.*, **32**, 121–30.

Orlandi, C., Humphrey, W. R., Hollenberg, N. K., and Schaub, R. G. (1990). In vivo demonstration of enhanced arterial constrictor response to serotonin following focal endothelial cell loss. *Exp. Mol. Pathol.*, **52**, 192–201.

Paskins-Hurlburt, A. J. and Hollenberg, N. K. (1992). "Tissue need" and limb collateral arterial growth. Skeletal contractile power and perfusion during collateral development in the rat. *Circ. Res.*, **70**, 546–53.

Pedersen, A. K. and FitzGeraid, G. A. (1984). Dose-related kinetics of aspirin: Presystemic acetylation of platelet cycloxygenase. *N. Engl. J. Med.*, **311**, 1206–11.

Randall, M. D. and Griffith, T. M. (1992). EDRF plays central role in collateral flow after arterial occlusion in rabbit ear. *Am. J. Physiol.*, **263**, H752–60.

Rosendorff, C. Hoffman, J. I. E., Verrier, E. D., Rouleau, J., and Boerboom, L. E. (1981). Cholesterol potentiates the coronary artery response to norepinephrine in anesthetized and conscious dogs. *Circ. Res.*, **48**, 320–9.

Ross, R. (1986). The pathogenesis of atherosclerosis: an update. *N. Engl. J. Med.*, **314**, 488–500.

Schaper, W., Bernotat-Danielowski, S., Nienaber, C., and Schaper, J. (1992). In *The heart and cardiovascular system*. (ed. H. A. Fozzard et al.), pp. 1427–64. Raven Press, Ltd., New York.

Schaub, R. G., Meyers, K. M., Sande, R., and Hamilton, G. (1976). Inhibition of feline collateral vessel development following thrombotic occlusion. *Circ. Res.*, **39**, 736–43.

Schaub, R. G., Meyers, K. M., and Sande, R. (1977). Serotonin as a factor in depression of collateral blood flow following experimental arterial thrombosis. *J. Lab. Clin. Med.*, **90**, 645–53.

Sellke, F. W., Quillen, J. E., Brooks, L. A., and Harrison, D. G. (1990). Endothelial modulation of the coronary vasculature in vessels perfused via mature collaterals. *Circulation*, **81**, 1938-47.

Simon, B. C., Cunningham, L. D., and Cohen, R. A. (1990). Oxidized low density lipoproteins cause contraction and inhibit endothelium-dependent relaxation in the pig coronary artery. *J. Clin. Invest.*, **86**, 750-9.

Somlyo, A. P. and Somlyo, A. V. (1970). Vascular smooth muscle. II. Pharmacology of normal and hypertensive vessels. *Pharmacol. Rev.*, **22**, 249-353.

Stamler, J. S., Osborne, J. A., Jaraki, O., Rabbani, L. E., Mullins, M., Singel, D., *et al.* (1993). Adverse vascular effects of homocysteine are modulated by endothelium-derived relaxing factor and related oxides of nitrogen. *J. Clin. Invest.*, **9**, 308-18.

Tanner, F., Noll, G., Boulanger, C. M., Luscher, T. F. (1991). Oxidized low-density lipoproteins inhibit relaxations of porcine coronary arteries: role of scavenger receptor and endothelium derived nitric oxide. *Circulation*, **83**, 2012-20.

Tesfamariam, B., Brown, M. L., and Cohen, R. A. (1991). Elevated glucose impairs endothelium-dependent relaxation by activating protein kinase C. *J. Clin. Invest.*, **87**, 1643-8.

Thoma, R. (1983). Untersuchungen uber die Histogenase und Histomechanik des Gefassystems. Stuttgart: Enke.

Thulesius, O. (1962). Hemodynamic studies on experimental obstruction on the femoral artery of the cat with special references to the peripheral action of vasoactive substances. *Acta Physiol. Scand.*, **199**, 1-95.

Van Nueten, J. M. and Vanhoutte, P. M. (1981). Selectivity of calcium antagonism and serotonin antagonism with respect to venous and arterial tissues. *Angiology*, **32**, 476-84.

Verbeuren, T. J., Coene, M.-C., Jordaens, F. H., Van Hove, C. E., Zonnekeyn, L. L., and Herman, A. G. (1986). Effect of hypercholesteremia in vascular reactivity in the rabbit: II: influence of treatment with dipyridamole on endothelium-dependent and endothelium-independent responses in isolited aortas of control and hypercholesterolemic rabbits. *Circ. Res.*, **59**, 496-504.

Verheyen, A., Vlaminckx, E., Lauwers, F., Van Den Broeck, C., and Wouters, L. (1984). Serotonin-induced blood flow changes in the rat hind legs after unilateral ligation of the femoral artery. Inhibition by the S2 receptor antagonist ketanserin. *Arch. Int. Pharmacodyn. Ther.*, **270**, 280-98.

Verheyen, A., Lauwers, F., Vlaminckx, E., Wouters, L., and DeClerck, F. (1987). Effects of vasoactive agonists on peripheral collateral arteries *in situ* perfused rat hind quarters. Anstract. *Belg. Cardiol. Soc.*, A7.

Vita, J. A., Treasure, C. B., Nabel, E. G., McLenachan, J. M., Fish, R. D., Yeung, A. C., *et al.* (1990). Coronary vasomotor response to acetylcholine relates to risk factors for coronary artery disease. *Circulation*, **81**, 491-7.

Ware, J. A., and Heistad, D. D. (1993). Platelet-endothelium interactions. *N. Engl. J. Med.*, **328**, 628-35.

Weidinger, F. F., McLenachan, J. M., Cybulsky, M. I., Gordon, J. B., Rennke, H. G., Hollenberg, N. K., *et al.* (1990). Persistent dysfunction of regenerated endothelium after balloon angioplasty of rabbit iliac artery. *Circulation*, **81**, 1667-79.

Weldinger, F. F., McLenachan, J. M., Cybulsky, M. I., Fallon, J. T., Hollenberg, N. K., Cooke, J. P., *et al.* (1991). Hypercholesterolemia enhances macrophage recruitment and dysfunction of regenerated endothelium after balloon injury of the rabbit iliac artery. *Circulation*, **84**, 755-67.

Williams, J. K., Adams, M. R., and Klopfenstein, H. S. (1990). Estrogen modulates responses of atherosclerotic coronary arteries. *Circulation*, **81**, 1680-7.

Wright, C. E. and Angus, J. A. (1986). Effects of hypertension and hypercholesterolemia on vasodilatation in the rabbit. *Hypertension*, **8**, 361-71.

Yokoyama, M., Akita, H., Mizutani, T., Fukazaki, H., and Watanabe, Y. (1993). Hyperreactivity of coronary arterial smooth muscles in response to ergonovine from rabbits with hereditary hyperlipidemia. *Circ. Res.*, **53**, 63-71.

Young, M. S., Iwanov, V., and Moulds, R. F. W. (1986). Interaction between platelet-released serotonin and thromboxane A_2 on human digital arteries. *Clin. Exp. Pharmacol. Physiol.*, **13**, 143-52.

16. The cerebral microvascular endothelium in ischaemia

A. Lorris Betz and Fausto Iannotti

INTRODUCTION

A sudden interruption in the blood supply to the brain triggers a cascade of events which ultimately results in cell death. While neurones are particularly vulnerable to ischaemia, extreme or prolonged oxygen deprivation can also injure the microvasculature. This microvascular injury can produce further neuronal damage as a result of accelerated influx of electrolytes, water, and other blood-borne substances. Thus, 'neuroprotection' in ischaemia must be directed not only at the neurone, but also at the cerebral microvasculature.

Some of the processes that produce cellular damage during cerebral ischaemia injure both neurones and microvascular cells. Others are more selective. For example, free radicals may produce non-selective injury to any cell which is in the vicinity of their site of production (Betz 1993). In contrast, glutamate has been implicated in the selective neuronal vulnerability of those neurones that have receptors for excitatory amino acids (Rothman and Olney 1986), but there is no evidence for direct injury of the microvasculature by glutamate. Microvascular cells, on the other hand, contain receptors which may predispose them to a different pattern of selective injury. Thus, pharmacologic approaches to microvascular injury in cerebral ischaemia could be directed at both the receptor-mediated and the non-selective injury mechanisms.

It is important to recognize that the brain microvasculature is composed of smooth muscle cells, endothelial cells, and pericytes and each of these is subject to injury in ischaemia. A discussion of pharmacologic regulation of cerebral vascular smooth muscle cells is presented in Chapter 11. The function of the pericyte and its response to disease is largely unknown. Therefore, we will have nothing to say about pharmacologic control of the pericyte in ischaemia. The present discussion will focus on the microvascular endothelial cell in brain, how its function is regulated, and the mechanisms by which its function is altered in ischaemia. Although to date there are few examples of pharmacological agents which have been shown to attenuate ischaemic damage to the cerebral microvasculature, we believe that, with an understanding of the mechanisms which produce injury to endothelial cells, it should be possible to develop effective therapeutic interventions.

Table 16.1 Multiple functions of the BBB

- Provide a barrier to the passive diffusion of polar substances between blood and brain
- Facilitate the equilibration of metabolic substrates through carrier-mediated transport
- Actively pump ions and wastes into or out of the brain via active transport
- Metabolize substances that are potentially toxic to the brain
- Produce paracrine substances that influence other cells

THE BLOOD-BRAIN BARRIER

In brain, the microvascular endothelial cells form a blood-brain barrier (BBB) which controls the exchange of solutes between the blood and the brain (Table 16.1) (reviewed in detail elsewhere: (Bradbury 1979; Betz et al. 1989b)). For many polar solutes, the BBB forms an impermeable wall that isolates the brain from the blood. This passive barrier results from the continuous tight junctions that seal the endothelial cells together and the absence of transcellular vesicular transport and fenestrations. In order to enhance brain uptake of compounds which are essential for brain function, specific carrier-mediated transport systems are present in the luminal and abluminal membranes of the endothelial cell. Thus, metabolic substrates such as glucose and large neutral amino acids readily enter brain from the blood via these transporters. Some compounds are pumped into or out of the brain by active transport systems that are present on either the luminal or abluminal side of the endothelial cell. Because of this epithelium-like property (Betz 1985), the brain capillary endothelial cell can secrete fluid into the brain and regulate the concentration of potassium and metabolites in the brain's interstitial fluid. Finally, the brain capillary endothelial cell is a metabolically active tissue containing enzymes that can metabolize toxins as they traverse through the cell or produce substances which influence neighbouring cells (e.g. nitric oxide). Taken together, these various properties permit the microvascular endothelial cell in brain to maintain a relatively constant extracellular environment which is optimal for neuronal function.

REGULATION OF THE BLOOD-BRAIN BARRIER

BBB function is not static, but rather, it is regulated by a wide variety of neurotransmitters, hormones, growth factors, and cytokines. It is now known that brain microvessels are richly endowed with a wide variety of receptors (Table 16.2) and each of these receptors presents a potential target for pharmacologic manipulation of BBB function. Since there is experimental evidence for reversible alterations of BBB permeability under various conditions, it seems likely that receptor-mediated processes are involved. In theory, the passive permeability of

Table 16.2 Receptors on brain microvessels

β-Adrenergic
α-Adrenergic
Dopamine
Histamine
Adenosine
Prostaglandins
Leukotrienes
Bradykinin
Insulin
Glucocorticoid
Mineralocorticoid
Vasoactive intestinal peptide
Parathyroid hormone
Vasopressin
Angiotensin II
Atrial natriuretic factors
Endothelin

the BBB could be altered in a number of different ways including activation of vesicular transport, regulation of the tight junctions, or disruption of membrane integrity (Fig. 16.1).

The rate of transcellular vesicular transport at the normal BBB is very low and, therefore, activation of this pathway could enhance BBB permeability. Although the role of endothelial cell vesicles in capillary permeability is uncertain (Bundgaard 1980), a large number of vesicles are seen in brain endothelial cells in diseases that are associated with increased BBB permeability, including ischaemia (Westergaard 1977; Petito 1979). This may result from stimulation by histamine (Joó et al. 1981; Dux and Joó 1982) or noradrenaline (Sarmento et al. 1991), and increases in intracellular cGMP (Joó et al. 1983), cAMP (Joó 1972), or polyamines (Trout et al. 1986).

The tightness of the tight junctions may also be actively regulated by neurotransmitters and hormones (Fig. 16.1). The BBB in normal animals becomes tighter following treatment with dexamethasone (Ziylan et al. 1988, 1989; Betz and Coester 1990), progesterone (Betz and Coester 1990), and corticotrophin (Ziylan et al. 1993). Increases in intracellular cAMP tighten the BBB in vitro (Rubin et al. 1991) and in vivo (Easton and Fraser 1993a), although one study has reported the opposite effect (Joó et al. 1974). In contrast, raising the intracellular calcium concentration increases BBB permeability (Olesen 1985; Olesen and Crone 1986) and this appears to be the mechanism by which 5-HT (Olesen 1985) opens the barrier. Histamine also opens the barrier by acting at H_2-histaminergic receptors (Gross et al. 1981; Dux and Joó 1982; Butt and Jones 1992; Easton and Fraser 1993b) while bradykinin increases BBB permeability through the activation of B_2-kininergic receptors (Unterberg et al. 1984; Olesen and Crone 1986). Increases in intracellular calcium may mediate these increases in permeability (Revest et al. 1991).

Regulation of BBB Permeability

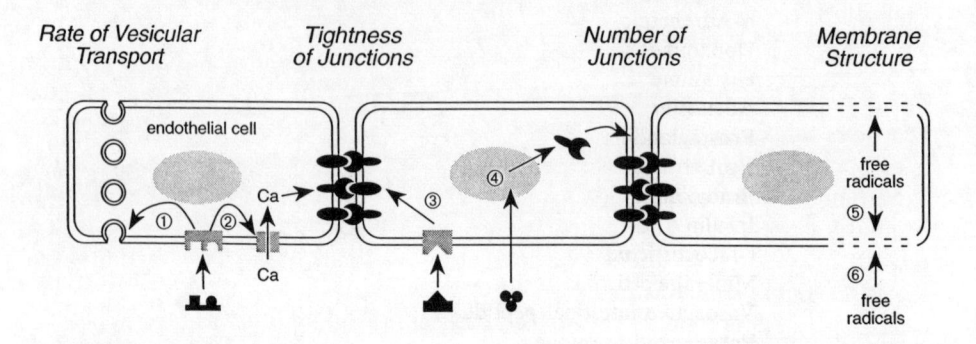

Fig. 16.1 The passive permeability of the BBB may be controlled through a number of different mechanisms. Specific interactions of hormones or neurotransmitters with endothelial cell receptors could increase the rate of vesicular transport (①), or alter the tightness of the tight junctions through changes in intracellular calcium concentration (②), or other second messengers (③). The number of the junctions might be altered by regulation of gene expression (④). Frank disruption of the endothelial cell membrane could be mediated by the release of toxins such as free radicals, produced either by the endothelial cell itself (⑤), or by other cells in the brain or blood (⑥).

In isolated brain capillaries, B_2 receptors are also linked to phosphoinositide hydrolysis (Homayoun and Harik 1991).

Finally, the passive permeability of the BBB is increased when the endothelial cell membrane is disrupted (Fig. 16.1). Arachidonic acid causes BBB opening when it is injected into the brain (Wakai *et al.* 1982; Chan *et al.* 1983; Black and Hoff 1985) or superfused over the brain's surface (Kontos *et al.* 1980; Unterberg *et al.* 1987). Exposure to arachidonic acid is associated with destruction of the luminal membrane of the endothelial cell (Wakai *et al.* 1982), perhaps mediated by circulating neutrophils (Unterberg *et al.* 1987). Some studies suggest that metabolism of the arachidonate to prostaglandins (Kontos *et al.* 1980; Ellis *et al.* 1981; Wei *et al.* 1981) or leukotrienes (Black and Hoff 1985) is required since the damaging effects could be prevented by systemic administration of inhibitors of the respective biosynthetic pathways. Other investigators were unable to attenuate arachidonic acid-induced injury with inhibitors of arachidonic acid metabolism (Unterberg *et al.* 1987). The studies of Wei *et al.* (1986) support the idea that arachidonate toxicity is mediated through oxygen free radicals. Chan *et al.* (1983) found that the intracerebral injection of polyunsaturated fatty acids also causes BBB breakdown, an effect they attributed to free radicals (Chan and Fishman 1980). Direct injection of free radical-generating reagents into the brain (Chan *et al.* 1984) or superfusion over the cerebral surface (Olesen 1987) increases BBB permeability and causes localized destruction of the luminal membrane of the endothelial cell (Wei *et al.* 1986). Although free radicals are often considered to be highly toxic, their effect on the BBB may be more subtle and reversible. For example, inflamed cerebral microvessels exhibit a fluctuating increase in permeability which appears to result from the opening of 22 nm gaps, possibly at the tight junctions (Easton and Fraser 1994). These fluctuations in permeability can be blocked by catalase (Easton and Fraser 1993b).

Recent studies indicate that various cytokines may produce BBB disruption. For example, injection of tumour necrosis factor alpha (TNF-α) into the cerebral ventricles causes an increase in BBB permeability after three to four hours which is associated with an increase in the number of leucocytes in the cerebrospinal fluid (Quagliarello *et al.* 1991; Kim *et al.* 1992; Megyeri *et al.* 1992). A similar response is seen after the intraventricular administration of interleukin-1 beta (IL-1β) (Quagliarello *et al.* 1991) although IL-1β does not appear to acutely disrupt the BBB (Banks and Kastin 1992). In cultured brain microvascular endothelial cells, both TNF-α and IL-1β induce the expression of intercellular adhesion molecule-1 (ICAM-1), a glycoprotein on the cell surface that mediates leucocyte adhesion to the endothelial cell (Wong and Dorovini Zis 1992). Thus, it is possible that the BBB injury which follows injection of these cytokines *in vivo* is the result of the induction of ICAM-1 expression on the endothelium and attachment and migration of leucocytes from blood to brain.

The preceding discussion emphasized regulation of the passive permeability of the BBB. Perhaps equally important, although less well studied, is the regulation of the transport and enzymatic functions (Table 16.1) of the brain microvascular endothelium. One of the first examples of a neurotransmitter-mediated alteration of BBB function was the study of Raichle *et al.* (1975) showing that noradrenergic innervation from the locus coeruleus altered BBB permeability to water. Subsequently, Harik (1986) showed that ablation of the locus coeruleus results in loss of Na,K-ATPase activity in brain capillaries. Thus, it appears that ion transport across the BBB is regulated by the sympathetic nervous system in the brain. The activity of Na,K-ATPase of brain capillaries can also be influenced by changes in extracellular potassium concentration (Goldstein 1979; Schielke *et al.* 1990) and exposure to free radicals (Lo and Betz 1986). Other examples of hormonal control of BBB transport include the modulation of a sodium channel (Ibaragi *et al.* 1989) and increased BBB permeability to water (Brust *et al.* 1991) induced by atrial natriuretic peptide, the activation of Na/H exchange by endothelin (Frelin *et al.* 1992), and the inhibition of neutral amino acid transport by vasopressin (Brust 1986; Brust and Diemer 1990). Finally, brain microvascular endothelial cells in culture secrete endothelin when exposed to angiotensin II or vasopressin (Spatz *et al.* 1992) while interferon and TNF-α induce the synthesis of nitric oxide (Gross *et al.* 1991).

ALTERATION OF BLOOD-BRAIN BARRIER FUNCTION IN ISCHAEMIA

Breakdown of the BBB is a commonly observed consequence of cerebral ischaemia. However, as discussed above, it is important to recognize that the BBB is more than just an impermeable wall. The other functions of the BBB (Table 16.1) are also susceptible to damage in ischaemia and these may contribute significantly to brain injury. For example, the transport of sodium from blood to brain is stimulated during the first several hours of ischaemia (Betz *et al.* 1989a, 1994; Betz and Coester 1990; Ennis *et al.* 1990; Schielke *et al.* 1991) probably as a result of the increase in extracellular potassium concentration (Schielke *et al.* 1990, 1991). Since the rate of sodium entry into brain may control the rate at which oedema forms (Betz *et al.* 1989a), this acceleration in sodium entry allows oedema to accumulate at an excessive rate. In agreement with this proposal, inhibition of Na,K-ATPase by intravascular infusion of ouabain attenuates ischaemic oedema formation (Shigeno *et al.* 1989). In contrast to sodium, BBB transport of potassium (Betz *et al.* 1994) and glucose (Betz *et al.* 1983) are reduced in cerebral ischaemia.

Although there have been over 100 reports of BBB breakdown during ischaemia or following reperfusion of ischaemic brain, there are few studies of the mechanisms involved. In general, BBB opening during focal ischaemia does not occur immediately, but rather, it requires three to six hours of a continuous reduction in blood flow (Olsson *et al.* 1971; Tyson *et al.* 1982; Shigeno *et al.* 1984; Kuroiwa *et al.* 1986; Rubino and Young 1988; Hatashita and Hoff 1990; Menzies *et al.* 1993). The greater the reduction in blood flow, the earlier the BBB opens, but the barrier may open in moderately ischaemic tissue if the reduction in blood flow is prolonged (Menzies *et al.* 1993). After about three weeks of continuous ischaemia, BBB permeability returns to normal, coincident with involution and removal of the infarcted tissue (Menzies *et al.* 1993).

The delay in appearance of BBB disruption during continuous focal ischaemia suggests that the mechanism requires either a cumulative toxic effect (e.g. through continued attack by free radicals) or the induction of an injurious mediator (e.g. ICAM-1 or NO synthase induction). The involvement of free radicals is a strong possibility since they have been implicated in ischaemic brain injury during the first four hours of focal ischaemia (Martz *et al.* 1989, 1990). Nevertheless, in one study, treatment with a free radical scavenger did not attenuate the BBB opening that was seen after 24 hours of ischaemia (Martz *et al.* 1990). In other types of brain injury, arachidonic acid-derived free radicals have been shown to be responsible for BBB opening (Wei *et al.* 1981; Kontos 1985). Furthermore, there is increased activity of the cyclo-oxygenase and lipoxygenase pathways in capillaries isolated from ischaemic brain (Koide *et al.* 1985).

In contrast to the change in BBB permeability seen in continuous ischaemia, reperfusion of ischaemic brain produces a biphasic change with an early, transient increase followed by a delayed, persistent opening (Suzuki *et al.* 1983; Sage *et al.* 1984; Kuroiwa *et al.* 1985; Dobbin *et al.* 1989). The early opening appears to be related to post-ischaemic hyperemia and can be attenuated by hypotension (Ting *et al.* 1986) and increased by hypertension (Ito *et al.* 1980; Cole *et al.* 1991). While this might suggest that it is due to over-distention of the vasculature and mechanical disruption of the endothelial cell membrane when flow is re-established, it seems unlikely that significant membrane disruption would be so readily reversible. Furthermore, hypothermia (Dietrich *et al.* 1990) or pre-treatment with polyethylene glycol-conjugated superoxide dismutase and catalase (Armstead *et al.* 1992) reduce this early opening of the BBB. As an alternative explanation, we speculate that neurotransmitters and/or hormones are released and intraendothelial calcium increases during the ischaemic phase and these cause separation of the tight junctions. If this hypothesis is true, it may be possible to prevent the early reperfusion-induced opening of the BBB with receptor antagonists. The mechanism responsible for the later opening of the BBB following ischaemia and reperfusion is probably similar to that which causes barrier damage in continuous ischaemia, i.e. the cumulative effect of a toxin or the induction of an injurious mediator.

CONCLUSION

In the past decade, there has been an enormous increase in our understanding of the multiple functions of the microvascular endothelium in brain. Although studies of the normal physiological regulation of the endothelium have moved towards biochemistry and cell biology, studies of the BBB in ischaemia remain largely descriptive. It should now be possible to utilize our knowledge of the regulatory processes pharmacologically to modify the response of the brain microvasculature to ischaemia. In so doing, a more complete understanding of the mechanisms that produce ischaemic damage to the cerebrovascular endothelium will be achieved.

ACKNOWLEDGEMENTS

Supported by grants NS-23870, HL-18575, and NS-17760 from the National Institutes of Health and by the Wessex Medical Trust.

REFERENCES

Armstead, W. M., Mirro, R., Thelin, O. P., Shibata, M., Zuckerman, S. L., Shanklin, D. R., *et al.* (1992). Polyethylene glycol superoxide dismutase and catalase attenuate increased blood–brain barrier permeability after ischemia in piglets. *Stroke*, **23**, 755–62.
Banks, W. A. and Kastin, A. J. (1992). The interleukins-1alpha, -1beta, and -2 do not acutely disrupt the murine blood–brain barrier. *Int. J. Immunopharmacol.*, **14**, 629–36.
Betz, A. L. (1985). Epithelial properties of brain capillary endothelium. *Fed. Proc.*, **44**, 2614–15.
Betz, A. L. (1993). Oxygen free radicals and the brain microvasculature. In *The blood–brain barrier, cellular and molecular biology* (ed. W. M. Pardridge), pp. 303–21. Raven Press, New York.
Betz, A. L. and Coester, H. C. (1990). Effect of steroids on edema and sodium uptake of the brain during focal ischemia in rats. *Stroke*, **21**, 1199–204.
Betz, A. L., Iannotti, F., and Hoff, J. T. (1983). Ischemia reduces blood-to-brain glucose transport in the gerbil. *J. Cereb. Blood Flow Metab.*, **3**, 200–6.

Betz, A. L., Ennis, S. R., and Schielke, G. P. (1989a). Blood-brain barrier sodium transport limits development of brain edema during partial ischemia in gerbils. *Stroke*, **20**, 1253-9.

Betz, A. L., Goldstein, G. W., and Katzman, R. (1989b). Blood-brain-cerebrospinal fluid barriers. In *Basic neurochemistry* (ed. G. J. Siegel, B. Agranoff, R. W. Albers, and P. Molinoff), pp. 591-606. Raven Press, New York.

Betz, A. L., Keep, R. F., Beer, M. E., and Ren, X.-D. 1994. Blood-brain barrier permeability and brain content of sodium, potassium and chloride during focal ischemia. *J. Cereb. Blood Flow Metab.*, **14**, 29-37.

Black, K. L. and Hoff, J. T. (1985). Leukotrienes increase blood-brain barrier permeability following intraparenchymal injections in rats. *Ann. Neurol.*, **18**, 349-51.

Bradbury, M. (1979). *The concept of a blood-brain barrier.* John Wiley & Sons, Chichester.

Brust, P. (1986). Changes in regional blood-brain transfer of L-leucine elicited by arginine-vasopressin. *J. Neurochem.*, **46**, 534-41.

Brust, P. and Diemer, N. H. (1990). Blood-brain transfer of L-phenylalanine declines after peripheral but not central nervous administration of vasopressin. *J. Neurochem.*, **55**, 2098-104.

Brust, P., Baethmann, A., Gjedde, A., and Ermisch, A. (1991). Atrial natriuretic peptide augments the blood-brain transfer of water but not leucine and glucose. *Brain Res.*, **564**, 91-6.

Bundgaard, M. (1980). Transport pathways in capillaries-in search of pores. *Ann. Rev. Physiol.*, **42**, 325-36.

Butt, A. M. and Jones, H. C. (1992). Effect of histamine and antagonists on electrical resistance across the blood-brain barrier in rat brain-surface microvessels. *Brain Res.*, **569**, 100-5.

Chan, P. H. and Fishman, R. A. (1980). Transient formation of superoxide radicals in polyunsaturated fatty acid-induced brain swelling. *J. Neurochem.*, **35**, 1004-7.

Chan, P. H., Fishman, R. A., Caronna, J., Schmidley, J. W., Prioleau, G., and Lee, J. (1983). Induction of brain edema following intracerebral injection of arachidonic acid. *Ann. Neurol.*, **13**, 625-32.

Chan, P. H., Schmidley, J. W., Fishman, R. A., and Longar, S. M. (1984). Brain injury, edema, and vascular permeability changes induced by oxygen-derived free radicals. *Neurology*, **34**, 315-20.

Cole, D. J., Matsumura, J. S., Drummond, J. C., Schultz, R. L., and Wong, M. H. (1991). Time- and pressure-dependent changes in blood-brain barrier permeability after temporary middle cerebral artery occlusion in rats. *Acta Neuropathol.*, **82**, 266-73.

Dietrich, W. D., Busto, R., Halley, M., and Valdes, I. (1990). The importance of brain temperature in alterations of the blood-brain barrier following cerebral ischemia. *J. Neuropathol. Exp. Neurol.*, **49**, 486-97.

Dobbin, J., Crockard, H. A., and Ross-Russell, R. (1989). Transient blood-brain barrier permeability following profound temporary global ischaemia: an experimental study using ^{14}C-AIB. *J. Cereb. Blood Flow Metab.*, **9**, 71-8.

Dux, E. and Joé, F. (1982). Effects of histamine on brain capillaries. *Exp. Brain Res.*, **47**, 252-8.

Easton, A. S. and Fraser, P. A. (1993a). CGRP reduces leaky venular permeability in the anaesthetized rat. *J. Physiol.*, **459**, 361P.

Easton, A. S. and Fraser, P. A. (1993b). Histamine increases and reduces the permeability of cerebral venules of the anaesthetized rat. *J. Physiol.*, **467**, 40P.

Easton, A. S. and Fraser, P. A. (1994). Variable restriction of albumin diffusion across inflammed cerebral microvessels. *J. Physiol.*, **475**, 147-57.

Ellis, E. F., Wright, K. F., Wei, E. P., and Kontos, H. A. (1981). Cyclooxygenase products of arachidonic acid metabolism in cat cerebral cortex after experimental concussive brain injury. *J. Neurochem.*, **37**, 892-6.

Ennis, S. R., Keep, R. F., Schielke, G. P., and Betz, A. L. (1990). Decrease in perfusion of cerebral capillaries during incomplete ischemia and reperfusion. *J. Cereb. Blood Flow Metab.*, **10**, 213-20.

Frelin, C., Ladoux, A., Marsault, R., and Vigne, P. (1992). Function of vasoactive factors in the cerebral microcirculation. *J. Cardiovasc. Pharmacol.*, **20**(Suppl. 12), S94-6.

Goldstein, G. W. (1979). Relation of potassium transport to oxidative metabolism in isolated brain capillaries. *J. Physiol.*, **286**, 185-95.

Gross, P. M., Teasdale, G. M., Angerson, W. J., and Harper, A. M. (1981). H_2-receptors mediate increases in permeability of the blood-brain barrier during arterial histamine infusion. *Brain Res.*, **210**, 396-400.

Gross, S. S., Jaffe, E. A., Levi, R., and Kilbourn, R. G. (1991). Cytokine-activated endothelial cells express an isotype of nitric oxide synthase which is tetrahydrobiopterin-dependent, calmodulin-independent and inhibited by arginine analogs with a rank-order of potency characteristic of activated macrophages. *Biochem. Biophys. Res. Commun.*, **178**, 823-9.

Harik, S. I. (1986). Blood-brain barrier sodium/potassium pump: modulation by central noradrenergic innervation. *Proc. Natl. Acad. Sci. USA*, **83**, 4067-70.

Hatashita, S. and Hoff, J. T. (1990). Brain edema and cerebrovascular permeability during cerebral ischemia in rats. *Stroke*, **21**, 582-8.

Homayoun, P. and Harik, S. I. (1991). Bradykinin receptors of cerebral microvessels stimulate phosphoinositide turnover. *J. Cereb. Blood Flow Metab.*, **11**, 557-66.

Ibaragi, M.-A., Niwa, M., and Ozaki, M. (1989). Atrial natriuretic peptide modulates amiloride-sensitive Na^+ transport across the blood-brain barrier. *J. Neurochem.*, **53**, 1802-6.

Ito, U., Ohno, K., Yamaguchi, T., Takei, H., Tomita, H., and Inaba, Y. (1980). Effect of hypertension on blood-brain barrier change after restoration of blood flow in post-ischemic gerbil brains. *Stroke*, **11**, 606-11.

Joó, F. (1972). Effect of N^6O^2-dibutyryl cyclic $3',5'$-adenosine monophosphate on the pinocytosis of brain capillaries of mice. *Experientia*, **28**, 1470-1.

Joó, F., Rakonczay, Z., and Wollemann, M. (1974). cAMP-mediated regulation of the permeability in the brain capillaries. *Experientia*, **31**, 582-4.

Joó, F., Dux, E., Karnushina, I. L., Halász, N., Gecse, A., Ottlecz, A., et al. (1981). Histamine in brain capillaries. *Agents Actions*, **11**, 129-34.

Joó, F., Temesvári, P., and Dux, E. (1983). Regulation of the macromolecular transport in the brain microvessels: the role of cyclic GMP. *Brain Res.*, **278**, 165-74.

Kim, K. S., Wass, C. A., Cross, A. S., and Opal, S. M. (1992). Modulation of blood-brain barrier permeability by tumor necrosis factor and antibody to tumor necrosis factor in the rat. *Lymphokine Cylokine Res.*, **11**, 293-8.

Koide, T., Gotoh, O., Asano, T., and Takakura, K. (1985). Alterations of the eicosanoid synthetic capacity of rat brain microvessels following ischemia: relevance to ischemic brain edema. *J. Neurochem.*, **44**, 85-93.

Kontos, H. A. (1985). George E. Brown memorial lecture. Oxygen radicals in cerebral vascular injury. *Circ. Res.*, **57**, 508-16.

Kontos, H. A., Wei, E. P., Povlishock, J. T., Dietrich, W. D., Magiera, C. H., and Ellis, E. F. (1980). Cerebral arteriolar damage by arachidonic acid and prostaglandin G2. *Science*, **209**, 1242-5.

Kuroiwa, T., Ting, P., Martinez, H., and Klatzo, I. (1985). The biphasic opening of the blood–brain barrier to proteins following temporary middle cerebral artery occlusion. *Acta Neuropathol.*, **68**, 122–9.

Kuroiwa, T., Seida, M., Tomida, S., Hiratsuka, H., Okeda, R., and Inaba, Y. (1986). Discrepancies among CT, histological, and blood–brain barrier findings in early cerebral ischemial. *J. Neurosurg.*, **65**, 517–24.

Lo, W. D. and Betz, A. L. (1986). Oxygen free-radical reduction of brain capillary rubidium uptake. *J. Neurochem.*, **46**, 394–8.

Martz, D., Rayos, G., Schielke, G. P., and Betz, A. L. (1989). Allopurinol and dimethylthiourea reduce brain infarction following middle cerebral artery occlusion in rats. *Stroke*, **20**, 488–94.

Martz, D., Beer, M., and Betz, A. L. (1990). Dimethylthiourea reduces ischemic brain edema without affecting cerebral blood flow. *J. Cereb. Blood Flow Metab.*, **10**, 352–7.

Megyeri, P., Abrahám, C. S., Temesvári, P., Kovács, J., Vas, T., and Speer, C. P. (1992). Recombinant human tumor necrosis factor alpha constricts pial arterioles and increases blood–brain barrier permeability in newborn piglets. *Neurosci. Lett.*, **148**, 137–40.

Menzies, S. A., Betz, A. L., and Hoff, J. T. (1993). Contributions of ions and albumin to the formation and resolution of ischemic brain edema. *J. Neurosurg.*, **78**, 257–66.

Olesen, S.-P. (1985). A calcium-dependent reversible increase in microvessels in frog brain induced by serotonin. *J. Physiol.*, **361**, 103–13.

Olesen, S.-P. (1987). Free oxygen radicals decrease electrical resistance of microvascular endothelium in brain. *Acta Physiol. Scand.*, **129**, 181–7.

Olesen, S.-P. and Crone, C. (1986). Substances that rapidly augment ionic conductance of endothelium in cerebral venules. *Acta Physiol. Scand.*, **127**, 233–41.

Olsson, Y., Crowell, R. M., and Klatzo, I. (1971). The blood–brain barrier to protein tracers in focal cerebral ischemia and infarction caused by occlusion of the middle cerebral artery. *Acta Neuropathol.*, **18**, 89–102.

Petito, C. K. (1979). Early and late mechanisms of increased vascular permeability following experimental cerebral infarction. *J. Neuropathol. Exp. Neurol.*, **38**, 222–34.

Quagliarello, V. J., Wispelwey, B., Long, W. J. Jr., and Scheld, W. M. (1991). Recombinant human interleukin-1 induces meningitis and blood–brain barrier injury in the rat. Characterization and comparison with tumor necrosis factor. *J. Clin. Invest*, **87**, 1360–6.

Raichle, M. E., Hartman, B. K., Eichling, J. O., and Sharpe, L. G. (1975). Central noradrenergic regulation of cerebral blood flow and vascular permeability. *Proc. Natl. Acad. Sci. USA*, **72**, 3726–30.

Raymond, J. J., Robertson, D. M., and Dinsdale, H. B. (1986). Pharmacological modification of bradykinin induced breakdown of the blood–brain barrier. *Can. J. Neurol. Sci.*, **13**, 214–20.

Revest, P. A., Abbott, N. J., and Gillespie, J. I. (1991). Receptor-mediated changes in intracellular [Ca^{2+}] in cultured rat brain capillary endothelial cells. *Brain Res.*, **549**, 159–61.

Rothman, S. M. and Olney, J. W. (1986). Glutamate and the pathophysiology of hypoxic-ischemic brain damage. *Ann. Neurol.*, **19**, 105–11.

Rubin, L. L., Hall, D. E., Porter, S., Barbu, K., Cannon, C., Horner, H. C., et al. (1991). A cell culture model of the blood–brain barrier. *J. Cell Biol.*, **115**, 1725–35.

Rubino, G. J. and Young, W. (1988). Ischemic cortical lesions after permanent occlusion of individual middle cerebral artery branches in rats. *Stroke*, **19**, 870–7.

Sage, J. I., Van Uitert, R. L., and Duffy, T. E. (1984). Early changes in blood brain barrier permeability to small molecules after transient cerebral ischemia. *Stroke*, **15**, 46–50.

Sarmento, A., Borges, N., and Azevedo, I. (1991). Adrenergic influences on the control of blood-brain barrier permeability. *Naunyn Schmiedebergs Arch. Pharmacol.*, **343**, 633-7.

Schielke, G. P., Moises, H. C., and Betz, A. L. (1990). Potassium activation of the Na,K-pump in isolated brain microvessels and synaptosomes. *Brain Res.*, **524**, 291-6.

Schielke, G.P., Moises, H. C., and Betz, A. L. (1991). Blood to brain sodium transport and interstitial fluid potassium concentration during focal ischemia in the rat. *J. Cereb. Blood Flow Metab.*, **11**, 466-71.

Shigeno, T., Graham, D. I., McCulloch, J., and Teasdale, G. M. (1984). Cerebrovascular permeability and ischemic brain damage following MCA occlusion in the rat: A comparative study with C^{14}-AIB transfer, enzyme histochemistry, and neuropathology. In *Brain edema* (ed. Y. Inaba, I. Klatzo, and M. Spatz), pp. 403-9. Springer-Verlag, Berlin.

Shigeno, T., Asano, T., Mima, T., and Takakura, K. (1989). Effect of enhanced capillary activity on the blood-brain barrier during focal cerebral ischemia in cats. *Stroke*, **20**, 1260-6.

Spatz, M., Stanimirovic, D. B., Bacic, F., Uematsu, S., Bembry, J., and McCarron, R. M. (1992). Peptidergic induction of endothelin 1 and prostanoid secretion in human cerebromicrovascular endothelium. In *Frontiers in cerebral vascular biology* (ed. L. R. Drewes and A. L. Betz), pp. 165-70. Plenum, New York.

Suzuki, R., Yamaguchi, T., Kirino, T., Orzi, F., and Klatzo, I. (1983). The effects of 5-minute ischemia in mongolian gerbils: I. Blood-brain barrier, cerebral blood flow, and local cerebral glucose utilization changes. *Acta Neuropathol.*, **60**, 207-16.

Ting, P., Masaoka, H., Kuroiwa, T., Wagner, H., Fenton, I., and Klatzo, I. (1986). Influence of blood-brain barrier opening to proteins on development of post-ischemic brain injury. *Neurol. Res.*, **8**, 146-51.

Trout, J. J., Koenig, H., Goldstone, A. D., and Lu, C. Y. (1986). Blood-brain barrier breakdown by cold injury. Polyamine signals mediate acute stimulation of endocytosis, vesicular transport, and microvillus formation in rat cerebral capillaries. *Lab. Invest.*, **55**, 622-31.

Tyson, G. W., Teasdale, G. M., Graham, D. I., and McCulloch, J. (1982). Cerebrovascular permeability following MCA occlusion in the rat. The effect of halothane-induced hypotension. *J. Neurosurg.*, **57**, 186-96.

Unterberg, A., Wahl, M., and Baethmann, A. (1984). Effects of bradykinin on permeability and diameter of pial vessels *in vivo*. *J. Cereb. Blood Flow Metab.*, **4**, 574-85.

Unterberg, A., Wahl, M., Hammersen, F., and Baethmann, A. (1987). Permeability and vasomotor response of cerebral vessels during exposure to arachidonic acid. *Acta Neuropathol.*, **73**, 209-19.

Wakai, S., Aritake, K., Asano, T., and Takakura, K. (1982). Selective destruction of the outer leaflet of the capillary endothelial membrane after intracerebral injection of arachidonic acid in the rat. *Acta Neuropathol.*, **58**, 303-6.

Wei, E. P., Kontos, H. A., Dietrich, W. D., Povlishock, J. T., and Ellis, E. F. (1981). Inhibition by free radical scavengers and by cyclooxygenase inhibitors of pial arteriolar abnormalities from concussive brain injury in cats. *Circ. Res.*, **48**, 95-103.

Wei, E. P., Ellison, M. D., Kontos, H. A., and Povlishock, J. T. (1986). O_2 radicals in arachidonate-induced increased blood-brain banner permeability to proteins. *Am. J. Physiol.*, **251**, H693-9.

Westergaard, E. (1977). The blood-brain barrier to horseradish peroxidase under normal and experimental conditions. *Acta Neuropathol.*, **39**, 181-7.

Wong, D. and Dorovini Zis, K. (1992). Upregulation of intercellular adhesion molecule-1 (ICAM-1) expression in primary cultures of human brain microvessel endothelial cells by cytokines and lipopolysaccharide. *J. Neuroimmunol.*, **39**, 11-22.

Ziylan, Y. Z., LeFauconnier, J. M., Bernard, G., and Bourre, J. M. (1988). Effect of dexamethasone on transport of α-aminoisobutyric acid and sucrose across the blood-brain barrier. *J. Neurochem.*, **51**, 1338-42.

Ziylan, Y. Z., Lefauconnier, J. M., Bernard, G., and Bourre, J. M. (1989). Regional alterations in blood-to-brain transfer of α-aminoisobutyric acid and sucrose, after chronic administration and withdrawal of dexamethasone. *J. Neurochem.*, **52**, 684-9.

Ziylan, Y. Z., Lefauconnier, J. M., Bernard, G., and Bourre, J. M. (1993). Hormonal influence on the permeability of the blood-brain barrier: corticotrophin. *Neurosci. Lett.*, **151**, 59-63.

17. Regulation of vascular smooth muscle tone in sepsis

Richard G. Bogle and Patrick Vallance

INTRODUCTION

Clinical features of septic shock include a gradual fall in mean arterial blood pressure with peripheral arteriolar vasodilatation. There is a hyperdynamic state with low systemic vascular resistance, high cardiac output, hypotension, and inadequate tissue perfusion. Reduced flow to metabolically active tissues leads to lactic acidosis, and oxygen delivery and/or cellular oxygen utilization are often impaired. The major histopathological findings are cell necrosis, tissue haemorrhage, oedema, and fibrin deposits. These abnormalities are present in most tissues although they are most marked in lung and liver. Within the vasculature there is global loss of cardiovascular control with regional vasodilatation and vasoconstriction although the net effect is a fall in overall vascular resistance. There is extensive evidence from studies in animals and humans that many of the cardiovascular features of sepsis are due to the presence of endotoxin and the subsequent release of cytokines. This chapter will focus on the pharmacology of changes in vascular tone in septic shock and the acute and chronic effects of endotoxin and certain cytokines in mediating these changes.

PRODUCTS OF INFECTION AS INITIATORS OF CYTOKINE PRODUCTION

For many years it has been known that endotoxin (otherwise known as bacterial lipopolysaccharide) is present in the outer membrane of Gram-negative bacteria and that it can induce a clinical syndrome similar to that observed in septic shock (Hale et al. 1986; Michie et al. 1988; Suffrendini et al. 1989; Cannon et al. 1990). Recently, it has become clear that many of the cardiovascular features of septic shock result from a complex cascade of endogenous mediators whose release is triggered by endotoxin (Filkins 1985; Buetler and Cerami 1987; Tracey et al. 1987).

Endotoxin is a potent stimulus for the production of cytokines from a variety of cells including macrophages/monocytes, lymphocytes, natural killer cells, astrocytes, microglial cells, Kupffer cells, and vascular endothelial and smooth muscle cells (Fig. 17.1). Production of cytokines is increased also by other products of infection including staphylococcal and streptococcal exotoxins, enterotoxins

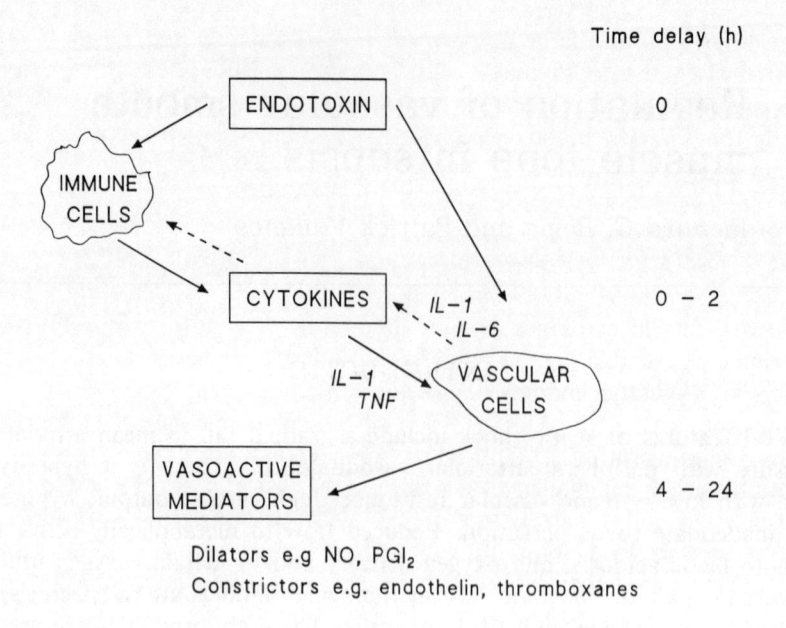

```
                                              Time delay (h)

              ┌─────────────┐
              │  ENDOTOXIN  │                      0
              └─────────────┘
             ↙              ↘
   ╱IMMUNE╲                   ↓
   ╲CELLS ╱ ←- - - - - -
             ↘              ↓
              ┌───────────┐  IL-1
              │ CYTOKINES │ ←----                  0 - 2
              └───────────┘  IL-6
                       ↘     ↑
                    IL-1    ╱VASCULAR╲
                    TNF     ╲ CELLS  ╱
                            ↙
              ┌─────────────┐
              │  VASOACTIVE │ ←
              │  MEDIATORS  │                      4 - 24
              └─────────────┘
```

Dilators e.g NO, PGI$_2$
Constrictors e.g. endothelin, thromboxanes

Fig. 17.1 Infection and vasodilatation. Endotoxin acts on immune cells and vascular cells to stimulate cytokine production. Endotoxin and certain cytokines (e.g. TNF and IL-1) increase mediator production from endothelial and smooth muscle cells and the net result is vasodilatation. Cytokines produced by immune cells or vascular cells may up-regulate or down-regulate the overall process.

(Augert *et al.* 1992; Zembowicz and Vane 1992), viruses, and fungal or parasitic antigens (Fast *et al.* 1989; Ikejima *et al.* 1989; Fischer *et al.* 1990). In addition, infection by these agents may also increase absorption of endotoxin from the gut or interfere with its removal by the liver. These observations suggest possible mechanism(s) by which Gram-positive organisms and other infective agents that do not contain endotoxin are able to lead to septic shock indistinguishable from classical shock produced by Gram-negative infection.

Infusion of endotoxin or Gram-negative bacteria into animals or human volunteers causes an increase in the plasma concentration of certain cytokines. The kinetics of release of these substances have been investigated, and although many are elevated in septic shock the time course of the increases differs between cytokines. Following endotoxin injection, tumour necrosis factor (TNF) reaches a peak at 90 minutes and then declines promptly (Michie *et al.* 1986, 1988; Cannon *et al.* 1990). Infused TNF has a half-life in plasma of 15–20 min (Chapman *et al.* 1987) and is rapidly cleared from the circulation. In contrast, plasma concentrations of interleukin-1 (IL-1) and interleukin-6 (IL-6) are elevated three to four hours after endotoxin injection (Cannon *et al.* 1990), although these increases are variable and usually less than those with TNF (Michie *et al.* 1988). The major source of cytokines is thought to be the macrophage, however, endotoxin and/or IL-1 have also been shown to stimulate production of IL-1 and TNF (Warner and Libby 1990) and large amounts of IL-6 (Loppnow and Libby 1990) from cultured vascular smooth muscle cells. Similarly, in isolated rat aortic rings, cytokines are produced in response to low levels of endotoxin (McKenna 1990), suggesting that *in vivo* blood vessels themselves may contribute to the increased plasma levels of cytokines.

CYTOKINES MEDIATING THE EFFECTS OF ENDOTOXIN

The evidence that cytokines mediate the effects of endotoxin is exemplified by experimental data relating to TNF. First, TNF levels are elevated in the early phase of sepsis. Secondly, endotoxin infusion stimulates TNF production. Thirdly, administration of TNF results in a similar biological response to endotoxin, and finally, administration of antibodies directed against TNF protects animals against a subsequent challenge with endotoxin. Similar cases can be presented for IL-1 and IL-6 and it is likely that the biological effects of endotoxin *in vivo* can be accounted for by a 'soup' of cytokines acting in concert (Fig. 17.1). However, it should be noted that cytokines are not the only mediators synthesized and released in response to endotoxin. Endotoxin stimulates the production of a variety of agents derived both from vascular smooth muscle and endothelial cells. These include anaphylotoxins, complement factors C3a and C5a, arachidonic acid derivatives, reactive oxygen intermediates, endorphins, coagulation factors, platelet activating factor, and nitric oxide (NO). Furthermore, procoagulant molecules including tissue factor and intercellular adhesion molecule-1 (ICAM-1) are synthesized and expressed on the surface of endothelial cells, and this is likely to contribute to increased leucocyte adhesion and extravasation, and the development of disseminated intravascular coagulation which is a common occurrence in sepsis. It is not yet clear which of these mediators are released directly by endotoxin and which require cytokines as intermediaries.

CHANGES IN VASCULAR TONE INDUCED BY ENDOXIN AND CYTOKINES

Administration of endotoxin to experimental animals results in a biphasic cardiovascular response. Initially, there is a rapid and transient fall in mean blood pressure which recovers within 30 min. This is followed over the next two to three hours by a slow decrease in blood pressure which is due to a fall in peripheral vascular resistance. Thus the effects of endotoxin can be divided into two phases — acute and chronic.

Acute effects

The acute effects of endotoxin appear to be mediated by the production of vasoactive substances from endothelial cells. The mechanisms are not fully understood although both nitric oxide (NO) and vasodilator prostaglandins such as prostacyclin have been implicated. Endotoxin stimulates the immediate release of a nitric oxide-like factor from cultured bovine aortic endothelial cells (Salvemini *et al.* 1990) and produces an endothelium-dependent fall in resistance in the rat isolated perfused heart (Baydoun *et al.* 1993). However, this effect appears to be variable (Myers *et al.* 1992) and inhibition of nitric oxide synthesis does not affect the transient fall in blood pressure produced by administration of endotoxin to rabbits (Wright *et al.* 1992). Furthermore, the rapid relaxation of rabbit mesenteric artery produced by IL-1 is independent of nitric oxide synthesis but blocked by the cyclo-oxygenase inhibitor indomethacin (Marceau *et al.* 1991) as is the initial rapid decrease in blood pressure following endotoxin challenge in cats (Parratt and Sturgess 1974, 1975). Thus, the mechanisms underlying the initial dilator effect of endotoxin appear to vary between species and between vascular beds. One possibility is that endotoxin or cytokines stimulate the immediate release of mediators such as platelet activating factor and/or kinins from endothelial cells and these act to stimulate production of either nitric oxide or vasodilator prostaglandins depending on the receptors present and the coupling of these receptors to their respective effector systems (Katori *et al.* 1989; Fleming *et al.* 1992; Baydoun *et al.* 1993). The significance of this initial endotoxin- and cytokine-evoked hypotension for the pathophysiology of septic shock in patients is not clear, and it is likely that the acute vasodilatation evoked by endotoxin is less important than the chronic effects.

Chronic effects

Chronic hypotension develops two to three hours after administration of endotoxin or certain cytokines and this is seen in animals and humans. One of the features of the hypotension observed during this phase is that it is accompanied by loss of vascular responsiveness to vasoconstrictor agents including α-adrenoceptor agonists, thromboxane, vasopressin, and 5-hydroxytryptamine (Parratt 1973). This hyporesponsiveness can be demonstrated *in vitro* and *in vivo*. Vessels isolated from endotoxin-treated animals demonstrate impaired vasoconstrictor responses to noradrenaline or phenylephrine and this effect is endothelium-independent (Julou-Schaeffer *et al.* 1990). Injection of TNF, IL-1, or interleukin-2 into animals produces a similar effect. The response is impaired to a wide variety of constrictor agents which act through different receptors and second messenger systems, and the most straightforward explanation of the changes seen is that there is increased production of a dilator substance within the smooth muscle itself that opposes vasoconstriction.

The lag before the onset of persistent hypotension suggests that endotoxin or cytokines mediate their effects indirectly. This idea is strengthened by the observation that antibodies that neutralize endotoxins or cytokines have little effect on vascular reactivity or hypotension if given after the hypotension has developed. Furthermore, the changes can be prevented *in vitro* by cycloheximide, suggesting that during the delay protein synthesis occurs and the products of this synthesis after vascular reactivity (Fig. 17.1). For the pathogenesis of vasodilatation, two proteins induced by endotoxin/cytokines are of particular interest: the inducible forms of nitric oxide synthase and cyclo-oxygenase.

Nitric oxide

In healthy vessels, production of NO in the cardiovascular system occurs mainly from endothelial cells (see Chapter 10). In these cells, NO is synthesized from the semi-essential amino acid L-arginine by the action of a calcium/calmodulin-dependent, constitutive NO synthase (see Fig. 17.2A) (Palmer and Moncada 1989). However endotoxin, cytokines including IL-1 and TNF, and products of Gram-positive bacteria including muramyl dipeptide and staphylococcal toxin (Fleming *et al.* 1991*a,b*; Zembowicz and Vane 1992) induce the expression, in endothelial cells (Kilbourn and Belloni 1990; Radomski *et al.* 1991) **and** smooth muscle (see Fig. 17.2B) Busse and Mulsch 1990; Beasley *et al.* 1991; Durante *et al.* 1991; Schini *et al.* 1991; Gross and Levi 1992) of a distinct isoform of nitric oxide synthase that is functionally calcium-independent. Induction of calcium-insensitive nitric oxide synthase been demonstrated in arteries (Fleming *et al.* 1990; Rees *et al.* 1990; Shibano and Vanhoutte 1993), arterioles (Schneider *et al.* 1992*a*), and veins (Vallance *et al.* 1992) derived from animals and also in **human** endothelial cells (Radomski *et al.* 1993), smooth muscle cells (Junquero *et al.* 1992), and hepatocytes (Geller *et al.* 1993). In endotoxic shock, the induction of NO synthase is widespread and has been demonstrated in pulmonary, renal, cardiac, mesenteric, and skeletal muscle circulations.

Induction of nitric oxide synthase involves protein synthesis and is inhibited by glucocorticoids including dexamethasone (Rees *et al.* 1990). The level of induction of nitric oxide synthase may be regulated by the balance of local cytokines; IL-1 and TNF induce nitric oxide synthase whereas interleukin-4 and interleukin-10 (Cunha *et al.* 1992), transforming growth factor β (Junquero *et al.* 1992), and platelet-derived growth factor$_{AB}$ inhibit induction (Schultz *et al.* 1992). Furthermore, plasmin potentiates induction of NO synthase by IL-1 whereas thrombin inhibits it (Schini *et al.* 1993). Interestingly, the production of NO via the constitutive NO synthase appears to be inhibited following induction of inducible NO synthase and this effect is mediated by a decrease in the stability of the RNA encoding for constitutive NO synthase messenger (Yoshizumi *et al.* 1993). Thus, whereas in the healthy vessel the endothelium is the major vascular source of nitric oxide, in sepsis the whole vessel wall synthesizes this mediator.

There is also strong evidence that induction of NO synthase occurs *in vivo*. Nitrite and nitrate (breakdown products of NO) levels in plasma are elevated after injection of endotoxin (Wagner *et al.* 1983) and/or cytokines (Kilbourn *et al.* 1990), and calcium-independent conversion of radiolabelled L-arginine to L-citrulline (indicative of inducible NO synthase activity) can be demonstrated in vessels obtained from rats treated with endotoxin (Knowles *et al.* 1990; Rees *et al.* 1990).

Once expressed, the inducible NO synthase synthesizes large amounts of NO

A Constitutive NO Pathway

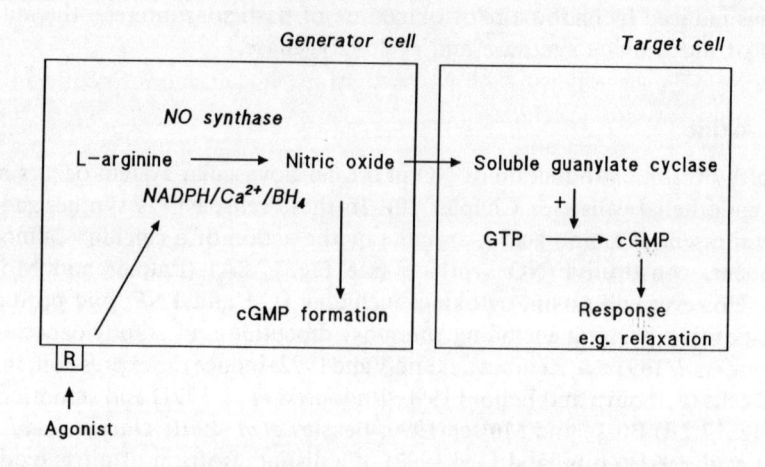

```
                    Generator cell                          Target cell
    ┌──────────────────────────────────┐  ┌──────────────────────────────────┐
    │           NO synthase            │  │                                  │
    │   L-arginine ──────→ Nitric oxide│──→│ Soluble guanylate cyclase        │
    │   NADPH/Ca²⁺/BH₄                 │  │          +  │                    │
    │              ↗         │         │  │   GTP ─────→ cGMP                │
    │             ↑          ↓         │  │              │                   │
    │                  cGMP formation  │  │              ↓                   │
    │                                  │  │         Response                 │
    │  R                               │  │         e.g. relaxation          │
    └──────────────────────────────────┘  └──────────────────────────────────┘
      ↑
    Agonist
```

B Inducible NO Pathway

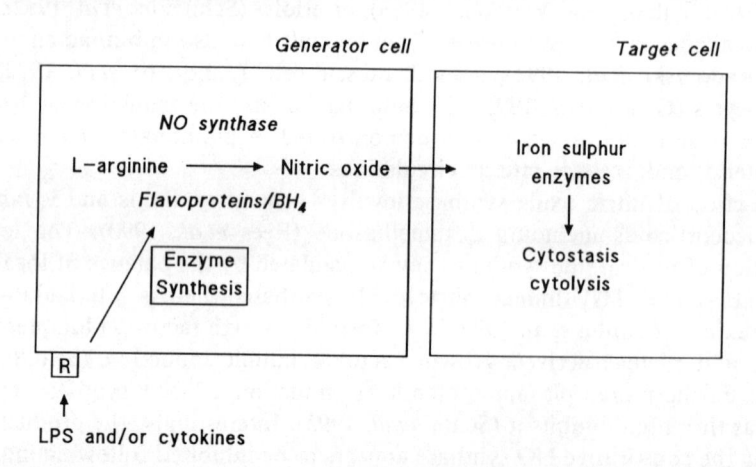

```
                    Generator cell                          Target cell
    ┌──────────────────────────────────┐  ┌──────────────────────────────────┐
    │           NO synthase            │  │                                  │
    │   L-arginine ──────→ Nitric oxide│──→│      Iron sulphur               │
    │   Flavoproteins/BH₄              │  │        enzymes                   │
    │         ┌─────────┐              │  │          │                       │
    │         │ Enzyme  │              │  │          ↓                       │
    │         │Synthesis│              │  │      Cytostasis                  │
    │         └─────────┘              │  │       cytolysis                  │
    │  R                               │  │                                  │
    └──────────────────────────────────┘  └──────────────────────────────────┘
      ↑
    LPS and/or cytokines
```

Fig. 17.2 The L-arginine:nitric oxide pathways. (A) The constitutive pathway present in endothelium. The NO synthesized acts on adjacent smooth muscle to cause tightly regulated physiological vasodilatation. (B) The inducible pathway which is expressed in endothelium and smooth muscle after exposure to endotoxin or certain cytokines. The large quantities of NO synthesized cause profound vasodilatation, hyporesponsiveness to constrictors, and tissue damage.

over long time periods. The consequences of NO synthase induction in the vessel wall are vascular relaxation and hyporesponsiveness to vasoconstrictors or sympathetic stimulation (Gonzalez et al. 1992). These effects appear to be mediated by cyclic GMP, although the large quantities of NO produced by inducible NO synthase also have toxic effects by interfering with the activity of iron–sulfur containing enzyme systems and may contribute to vascular damage (see below).

It is possible to inhibit NO synthesis with guanidine-substituted analogues of L-arginine including N^G-monomethyl-L-arginine (L-NMMA) and nitro-L-arginine (Rees et al. 1989; Chapters 4 + 10) and these agents are useful tools with which to study the effects of NO *in vivo* and *in vitro*. Inhibition of NO synthesis increases blood pressure in endotoxin or cytokine-induced shock and restores the vascular responsiveness to noradrenaline and sympathetic stimulation.

Dilator prostaglandins

An enhanced formation of vasodilator prostaglandins has also been implicated in the chronic haemodynamic changes in endotoxin shock (Collier et al. 1973; Parratt and Sturgess 1974; Feuerstein et al. 1981; Gray et al. 1991; Mozes et al. 1991). Cyclo-oxygenase, like NO synthase, exists in at least two isoforms, one of which is present as a normal constituent of healthy endothelium (COX-I) and the other which is induced in response to endotoxin and cytokines (COX-II) (Fu et al. 1990; Masferrer et al. 1992). Similarly, IL-1 increases synthesis of prostacyclin from endothelial and smooth muscle cells (Rossi et al. 1985; Breviario et al. 1990). The products of COX-II enzyme include prostacyclin and other dilator prostaglandins which act by stimulating adenylate cyclase in target cell which results in a increased cyclic AMP production and vascular relaxation. Cyclo-oxygenase can be inhibited by non-steroidal anti-inflammatory drugs including aspirin and indomethacin. A role for this enzyme and its products in the pathogenesis of septic shock is supported by the finding that cyclo-oxygenase inhibitors restore blood pressure in certain animal models (Parratt and Sturgess 1974).

Platelet activating factor and kinins

Platelet activating factor (PAF) is released in response to endotoxin in the pig (Mozes et al. 1991), and the rat (Rabinovici et al. 1991), and there is a correlation between the severity of shock and the release of PAF. Furthermore, PAF antagonists have some beneficial effects in certain animal models of shock. Similar data suggests a role for kinins including bradykinin, however, kinin antagonists produce variable protection against the hypotensive response to endotoxin (Berg et al. 1990). Recently, it has become clear that the vascular effects of PAF and bradykinin may not be direct and appear to be mediated largely by stimulation of NO or prostaglandin production. In addition PAF leads to expression of NO synthase in certain cells.

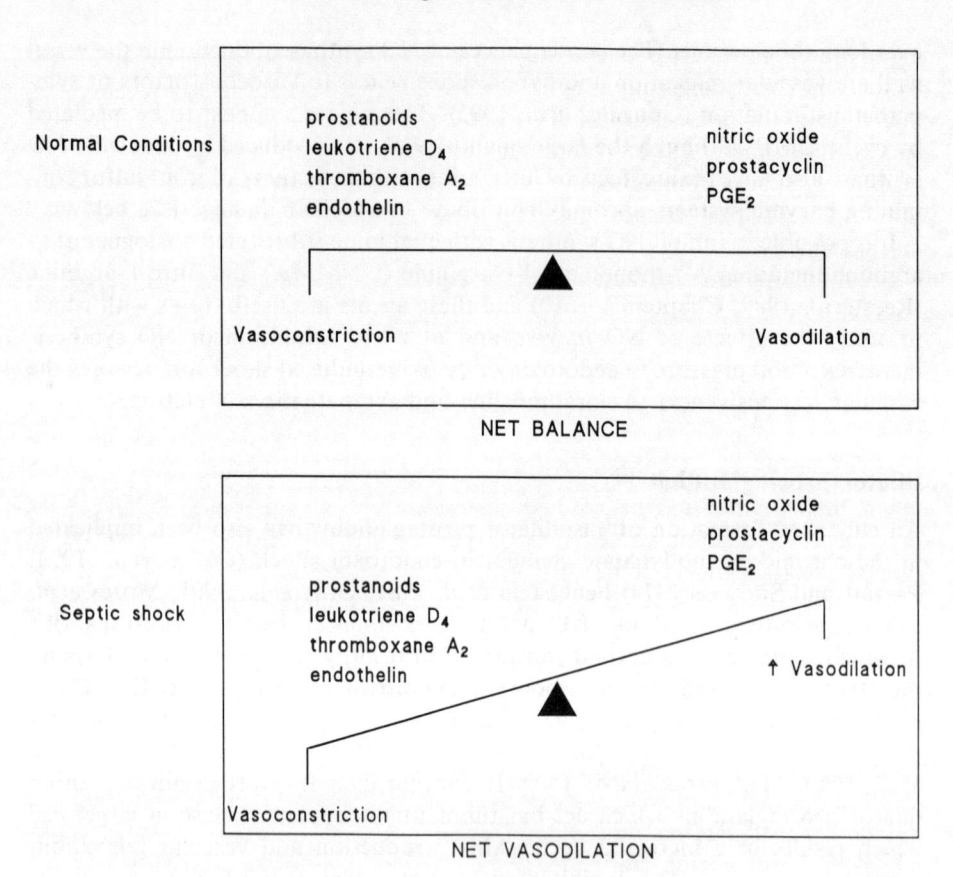

Fig. 17.3 The balance of vasoconstrictors and vasodilators in the cardiovascular system. Although endotoxin increases the production of constrictor and dilator mediators, nitric oxide causes hyporeactivity to the constrictors and the balance changes in favour of vasodilatation.

Vasoconstrictors

The hallmark of sepsis is vasodilatation, however, endogenous production of vasoconstrictor substances, including catecholamines, endothelin, vasopressin, and thromboxane is increased in septic shock or following endotoxin injection (Voerman *et al.* 1992). This may be seen as an attempt to overcome the effects of increased production of dilators and restore arterial pressure. However, the tone of vessels will depend on the balance of constrictors and dilators (see Fig. 17.3) and in some beds the net result is a distinct increase in vascular tone. Constriction of pulmonary, splanchnic, and renal arterioles occurs during sepsis and has been implicated in the pathogenesis of lung injury, gut ischaemia, and renal failure. In the mesenteric circulation, a relative insensitivity to the effects of induction of NO synthase has been demonstrated (Mitchell *et al.* 1993) and, in the presence of increased levels of circulating constrictors, or enhanced activity of the sympathetic nervous system, this would lead to constriction. In the renal bed a role for increased production of the potent vasoconstrictor peptide endothelin (Chapter 13) has been suggested and endothelin antagonists might be beneficial. Regional imbalance in constriction and dilation may lead to shunting of blood to bypass tissues and this could contribute to tissue hypoxia. The mechanisms controlling the production and effects of constrictor factors in sepsis is becoming an area of increasing importance for research.

PREVENTING AND TREATING VASCULAR HYPORESPONSIVENESS

In the previous section some of the pathways involved in the induction and subsequent maintenance of the vascular complications of septic shock have been described. Therapeutic strategies have been developed which interfere with certain of these pathways some with more success than others.

Antibodies against endotoxin and cytokines

Several studies have shown that neutralizing antibodies to endotoxin or TNF prevent the lethal action of endotoxin in different species (Buetler *et al.* 1985; Sheehan *et al.* 1989). More recently it has been demonstrated that experimental septic shock can be prevented by neutralizing IL-1 or by giving an IL-1 receptor antagonist protein (Ohlsson *et al.* 1990). However, this approach is most effective when the neutralizing antibody (or antagonist) is administered before the endotoxin/cytokine and is relatively ineffective at reversing established hypotension and vasodilatation. These findings are consistent with the observation that endotoxin and cytokines trigger a cascade of mediators which alter vascular tone (Figs. 17.1 and 17.3) and that once induced, NO synthase and cyclo-oxygenase II do not require continued stimulation with the inflammatory signal.

Inhibition of mediator production or effect

An alternative approach to restoring cardiovascular normality is to interfere with the mediators producing direct effects on vascular tone.

Nitric oxide
Currently there are three major approaches to the inhibition of nitric oxide-mediated vasodilatation in endotoxin and cytokine-induced shock: inhibition of the enzyme with substrate analogues (NO synthase inhibitors), inhibition of enzyme activity by depleting essential substrates, and attenuation of the effector molecule, guanylate cyclase (see Fig. 17.4)

NO synthase inhibitors have been administered to experimental animals

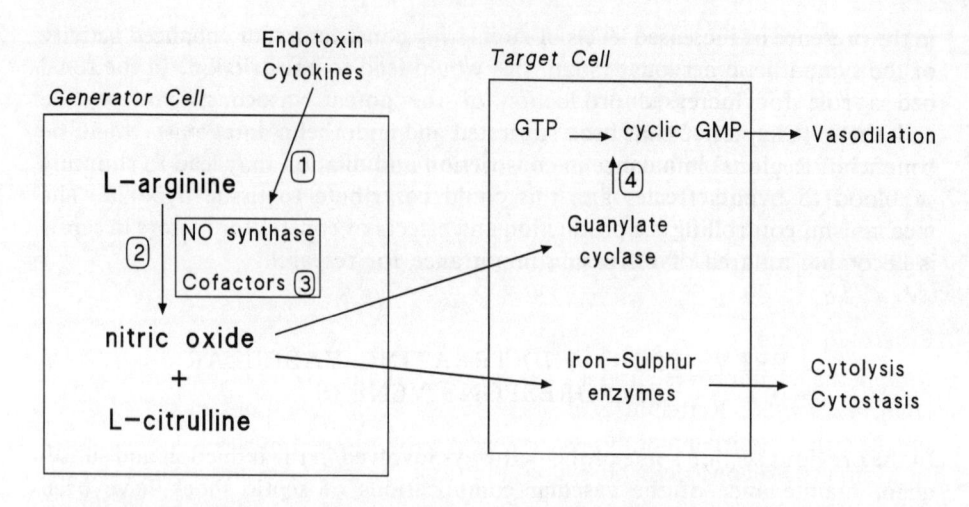

```
                    Endotoxin
                    Cytokines              Target Cell
    Generator Cell
                                          GTP ──→ cyclic GMP ──→ Vasodilation
     L-arginine      ①
                                                 ↑④
                    NO synthase                 Guanylate
              ②                                  cyclase
                    Cofactors ③

     nitric oxide
         +                                   Iron–Sulphur          Cytolysis
     L-citrulline                              enzymes             Cytostasis
```

1 Inhibitors of NO synthase induction e.g. glucocorticoids
2 Substrate analogue inhibitors of NO synthase e.g. L-NMMA
3 Inhibitors of cofactor biosynthesis or function
4 Inhibitors of soluble guanylate cyclase

Fig. 17.4 Inhibition of the L-arginine:nitric oxide pathway. Possible sites of inhibition include (1) inhibitors of induction of NO synthase (e.g. glucocorticoids); (2) substrate analogue inhibitors (e.g. L-NMMA); (3) inhibitors of cofactor biosynthesis or function (e.g. methotrexate); (4) inhibitors of soluble guanylate cyclase (e.g. methylene blue).

(Thiemermann and Vane 1990; Nava *et al.* 1991; Wright *et al.* 1992) and their effects on vascular reactivity and blood pressure are well established. Inhibition of nitric oxide synthesis increases blood pressure in endotoxin- or cytokine-induced shock and restores vascular responsiveness to noradrenaline (Kilbourn *et al.* 1990; Gray *et al.* 1991). Hence inhibition of the L-arginine–NO pathway appears to return the cardiovascular system towards a state of normality. A selective inhibitor of the inducible isoform of the enzyme offers theoretical advantages and one such compound, aminoguanidine, is currently under investigation.

In smooth muscle cells the induction of NO synthase is accompanied by induction of tetrahydrobiopterin synthesis and this essential cofactor is an absolute requirement for NO generation by smooth muscle cells following endotoxin treatment (Gross and Levi 1992). Inhibition of tetrahydrobiopterin synthesis can be achieved *in vitro* by methotrexate and this might provide a useful way to limit selectively the synthesis of NO by the inducible NO synthase (see Fig. 17.4).

Many of the immunological effects of NO are mediated via its ability to inhibit cellular respiration and cell division by inactivation of iron–sulfur centre-containing enzymes whereas the vascular effects of NO on smooth muscle cells are mediated by stimulation of cyclic GMP production (see Moncada *et al.* 1991). Therefore, selective inhibition of guanylate cyclase would be a possible strategy for the inhibition of NO action within the cardiovascular system. Methylene blue inhibits guanylate cyclase and restores blood pressure and vascular tone in experimental shock (Schneider *et al.* 1992*b*). However, this compound has many other actions including generation of free radicals and direct inhibition of NO synthase, and it is not possible to be certain that the effects seen are due solely to inhibition of guanylate cyclase. Clearly an inhibitor of guanlyate cyclase will not affect the toxic effects of NO which are independent of cyclic GMP formation and moreover will inhibit the vasodilator actions of both the constitutive as well as inducible NO synthase.

Prostaglandins

Indomethacin improves survival in endotoxin- and TNF-induced shock in rats (Ball *et al.* 1986; Kettelhut *et al.* 1987; Goto *et al.* 1989) and increases blood pressure in certain animal models. However, certain of these effects may relate to a direct vasoconstrictor action of the drug unrelated to inhibition of cyclo-oxygenase (Mozes *et al.* 1991), and the precise effects of cyclo-oxygenase inhibitors in shock remain to be established. Furthermore, there appear to be a large interspecies variation in the relative importance of prostanoids in the vascular changes.

Vascular damage

Altered vascular tone is a major feature of sepsis, however equally important may be vascular damage. This could contribute to altered reactivity and also lead to vascular leakage and oedema formation. The mechanisms are not fully understood, but might be linked to vasoactive mediators. Endotoxin and cytokines (e.g. TNF) cause damage to endothelial cells in culture (Palmer *et al.* 1991; Estrada *et al.* 1992) and the cytotoxic effects of these agents are mediated in part by induction of nitric oxide synthesis. It is proposed that the large amounts of nitric oxide produced inhibit cellular function and lead to endothelial damage. It is unlikely that this is the sole mechanism, however, this would provide a link between hypotension and vascular damage.

Septic shock in patients

The identification of endotoxin as an initiator, and the cytokines as mediators involved in the pathogenesis of sepsis, has lead to the development of antibodies designed to selectively neutralize these agents. Initial results in animal models of sepsis have been encouraging, and there are many theoretical advantages to this approach in treatment of human sepsis. At least two immunoglobulin (IgM) monoclonal antibodies to the conserved region of lipid A of endotoxin have been developed. These antibodies have undergone phase 3 clinical trials and although in certain subgroups of patients this therapy may have been of benefit, overall no significant reduction in mortality was observed. Similarly, although experiments in animals appeared promising, there is no evidence yet that antibodies

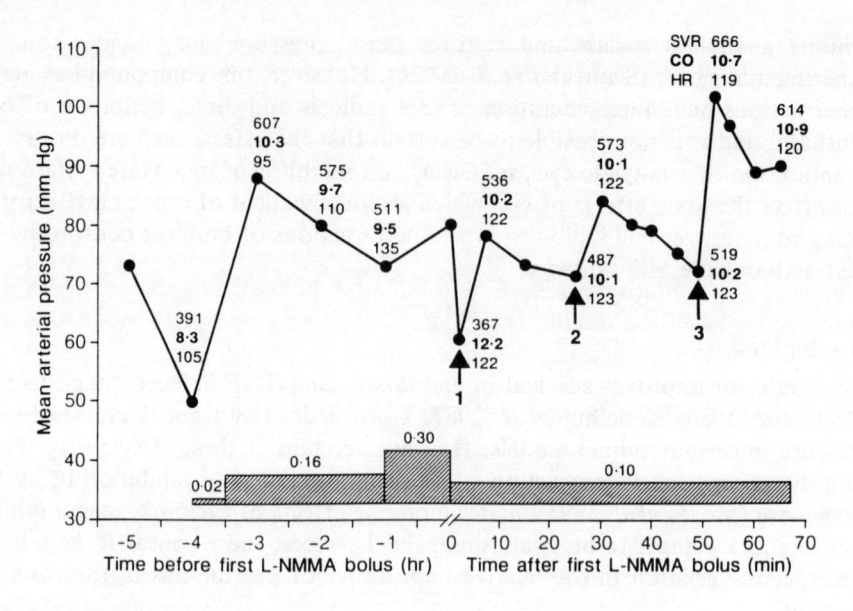

Fig. 17.5 Effects of N^G-monomethyl-L-arginine (L-NMMA) on mean arterial blood pressure, cardiac output (CO, Litre/min), heart rate (HR, beats/min), and systemic vascular resistance (SVR, dyne. s/cm^5) in a patient with septic shock. *Arrows* show bolus injections of L-NMMA: 1, 0.3 mg/kg; 2, 0.3 mg/kg; 3, 1 mg/kg. Hatched columns indicate noradrenaline infusions (μg/kg/min shown above columns). Reproduced from Petros *et al.* (1991).

against TNF or neutralizing IL-1 improves outcome in patients. In terms of the cardiovascular system it is not surprising that these agents do not produce immediate changes, since the vasodilatation is mediated by the induction of vasoactive agents. An alternative therapeutic strategy is the inhibition of these secondary mediators.

There is accumulating evidence for a role for nitric oxide in the pathogenesis of human sepsis. Biochemical evidence for increased production of nitric oxide in sepsis is provided by studies showing increased plasma concentrations of nitrite and nitrate in patients with septic shock (Ochoa *et al.* 1991) or those receiving therapy with interleukin-2 (Hibbs *et al.* 1992; Ochoa *et al.* 1992). In addition, the plasma concentration of arginine (the substrate for NO synthesis) is reduced in patients with sepsis, although other amino acids are also depleted (Freund *et al.* 1979; Vente *et al.* 1989). Functional evidence for a role for nitric oxide in human sepsis has also been obtained by examining the effects of nitric oxide synthase inhibitors in patients with severe hypotension (Petros *et al.* 1991) (Fig. 17.5). In such patients, L-NMMA elevates blood pressure by increasing peripheral arterioler resistance. Although a role for nitric oxide in mediating the cardiovascular dysfunction observed is human sepsis has been defined, further studies will be necessary to determine whether this mediator is also responsible for the tissue damage observed in this condition. Trials of L-NMMA in septic shock are now underway and it seems likely that this will be the first drug based specifically on the L-arginine–NO pathway to be used clinically. In contrast, inhibitors of cyclooxygenase do not have a major effect in patients with sepsis and may precipitate renal failure.

CONCLUDING REMARKS

Septic shock is a multisystem disorder, often initiated by the binding of endotoxin to receptors found on monocytes, macrophages, and other cells and associated with the secretion of cytokines. Endotoxin and cytokines lead to vascular relaxation and this effect is produced by vasoactive mediators including nitric oxide, prostaglandins, and other arachidonic acid derivatives. The overall effect of sepsis on vascular tone varies between vascular beds and depends on the local balance of constrictor and dilator mediators produced and the sensitivity of the smooth muscle to these agents. Over-production of nitric oxide accounts for much of the vasodilatation, and inhibitors of nitric oxide synthase effectively restore blood pressure in patients. The mechanisms underlying the regional vasoconstriction in patients remain to be established and the complex interaction between vasoactive agents is incompletely understood. Drugs based on restoring vascular reactivity are currently in development and it seems likely that inhibition of the L-arginine–NO pathway will become a major therapeutic target. What remains to be determined is whether restoring vascular function by inhibiting mediator production will lead to improved survival.

REFERENCES

Auguet, M., Lonchampt, M.-O., Delaflotte, S., Goulin-Schilz, J., Chabrier, P. E., and Braquet, P. (1992). Induction of nitric oxide synthase by lipoteichoic acid from staphylococcus aureaus in vascular smooth muscle cells. *FEBS Lett.*, **297**, 183–5.

Ball, H. A., Cook, J. A., Wise, W. C., and Halushka, P. V. (1986). Role of thromboxane, prostaglandins and leukotrienes in endotoxic and septic shock. *Int. Care Med.*, **12**, 116–26.

Baydoun, A. R., Foale, R. D., and Mann, G. E. (1993). Bacterial endotoxin causes a rapid reduction in vascular tone in the rat isolated perfused heart. *Br. J. Pharmacol.*, **109**, 987–91.

Beasley, D., Schwartz, J. H., and Brenner, B. M. (1991). Interleukin-1 induces prolonged L-arginine dependent cyclic guanosine monophosphate and nitrite production in rat vascular smooth muscle cells. *J. Clin. Invest.*, **87**, 602–8.

Berg, T., Schlichting, E., Ishida, H., and Carretero, D. A. (1990). Kinin antagonist does not protect against the hypotensive response to endotoxin, anaphylaxis or acute pancreatitis. *J. Pharmacol. Exp. Ther.*, **251**, 731–41.

Breviario, F., Proserpio, P., Bertocchi, F., Lampugnani, M. G., Mantovani, A., and Dejani, E. (1990). Interleukin-1 stimulates prostacyclin production by cultured human endothelial cells by increasing arachidonic acid mobilization and conversion. *Atherosclerosis*, **10**, 129–34.

Buetler, B. and Cerami, A. (1987). The endogenous mediator of septic shock. *Clin. Res.*, **35**, 192–7.

Buetler, B., Milsark, I. W., and Cerami, A. (1985). Passive immunization against cachectin/tumour necrosis factor protects mice from lethal effects of endotoxin. *Science*, **229**, 869-71.

Busse, R. and Mülsch, A. (1990). Induction of nitric oxide synthase by cytokines in vascular smooth muscle cells. *FEBS Lett.*, **275**, 87-90.

Cannon, J. G., Tompkins, R. G., and Gelfland, J. A. (1990). Circulating interleukin-1 and tumour necrosis factor in experimental endotoxin fever. *J. Infect. Dis.*, **161**, 79-84.

Chapman, P. B., Lester, T. J., Cooper, E. S., Gabrilove, J. L., Wong, G. Y., and Kempin, S. J. (1987). Clinical pharmacology of recombinant human tumour necrosis factor in patients with advanced cancer. *J. Clin. Oncol.*, **5**, 1942-51.

Collier, J. G., Herman, A. G., and Vane, J.R. (1973). Appearance of prostaglandins in the renal venous blood of dogs in response to acute systemic hypotension produced by bleeding or endotoxin. *J. Physiol.*, **230**, 19-20P.

Cunha, F. Q., Moncada, S., and Liew, F. Y. (1992). Interleukin-10 (IL-10) inhibits the induction of nitric oxide synthase by interferon-γ in murine macrophages. *Biochem. Biophys. Res. Commun.*, **182**, 1155-9.

Durante, W., Schini, V. B., Scott-Burden, T., Junquero, D. C., Kroll, M. H., Vanhoutte, P. M., et al. (1991). Platelet inhibition by an L-arginine-derived substance release by IL-1β treated vascular smooth muscle cells. *Am. J. Physiol.*, **261**, H2024-30.

Estrada, C., Gomez, C., and Martin, C. (1992). Nitric oxide mediates tumour necrosis factor-α cytotoxicity in endothelial cells. *Biochem. Biophys. Res. Commun.*, **186**, 475-82.

Fast, D. J., Schlievert, P. M., and Nelson, R. D. (1989). Toxic-shock syndrome associated staphylococcal and streptococcal pyrogenic toxins are potent inducers of tumour necrosis factor production. *Infect. Immun.*, **57**, 291-4.

Feuerstein, G., Dimicco, J. A., Ramu, A., and Kopin, I. J. (1981). Effect of indomethacin on the blood pressure and plasma catecholamine responses to acute endotoxaemia. *J. Pharm. Pharmacol.*, **33**, 576-9.

Filkins, J. P. (1985). Monokines and metabolic pathophysiology of septic shock. *Fed. Proc.*, **44**, 300-4.

Fischer, H., Dohlstein, M., Andersson, U., Hedlund, G., Ericsson, P., Hansson, J., and Sjogren, H. O. (1990). Production of TNF-alpha and TNF-beta by staphylococcal enterotoxin and activated human T-cells *J. Immunol.*, **144**, 4663-9.

Fleming, I., Gray, G. A., Julou-Schaefer, G., Parratt, J. R., and Stocklet, J.-C. (1990). Incubation with endotoxin activates the L-arginine pathway in vascular tissue. *Biochem. Biophys. Res. Commun.*, **168**, 458-65.

Fleming, I., Gray, G. A., and Stocklet, J.-C. (1991a). Inducible by not constitutive production of NO by vascular smooth muscle cells. *Eur. J. Pharmacol.*, **200**, 375-6.

Fleming, I., Julou-Schaeffer, G., Gray, G. A., Parratt, J. R., and Stoclet, J.-C. (1991b). Evidence than an L-arginine/nitric oxide dependent elevation of tissue cyclic GMP content is involved in depression of vascular reactivity by endotoxin. *Br. J. Pharmacol.*, **103**, 1047-52.

Fleming, I., Dabmacher, T., and Busse, R. (1992). Endothelium-derived kinins account for the immediate response of endothelial cells to bacterial lipopolysaccharide. *J. Cardiovasc. Pharmacol.*, **20(Suppl. 12)**, S135-8.

Freund, H., Atamian, S., and Holroyde, J. (1979). Plasma amino acios as predictors of the severity and outcome of sepsis. *Ann. Surg.*, **190**, 571-6.

Fu, J. Y., Masferrer, J. L., Seibert, K., Raz, A., and Needleman, P. (1990). The induction and suppression of prostaglandin H_2 synthase (cycloxygenase) in human monocytes. *J. Biol. Chem.*, **265**, 16737-40.

Geller, D. A., Lowenstein, C. J., Shapiro, R. A., Nussler, A. K., DiSilvio, M., Wang,

S. C., *et al.* (1993). Molecular cloning and expression of inducible nitric oxide synthase from human hepatocytes. *Proc. Acad. Sci. USA*, **90**, 3491-5.

Gonzalez, C., Fernandez, A., Martin, C., Moncada, S., and Estrada, C. (1992). Nitric oxide from endothelium and smooth muscle modulates responses to sympathetic nerve stimulation: implications for endotoxic shock. *Biochem. Biophys. Res. Commun.*, **186**, 150-6.

Goto, F., Watranabe, E., Maruyama, N., and Fujita, T. (1989). Prevention of the toxic action of tumour necrosis factor by cyclooxygenase inhibitors and leukopaenia. *Circulat. Shock*, **29**, 175-80.

Gray, G. A., Schott, C., Julou-Scaeffer, G., Fleming, I., Parratt, J. R., and Stoclet, J.-C. (1991). The effect of inhibitors of the L-arginine/nitric oxide pathway on endotoxin-induced loss of vascular responsiveness in enaesthetized rats. *Br. J. Pharmacol.*, **103**, 1218-24.

Gross, S. S. and Levi, R. (1992). Tetrahydrobiopterin synthesis: An absolute requirement for cytokine-induced nitric oxide generation by vascular smooth muscle. *J. Biol. Chem.*, **267**, 25722-9.

Hale, D. J., Robinson, J. A., Loeb, H. S., and Gunnar, R. M. (1986). Pathophysiology of endotoxin shock in man. In *Handbook of endotoxin* (ed. R. A. Protoc), pp. 1-17. Elsevier, Amsterdam.

Hibbs, J. B., Westenfelder, C., and Taintor, R. (1992). Evidence for a cytokine-inducible nitric oxide synthesis from L-arginine in patients receiving interleukin-2 therapy. *J. Clin. Invest.*, **89**, 867-77.

Ikejima, T., Okusawa, S., van der Meer, J. V., and Dinarello, C. A. (1989). Induction by toxic-shock-syndrome-toxin-1 of a circulating tumour necrosis factor like substance in rabbits and of immunoreactive tumour necrosis factor and interleukin-1 from human mononuclear cells. *J. Infect. Dis.*, **158**, 1017-25.

Julou-Schaeffer, G., Gray, G. A., Fleming, I., Schott, C., Parratt, J. R., and Stoclet, J. C. (1990). Loss of vascular responsiveness induced by endotoxin involved L-arginine pathway. *Am. J. Physiol.*, **259**, H1038-43.

Junquero, D. C., Scott-Burden, T., Schini, V. B., and Vanhoutte, P. M. (1992). Inhibition of cytokine-induced nitric oxide production by transforming growth factor-$\beta 1$ in human smooth muscle cells. *J. Physiol.*, **454**, 451-65.

Katori, M., Majina, M., Odoi-Adome, R., Sunahara, N., and Uchida, Y. (1989). Evidence for an involvement of a plasma kallikrein-kinin system in the immediate hypotension produced by endotoxin in anaesthetized rats. *Br. J. Pharmacol.*, **98**, 1383-91.

Kettelhut, I. C., Fiers, W., and Goldberg, A. L. (1987). The toxic effects of tumour necrosis and their prevention by cyclooxygenase inhibitors. *Proc. Natl Acad. Sci. USA*, **84**, 4273-7.

Kilbourn, R. G. and Belloni, B. (1990). Endothelial cell production of nitrogen oxides in response to interferon-γ in combination with tumour necrosis factor, interleukin-1, or endotoxin. *J. Nat. Cancer Inst.*, **82**, 772-6.

Kilbourn, R. G., Gross, S. S., Jubran, A., Adams, J. Griffith, O. W., Levi, R., *et al.* (1990). N^G-methyl-L-arginine inhibits tumour necrosis factor induced hypotension: implications for the involvement of nitric oxide. *Proc. Nat. Acad. Sci. USA*, **87**, 3629-32.

Knowles, R. G., Salter, M., Brooks, S. L., and Moncada, S. (1990). Anti-inflammatory glucorticoids inhibit the induction by endotoxin of nitric oxide synthase in lung, liver and aorta of the rat. *Biochem. Biophys. Res. Commun.*, **172**, 1042-8.

Loppnow, H. and Libby, P. (1990). Proliferating or IL-1 activated human smooth muscle cells secrete copious IL-6. *J. Clin. Invest.*, **85**, 731-8.

McKenna, T. M. (1990). Prolonged exposure of rat aorta to low levels of endotoxin results in impaired contractility: association with vascular cytokine release. *J. Clin. Invest.*, **86**, 160-8.

Marceau, F., Petitclerc, E., DeBlois, D., Pradelles, P., and Poubelle, P. (1991). Human interleukin-1 induces a rapid relaxation of the rabbit isolated mesenteric artery. *Br. J. Pharmacol.*, **103**, 1367-72.

Masferrer, J. L., Zweifel, B. S., Seibert, K., and Needleman, P. (1992). Selective regulation of cellular cycloxygenase by dexamethasone and endotoxin in mice. *J. Clin. Invest.*, **86**, 1375-9.

Michie, H. R., Manogue, K. R., Spriggs, D. R., Revhaug, A., O'Dwyer, S., Dinarello, C. A., et al. (1986). Detection of circulating tumour necrosis factor after endotoxin administration. *New Engl. J. Med.*, **318**, 1481-6.

Michie, H. R., Spriggs, D. R., and Manogue, K. R. (1988). Tumour necrosis factor and endotoxin induce similar metabolic responses in human beings. *Surgery*, **104**, 280-6.

Mitchell, J. A., Kohnhas, K. L., Sorrentino, R., Warner, T. D., Murad, F., and Vane, J. R. (1993). Induction by endotoxin of nitric oxide synthase in the rat mesentery: lack of effect on action of vasoconstriction. *Br. J. Pharmacol.*, **109**, 265-70.

Moncada, S., Palmer, R. M. J., and Higgs, E. A. (1991). Nitric oxide: Physiology, pathophysiology and pharmacology. *Pharmacol. Rev.*, **43**, 109-42.

Mozes, T., Zijlstra, F. J., Heiligers, J. P. C., Tak, C. J. A. M., Ben-Efraim, S., Bonta, I. L., et al. (1991). Sequential release of tumour necrosis factor, platelet activating factor and eicosanoids during endotoxin shock in anaesthetized pigs; protective effects of indomethacin. *Br. J. Pharmacol.*, **104**, 691-9.

Myers, P. R., Wright, T. F., Tanner, M. A., and Adams, H. R. (1992). EDRF and nitric oxide production by cultured endothelial cells: direct inhibition by *E. coli* endotoxin. *Am. J. Physiol.*, **262**, H710-18.

Nava, E., Palmer, R. M. J., and Moncada, S. (1991). Inhibition of nitric oxide synthesis in septic shock: how much is beneficial? *Lancet*, **388**, 1555-7.

Ochoa, J. B., Udekwu, A. O., and Billiar, T. R. (1991). Nitrogen oxide levels in patients following trauma and during sepsis. *Ann. Surg.*, **214**, 621-6.

Ochoa, J. B., Curti, B., and Peitzmann, A. B. (1992). Increased circulating nitrogen oxide after human tumour immunotherapy: correlation with toxic hemodynamic changes. *J. Nat. Cancer Inst.*, **84**, 864-7.

Ohlsson, K., Bjork, P., Bergenfeldt, M., Hageman, R., and Thompson, R. C. (1990). Interleukin-1 receptor antagonist reduces mortality from endotoxin shock. *Nature*, **348**, 550-2.

Palmer, R. M. J. and Moncada, S. (1989). A novel citrulline-forming enzyme implicated in the formation of nitric oxide by vascular endothelial cells. *Biochem. Biophys. Res. Commun.*, **158**, 348-52.

Palmer, R. M. J., Bridge, L., Foxwell, N. A., and Moncada, S. (1991). The role of nitric oxide in endothelial damage and its inhibition by glucocorticoids. *Br. J. Pharmacol.*, **105**, 11-12.

Parratt, J. R. (1973). Myocardial and circulatory effects of *E. coli* endotoxin: modification of responses to endotoxin. *Br. J. Pharmacol.*, **47**, 12-25.

Parratt, J. C. and Sturgess, R. M. (1974). The effect of indomethacin on the cardiovascular and metabolic responses to *E. coli* in the cat. *Br. J. Pharmacol.*, **50**, 177-83.

Parratt, J. C. and Sturgess, R. M. (1975). *E. coli* endotoxin shock in the cat: treatment with indomethacin. *Br. J. Pharmacol.*, **53**, 485-8.

Petros, A. J., Bennett, D., and Vallance, P. (1991). Effect of nitric oxide synthase inhibitors on hypotension in patients with septic shock. *Lancet*, **338**, 1558-60.

Rabinovici, R., Yue, T. C., and Feuerestein, G. (1991). Platelet activating factor in cardiovascular stress situations. *Lipids*, **26**, 1257–63.

Radomski, M. W., Palmer, R. M. J., and Moncada, S. (1991). Glucorticoids inhibit the expression of an inducible, but not the constitutive, nitric oxide synthase in vascular endothelial cells. *Proc. Nat. Acad. Sci. USA*, **87**, 10043–7.

Radomski, M. W., Vallance, P., Whitley, G., Foxwell, N., and Moncada, S. (1993). Platelet adhesion to human vascular endothelium is modulated by constitutive and inducible nitric oxide. *Cardiovasc. Res.*, **27**, 1380–2.

Rees, D. D., Palmer, R. M. J., Hodson, H. F., and Moncada, S. (1989). A specific inhibitor of nitric oxide formation from L-arginine attenuates endothelium-dependent relaxation. *Br. J. Pharmacol.*, **96**, 418–24.

Rees, D. D., Cellek, S., Palmer, R. M. J., and Moncada, S. (1990). Dexamethasone prevents the induction by endotoxin of a nitric oxide synthase and the associated effects on vascular tone. An insight into endotoxin shock. *Biochem. Biophys. Res. Commun.*, **173**, 541–7.

Rossi, V., Breviario, F., Ghezzi, P., Dejana, E., and Mantovani, A. (1985). Prostacyclin synthesis induced in vascular cells by interleukin-1. *Science*, **229**, 174–6.

Salvement, D. D., Korbut, R., Anggard, E., and Vane, J. (1990). Immediate release of a nitric oxide like factor from bovine aortic endothelial cells by *Escherichia coli* lipopolysaccharide. *Proc. Natl. Acad. Sci. USA*, **87**, 2593–7.

Schini, V. B., Junquero, D. C., Scott-Burden, T., and Vanhoutte, P. M. (1991). Interleukin-1β induces the production of an L-arginine-derived relaxing factor from cultured smooth muscle cells from rat aorta. *Biochem. Biophys. Res. Commun.*, **176**, 114–21.

Schini, V. B., Catovsky, S., Durante, W., Scott-Burden, T., Schafer, A. I., and Vanhoutte, P. M. (1993). Thrombin inhibits induction of nitric oxide synthase in vascular smooth muscle cells. *Am. J. Physiol.*, **264**, H611–16.

Schneider, F., Schott, C., Stoclet, J.-C., and Julou-Schaeffer, G. (1992a). L-arginine induces relaxation of small mesenteric arteries from endotoxin treated rats. *Eur. J. Pharmacol.*, **211**, 269–72.

Schneider, F., Lutun, P., Hasselmann, M., Stoclet, J.-C., and Tempe, J. D. (1992b). Methylene blue increases systemic vascular resistance in human septic shock. *Inten. Care Med.*, **18**, 309–11.

Schulz, R., Nava, E., and Moncada, S. (1992). Induction and potential biological relevance of a Ca^{2+}-independent nitric oxide synthase in the myocardium. *Br. J. Pharmacol.*, **105**, 575–80.

Sheehan, K. C., Ruddle, N. H., and Schreiber, R. D. (1989). Generation and characterization of hamster monoclonal antibodies to murine tumour necrosis factor. *J. Immunol.*, **142**, 3884–93.

Shibano, T. and Vanhoutte, P. M. (1993). Induction of NO production by TNF-α and lipopolysaccharide in porcine coronary arteries. *Am. J. Physiol.*, **264**, H403–7.

Suffredini, A. F., Fromm, R. E., Parker, M. M., Brenner, M., Kovacs, J. A., Wesley, R. A., *et al.* (1989). The cardiovascular response of normal humans to the administration of endotoxin. *N. Engl. J. Med.*, **321**, 280–7.

Thiemermann, C. and Vane, J. (1990). Inhibition of nitric oxide synthesis reduces the hypotension induced by bacterial lipopolysaccharides in the rat *in vivo*. *Eur. J. Pharmacol.*, **182**, 591–5.

Tracey, K. J., Fong, Y., Hesse, D.G., Manogue, K.R., Lee, A. T., Kuo, G. C., *et al.* (1987). Anti-cachectin/TNF monoclonal antibodies prevent septic shock during lethal bacteraemia. *Nature*, **330**, 662–4.

Vallance, P., Palmer, R. M. J., and Moncada, S. (1992). The role of induction of nitric oxide synthesis in the altered response of jugular veins from endotoxaemic rabbits. *Br. J. Pharmacol.*, **106**, 459-63.

Vente, J. P., Von Meyenfeldt, M., Van Eijk, H. M. H., van, Berbo, C. L., Gouma, D. J., van der Linden, C. J., and Soeters, P. B. (1989). Plasma amino acid profiles in sepsis and stress. *Ann. Surg.*, **209**, 57-62.

Voerman, H. J., Stenhouwer, C. D., van Kepm, G. J., Strack van Schijndel, R. J., Groeneveld, A. B., and Thijs, L. G. (1992). Plasma endothelin levels are increased in septic shock. *Crit. Care Med.*, **20**, 1097-101.

Wagner, D. A., Young, V. R., and Tannembaum, S. R. (1983). Mammalian nitrate biosynthesis: Incorporation of $^{15}NH_3$ into nitrate is enhanced by endotoxin treatment. *Proc. Natl. Acad. Sci. USA*, **80**, 4518-21.

Warner, S. J. C. and Libby, P. (1990). Human vascular smooth muscle cells: Target for and source of tumour necrosis factor. *J. Immunol.*, **142**, 100-9.

Wright, C. E., Rees, D. D., and Moncada, S. (1992). Protective and pathological roles of nitric oxide in endotoxin shock. *Cardiovasc. Res.*, **26**, 48-57.

Yoshizumi, M., Perrella, M. A., Burnett, J. C., and Lee, M.-E. (1993). Tumour necrosis factor downregulates an endothelial nitric oxide synthase mRNA by shortening its half-life. *Circ. Res.*, **73**, 205-9.

Zembowicz, A. and Vane, J. R. (1992). Induction of nitric oxide synthase activity by toxic shock syndrome toxin 1 in a macrophage/monocyte cell line. *Proc. Natl. Acad. Sci. USA.* **89**, 2051-5.

18. Hypertension

Jaye P. F. Chin and Anthony M. Dart

INTRODUCTION

Hypertension, a state in which the systemic arterial pressure is inappropriately elevated, is a prevalent cardiovascular condition in Westernized communities, and contributes to mortality and morbidity as a major risk factor for stroke and coronary heart disease. The aetiology of hypertension remains obscure in the majority of cases, and treatment, therefore, somewhat empirical. However, abnormalities in the structure and function of the vasculature are increasingly recognized as contributing to the hypertensive state by increasing total peripheral resistance. This chapter will briefly review some of these abnormalities with particular regard to the way in which they influence treatment, and suggest new therapeutic strategies. A minority of hypertensive individuals have a clearly identified hormonal or structural cause for their elevated pressure ('secondary hypertension') and will not be specifically considered further, although some animal models rely on such aetiologies to produce hypertension for experimental purposes.

ABNORMALITIES OF THE VASCULATURE

Functional changes

In general, vasoconstrictor drugs are reported to be more potent in blood vessels from hypertensive subjects or animals compared with those from matched normotensive controls (Griendly and Alexander 1990). The increased reactivity is of a non-specific type in that agonists which act via different receptors and/or modes of action (sympathomimetics, angiotensin II, 5-HT, vasopressin) have all been reported to elicit a more constrictive effect in hypertensives. Alterations in the biochemical signalling pathway have been reported at almost every step in the transduction of agonist stimulation into contractile activity. Vascular smooth muscle cells cultured from the mesenteric bed of spontaneously hypertensive rats (SHR) show an augmentation of angiotensin II and thromboxane A_2-induced enhancement of intracellular calcium and accumulation of inositol phosphate when compared with cells from normotensive controls. These differences could not be accounted for by changes in receptor number or affinity (Osanai and Dunn 1992). Functional studies using vascular strips (aorta and portal vein) from SHR also indicate an increase in calcium sensitivity, that can be linked to an increase in the protein kinase C activity of these vessels (Soloviev and Bershtein 1992). In addition, increased activation of phospholipase C has been shown to be responsible for increased accumulation of the second messengers inositol 1,4,5-triphosphate and diacylglycerol in aortas of SHR (Kato *et al.* 1992). Although similar studies are scarce in vascular smooth muscle from man, platelets from hypertensive patients demonstrate increased basal and stimulated calcium levels (Lechi *et al.* 1987). Another, quite separate issue, is the finding that vascular distending pressure can increase the number of intermediate and actin filaments in proportion to cell volume (Berner *et al.* 1981), suggesting that a change in contractile proteins may also contribute to enhanced vascular hyperreactivity.

A current popular hypothesis for the enhanced vasoconstriction seen in hypertensives is endothelial cell dysfunction. During the past decade, it has become increasingly clear that the endothelium, the single cell, innermost layer of blood vessels, is more than a passive barrier between the blood and the vascular smooth muscle. We now know that the endothelium plays a crucial role in circulatory homeostasis responding not only to humoral and chemical signals, but also to changes in the haemodynamics of blood flow such as shear stress. Endothelial cells release chemical mediators that modulate the responses of numerous cells including vascular smooth muscle, platelets, and leucocytes (Luscher *et al.* 1990). Such vasoactive mediators include prostaglandins (in particular prostacyclin), endothelium-derived relaxing factor (EDRF), now widely accepted to be nitric oxide (NO), and endothelin, a 21-amino acid vasoactive peptide, the most potent endogenous vasoconstrictor so far identified (Fig. 18.1). Endothelial cell dysfunction in hypertension has been reported in various forms. Plasma levels of endothelin, for example, have been reported to be significantly higher in patients with essential hypertension (Naruse *et al.* 1991). In addition, both chemical-stimulated and basal release of EDRF has been shown to be severely attenuated in hypertensive patients (Panza *et al.* 1990) as well as in experimental models of hypertension (Van de Voorde and Leusen 1986). Either, or both of these abnormalities could contribute to increased vasomotor tone, leading to elevated total peripheral resistance, and hence increased blood pressure. A role for increased activity of oxygen-derived free radicals (ODFRs) in the pathogenesis of hypertension (Nakazono *et al.* 1991) has also been suggested since EDRF is known to be inactivated by such radicals. An underlying abnormality in blood vessels from hypertensives is thus thought to be increased superoxide production or a decreased action of superoxide dismutase (an enzyme responsible for superoxide breakdown), rather than impaired EDRF synthesis or release (Fig. 18.1).

Another abnormality in the biology of vascular smooth muscle cells that may account for increased vasotone of hypertensives, is a disturbance in the physicochemical properties of the cell membrane leading to abnormalities in ion handling (Swales 1991). Reported abnormalities of cellular electrolyte homeostasis include increased sodium influx due to elevation of sodium–hydrogen exchange activity (Inariba *et al.* 1992), decreased sodium–potassium cotransport (Adragna *et al.* 1982), increased lithium–sodium countertransport (Bing *et al.* 1987), decreased red cell membrane binding of calcium (Bing *et al.* 1987), increased voltage operated

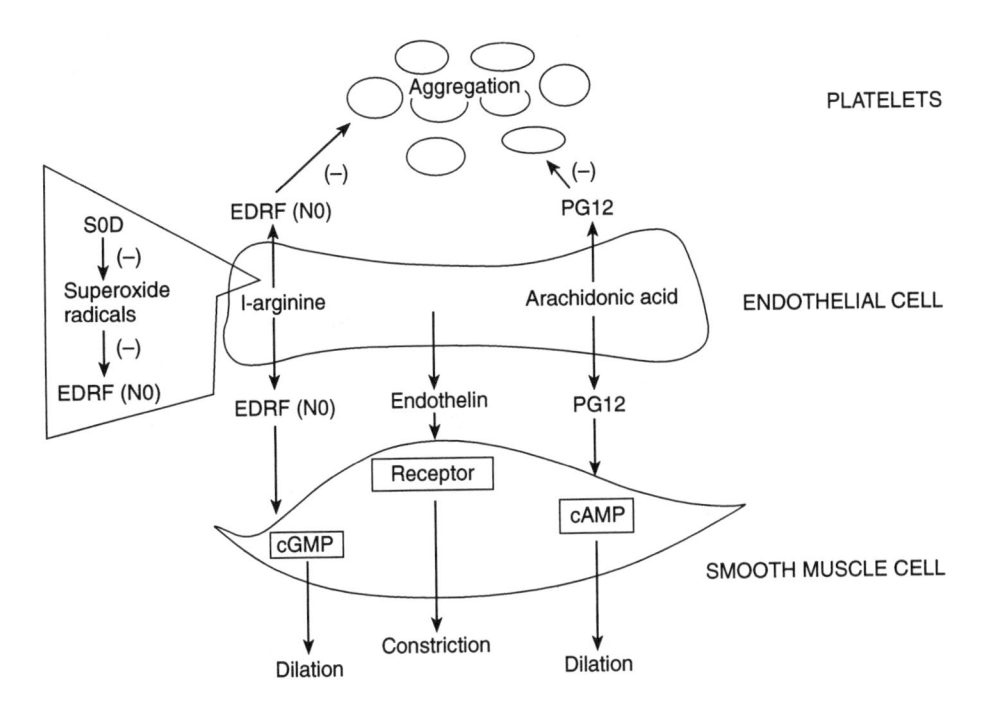

Fig. 18.1 Endothelial cells release chemical mediators such as the anti-platelet aggregators, and vasodilators prostacyclin and endothelium-derived relaxing factor (EDRF), and the potent vasoconstrictor endothelin. EDRF is derived from L-arginine and can be inactivated by superoxide radicals. Endothelial cell dysfunction in hypertension may lead to increased release of endothelin, decreased release of EDRF, and increased superoxide production or decreased superoxide dismutase (SOD).

as well as nifedipine-resistant calcium mobilization (Kurahashi *et al.* 1992), an intrinsic defect in the regulation of intracellular magnesium (Ng *et al.* 1992), and a decreased rate constant for sodium efflux in the leucocyte (Swales 1991). Family studies show similar abnormalities in ion transport in the normotensive offspring of hypertensive parents (Swales 1991; Yamakawa *et al.* 1992) so it is unlikely that the observed changes are merely the consequence of elevated blood pressure. Three favoured explanations as to how abnormal ion handling might contribute to an elevation of blood pressure are:

(a) That sodium (and hence fluid) retention occurs within the arteriole smooth muscle and results in a reduction in luminal area and an elevation of peripheral resistance (Simon 1990).

(b) That inhibition of a vascular sodium–calcium exchange mechanism produces an increase in intracellular calcium acting as a second messenger for contraction, leading to an increase in vasomotor tone (Jones 1982).

(c) That a primary disturbance in cell membrane permeability gives rise to depolarization, increased calcium influx, and thus enhanced vasotone (Jones 1982).

It is also possible, however, that ion transport abnormalities are an epiphenomenon, linked genetically to some other, as yet unidentified, causal mechanism.

Structural changes

In parallel with studies on the function of vascular smooth muscle in the hypertensive state, considerable attention has been given to the importance of structural changes. The change in the geometry of the vessel wall that results in an increased vasoconstrictor response with the same degree of shortening of vascular smooth muscle is a decrease in the lumen (internal radius of the vessel). This can result from an increase in wall thickness either due to medial smooth muscle cell proliferation, accumulation of glycoaminoglycans, or vascular 'remodelling'. The foremost proponent of the structural aetiology of hypertension (Folkow 1990), has argued that the ability of a resistance vessel to restrict blood flow depends on the relative thickness of the vessel wall to the size of the vessel lumen. The hypothesis is that the greater the relative thickness of the wall the greater the amplifier properties of that wall, such that an equivalent stimulus would produce greater narrowing of the lumen. Resistance vessels from animal models and humans with hypertension show an increase in media to lumen ratio. Present evidence suggests that although there is no increase in vascular smooth muscle mass in essential hypertension (Angus *et al.* 1992), there is an increase in media thickness to lumen diameter ratio (Aalkjaer *et al.* 1987) suggesting that the altered structure is due to 'remodelling,' i.e. an abnormal arrangement of a normal amount of normal material (Mulvany 1992). This increase in wall to lumen ratio could be pressure related and result from the increased load imposed on the resistance vessels or to enhanced smooth muscle trophic response to a given pressor load. There is evidence, however, that structural changes precede any elevation in blood pressure (Gray 1982; Adams *et al.* 1989). Indeed the postulate that the early development of cardiovascular structure has a major influence on blood pressure in later life, raises the possibility that non-pressor factors may be responsible for excessive growth of the heart and vessels (Lever and Harrap 1992; Lever *et al.* 1992). In this hypothesis, the primary disturbance in essential hypertension is considered to be growth regulation rather than contractility. Smooth muscle cell proliferation has been attributed to growth factors, hormones with growth regulatory properties, and intracellular mediators of replication. The relation of smooth muscle proliferation to the first clinical event (vascular narrowing) has, however, not been clearly established. A further consequence of a thicker media is the added difficulty of penetration and hence accessibility of EDRF from the endothelium leading to blunted vasorelaxation (Van de Voorde and Leusen 1986).

HYPERTENSION AND OTHER DISEASE STATES

In discussing the pharmacology and therapeutics of hypertension it is important to consider the frequent coexistence and interaction of hypertension with other disease states. Thus, hypertension frequently occurs in conjunction with coronary heart disease, peripheral vascular disease, early cardiac failure, and diabetes mellitus. These disease states may be causally linked, share common aetiologies, and have pathophysiological consequences amplified by their common occurrence. In addition, therapeutic strategies used for one condition may impact, favourably or unfavourably, on another.

Although diabetes mellitus is by itself associated with a considerable increase in cardiovascular risk, the presence of hypertension markedly increases morbidity and mortality in these patients (Fuller 1985). Type 1, insulin-dependent diabetic patients are twice as likely to suffer from hypertension as are non-diabetic patients. Following the compelling evidence for an interrelationship between hypertension and diabetes mellitus, attention has been given to the possible role of hyperinsulinaemia, insulin resistance, and hyperglycaemia in the pathogenesis of hypertension, not only in relation to diabetes but more generally. The enhanced vascular contractility seen in the hypertensive state also appears to be a hallmark of the diabetic state (Weidman et al. 1985). Since insulin is known to regulate both the Ca^{2+}-ATPase (Levy et al. 1989) and Na^+, K^+-ATPase (Lytton et al. 1985) pumps, it is likely that insulin deficiency or resistance results in decreased activity of these pumps leading to increases in intracellular levels of Ca^{2+} and enhanced contractility. Such abnormalities in vascular smooth muscle in states of decreased cellular insulin action may play a pivotal role in the increased peripheral resistance that contributes to high blood pressure in these patients. Other coexisting factors such as increased plasma endothelin levels (Takahashi et al. 1990) and increased exchangeable sodium levels (Weidman and Ferrari 1991) may also play a major role in linking the two diseases. Chronic hyperglycaemia per se has been postulated to contribute to the pathogenesis of hypertension in diabetics through increased sodium retention (Weidman and Ferrari 1991), by increasing vascular rigidity through over-expression of fibronectin (Roy et al. 1990) and collagen IV, and by enhanced secretion of the smooth muscle cell proliferates, interleukin-1 and tumour necrosis factor (Vlassara et al. 1988). At high concentrations, glucose has also been reported to have a toxic effect on endothelial cells resulting in endothelial cell dysfunction as observed in the hypertensive state (Lorenzi et al. 1985).

Atherosclerosis is another condition characterized by many changes similar to those seen in hypertension. Although hypertension is identified as a 'risk factor' for the development of atherosclerosis it is not clear to what extent this relationship describes a causal mechanism as opposed to certain individuals being susceptible to both states. Treatment of hypertension has been less successful in preventing coronary heart disease than theoretically expected from epidemiological considerations, although this may be due to adverse effects on other risk factors (e.g. serum lipids) resulting from antihypertensive therapy. Whilst in hypertension, smooth muscle cell proliferation leads to an increase in vessel wall mass, in atherosclerosis there is pronounced intimal hyperplasia. Both are characterized by abnormal smooth muscle structure and function, endothelial cell dysfunction, and other disturbances that affect cellular responses to various external stimuli (Bondjers et al. 1991). Although reduction of high blood pressure has by itself anti-atherogenic effects, there is experimental and clinical evidence that some antihypertensive drugs are independently anti-atherogenic as well. The INTACT trial showed that the development of new atherosclerotic lesions in the coronary circulation can be delayed by nifedipine (Lichtlein et al. 1990) while anti-atherogenic effects of ACE inhibitors have been documented in studies with the rabbit and monkey (see Correia 1992).

OTHER STRUCTURAL CHANGES

Another, quite separate issue to be considered in discussing future therapeutic control of hypertension, are the changes outside those which occur in resistance arteries. The presence of cardiac left ventricular hypertrophy in hypertension, for example, carries a greatly increased risk independent of the level of blood pressure (Levy et al. 1980). Although haemodynamic afterload is a major determinant of left ventricular wall thickness, factors that affect hypertrophy of vascular smooth muscle may also contribute to thickening of the left ventricular wall. Animal studies show that non-hypotensive doses of ACE inhibitors are able to regress left ventricular hypertrophy in hypertensive rats (Linz and Scholkens 1992). This effect was blocked by the selective bradykinin antagonist HOE 140, suggesting that inhibition of the degradation of bradykinin (most likely leading to enhancement of the autacoids nitric oxide and prostacyclin), and not angiotensin, is responsible. In man, drug therapy equivalent in terms of lowering blood pressure is not necessarily equivalent in effect on left ventricular hypertrophy (Cruickshank et al.1992).

Reduction of large artery compliance (increased stiffness) is another structural change that can exert deleterious effects on the cardiovascular system (Randall 1982). Mortality and morbidity in hypertension are better correlated with systolic than diastolic blood pressure, indicating a pulsatile stress effect. Both distensibility and compliance are large artery properties and important determinants of pulsatile stress effect (Van Bortel et al. 1992). Since large artery compliance is dependent on arterial blood pressure — the lower the pressure, the higher the compliance — it is difficult to ascertain the effects of antihypertensive drugs on compliance. In an attempt to dissociate the passive effect of antihypertensive drugs on large arteries, i.e. the changes due to changes in blood pressure, from the drug action *per se*, Chau et al. (1992) used a simple non-linear arterial diameter — blood pressure model which concluded that not all antihypertensive drugs have acute active effects on large artery compliance, but those that did, including nitrendipine and captopril, strongly potentiated the passive effect. An emerging issue of interest is the study of small vessel compliance and its role in the pathophysiology of the microcirculation.

ANTIHYPERTENSIVE THERAPY: CURRENT AND FUTURE

The two physiological ways of lowering mean blood pressure are first by reducing peripheral resistance, and secondly by reducing cardiac output (Man in't Veld and Van der Meirecker 1990). In addition, systolic blood pressure is lowered by increasing large artery compliance. Reduction of peripheral resistance can be achieved by reducing sympathetic vasomotor tone, decreasing vascular reactivity, decreasing endogenous, humorally-mediated vasoconstriction, and/or reducing vascular hypertrophy. Reduction of cardiac output can also be achieved by reducing sympathetic cardiac tone, by depressing myocardial contractility directly, and by decreasing cardiac venous return. The latter can be achieved by increasing venous capacitance, by lowering venomotor tone, or by decreasing circulating fluid volume. However, none of the antihypertensive drugs currently used act solely through a single one of these actions. Nevertheless, combinations of drugs are often used to provide therapeutic synergism without producing undue side-effects.

The following account of therapeutic considerations will focus on effects on vascular smooth muscle and is not intended as a comprehensive review of antihypertensive therapy.

Non-pharmacological therapy

Obesity, diet, and alcohol consumption have all been shown to be major environmental determinants of blood pressure elevation (see Beilin 1989). An average fall of 1 mmHg systolic and diastolic per kilogram weight loss has been reported for middle aged obese hypertensives (average weight loss 7.7 kg over five months) — a fall greater than that seen with a beta-blocker (MacMahon *et al.* 1984). An improvement in blood lipid profiles and a reduction of left ventricular hypertrophy has also been associated with weight reduction in hypertensives. Vascular responses to phenylephrine and 5-HT have been shown to be enhanced in insulin resistant Zucker obese rats (Ambrozy *et al.* 1991), perhaps accounting for the greater propensity to hypertension seen in these animals.

The effect of alcohol on blood pressure appears to be independent of, but additive to, that of obesity (Arkwright *et al.* 1982). The 'pressor' effect of regular alcohol consumption appears to be unrelated to the type of alcoholic beverage drunk and is presumed to be the ethanol *per se*. Although acute administration of ethanol causes vasodilatation which may be due to an inteference with the availability of intracellular calcium, as seen in rat cultured aortic smooth muscle cells (Zhang *et al.* 1992), chronic ethanol consumption has been reported to heighten heart rate reactivity to stress (Beilin *et al.* 1992). Vascular neuroeffector characteristics in these chronically treated spontaneously hypertensive rats (SHR) were, however, not apparent. This may indicate that the effect of ethanol is a central one, caused by suppression of central nervous inhibitory systems.

Dietary salt (NaCl) intake remains a controversial focus of attention in relation to hypertension, since randomized controlled trials of reduction in sodium intake have often used complex dietary manoeuvres to achieve their goal, thereby rendering interpretation of results difficult. On the other hand, trials of low NaCl diets (70 mmol/day) with comparison of replacement by placebo have shown significant blood pressure reduction in untreated hypertensives (see Beilin 1989). This may be due to a decrease in sympathetic tone, since low sodium diets are able to significantly decrease potassium-induced release of ^{3}H-noradrenaline in caudal arteries from both the SHR and WKY (Meldrum and Glenton 1992). In addition, a low sodium intake has been correlated to a larger brachial artery diameter in hypertensives and sodium overload, particularly in elderly hypertensives, reduces arterial compliance and distensibility independently of blood pressure changes (Safar et al. 1992).

In an attempt to identify specific nutrients responsible for blood pressure changes, most studies have failed to show any effect of increasing P/S ratio, dietary fibre or meat versus vegetable protein (see Beilin 1989). On the other hand, a combination of nutrient changes may be required to achieve blood pressure reduction and to this end blood pressure has been shown to be lowered by reducing saturated fat intake, in combination with increased fruit and vegetable and decreased total energy consumption (Puska et al. 1983). A number of controlled studies have suggested a mild hypotensive effect of fish oil supplements. We have provided evidence that the antihypertensive effect of fish oils during the resting state is not due to changes in the activity of the sympathetic nervous system (Dart et al. 1993) but rather that it may be due to their blunting effects on the direct postsynaptic pressor effects of noradrenaline and angiotensin II (Chin et al. 1993).

Another method for the non-pharmacological manipulation of resting blood pressure is exercise. Increasing levels of physical activity have a lowering effect on blood pressure (Nelson et al. 1986). These beneficial effects are unlikely to be due to restoration of endothelial function, evidenced by the failure of exercise training to improve dilator responses to acetylcholine in aortic rings from rats with cardiac heart failure (Lindsay et al. 1992). Rather, chronic exercise training induced selective alterations in response to various constrictor and dilator agonists in pig coronary arterial rings, independent of the endothelium (Oltman et al. 1992). There is also some evidence that aerobic exercise training can greatly increase functional vasodilatation, with arterioles dilating proportionately more in trained than sedentary rats during 1-8 Hz skeletal muscle contraction (Lash and Bohlen 1992). With the use of vascular casts, these authors also demonstrated a trend for an increase in vascular density in skeletal muscle tissues, even though the oxidative capacity of these tissues was not increased by the training regimen.

Pharmacological therapy

Diuretics

Diuretics act by their natriuretic action, increasing the quantity of sodium in the urine — the increased salt excretion being accompanied by an increased water excretion to maintain osmotic balance. Sodium-depleting diuretics produce a fall in blood pressure by initiating and maintaining a fall in extracellular fluid volume, leading to decreased venous return and hence decreased cardiac output (Frochlich *et al.* 1960). Diuretics may also cause a decrease in peripheral resistance directly, since loss of fluid from the smooth muscle of small resistance arteries can decrease the ratio of wall thickness to lumen radius, thereby lowering resistance and perhaps also their reactivity (Haddy *et al.* 1985). In animal studies, the diuretic compounds cycletanine and indapamide increase systemic and carotid compliance independently of blood pressure changes (Safar *et al.* 1992).

β-Adrenoceptor antagonists

The vascular effects of β-adrenoceptor blockers apparently have little to do with their antihypertensive action. Indeed, the blockade of vasodilatory responses mediated by $β_2$-adrenoceptors in the vascular smooth muscle can in fact acutely increase total peripheral resistance, resulting in some instances in an increase in blood pressure (Schulte *et al.* 1992). This effect is absent with cardioselective ($β_1$-adrenoceptor) blocking drugs. On the other hand, an important mechanism for antihypertensive action is the negative inotropic and chronotropic effect of this class of drugs. β-Blocking (atenolol) does not appear to have any active effect on arterial compliance (De Cesaris *et al.* 1992). The incidence of non-fatal reinfarctions and sudden death rates have, however, been reported to be significantly reduced in patients on β-blocking therapy (the BHAT research group 1983).

Calcium antagonists

Since increased calcium influx is the final common pathway in eliciting an increased systemic peripheral resistance, drugs preventing intracellular calcium accumulation make potent vasodilators and logical antihypertensive agents. In addition, some calcium antagonists have been reported to have a natriuretic effect. Renal haemodynamic responses to calcium antagonists greatly depend on the prevailing neural and hormonal determinants of renal vascular tone which are differently sensitive to these drugs (Loutzenhiser and Epstein 1985). Their common renal effect is to reduce (elevated) preglomeruler resistance and to maintain or increase the glomerular filtration rate. In addition to their effect in producing vasodilatation and thereby lowering blood pressure, experimental and clinical evidence suggests that the progression of atheroma can also be modified by this class of drugs. Thus, in the INTACT study (Lichtlein *et al.* 1990) although nifedipine did not affect the progression of established coronary stenoses, it did significantly reduce the number of new lesions appearing during a two year follow-up period. Similarly, isradipine has been shown to be an effective antihypertensive agent that also has beneficial effects on platelet aggregation and lipids (Ding *et al.* 1992). In addition, some calcium antagonists have been shown to increase significantly arterial diameter and compliance (Ko *et al.* 1992), as well as to possess anti-mitogenic potential, thus potentially contributing to the regression of the structural changes of blood vessels seen with hypertension (Ko *et al.* 1992). Caution is necessary, however, in extrapolating these benefits in view of some of the neutral or unfavourable effects of calcium antagonists on clinical end-points in ischaemic heart disease (Wilcox *et al.* 1986; Lichtlein *et al.* 1990).

ACE inhibitors

ACE inhibitors inhibit the generation of angiotensin II and are thereby able to chronically block the renin-angiotensin system (RAS). ACE inhibitors therefore lower blood pressure by reducing the direct effect of angiotensin II on vascular tone, and by reducing its effects on the release and/or action of a variety of other vasoactive agents. In addition, ACE inhibition will block the degradation of the potent vasodilator, bradykinin. Angiotensin II has also been shown to be a growth promoting hormone and ACE inhibitors have been postulated, and in some experimental models proven, to decrease vascular smooth muscle cell proliferation (Dzau 1987). Some of the effects of AII, and therefore some of the consequences of ACE inhibition, may depend on local tissue generation of AII at non-renal sites which may contribute, for example, to LVH independently of any hypertensive effect (Dunn *et al.* 1984). The ability of non-hypotensive doses of ACE inhibitors to regress LVH in some species may be an indication of these actions (Linz and Scholkens 1992). Recent studies in the human heart, however, have shown a rather low level of ACE activity, but high activity for a human heart chymase which is only minimally inhibited by ACE inhibitors (Husain *et al.* 1992).

Current trends in the development of RAS inhibition include approaches aimed at inhibition of RAS at the renin level (Haber and Hui 1990) and at the angiotensin II receptor level (Timmermans *et al.* 1990). The former is of special interest following evidence that while renin is synthesized locally in the vasculature, this may not be the case for the converting enzyme.

α-Adrenoceptors

Centrally acting α_2-adrenoceptor agonists like clonidine and rilminidine depress sympathetic activity to the periphery thus decreasing peripheral resistance. Currently, studies on selective imidazoline receptor agonists are being pursued as alternative centrally acting sympathodepressants. The vasodilating properties of α_1-adrenoceptor antagonists are also of some use in the treatment of hypertension.

Endothelial hormones

Endothelial dysfunction is a major feature of the vasculature in both hypertension and a number of related conditions such as atherosclerosis and diabetes. The abnormalities so far identified suggest a number of therapeutic avenues, although none are yet at the stage of routine clinical use. Substantial information suggests a relative deficiency of EDRF and possible strategies to overcome this include the use of precursor compounds, such as L-arginine, to promote its synthesis and release. NO has been used, by inhalation, in the treatment of pulmonary hypertension with some success reported. The development of selective anatagonists to endothelin, either at the level of synthesis or effect, would also be expected to open up new therapeutic possibilities.

REFERENCES

Aalkjaer, C., Heagerty, A. M., Peterson, K., Swales, J. D., and Mulvany, M. J. (1987). Evidence for increased media thickness, increased neuronal amine uptake, and depressed excitation-contraction coupling in isolated resistance vessels from essential hypertensives. *Circ. Res.*, **61**, 181-6.

Adams, M. A., Bobik, A., and Korner, P. I. (1989). Differential development of vascular and cardiac hypertrophy in genetic hypertension. Relation to sympathetic function. *Hypertension*, **14**, 191-202.

Adragna, N. C., Canessa, M. L., Solomon, H., Slater, E., and Tosteson, D. C. (1982). Red cell lithium-sodium counter transport and sodium-potassium co-transport in patients with essential hypertension. *Hypertension*, **4**, 795-804.

Ambrozy, S. L., Shehin, S. E., Chiou, C. Y., Sowers, J. R., and Zemel, M. B. (1991). Effects of dietary calcium on blood pressure, vascular reactivity and vascular smooth muscle calcium efflux in Zucker rats. *Am. J. Hypertens.*, **47**, 592-6.

Angus, J. A., Jennings, G. L., and Sudhir, K. (1992). Enhanced contraction to noradrenaline, serotonin and nerve stimulation but normal endothelium-derived relaxing factor response in skin small arteries in human primary hypertension. *Clin. Exp. Pharmacol. Physiol.*, **19**, 39-47.

Arkwright, P. D., Beilin, L. J., Rouse, I., Armstrong, B. K., and Vandongen, R. (1982). Effects of alcohol use and other aspects of life-style on blood pressure levels and prevalence of hypertension in a working population. *Circulation*, **66**, 60-6.

Beilin, L. J. (1989). Diet, alcohol and hypertension. *Clin. Exp. Hyper.-Theory and Practice*, **A11 (5&6)**, 991-1010.

Beilin, L. J., Hoffman, P., Nilsson, H., Skarphedinsson, J., and Folkow, B. (1992). Effect of chronic ethanol consumption upon cardiovascular reactivity, heart rate and blood pressure in spontaneously hypertensive and Wistar-Kyoto rats. *J. Hypertens.*, **10**, 645-50.

Berner, P. F., Somlyo, A. V., and Somlyo, A. P. (1981). Hypertrophy induced increase of intermediate filaments in vascular smooth muscle. *J. Cell Biol.*, **88**, 96-101.

Bing, R. F., Heagerty, A. M., and Swales, J. D. (1987). Membrane handling of calcium in essential hypertension. *J. Hypertens.*, **5**, S29-35.

Bondjers, G., Glukhova, M., Hanssen, G. K., Postnov, Y. V., Reidy, M. A., and Schwartz, S. M. (1991). Hypertension and Atherosclerosis. Cause and Effect, or two effects with one unknown cause? *Circulation*, **84**, VI 2-16.

Chau, N. P., Simon, A., Vilar, J., Cabrera-Fischer, E., Pithois-Merli, I., and Levenson, J. (1992). Active and passive effects of antihypertensive drugs on large artery diameter and elasticity in human essential hypertension. *J. Cardiovasc. Pharmacol.*, **19**, 78-85.

Chin, J. P. F., Gust, A. P., Nestel, P. J., and Dart, A. M. (1993). Marine oils dose-dependently inhibit vasoconstriction of forearm resistance vessels in humans. *Hypertension*, **21**, 22-8.

Correia, J. F. (1992). Antihypertensive treatment and regression of atherosclerosis. *Rev. Port. Cardiol.*, **11**, 623-30.

Cruickshank, J. M., Lewis, J., Moore, V., and Dodd, C. (1992). Reversibility of left ventricular hypertrophy by differing types of antihypertensive therapy. *J. Hum. Hypertens.*, **6**, 85-90.

Dart, A. M., Chin, J. P. F., and Esler, M. D. (1993) Effects of dietary supplementation with n-3 polyunsaturated fatty acids on sympathetic and haemodynamic responses to stress in man. *Nutr. Metab. Cardiovasc. Dis.*, **3**, 105–111.

De Cesaris, R., Ranieri, G., Filitti, V., and Andriani, A. (1992). Large artery compliance in essential hypertension. Effects of calcium antagonism and beta-blocking. *Am. J. Hypertens.*, **5**, 624–8.

Ding, Y. A., Han, C. L., Chou, T. C., Lai, W. Y., and Shiao, M. F. (1992). Effects of the calcium antagonist isradipine on 24-hour ambulatory blood pressure, platelet aggregation and neutrophil oxygen free radicals in hypertension. *J. Cardiovasc. Pharmacol.*, **19**, S32–7.

Dunn, F. G., Oigman, W., Ventura, H. O., Messuli, F. H., Kobrin, I., and Frohlich, E. D. (1984). Enalapril improves systemic and renal hemodynamics and allows regression of left ventricular mass in essential hypertension. *Am. J. Cardiol.*, **53**, 105–8.

Dzau, V. J. (1987). Vascular angiotensin pathways: a new therapeutic target. *J. Cardiovasc. Pharmacol.*, **10**, 9–16.

Folkow, B. (1990). 'Structural Factor' in primary and secondary hypertension. *Hypertension*, **16**, 89–101.

Frochlich, E. D., Schnaper, H. W., Wilson, I. M., and Freis, E. (1960). Hemodynamic alterations in hypertensive patients due to chlorothiazide. *N. Engl. J. Med.*, **262**, 1261–3.

Fuller, J. H. (1985). Epidemiology of hypertension associated with diabetes mellitus. *Hypertension*, **2**, 113–17.

Gray, S. D. (1982). Anatomical and physiological aspects of cardiovacular function in Wistar-Kyoto and spontaneously hypertensive rats at birth. *Clin. Sci.*, **63**, 383s–5.

Griendly, K. K. and Alexander, R. W. (1990). Angiotensin, other pressors and the transduction of vascular smooth muscle contraction. In *Hypertension: pathophysiology, diagnosis and management* (ed. J. H. Laragh and B. M. Brenner), pp. 583–600. Raven Press Ltd, New York.

Haber, E. and Hui, K. Y. (1990). Specific renin inhibitors. The concept and the prospects. In *Hypertension: pathophysiology, diagnosis and management* (ed. J. H. Laragh and B. M. Brenner), pp. 2343–50. Raven Press Ltd, New York.

Haddy, F. J., Pammani, M. B., Swindall, B. T., Johnton, J., and Cragoe, E. J. (1985). Sodium channel blockers are vasodilators as well as natriuretic and diuretic agents. *Hypertension*, **7**, I121–6.

Husain, A., Urata, H., Kinoshita, A., and Merlin Bumpus, F. (1992). A novel angiotensin II-forming pathway in the human heart. *J. Mol. Cell Cardiol.*, **24**, S18.

Inariba, H., Kanayama, Y., Takaori, K., Negoro, N., Inoue, T., and Takeda, T. (1992). Increased Na^+/H^+ exchange activity in vascular smooth muscle cells of spontaneously hypertensive rats and possible involvement of protein kinase C. *Clin. Exp. Pharmacol. Physiol.*, **19**, 171–6.

Jones, A. W. (1982). Ionic dysfunction and hypertension. *Ad. Microcirc.*, **2**, 134–59.

Kato, H., Fukami, K., Shibasaki, F., Homma, Y., and Takenawa, T. (1992). Enhancement of phospholipase C delta 1 activity in the aortas of spontaneously hypertensive rats. *J. Biol. Chem.*, **267**, 6483–7.

Ko, Y. D., Sachinis, A., Graack, G. H., Appenheimer, M., Wieczorek, A. J., Dusing, R., et al. (1992). Inhibition of angiotensin II and platelet-derived growth factor-induced vascular smooth muscle cell proliferation by calcium entry blockers. *Clin. Invest.*, **70**, 113–17.

Kurahashi, K., Akimoto, Y., Usui, H., and Jino, H. (1992). Nifedipine-resistant $Ca(++)$-induced contraction in tail artery of spontaneously hypertensive rats. *Life Sci.*, **51**, 695–702.

Lash, J. M. and Bohlen, H. G. (1992). Functional adaptations of rat skeletal muscle arterioles to aerobic exercise training. *J. Appl. Physiol.*, **72**, 2052-62.

Lechi, A., Lechi, C., Bonadonna, G., Sinigaglia, D., Corradini, P., Polignano, R., *et al.* (1987). Increased basal and thrombin-induced free calcium in platelets of essential hypertensive patients. *Hypertension*, **9**, 230-5.

Lever, A. F. and Harrap, S. B. (1992). Essential hypertension: a disorder of growth with origins in childhood? *J. Hypertens.*, **10**, 101-20.

Lever, A. F., Lyall, F., Morton, J. J., and Folkow, B. (1992). Angiotensin II, vascular structure and blood pressure. *Kidney Int.*, **37**, S51-5.

Levy, D., Garrison, R. J., Savage, D. D., Kannel, W. B., and Castelli, W. P. (1980). Prognostic implications of echocardiographically determined left ventricular mass in the Framingham study. *N. Engl. J. Med.*, **332**, 1561-6.

Levy, J., Zemel, M. B., and Sowers, J. R. (1989). Role of cellular calcium metabolism in abnormalities in glucose metabolism and diabetic hypertension. *Am. J. Med.*, **87**, 7-16.

Lichtlein, P. R., Hugenholtz, P. G., Rafflenbeul, W., Hecker, H., Jost, S., and Deckers, J. W. (1990). Retardation of angiographic progression of coronary artery disease by nifedipine. Results of the International Nifedipine Trial on Antiatherosclerotic Therapy (INTACT). *Lancet*, **335**, 1109-13.

Lindsay, D. C., Jiang, C., Brunotte, F., Adamopoulos, S., Coats, A. J., Rajagopalan, B., *et al.* (1992). Impairment of endothelium dependent responses in a rat model of chronic heart failure: effects of an exercise training protocol. *Cardiovasc. Res.*, **26**, 694-7.

Linz, W. and Scholkens, B. A. (1992). The role of bradykinin for the cardiac actions of angiotensin converting enzyme inhibitors. *J. Mol. Cell Cardiol.*, **24**, S19.

Lorenzi, M., Cagliero, E., and Toledo, S. (1985). Glucose toxicity for human endothelial cells in culture: delayed replication, disturbed cell cycle and accelerated death. *Diabetes*, **34**, 621-7.

Loutzenhiser, R. and Epstein, M. (1985). Effects of calcium antagonists on renal haemodynamics. *Am. J. Physiol.*, **249**, F619-29.

Luscher, T. F., Diederich, D., Buhler, F. R., and Vanhoutte, P. M. (1990). Interactions between platelets and the vessel wall. Role of endothelium-derived vasoactive substances. In *Hypertension: pathophysiology, diagnosis and management* (ed. J. H. Laragh and B. M. Brenner), pp. 637-48. Raven Press Ltd, New York.

Lytton, J., Lin, J. C., and Guidotti, G. (1985). Identification of two molecular forms of (Na^+,K^+)-ATPase in rat adipocytes: Relation to insulin stimulation of the enzyme. *J. Biol. Chem.*, **249**, C166-71.

MacMahon, S. W., Blacket, R. B., MacDonald, G. J., and Hall, W. (1984). Obesity, alcohol consumption and blood pressure in Australian men and women. The National Heart Foundation of Australia Risk Factor Prevalence Study. *J. Hypertens.*, **2**, 85-91.

Man in't Veld, A. J., and van der Meirecker, A. H. (1990). Effects of antihypertensive drugs on cardiovascular haemodynamics. In *Hypertension: pathophysiology, diagnosis and management* (ed. J. H. Laragh and B. M. Brenner), pp. 2117-31. Raven Press Ltd, New York.

Meldrum, M. J. and Glenton, P. (1992). ^{3}H-norepinephrine release in caudal artery of spontaneously hypertensive and Wistar-Kyoto rats: effects of altered salt diets. *Pharmacology*, **44**, 19-25.

Mulvany, M. J. (1992). The development and regression of vascular hypertrophy. *J. Cardiovasc. Pharmacol.*, **19**, S22-7.

Nakazono, K., Watanabe, N., Matsuno, K., Sasaki, J., Sato, T., and Inoue, M. (1991). Does superoxide underlie the pathogenesis of hypertension? *Proc. Natl. Acad. Sci. USA*, **88**, 10045-8.

Naruse, M., Kawana, M., Hifuni, S., Naruse, K., Yoshihara, I., Oka, T., *et al.* (1991). Plasma immunoreactive endothelin, but not thrombomodulin, is increased in patients with essential hypertension and ischaemic heart disease. *J. Cardiovasc. Pharmacol.*, **17**, S471-4.

Nelson, L., Jennings, G. L., Esler, M. D., and Korner, P. I. (1986). Effect of changing levels of physical activity on blood pressure and haemodynamics in essential hypertension. *Lancet*, **i**, 473-6.

Ng, L. L., Davies, J. E., and Ameen, M. (1992). Intracellular free-magnesium levels in vascular smooth muscle and striated muscle cells of the spontaneously hypertensive rat. *Metabolism*, **41**, 772-7.

Oltman, C. L., Paker, J. L., Adams, H. R., and Laughlin, M. H. (1992). Effects of exercise training on vasomotor reactivity of porcine coronary arteries. *Am. J. Physiol.*, **263**, H372-82.

Osanai, T. and Dunn, M. J. (1992). Phospholipase C responses in cells from spontaneously hypertensive rats. *Hypertension*, **19**, 446-55.

Panza, J. A., Quyyumi, A. A., Brush, J. E., and Epstein, S. E. (1990). Abnormal endothelium-dependent vascular relaxation in patients with essential hypertension. *N. Engl. J. Med.*, **323**, 22-7.

Puska, P., Iacono, J. M., Nissinen, A., Korbonen, H. J., Vortionen, E., Pietinen, P., *et al.* (1983). Controlled randomized trial of the effect of dietary fat on blood pressure. *Lancet*, **i**, 1-5.

Randall, O. S. (1982). Effect of arterial compliance on systolic blood pressure and cardiac function. *Clin. Exp. Hypertens.*, **4**, 1045-57.

Roy, S., Sala, R., Cagliero, E., and Lorenzi, M. (1990). Overexpression of fibronectin induced by diabetes or high glucose: Phenomenon with a memory. *Proc. Natl. Acad. Sci. USA*, **87**, 404-8.

Safar, M. W., Asmar, R. G., Benetos, A., London, G. M., and Levy, B. I. (1992). Sodium, large arteries and diuretic compounds in hypertension. *J. Hypertens.*, **10**, 133-6.

Schulte, W., Ruddel, H., Schmieder, R., Schachinger, H., Brautigam, M., and Weizel, D. (1992). Pharmacological modulation of stress-induced hyperreactivity in essential hypertension. *J. Cardiovasc. Pharmacol.*, **19**, S70-3.

Simon, G. (1990). Increased vascular wall sodium in hypertension, where is it, how does it get there and what does it do there? *Clin. Sci.*, **78**, 533-40.

Soloviev, A. I., and Bershtein, S. A. (1992). The contractile apparatus in vascular smooth muscle cells of spontaneously hypertensive rats possess increased calcium sensitivity: the possible role of protein kinase C. *J. Hypertens.*, **10**, 131-6.

Swales, J. D. (1991). Is there a cellular abnormality in hypertension? *J. Cardiovasc. Pharmacol.*, **18**, S39-44.

Takahashi, K., Ghatei, M. A., Lam, H.-C., O'Halloran, D. J., and Bloom, S. R. (1990). Elevated plasma endothelin in patients with diabetes mellitus. *Diabetologia*, **33**, 306-10.

The BHAT research group. (1983). A randomized trial of propranolol in patients with acute myocardial infarction. *JAMA*, **250**, 2814-19.

Timmermans, P. B. M. W. M., Carini, D. J., Chiu, A. T., Duncia, J. V., Price, W. A., Wells, G. J., *et al.* (1990). The discovery and physiological effects of a new class of highly specific angiotensin II receptor antagonists. In *Hypertension: pathophysiology, diagnosis and management* (ed. J. H. Laragh and B. M. Brenner), pp. 2351-60. Raven Press Ltd, New York.

Van Bortel, L. M., Hoeks, A. P., Kool, M. J., and Struijker-Boudier, H. A. (1992). Introduction to large artery properties as a target for risk reduction by antihypertensive therapy. *J. Hypertens.*, **10**, S123-6.

Van de Voorde. J., and Leusen, I. (1986). Endothelium dependent and independent relaxation of aortic rings from hypertensive rats. *Am. J. Physiol.*, **250**, H711-17.

Vlassara, H., Brownlee, M., Manaque, K., Pasagian. A., and Cerami, A. (1988). Cachetin/TNF and IL-2 synthesis and secretion are induced by glucose-modified protein binding to a high affinity macrophage receptor. *Science*, **240**, 1546-8.

Weidman, P. and Ferrari, P. (1991). Central role of sodium in hypertension in diabetic subjects. *Diabetes Care*, **14**, 220-32.

Weidman, P., Beretta-Piccoli, C., and Trost, B. N. (1985). Pressor factors and responsiveness in hypertension accompanying diabetes mellitus. *Hypertension*, **7**, 33-42.

Wilcox, R. G., Hampton, J. R., Banks, D. C., Birkhead, J. S., Brooksby, I. A. B., Burns-Cox, C. J., *et al.* (1986). Trial of early nifedipine in acute myocardial infarction: the Trent study. *Br. Med. J.*, **293**, 1204-8.

Yamakawa, H., Suzuki, H., Nakamura, M., Ohno, Y., and Saruta, T. (1992). Disturbed calcium metabolism in offspring of hypertensive parents. *Hypertension*, **19**, 528-34.

Zhang, A., Cheng, T. P., and Altura, B. M. (1992). Ethanol decreases cytosolic-free calcium ions in vascular smooth muscle cells as assessed by digital image analysis. *Alcohol Clin. Exp. Res.*, **16**, 55-7.

19. Pulmonary hypertension

George Cremona and Tim Higenbottam

INTRODUCTION

Over the last 50 years information has been steadily accumulating demonstrating the astonishingly complex systems for active regulation of blood flow in the lung and refuting the earlier notions regarding the pulmonary circulation simply as a passive conduit for the flow of blood to and from the alveoli. The emerging evidence of the endocrine and paracrine role of the endothelium has had a major impact on the understanding of local mechanisms of vascular control in the systemic circulation where the importance of the regulation of vascular tone has long been recognized. The aim of this chapter is to outline the unique characteristics of the pulmonary circulation and to present some of the information regarding the role of the endothelium in regulating pulmonary vascular tone and how this is altered in pulmonary hypertensive states.

ANATOMY OF THE NORMAL PULMONARY CIRCULATION

Considerable differences exist between the structure of systemic and pulmonary arteries which reflect the different function of the two circulations. The systemic circulation has to distribute blood flow through numerous organs separated by considerable vertical distances, thus necessitating a high blood pressure gradient. The resistance vessels are themselves under powerful active control mechanisms both local and central to maintain the necessary pressure. The pulmonary circulation, although having to accommodate the whole cardiac output, has to distribute flow over a much smaller hydrostatic distance.

The pulmonary arteries form a rapidly branching structure with daughter branches occurring generally at the distal end of parent vessels although an artery may have a number of side branches often coming off at right angles to the parent branch. The main pulmonary artery exhibits some degree of tapering up to the point of bifurcation. Using a system devised by Strahler for measuring river networks, Singhal *et al.* (1973) estimated 17 orders in the human pulmonary arterial and only 15 orders in the venous tree as the four lobar veins drain directly into the left atrium. Except for the primary branches of the pulmonary trunk, the pulmonary arterial tree rapidly increases in cross-section with an area coefficient of 1.15–1.3 (Singhal *et al.* 1973; Horsefield 1978) which is comparable to the systemic circulation. The largest pulmonary arteries, however, differ from the systemic vessels in having an elliptical cross-section which may affect the pressure–flow relationships considerably (Milnor 1989). Although most of the pulmonary arteries follow the branching pattern of the airways, some vessels near the hilum simply penetrate the lung parenchyma immediately after branching.

The pulmonary arteries from the main trunk down to a diameter of a millimetre or less have the structure of typical conducting arteries with a media consisting predominantly of elastic fibrils with a small quantity of smooth muscle fibres. These have been defined as *elastic* pulmonary arteries. In the systemic circulation, the transition from elastic to muscular arteries occurs in large vessels of the calibre of the common iliac artery whereas pulmonary arteries retain an elastic structure. In contrast, pulmonary arteries retain a predominantly elastic structure down to vessels of around 1 mm in diameter. Moreover, pulmonary arteries have internal and external laminae which are both well developed and a less distinct muscular media than that found in systemic arteries. The muscular arteries accompanying the terminal bronchioles have four to six layers of obliquely arranged smooth muscle. At the level of the respiratory bronchioles, this layer is abruptly reduced and in the more distal branches the arteries are only partially muscular or non-muscular (Meynick and Reid 1983). This is the region most significantly affected in pulmonary hypertension.

There is however considerable variation in the structure of pulmonary vessels not only between species (Kay 1983) but also within species (Heath and Williams 1981). In mammals such as sheep, cow, pig, and mouse, pulmonary veins follow the branching pattern of the bronchi and arteries, unlike in man where these vessels follow an independent course to the hilum. In some domestic and laboratory mammals, muscular pulmonary arteries extend to vessels of less than 100 μm in diameter. Whereas this is a normal finding in animals such as pig, cow, horse, and sheep, in man this pattern is found in the earliest stages of pulmonary hypertension. Indeed in native residents of high altitude, muscular pulmonary arterioles extend to more distal branches and there is an absolute increase in the amount of arterial muscle in the terminal portions of the pulmonary arterial tree (Heath and Williams 1981). The same phenomenon is seen in other mammalian species living at high altitude with the notable exception of the llama (Heath *et al.* 1974) which was found to have thin walled pulmonary arteries although the main pulmonary artery is more muscular.

Measurements of the elasticity of post-mortem human pulmonary vessels showed large arteries to be more compliant than small ones until about a diameter of approximately 500 μm when compliance increases markedly at capillary level (Yen and Sobin 1988; Yen *et al.* 1990). Small veins are significantly more compliant than large veins. This pattern is similar to that observed in the cat (Yen *et al.* 1980) in spite of differences in the extension of muscular pulmonary arteries.

PHYSIOLOGY OF THE NORMAL PULMONARY VASCULATURE

In order to perform its main function of gas exchange efficiently, the air-blood interface formed by the alveolar and pulmonary capillary walls must be thin. Perfusion of the capillaries must therefore be regulated to avoid excessive fluid leakage into the air-blood interface and interfere with oxygenation. The varying requirements of oxygen uptake from rest to exercise or environmental perturbations demands that this interface be expansible. Pulmonary capillary perfusion must be matched to regional ventilation as overperfusion of underventilated units impairs gas exchange and wastes respiratory effort. The main function of the pulmonary circulation is therefore to accommodate the entire right ventricular output while maintaining low constant pulmonary and capillary pressures. This adaptation is reasonably well preserved in the face of a cardiac output that can increase 20-fold.

The relationship between pressure and flow in the pulmonary circulation is generally linear in physiological ranges of flow although at low flow rates a curvilinear relationship with a concavity towards the flow axis is often seen. This is due to the distensibility of the pulmonary vascular bed and/or the opening of new capillaries (recruitment). The latter process may occur passively through increasing hydrostatic pressure in more dependent parts of the lung, or may be caused by vessels in a state of active tension requiring different critical closing pressures. The interplay of distensibility, collapsible capillaries, hydrostatic gradients, and vascular tone make it difficult to establish whether a given stimulus or drug has caused an active vasomotor change in the lung. Ideally it is better to measure pressure-flow relationships over a wide range, a procedure that is almost impossible in live humans. Changes in vascular resistance assessed from changes in the ratio of pressure to flow when both are changing can often be very misleading and results should be interpreted with caution.

Hypoxic pulmonary vasoconstriction

The pulmonary circulation is unique in exhibiting a vasoconstrictor response to hypoxic conditions. This phenomenon has been explained teleologically as a negative feedback mechanism for matching ventilation and perfusion and although different species show varying degrees of response (Peake *et al.* 1981), the effect is universal. Acute hypoxic vasoconstriction (HPV) seems to be mediated locally as it has been demonstrated in isolated lungs (Duke and Killick 1952) and in lung transplant recipients (Robin *et al.* 1987). Since its first description almost 50 years ago (Von Euler and Liljestrand 1946), efforts have been made to explain the sensor and effector mechanisms which however still elude identification. Alveolar hypoxia rather than mixed venous oxygen saturation seems to be the more important stimulus (Lloyd 1964; Hauge 1969) and the site of action seems to be in small but extra-alveolar vessels (Quebbeman and Dawson 1977), that is in vessels that are not affected by changes in alveolar pressure but enlarge during lung inflation.

The structure of the pulmonary vessels, while giving some idea of resistance and elastance of the vascular bed of the species, does not predict its physiological and pharmacological responses. There is little correlation between thickness and extension of muscular pulmonary arteries and their grade of acute hypoxic vasoconstriction. For example while pig and sheep pulmonary arteries both have well developed muscular arteries, pigs have a much more marked hypoxic response. Rats and ferrets although possessing relatively thin walled vessels differ greatly in the degree of response to acute hypoxia.

Recent work focusing on a direct effect of hypoxia on pulmonary vascular smooth muscle has implicated potassium channels (Robertson *et al.* 1989; Post *et al.* 1992) as a possible effector mechanism. These studies suggest that hypoxia may inhibit potassium channels producing membrane depolarization leading to an increased entry of calcium ions through voltage-dependent calcium channels. One of the exciting implications of the ion channel mechanism is that a protein may regulate the response to hypoxia. This would provide a direct link between the mechanism and the generic differences observed in HPV.

Vasomotor regulation

The pulmonary vascular bed seems to be well adapted to perform its function of gas exchange with very little evidence of active regulation under normal conditions. Through the peculiar vasoconstrictor response to hypoxia, oxygen regulates its own uptake by adjusting local perfusion to match local ventilation. However the pulmonary circulation is endowed with a rich neural and humoral regulatory mechanisms whose physiological significance remains to be fully ascertained.

Initial tone

Vasomotor tone is low in the normal lung and has been suggested to be mediated at least in part by active mechanisms (Weir 1978). The responsiveness of the pulmonary vasculature is determined to a great extent by the initial tone of the preparation. Attempts to vasodilate the normal pulmonary circulation result in very limited responses unless the initial tone is elevated artificially. Artificial experimental conditions have also been shown to alter responsiveness — perfusion with physiological saline has been shown to blunt the response to vasoconstrictors. More vigorous responses can generally be achieved by the addition of red blood cells (McMurtry *et al.* 1977) or endogenous vasoconstrictors such as angiotensin II (McMurtry 1984).

Another important element in establishing initial tone and therefore vascular responsiveness is the presence of biologically vasoactive substances that reach the lung from elsewhere in the body. Not only can these substances act directly on the vascular smooth muscle of the pulmonary vessels but a number of vasoactive substances are cleared in the lung itself. Others are converted to a vasoactive agents by the lung.

METHODS OF STUDY OF THE VASOACTIVE SUBSTANCES ON THE PULMONARY CIRCULATION

Isolated pulmonary vessels

Successful preparations for the study of isolated pulmonary vessels include the main pulmonary artery of the rabbit with an intact sympathetic nerve supply (Bevan 1993). A segment of this artery may be used either as a ring or spirally cut to a narrow strip and mounted in a tissue bath. The main pulmonary artery is a typical elastic artery and certainly not representative of intraparenchymal pulmonary arteries. By careful dissection it has been possible to isolate more distal arteries and veins from the first to the fourth generation of branches and study them with the same technique (Joiner et al. 1973). More recently, arteries with diameters less than 1 mm and therefore of muscular type have been studied on specially designed myographs (Madden et al. 1985).

Intact lungs

Changes in tension from a small ring suspended in a bath are not always representative of physiological conditions and for this reason various preparations have been set-up to study the effects of drugs on intact lungs. These have the advantage of allowing a more direct measurement of pulmonary vascular resistance. However, the number of variables which may affect the response is increased and interpretation of data is not devoid of difficulty. This is especially the case when the test drug acts also on cardiac function or even extravascular sites, e.g. 5-HT causes bronchoconstriction and collapses pulmonary capillaries altering haemodynamics (Robard and Kira 1972). Systemic and neural effects may be avoided by studying isolated lung preparations perfused at constant flow although care must be taken on the type of perfusate employed (see above).

In summary therefore, experimental conditions must take into account a wide range of passive and active effects that could affect the response to a vasoactive stimulus. It is also essential to distinguish between the animal species studied and the types of preparation used.

NEURAL CONTROL OF THE PULMONARY CIRCULATION

The pulmonary vascular bed is richly supplied with motor nerve fibres of various types. Evidence has been provided showing that in some species at least, sympathetic fibres are predominantly vasoconstrictor but with some vasodilator effects (Ingram et al. 1968; Kadowitz et al. 1974) whereas parasympathetic cholinergic fibres are vasodilator (Kadowitz et al. 1964; Downing and Lee 1980; McMahon et al. 1992). Stimulation of the stellate ganglion increases pulmonary vascular resistance which is prevented by an α-adrenergic blocking agent (Hakim and Dawson 1979). This suggests that sympathetic innervation when activated acts in a similar way as in the systemic circulation but does not give evidence of the contribution to vasomotor tone *in vivo*. Likewise stimulation of discrete areas of the brain such as the medulla (Hyman *et al.* 1991) modulates pulmonary vascular resistance, but the physiological significance of this mechanism is still uncertain.

THE ENDOTHELIUM AND VASOACTIVE FUNCTION IN THE NORMAL PULMONARY CIRCULATION

The discovery of the endocrine role of the endothelium has generated a great interest in its potential regulatory role on the vascular tone of the pulmonary vascular bed and how this may be altered in pathologic conditions. Besides providing a physical barrier, the endothelium actively catabolizes vasoactive compounds as well as synthesizing and releasing numerous vasoactive and growth regulator substances.

Clearance of vasoactive substances by the pulmonary endothelium

The role of the lung in metabolizing vasoactive substances was identified almost 50 years ago (Rapport *et al.* 1948) when 5-HT was shown to be removed from serum perfused through a heart–lung preparation. The pulmonary endothelium, particularly at the level of pulmonary arterioles and capillaries, has been identified by autoradiographic and histochemical techniques as the site of uptake of substances such as 5-HT and noradrenaline (Strum and Junod 1972; Iwasawa and Gillis 1974; Gillis and Pitt 1982; Dawson *et al.* 1985). Specific active uptake mechanisms which are sodium-dependent and ouabain-sensitive are responsible and inactivation of these two amines is carried out by the monoamine oxidase and catechol-*O*-methyltransferase systems. The estimated degree of removal of 5-HT is up to 98% (Said 1983) and for noradrenaline up to 50% (Catravas and Gillis 1983). Histamine is also metabolized in the lung to some extent (Krell *et al.* 1978). Pulmonary endothelial cells contain a membrane bound enzyme, kininase II, which activates angiotensin I and metabolizes over half of the bradykinin present (Suzuki *et al.* 1984) in the blood. The presence of the enzymes 5′-nucleotidase and ATPase on the endothelial cell surface accounts for the clearance of ATP, ADP and AMP in the pulmonary circulation (Ryan 1990).

Prostanoids

A number of metabolites of arachidonic acid both through the cyclo-oxygenase and the lipoxygenase pathways have potent effects on the pulmonary circulation. Of the cyclo-oxygenase products $PGF_{2\alpha}$, PGE_2, thromboxanes, and endoperoxides are vasoconstrictors while prostacyclin (PGI_2) and PGE_1 are vasodilators. Leukotrienes produced via the lipoxygenase pathway have a vasoconstrictor action. The pulmonary endothelium can produce relatively large quantities of

PGI$_2$ (Gryglewski et al. 1978), thromboxane (Engineer et al. 1978), and leukotrienes (Morganroth et al. 1984), as well as clear a large part of the circulating arachidonic acid metabolites (Flower 1977) in a single pass. This complex system of synthesis and breakdown of potent vasoactive substances could theoretically provide a system of dynamic equilibrium involved in the maintenance of normal vascular tone. Both enzyme pathways have been implicated as mediators of HPV (Brigham 1987) but each has been proved to act as modulator than a unique mediator. Inhibition of the cyclo-oxygenase pathway by indomethacin or meclofenamate increase the pulmonary response to hypoxia and other vasoconstrictors suggesting a normalizing function of the metabolites of the cyclo-oxygenase pathway. This is probably due to the inhibition of PGI$_2$ (Weir et al. 1976) rather than the production of a vasoconstrictor. Hypoxia has also been shown to cause the degranulation of ovine mast cells presumably releasing leukotrienes and causing vasoconstriction (Martin et al. 1978). However the production of leukotrienes by various cell types and the lack of specificity of the inhibitors has weakened the evidence in favour of leukotrienes as mediators of HPV (Garrett et al. 1987; Lonigro et al. 1988). Also, not all the data is equivocal as in some species exogenous administration of arachidonic acid causes vasodilatation (Feddersen et al. 1990) while in others it causes vasoconstriction (Hyman et al. 1980).

EDRF/NO

Much of the initial research on EDRF/NO involved studies of systemic blood vessels, however more recently the role of stimulated as well as basal release of EDRF/NO has been investigated in a number of species in different experimental conditions.

Pharmacological stimulation of EDRF/NO in the pulmonary circulation

Endothelium-dependent relaxation has been demonstrated in conduit pulmonary arteries from isolated vessels in animals (Chand and Altura 1981) and man (Greenberg et al. 1987; Dinh-Xuan et al. 1990b) (Fig. 19.1). Similar results have been shown in isolated lung preparations (Cherry and Gillia 1987; Hyman and Kadowitz 1989) as well as in vivo (Fritts et al. 1958). As the vasorelaxant effects of acetylcholine are partly inhibited by pre-treatment with inhibitors of the release or action of EDRF/NO (Hyman et al. 1989; McMahon et al. 1991; Tseng and Mitzner 1992), it is likely that EDRF/NO also contributes at least in part to the endothelium-dependent relaxation of the pulmonary vascular bed. Other agonists of EDRF/NO have also been demonstrated to cause relaxation of preconstricted conduit pulmonary arteries (Table 19.1) as well as from more distal muscular arteries (Leach et al. 1992).

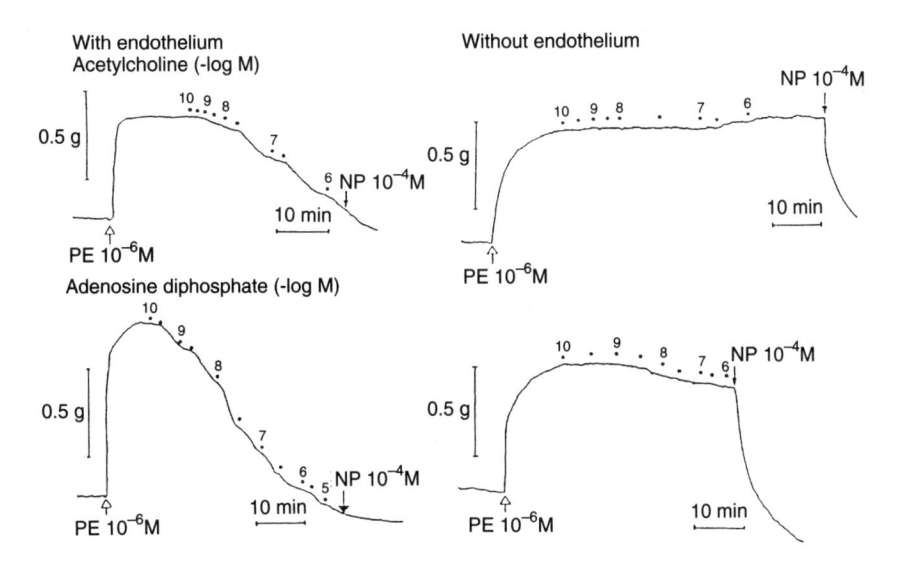

Fig. 19.1 Typical response of human pulmonary artery rings with (left curves) and without endothelium to acetylcholine and adenosine diphosphate. The rings are pre-contracted with phenylephrine (PE) 1 μM. Sodium nitroprusside (NP; 100 μM) added at the end of the experiment shows endothelium-independent relaxation. (Reproduced with kind permission from Dinh-Xuan et al. 1990b.)

Table 19.1 Pharmacological agents causing endothelium-dependent relaxation in pulmonary arteries

Agonist	Reference
Acetylcholine	Chand and Altura 1981a
Substance P	Bolton and Clapp 1986; Adnot et al. 1991
ADP, ATP	Christie et al. 1989; Dinh-Xuan et al. 1990b
Arachidonic acid	Chand and Altura 1981b
Leukotrienes	Sakuma et al. 1987
Histamine	Chen and Suzuki 1989
Thrombin	Christie et al. 1989
Bradykinin	Chand and Altura 1981a,b

Basal release of EDRF/NO

There is evidence in the systemic circulation, e.g. mesenteric (Randall and Hiley 1988), renal (Bhardwaj and Moore 1988), and hind limb (Forstermann et al. 1987; Gardiner et al. 1990a), as well as in human forearm (Vallance et al. 1989), that EDRF is continuously released and actively regulating basal vascular tone (Griffith et al. 1987a). The local action of EDRF/NO due to its rapid inactivation by haemoglobin (Rimar and Gillis 1993) would make it an ideal candidate for the active determinant of low basal pulmonary vascular tone.

Recent studies of immunohistochemical and cytochemical localization of nitric oxide synthase have evidenced the constitutive enzyme in the pulmonary endothelium (Sole et al. 1979). Studies of intact animals seem to support the role for basal release of EDRF/NO as a modulator of pulmonary vascular tone. Lobar infusion of methylene blue (Hyman et al. 1989) or N^G-nitro-L-arginine methyl ester (L-NAME) (McMahon et al. 1991) increased pulmonary vascular resistance in anaesthetized cats. Similar results have been observed in spontaneously breathing new-born lambs with both methylene blue (Fineman et al. 1991a) or L-NAME (Fineman et al. 1991b), and in anaesthetized but spontaneously breathing rabbits (Persson et al. 1990) with L-NAME. An increase in pulmonary vascular resistance has been reported following intravenous infusion of L-NMMA in healthy human adults (Stamler et al. 1994), and in children with congenital heart defects but normal pulmonary flow, L-NMMA decreased pulmonary blood flow velocity measured by quantitative angiography and intra-arterial Doppler catheters (Celermajer et al. 1994). However in experiments on intact animals other factors may influence the results. Simulation of pulmonary nerves may cause EDRF/NO release either directly (Liu et al. 1992) from non-adrenergic, non-cholinergic nerve endings or through the release of acetylcholine which in turn stimulates EDRF/NO secretion (McMahon et al. 1992). Inhibition of NO synthesis also induces increased release of prostacyclin (Tseng et al. 1993) and inhibits production of endothelin-1 (Boulanger and Luscher 1990; Luscher et al. 1990).

Isolated lungs and pulmonary arteries of the rat have been studied in detail but the evidence for continuous basal EDRF/NO production has been inconclusive in this species. Methylene blue (Rodman et al. 1990) and N^G-monomethyl-L-arginine (L-NMMA) (Archer et al. 1989) cause vasoconstriction of isolated rat pulmonary arteries. However, although methylene blue (Mazmanian et al. 1989) or L-NMMA (Liu et al. 1991; Barer et al. 1993) enhanced hypoxic pulmonary vasoconstriction in the isolated blood perfused rat lung, no change in baseline pulmonary vascular resistance was observed. Similarly methylene blue (Archer et al. 1990) and L-NMMA (Archer et al. 1989) failed to increase pulmonary vascular resistance in isolated rat lungs perfused with Earle's salt solution and 4% albumin. Modest increases in basal pulmonary vascular resistance (about 4%) have been reported with haemoglobin, L-canavanine, and L-NMMA (Hasunuma et al. 1991), but in the main there is little evidence of basal production of EDRF/NO in the rat isolated lung. A similar lack of increase in basal vascular tone has been observed in conscious dogs infused with N^G-nitro-L-arginine (L-NA) (Nishiwaki et al. 1992). A comparative study in isolated lungs of sheep, pig, dog, and man showed evidence of basal release of EDRF/NO in human, ovine, porcine, but not canine lungs (Cremona et al. 1994c) (Fig. 19.2). In dog lungs NO synthesis inhibitors only increased pulmonary vascular resistance when tone was increased by hypoxia and the findings were independent of the type of perfusate (blood or salt solution) used. This discrepancy may reflect an important difference between mammalian species in the regulation of basal pulmonary vascular tone. The site of action of endothelial EDRF/NO appears to be mainly in

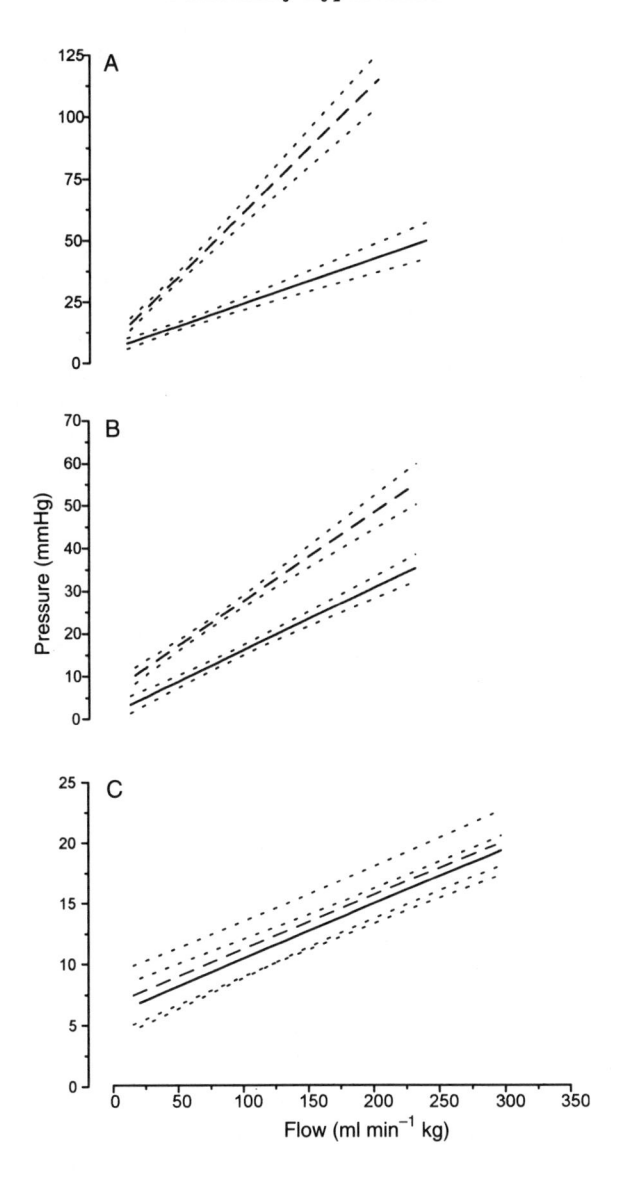

Fig. 19.2 Changes in pressure–flow relationships after L-NAME in isolated lungs perfused with Krebs–dextran solution. Mean pressure–flow lines in isolated (A) pig ($n = 6$); (B) sheep ($n = 4$); and (C) dog ($n = 3$) lungs perfused with Krebs–dextran solution before (solid line) and after (dashed line) L-NAME (10^{-5}M). Dotted lines show 95% confidence limits. (Reproduced with kind permission from Cremona *et al.* 1994c.)

the arterial segment of the pulmonary vascular bed although at a site quite distinct from hypoxia (Cremona et al. 1993; Gordon and Tod 1993).

ENDOTHELINS

This group of recently described peptides have been isolated from cultured porcine endothelial cells (Yanagisawa et al. 1988). The genes coding for three isoforms have been found to coexist on the human genome (Inoue et al. 1989) and the corresponding peptides called ET-1, ET-2, and ET-3. Although endothelin is the most potent known vasoconstrictor, intralobar administration of ET-1 to the conscious rats produces modest pulmonary vasconstriction (Raffestin et al. 1991) and even more modest pressor effects in the dog (Lippton et al. 1989). In vitro (de-Nucci et al. 1988) studies have shown that ET-1 releases thromboxane A_2 in the lung as well as PGI_2. In this study the lung was also found to metabolize 50% of ET-1 by first pass although studies in vivo have shown that the systemic vasodilator response to endothelin was not altered by first pass through the lung (Lippton et al. 1991). In this study carried out in intact rabbits, low doses of ET-1 and ET-3 caused modest vasoconstriction of the pulmonary vessels. Both peptides however caused modest contraction of isolated pulmonary conductance vessels with greater activity on venous than arterial segments. Similar results were reported in rat lungs with modest effects in vivo and more marked ones in isolated perfused preparations (Raffestin et al. 1991). In isolated rabbit lungs perfusion with a calcium-free buffer abolished the contractile response (Mann et al. 1991) and indomethacin blunted the effects of higher doses of ET-1. In the rat meclofenamate had no effect on ET-1-induced constriction which was enhanced in the presence of methylene blue or L-NMMA supporting the role of EDRF/NO attenuation of ET-1 activity. In pre-constricted cat lungs in a spontaneously breathing preparation, ET-1 caused a decrease in systemic and pulmonary vascular resistance. The vasodilator effects of ET-1 in the lung were diminished by cromakalim suggesting that ET-1 may act on potassium channels (Lippton et al. 1991). Overall it would seem that extracellular calcium entry and protein kinase C activation have an important role in mediating the vasoactive effect of ET-1 and consequently agents that block voltage-sensitive calcium channels or augment cAMP levels significantly reduce vasoconstriction (Mann et al. 1991). The effects of increases in cGMP levels are less remarkable.

PULMONARY HYPERTENSION

Pulmonary hypertension is a condition said to exist when pulmonary arterial pressure increases by 10–15 mmHg (Fishman 1985). Six potential mechanisms have been identified that may cause or contribute to the pathogenesis of pulmonary hypertension (Table 19.2). The main distinction is between those that cause a direct physical change in the pulmonary vascular bed due to structural or

Table 19.2 Potential aetiologic factors leading to pulmonary hypertension

Disease	Contributing factors
Primary pulmonary hypertension	Unknown
Eisenmenger's syndrome	Increased flow due to intracardiac shunt
Dietary pulmonary hypertension	Agents toxic to pulmonary endothelium
Chronic thromboembolic disease	Mechanical occlusion and vasoconstriction
Chronic hypoxia	Hypoxia and acidosis
Mitral stenosis	Increased post-capillary pressure
Pulmonary veno-occlusive disease	

functional causes and those which affect other determinants of pulmonary vascular resistance (such as flow and airway pressure) and contribute to exacerbate the process.

In most clinical situations, the reduction in cross-sectional area of the pulmonary vascular bed is not enough on its own to cause pulmonary hypertension. Raising pulmonary vascular resistance to pathological levels requires the removal of one lung plus a lobe of the remaining lung (Lategola 1958). Even in chronic destruction of small vessels such as occurs in emphysema, pulmonary hypertension is rarely found in the absence of chronic bronchitis. Rather it is the association of vasoconstriction and anatomical restriction to result in pulmonary hypertension.

Several experimental models have been used to produce chronic pulmonary hypertension. The most frequently used is the hypoxic one which uses normo- or hypobaric hypoxia to elicit pulmonary hypertension (Grover *et al.* 1988). This form of pulmonary hypertension actually exists in some residents of high altitudes (Heath and Williams 1981). Another model is known as dietary pulmonary hypertension which is provoked by the ingestion of leguminous plants containing the alkaloid monocrotaline (Olson *et al.* 1984). A spontaneous outbreak of dietary pulmonary hypertension occurred in Switzerland and Germany in the late 1960s as a result of the use of an appetite suppressant aminorex and more recently in Spain as a result of contaminated vegetable oil (Kilbourne *et al.* 1983). Monocrotaline does not act directly on the pulmonary circulation but is converted by the liver into a substance toxic to the pulmonary vasculature. The lesions are more similar to those seen in severe long standing mitral stenosis while those of Aminorex pulmonary hypertension are more typical of primary pulmonary hypertension.

Histopathology of pulmonary hypertension

Both primary (unexplained) and secondary pulmonary hypertension share several common histopathological features especially in the early stages of disease (Wagenvoort and Wagenvoort 1977).

The earliest change seen in pulmonary hypertension is the muscularization of the terminal portion of the pulmonary arterial tree due to hyperplasia of smooth muscle cells which extend distally in a layer internal to the original internal elastic lamina (Heath et al. 1987). The pattern of migration of smooth muscle cells from the media to the intima is different in hypoxic pulmonary hypertension and to that seen in plexogenic pulmonary hypertension (characteristic of primary pulmonary hypertension or Eisenmenger's syndrome) (Heath 1992). In the latter conditions the migration is more widespread and extends into the vascular lumen where the muscle fibres are transformed into myofibroblasts blocking up the vascular lumen. In hypoxic pulmonary hypertension there is a lack of occlusive lesions as the migration of smooth muscle fibres is more limited. However in this condition longitudinal muscle forms in the intima of pulmonary arteries and arterioles and is followed by the formation of an inner tube of circular smooth muscle. In both hypoxic and plexogenic pulmonary hypertension there is cellular intimal proliferation which may be concentric or eccentric.

The lesions evolve in a distinct manner. In hypoxic pulmonary hypertension, the intimal longitudinal muscle and inner muscular tubes become fibrosed (Wilkinson et al. 1988) whereas in plexogenic PH (Heath and Edwards 1958; Pietra et al. 1989), the invasion of myofibroblasts first form concentric rings, the so-called 'onion skin' layers. The thin walled branches of the muscular pulmonary arteries become dilated while the media of the parent vessels becomes constricted and undergoes patchy fibrinoid necrosis which liberates fibrin into the dilated branches. This stimulates a proliferation of undifferentiated cells from the media which form a plexiform pattern around the thin-walled branch. Eventually the fibrinoid necrosis becomes more widespread leading to narcotizing arteritis.

THE IMPORTANCE OF THE ENDOTHELIUM IN PULMONARY HYPERTENSION

The abundance of vasoactive substances released or metabolized by the pulmonary endothelium seems to leave little doubt on its importance in modulating vascular tone. This may be even more important in pathological conditions where structural and functional reserves may be impaired. The importance of the endothelium in disease has been underlined in a prospective morphometric analysis of open lung biopsies from 19 patients with primary pulmonary hypertension (Palevsky et al. 1989) which has shown that the degree of intimal thickening was the best predictor for survival. In this context another interesting association has been observed in the fawn-hooded rat which is affected with a hereditary disorder of platelet aggregation and which develops idiopathic pulmonary hypertension due to a genetic susceptibility but influenced by environmental conditions such as oxygen tension. The elevated levels of endothelin-1 found in these rats raises interesting questions about the role of the endothelium in the development of pulmonary hypertension (Sato et al. 1992; Stelzner et al. 1992).

FUNCTIONAL CHANGES IN THE ENDOTHELIUM IN PULMONARY HYPERTENSION

The metabolic functions of the pulmonary endothelium are affected in both experimental and clinical pulmonary hypertension. Isolated rat lungs treated with monocrotaline showed a reduced clearance of both and 5-HT and noradrenaline (Gillis *et al.* 1978). Similarly clearance of noradrenaline was reduced from 25% found in normotensive subjects to 0.02% in patients with primary or secondary pulmonary hypertension (Sole *et al.* 1979). The reduced clearance may enhance the vasoconstrictor effects of 5-HT which is released by activated platelets. Evidence for this has been suggested by the potentiation of the vasospastic response to coronary angioplasty in atherosclerotic rabbits treated with fluoxetine, an inhibitor of 5-HT clearance. A similar mechanism may also be involved in the reported cases of pulmonary hypertension in subjects using dexfenfluramine, an appetite suppressant which reduces 5-HT clearance (Buczko *et al.* 1975; Douglas *et al.* 1981; Powels *et al.* 1990).

The responses of the pulmonary vasculature to acute and chronic hypoxia have been suspected to involve related mechanisms (Fishman 1985). Evidence has been accumulating suggesting that the underlying mechanisms may well be quite dissimilar. HPV increases production of PGI_2 in canine lungs (Voelkel *et al.* 1981; Smith 1986) although this seems to be related to the increased tone rather than to hypoxia. Similarly, studies have shown that HPV is enhanced when the production (Archer *et al.* 1989; Hasunuma *et al.* 1991) or the effects (Mazmanian *et al.* 1989) of EDRF/NO are inhibited suggesting that EDRF/NO is modulating the response to hypoxia. This may also be due to the vasoconstriction rather than hypoxia *per se* as the same effect is seen when the pulmonary vascular bed is pharmacologically constricted with other agents (Barer *et al.* 1993). Taken together, these studies may just be illustrating the effects of two local systems in preserving low vascular tone.

Although these homeostatic systems may mitigate vasoconstriction in prolonged hypoxia, in the long-term they may become impaired. Evidence for this is suggested by studies carried out in models of systemic hypertension (Diederich *et al.* 1990; Dohi *et al.* 1990; Linder *et al.* 1990; Luscher *et al.* 1990). Hypoxic bovine lungs have been reported to produce less PGI_2 (Luscher *et al.* 1987; Diederich *et al.* 1990; Dohi *et al.* 1990; Linder *et al.* 1990) but cAMP-mediated relaxation was unimpaired in chronically hypoxic rats (Rodman 1992). However, chronic hypoxic rat pulmonary arteries showed an increase in PGI_2 production which was not accompanied by an increase in adenylate cyclase activity (Shaul *et al.* 1991). As stimulation of the enzyme with isoproterenol was similarly reduced, down-regulation of the receptor was postulated. Other models of pulmonary hypertension also provide contradictory results (Altiere *et al.* 1986; Rabinovitch 1987; Ito *et al.* 1988) and the role of PGl_2 in pulmonary hypertension remains unclear. Recent work in humans has evidenced an imbalance in the excretion of thromboxane and prostacyclin metabolites in patients will primary pulmonary hypertension and in patients with pulmonary hypertension secondary to hypoxia (Christman *et al.* 1992). This finding suggests that platelet activation and an abnormal pulmonary endothelial response may be present in pulmonary hypertensive states although whether this is a cause or an effect remains to be elucidated. Another role of prostaglandins may lie in the mediation of structural changes in pulmonary hypertension. Prostaglandins inhibit DNA synthesis (Huttner *et al.* 1977) and this mechanism may modulate some of the vascular changes in chronic hypoxia. Platelet-derived growth factor stimulates smooth muscle proliferation but releases both PGI_2 and PGE_2. This may be a negative feedback loop as both prostaglandins elevate cyclic AMP which inhibits DNA synthesis. Chronic infusion of indomethacin induces pulmonary hypertension in sheep but does not cause medial hypertrophy and increased muscularization of distal pulmonary arteries (Meyrick *et al.* 1985) suggesting that other factors may be involved. However, others (Rosenberg and Rabinovitch 1988) have shown that indomethacin can block the protective effects of angiotensin II on pulmonary hypertension in rats exposed to chronic hypoxia.

Endothelin levels have been reported to be elevated in patients with Eisenmenger's syndrome (Yoshibayashi *et al.* 1991) and increased production of endothelin-1 has been reported in fawn-hooded rats with idiopathic pulmonary hypertension (Stelzner *et al.* 1992). More recently, an increase in endothelin-1 immunoreactivity and endothelin-1 mRNA expression was observed in the lungs of both primary and secondary pulmonary hypertensives. The potent vasoconstricting effects of endothelin-1 as well as its mitogenic effect on smooth muscle cells make it an interesting potential mediator of the functional and morphological vascular abnormalities of pulmonary hypertension. The physiological significance of these increased levels has still to be fully determined as ET-1 vasodilates constricted pulmonary vascular beds (Hasunuma *et al.* 1990) although in chromic hypoxic rats endothelin-induced pulmonary vasodilatation is abolished (Eddahibi *et al.* 1993). The impairment of ET-1 and ET-3 induced vasodilatation in hypoxic rats is not due to alterations in receptor subtypes or to unresponsiveness of potassium channels and may be linked to other mediators such as EDRF/NO.

The changes in EDRF/NO pathway with pulmonary hypertension are equally equivocal. Early studies in humans with pulmonary hypertension secondary to mitral stenosis showed a decrease in pulmonary vascular resistance following infusion of acetylcholine (Wood *et al.* 1957). On the other hand prostacyclin and nitric oxide are both efficient vasodilators in pulmonary hypertension (Pepke-Zaba *et al.* 1991) (Fig. 19.3). Direct measurement of exhaled NO in patients with primary pulmonary hypertension was not lower than in healthy controls when corrected for diffusing capacity (Cremona *et al.* 1994*b*) suggesting that basal release of NO is sill intact. However, the study of endothelial EDRF/NO release from human lungs poses a number of problems. *In vivo* studies are compromised by the systemic effects of both L-arginine analogues (Gardiner *et al.* 1990*b*; Bower and Law 1993) and acetylcholine (Wood *et al.* 1957; Samet *et al.* 1960). Furthermore, the derivatives of L-arginine decrease coronary flow and depress cardiac output (Amezcua *et al.* 1989; Perrella *et al.* 1991). Neural stimulation of intact lungs may also cause NO release either directly from non-adrenergic non-

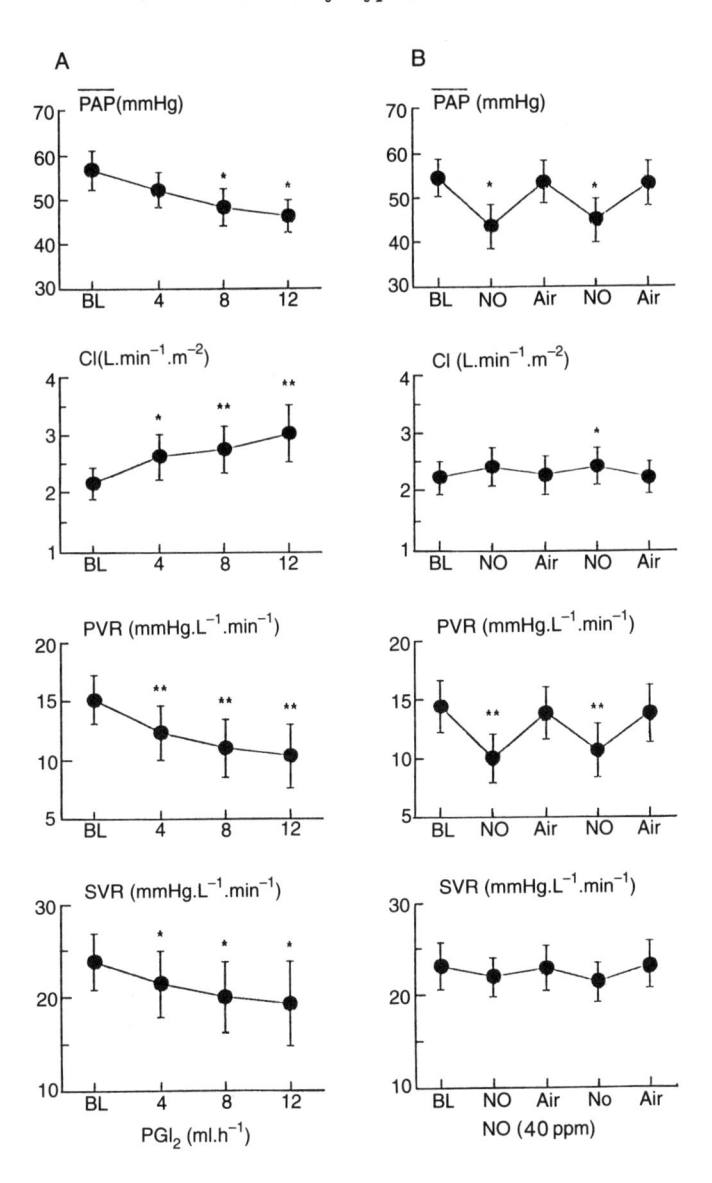

Fig. 19.3 Effect of inhaled nitric oxide (NO; 40 p.p.m.) on pulmonary (PVR) and systemic (SVR) vascular resistance in eight patients with primary pulmonary hypertension compared with infusion of prostacyclin (PGI$_2$; 4 ng/kg/min). Values are given as means ± s.e. (Reproduced with kind permission from Pepke-Zaba *et al.* 1991.)

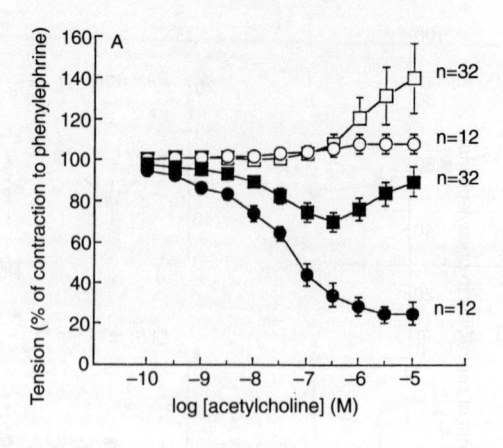

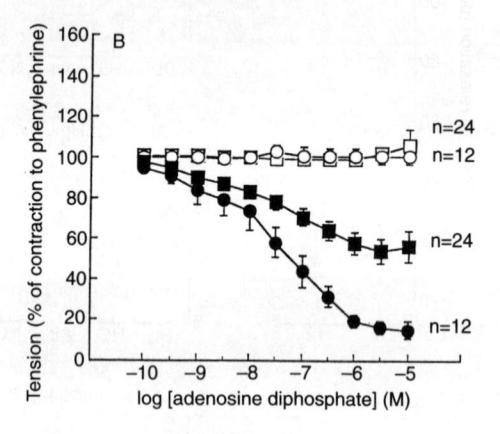

Fig. 19.4 Impaired relaxation to acetylcholine from pulmonary arteries from patients with chronic hypoxic lung disease (full squares) compared to controls (full circles). Open symbols represent the mean tension from endothelium denuded vessels. (Reproduced with kind permission from Dinh-Xuan *et al.* 1991.)

cholinergic nerve stimulation (Liu *et al.* 1992) or as a secondary consequence of the release of acetylcholine (McMahon *et al.* 1992).

Studies on isolated rings from patients undergoing heart–lung transplantation for Elsenmenger's syndrome (Dinh-Xuan *et al.* 1990*a*) or chronic obstructive lung disease (Dinh-Xuan *et al.* 1991) have reported diminished endothelium-dependent relaxation (Fig. 19.4). The degree of impairment correlated well with the amount of intimal thickening and with pre-operative levels of hypoxaemia (Fig. 19.5) and was not due to substrate deficiency as the addition of excess L-arginine did not normalize relaxation to acetylcholine or calcium ionophore A23187 (Dinh-Xuan *et al.* 1993). In isolated perfused human lungs with chronic obstructive lung disease due to cystic fibrosis or bronchiectasis basal release of EDRF/NO was intact but stimulated release of EDRF/NO with acetylcholine was impaired

Pulmonary hypertension

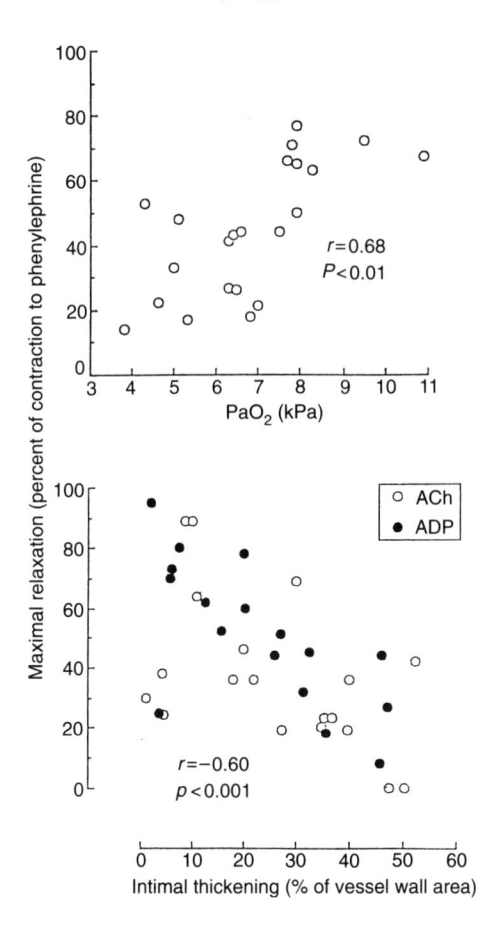

Fig. 19.5 Correlation between maximal relaxation to acetylcholine and adenosine diphosphate of pulmonary arterial rings from 22 patients with chronic obstructive disease and their prr-operative oxygen tension values. (Reproduced with kind permission from Dinh-Xuan *et al.* 1991.)

(Cremona *et al.* 1994*a,c*) (Figs 19.6 and 19.7). In both studies pulmonary vascular smooth muscle relaxed fully to sodium nitroprusside, a nitrovasodilator which acts independently of the endothelium indicating that the responsiveness of the vascular smooth muscle was still intact. The discrepancy between basal and simulated release of EDRF/NO could possibly be due to the different energy requirements of the two processes. Inhibitors of mitochondrial adenosine triphosphate (ATP) activity abolish stimulated (Griffith *et al.* 1986) but not basal (Griffith *et al.* 1987*b*) release of EDRF/NO. This may in turn be linked to the agonist-induced phosphorylation of the particulate NO synthase associated with translocation of the enzyme from membrane to cytosol (Michel *et al.* 1993).

Studies on animal models of hypoxic pulmonary hypertension have been carried out mainly in rat lungs and discordant results have been reported. In isolated

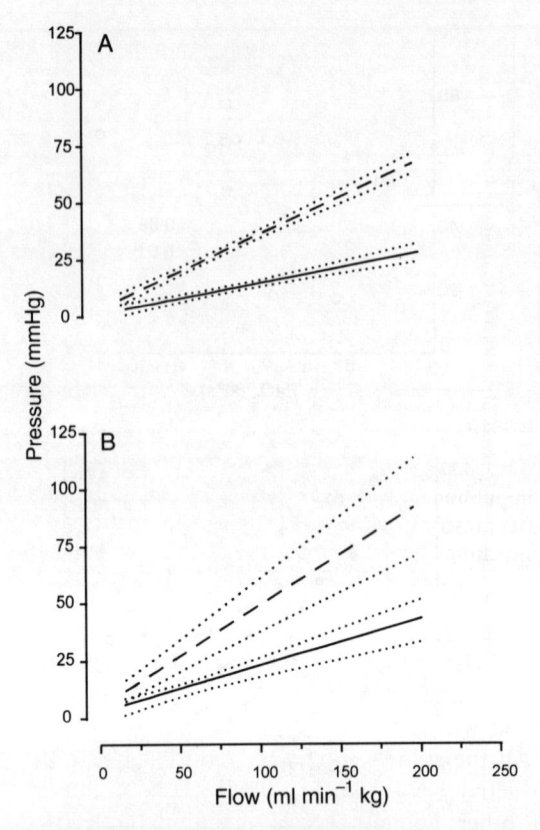

Fig. 19.6 Changes in pressure–flow relationships after L-NAME in human isolated lungs perfused with Krebs–dextran solution. Mean pressure flow lines in isolated human lungs perfused with Krebs–dextran solution before (solid line) and after (dashed line) L-NAME (10^{-5}M). (A) Lungs from cardiac donors ($n = 4$); (B) lungs from patients with cystic fibrosis ($n = 3$). Dotted lines show 95% confidence limits. (Reproduced with kind permission from Cremona et al. 1994a.)

salt perfused lungs, Russ and Walker (1993) showed that both basal and stimulated EDRF/NO activity was unchanged with chronic hypoxia, whereas other laboratories using a similar experimental set-up found evidence of enhanced EDRF/NO activity (Oka et al. 1993; Isaacson et al. 1994). In blood perfused rat lungs of a different strain, some laboratories reported a loss of EDRF/NO activity in chronic hypoxic rat lungs which was corrected by addition of L-arginine (Adnot et al. 1991; Eddahibi et al. 1992) whereas others have found evidence supporting an enhanced EDRF/NO activity with chronic hypoxia (Barer et al. 1993) which may be due to the higher levels of shear stress in the narrowed vessels of the hypertensive animals. Chronic ingestion of L-NAME did not cause pulmonary hypertension in rats (Hampl et al. 1993). The reason for the discrepancy between the different laboratories is not immediately obvious and may not be simply due to the particular strain of rat or type of perfusate used. In the same species,

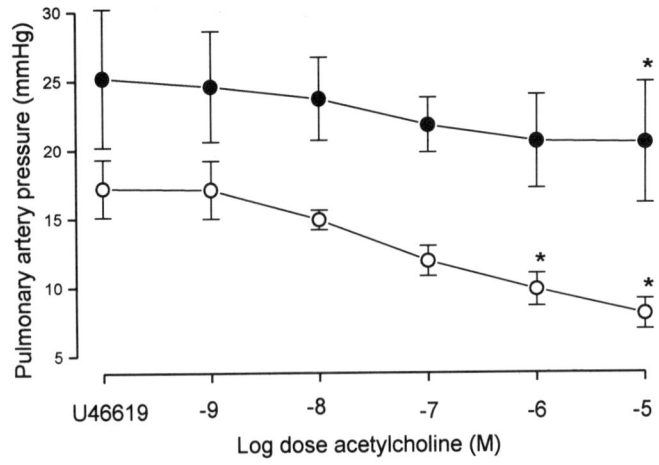

Fig. 19.7 The fall in pulmonary artery pressure in isolated human lungs perfused at constant flow is shown after pre-constriction with U46619 with cumulative doses of acetylcholine in normotensive donor lungs (○; $n = 7$) and COLD ●; $n = 6$) lungs.

hypertension due to monocrotaline treatment impaired relaxation to acetylcholine (Ito *et al.* 1988). The duration of exposure to hypoxia may be important as in rats studied at 72 h and after 4–5 weeks exposure to hypoxia, endothelium-dependent relaxation was found to be impaired only after prolonged exposure (Rodman 1992). All the studies, however, reported that in normoxic rat lungs basal EDRF/NO activity was almost absent. This is quite different from the results found in other animal species including man (Persson *et al.* 1990; McMahon *et al.* 1991; Cremona *et al.* 1994c), where basal EDRF/NO release is an important determinant of normoxic pulmonary vascular tone. This difference may limit the usefulness of the rat model in the interpretation of human disease. In hypoxic calves, Orton *et al.* (1988) found impaired relaxation to acetylcholine in isolated pulmonary artery ring studies, but an enhanced response *in vivo* and suggested that the experimental preparation should be taken into account when interpreting the results.

SUMMARY

Undoubtedly, the difference between various preparations, the aetiology and stage of pulmonary hypertension and the species studied account for a large part of the discrepancy in the results presented in this chapter. In spite of this, the overall picture that seems to emerge is that the endothelium has an important role in regulating pulmonary vascular tone and that it's homeostatic ability to modulate vascular tone is reduced in pulmonary hypertension. From the work done so far it is unlikely that any single mediator is solely responsible for the changes observed in pulmonary hypertension. The complex interactions of the vasodilator and vasoconstrictor products of the endothelium in the healthy and diseased pulmonary vascular bed need to be fully unravelled as well as the interaction between endothelium, platelets, and vascular smooth muscle in order to decipher whether endothelial dysfunction is a cause or a consequence of pulmonary hypertension.

REFERENCES

Adnot, S., Raffestin, B., Eddahibi, S., Braquet, P., and Chabrier, P. E. (1991). Loss of endothelium-dependent relaxant activity in the pulmonary circulation of rats exposed to chronic hypoxia. *J. Clin. Invest.*, **87**, 155-62.

Altiere, R. J., Olson, J. W., and Gillespie, M. N. (1986). Altered pulmonary vascular smooth muscle responsiveness in monocrotaline-induced pulmonary hypertension. *J. Pharmacol. Exp. Ther.*, **236**, 390-5.

Amezcua, J. L., Palmer, R. M., de-Souza, B. M., and Moncada, S. (1989). Nitric oxide synthesized from L-arginine regulates vascular tone in the coronary circulation of the rabbit. *Br. J. Pharmacol.*, **97**, 1119-24.

Archer, S. L., Tolins, J. P., Raij, L., and Weir, E. K. (1989). Hypoxic pulmonary vasoconstriction is enhanced by inhibition of the synthesis of an endothelium derived relaxing factor. *Biochem. Biophys. Res. Commun.*, **164**, 1198-205.

Archer, S. L., Rist, K., Nelson, D. P., DeMaster, E. G., Cowan, N., and Weir, E. K. (1990). Comparison of the hemodynamic effects of nitric oxide and endothelium-dependent vasodilators in intact lungs. *J. Appl. Physiol.*, **68**, 735-47.

Barer, G., Emery, C., Stewart, A., Bee, D., and Howard, P. (1993). Endothelial control of the pulmonary circulation in normal and chronically hypoxic rats. *J. Physiol.*, **463**, 1-16.

Bevan, J. A. (1993). Some chracteristics of the isolated sympathetic nerve-pulmonary artery preparation of the rabbit. *J. Pharmacol.*, **137**, 213-18.

Bhardwaj, R. and Moore, P. K. (1988). Increased vasodilator response to acetylcholine of renal blood vessels from diabetic rats. *J. Pharm. Pharmacol.*, **40**, 739-42.

Boulanger, C. and Luscher, T. F. (1990). Release of endothelin from the porcine aorta. Inhibition by endothelium-derived nitric oxide. *J. Clin. Invest.*, **85**, 587-90.

Bower, E. A. and Law, A. C. K. (1993). The effects of N^w-nitro-L-arginine methyl ester, sodium nitroprusside and noradrenaline on venous return in the anaesthetized cat. *Br. J. Pharmacol.*, **108**, 933-40.

Brigham, K. L. (1987). Conference summary: lipid mediators in the pulmonary circulation. *Am. Rev. Respir. Dis.*, **136**, 785-8.

Buczko, W., de Gaetano, G., and Garattini, S. (1975). Effect of fenfluramine on 5-hydroxytrptamine uptake and release by rat blood platelets. *Br. Cardiac Soc. Ann. Meet.*, **53**, 563.

Catravas, J. D. and Gillis, C. N. (1983). Single-pass removal of [^{14}C]-5-hydroxytryptamine and [^{3}H]norepinephrine by rabbit lung, *in vivo*: kinetics and sites of removal. *J. Pharmacol. Exp. Ther.*, **224**, 28-33.

Celermajer, D. S., Dollery, C., Burch, M., and Deanfield, J. E. (1994). Role of endothelium in the maintenance of low pulmonary vascular tone in normal children. *Circulation*, **89**, 2041-4.

Chand, N. and Altura, B. M. (1981). Acetylcholine and bradykinin relax intrapulmonary arteries by acting on endothelial cells: role in vascular disease. *Science*, **213**, 1376-9.

Cherry, P. D. and Gillis, C. N. (1987). Evidence for the role of endothelium-derived relaxing factor in acetylcholine-induced vasodilatation in the intact lung. *J. Pharmacol. Exp. Ther.*, **241**, 516–20.

Christman, B. W., McPherson, C. D., Newman, J. H., King, G. A., Bernard, G. R., Groves, B. M., *et al.* (1992). An imbalance between the excretion of thromboxane and prostacyclin metabolites in pulmonary hypertension. *N. Engl. J. Med.*, **327**, 70–5.

Cremona, G., Takao, M., and Higenbottam, T. W. (1993). Identification of site of action of nitric oxide in isolated pig lungs by occlusion technique. *Am. Rev. Respirat. Dis.*, **147**, A224.

Cremona, G., Bower, E. A., and Higenbottam, T. (1994*a*). Difference between basal release of nitric oxide and response to acetylcholine in isolated lungs from patients with chronic obstructive lung disease. *Thorax*, **49**, 425P–6.

Cremona, G., Higenbottam, T., Borland, C. D. R., and Mist, B. A. (1994*b*). Mixed expired nitric oxide in primary pulmonary hypertension in relation to lung diffusion capacity. *Q. J. Med.*, **87**, 547–51.

Cremona, G., Wood, A. M., Hall, L. W., Bower, E. A., and Higenbottam, T. W. (1994*c*). Effects of inhibitors of nitric oxide release and action on vascular tone in isolated lungs of pig, sheep, dog and man. *J. Physiol.*, **48**, 185–95.

Dawson, C. A., Christensen, C. W., Rickaby, D. A., Linehan, J. H., and Johnston, M. R. (1985). Lung damage and pulmonary uptake of serotonin in intact dogs. *J. Appl. Physiol.*, **58**, 1761–6.

de-Nucci, G., Thomas, R., D'Orleans-Juste, P., Antunes, E., Walder, C., Warner, T. D., *et al.* (1988). Pressor effects of circulating endothelin are limited by its removal in the pulmonary circulation and by the release of prostacyclin and endothelium-derived relaxing factor. *Proc. Natl. Acad. Sci. USA*, **85**, 9797–800.

Diederich, D., Yang, Z. H., Buhler, F. R. and Luscher, T. F. (1990). Impaired endothelium-dependent relaxations in hypertensive resistance arteries involve cyclooxygenase pathway. *Am. J. Physiol.*, **258**, H445–51.

Dinh-Xuan, A. T., Higenbottam, T. W., Clelland, C., Pepke-Zaba, J., Cremona, G., and Wallwork, J. (1990*a*). Impairment of pulmonary endothelium-dependent relaxation in patients with Eisenmenger's syndrome. *Br. J. Pharmacol.*, **99**, 9–10.

Dinh-Xuan, A. T., Higenbottam, T. W., Clelland, C., Pepke-Zaba, J., Wells, F., and Wallwork, J. (1990*b*). Acetylcholine and adenosine diphosphate cause endothelium-dependent relaxation of isolated human pulmonary arteries. *Eur. Res. J.*, **3**, 633–8.

Dinh-Xuan, A. T., Higenbottam, T. W., Clelland, C. A., Pepke-Zaba, J., Cremona, G., Butt, A. Y., *et al.* (1991). Impairement of endothelium-dependent pulmonary-artery relaxation in chronic obstructive lung disease. *N. Eng. J. Med.*, **324**, 1539–47.

Dinh-Xuan, A. T., Pepke Zaba, J., Butt, A. Y., Cremona, G., and Higenbottam, T. W. (1993). Impairment of pulmonary-artery endothelium-dependent relaxation in chronic obstructive lung disease is not due to dysfunction of endothelial cell membrane receptors nor to L-arginine deficiency. *Br. J. Pharmacol.*, **109**, 587–91.

Dohi, Y., Thiel, M. A., Buhler, F. R., and Luscher, T. F. (1990). Activation of endothelial L-arginine pathway in resistance arteries. Effect of age and hypertension. *Hypertension*, **16**, 170–9.

Douglas, J. G., Munro, J. F., Kitchen, A. H., Muir, A. L., and Proudfoot, A. T. (1981). Pulmonary hypertension and fenfluramine. *Br. Med. J.*, **283**, 881.

Downing, S. E. and Lee, J. C. (1980). Nervous control of the pulmonary circulation. *Annu. Rev. Physiol.*, **42**, 199–210.

Duke, H. N. and Killick, E. M. (1952). Pulmonary vasomotor responses of isolated perfused cat lungs to anoxia. *J. Physiol.*, **117**, 303–16.

Eddahibi, S., Adnot, S., Carville, C., Blouquit, Y., and Raffestin, B. (1992). L-Arginine restores endothelium-dependent relaxation in pulmonary circulation of chronically hypoxic rats. *Am. J. Physiol.*, **263**, L194-200.

Eddahibi, S., Springall, D., Mannan, M., Carville, C., Chabrier, P. E., Levame, M., *et al.* (1993). Dilator effect of endothelins in pulmonary circulation: changes associated with chronic hypoxia. *Am. J. Physiol.*, **265**, L571-80.

Engineer, D. M., Morris, H. R., Piper, P. J., and Sirois, P. (1978). The release of prostaglandins and thromboxanes from guinea pig lung by slow-reacting substance of anaphylaxis and its inhibition. *Br. J. Pharmacol.*, **64**, 211-18.

Feddersen, C. O., Chang, S., Czartalomna, J., and Voelkel, N. F. (1990). Arachidonic acid causes cyclooxygenase-dependent and -independent pulmonary vasodilation *J. App. Physiol.*, **68**, 1799-808.

Fineman, J. R., Crowley, M. R., Heymann, M. A., and Soifer, S. J. (1991a). In vivo attenuation of endothelium-dependent pulmonary vasodilation by methylene blue. *J. Appl. Physiol.*, **71**, 735-41.

Fineman, J. R., Heymann, M. A., and Soifer, S. J. (1991b). N^W-Nitro-L-arginine attenuates endothelium-dependent pulmonary vasodilation in lambs. *Am. J. Physiol.*, **260**, H1299-306.

Fishman, A. P. (1985). Pulmonary circulation. In *Handbook of physiology. Section 3 The respiratory system* (ed. A. P. Fishman and A. B. Fisher), pp. 93-166. American Physiological Society, Bethesda, MD.

Flower, R. J. (1977). Prostaglandin metabolism in the lung. In *Metabolic functions of the lung. Lung biology in health and disease*, (ed. Y. S. Bakhle and J. R. Vane), pp. 85-122. Dekker, New York.

Forstermann, U., Dudel, C., and Frolich, J. C. (1987). Endothelium-derived relaxing factor is likely to modulate the tone of resistance arteries in rabbit hindlimb *in vivo*. *J. Pharmacol. Exp. Ther.*, **243**, 1055-61.

Fritts, H. W., Harris, P., Claus, R. H., Odell, J. E., and Cournaud, A. (1958). The effect of acetylcholine on the human pulmonary circulation under normal and hypoxic conditions. *J. Clin. Invest.*, **379**, 99-110.

Gardiner, S. M., Compton, A. M., Bennett, T., Palmer, R. M., and Moncada, S. (1990a). Control of regional blood flow by endothelium-derived nitric oxide. *Hypertension*, **15**, 486-92.

Gardiner, S. M., Compton, A. M., Kemp, P. A., and Bennett, T. (1990b). Regional and cardiac haemodynamic effects of N^G-nitro-L-arginine methyl ester in conscious, Long Evans rats. *Br. J. Pharmacol.*, **101**, 625-31.

Garrett, R. C., Foster, S., and Thomas, H. M. (1987). Lipoxygenase and cyclooxygenase blockade by BW 755C enhances pulmonary hypoxic. *J. Appl. Physiol.*, **62**, 129-33.

Gillis, C. N. and Pitt, B. R. (1982). The fate of circulating amines within the pulmonary circulation. *Ann. Rev. Physiol.*, **44**, 269-83.

Gillis, C. N., Huxtable, R. J., and Roth, R. A. (1978). Effects of monocrotaline pretreatment of rats on removal of 5-hydroxytryptamine and noradrenaline by perfused lungs. *Br. J. Pharmacol.*, **63**, 435-43.

Gordon, J. B. and Tod, M. L. (1993). Effects of N^W-nitro-L-arginine on total and segmental vascular resistances in developing lamb lungs. *J. Appl. Physiol.*, **75**, 76-85.

Greenberg, B., Rhoden, K., and Barnes, P. J. (1987). Endothelium-dependent relaxation of human pulmonary arteries. *Am. J. Physiol.*, **252**, H434-8.

Griffith, T. M., Edwards, D. H., Newby, A. C., Lewis, M. J., and Henderson, A. H. (1986). Production of endothelium-derived relaxing factor is dependent on oxidative phosphorylation and extracellular calcium. *Cardiovasc. Res.*, **20**, 7-12.

Griffith, T. M., Edwards, D. H., Davies, R. L., Harrison, T. J., and Evans, K. T. (1987a). EDRF coordinates the behaviour of vascular resistance vessels. *Nature*, **329**, 442–5.

Griffith, T. M., Edwards, D. H., and Henderson, A. H. (1987b). Unstimulated release of endothelium derived relaxing factor is independent of mitochondrial ATP generation. *Cardiovasc. Res.*, **21**, 565–8.

Grover, R. F., Johnson, R. L. J., McCullough, R. G., McCullough, R. E., Hofmeister, S. E., Campbell, W. B., et al. (1988). Pulmonary hypertension and pulmonary vascular reactivity in beagles at high altitude. *J. App. Physiol.*, **65**, 2632–40.

Gryglewski, R. J., Korbut, R., and Ocetkiewicz, A. (1978). Generation of prostacyclin by the lungs *in vivo* and its release into the arterial circulation. *Nature*, **273**, 765–7.

Hakim, T. S. and Dawson, C. A. (1979). Sympathetic nerve stimulation and vascular resistance in a pump-perfused dog lung lobe. *Proc. Soc. Exp. Biol. Med.*, **160**, 38–41.

Hampl, V., Archer, S. L., Nelson, D. P., and Weir, E. K. (1993). Chronic EDRF inhibition and hypoxia: effects on pulmonary circulation and systemic blood pressure. *J. Appl. Physiol.*, **75**, 1748–57.

Hasunuma, K., Rodman, D. M., O'Brien, R. F., and McMurtry, I. F. (1990). Endothelin 1 causes pulmonary vasodilation in rats. *Am. J. Physiol.*, **259**, H48–54.

Hasunuma, K., Yamaguchi, T., Rodman, D. M., O'Brien, R. F., and McMurtry, I. F. (1991). Effects of inhibitors of EDRF and EDHF on vasoreactivity of perfused rat lungs. *Am. J. Physiol.*, **260**, L97–104.

Hauge, A. (1969). Hypoxia and pulmonary vascular resistance. The relative effects of pulmonary arterial and alveolar PO_2. *Acta Physiol. Scand.*, **76**, 121–30.

Heath, D. (1992). Pulmonary vascular remodelling in pulmonary hypertension. *App. Cardiopulmonary Pathophysiol.*, **4**, 205–11.

Heath, D. and Edwards, J. E. (1958). The pathology of hypertensive pulmonary vascular disease. A description of six grades of structural changes in the pulmonary arteries with special reference to congenital cardiac septal defects. *Circulation*, **18**, 533–47.

Heath, D. and Williams, D. R. (1981). *Man at high altitude. The pathophysiology of acclimatization and adaptation*. Churchill Livingstone, New York.

Heath, D., Smith, P., Williams, D., Harris, P., Arias-Stella, J., and Kruger, H. (1974). The heart and pulmonary vasculature of the llama (*Lama glama*). *Thorax*, **29**, 463–71.

Heath, D., Smith, P., Gosney, J., Mulcahy, D., Fox, K., Yacoub, M., et al. (1987). The pathology of the early and late stages of primary pulmonary hypertension. *Br. Heart, J.*, **58**, 204–13.

Horsefield, K. (1978). Morphometry of the small pulmonary arteries in man. *Circ. Res.*, **42**, 593–7.

Huttner, J. J., Gwebu, E. T., Panganamala, R. V., Milo, G. E., Coprnwell, D. G., Sharma, H. M., et al. (1977). Fatty acids and their prostaglandin derivatives: inhibitors of proliferation in aortic smooth muscle cells. *Science*, **197**, 289–91.

Hyman, A. L. and Kadowitz, P. J. (1989). Influence of tone on responses to acetylcholine in the rabbit pulmonary vascular bed. *J. Appl. Physiol.*, **67**, 1388–94.

Hyman, A. L., Spannhake, E. W., and Kadowitz, P. J. (1980). Disparate actions of arachidonic acid on feline pulmonary vascular bed. *Adv. Prostaglandin Thromboxane Res.*, **7**, 765–7.

Hyman, A. L., Kadowitz, P. J., and Lippton, H. L. (1989). Methylene blue selectively inhibits pulmonary vasodilator responses in cats. *J. Appl. Physiol.*, **66**, 1513–17.

Hyman, A. L., Dempesy, C. W., Richardson, D. E., and Lippton, H. L. (1991). Neural control. In *The lung: scientific foundations* (ed. R. G. Crystal and J. B. West), pp. 1087–103. Raven Press, New York.

Ingram, R. H., Szidon, J. P., Skalak, R., and Fishman, A. P. (1968). Effects of sympathetic nerve stimulation on the pulmonary arterial tree of the isolated lobe perfused *in situ*. *Circ. Res.*, **22**, 801-15.

Inoue, A., Yanagisawa, M., Kimura, S., Kasuya, Y., Miyauchi, T., Goto, K., *et al.* (1989). The human endothelin family: three structurally and pharmacologically distinct isopeptides predicted by three separate genes. *Proc. Natl. Acad. Sci. USA*, **86**, 2863-7.

Isaacson, T. C., Hampl, V., Weir, E. K., Nelson, D. P., and Archer, S. L. (1994). Increased endothelium-derived NO in hypertensive pulmonary circulation of chronically hypoxic rats. *J. Appl. Physiol.*, **76**, 933-40.

Ito, K., Nakashima, T., Murakami, K., and Murakami, T. (1988). Altered function of pulmonary endothelium following monocrotaline-induced lung vascular injury in rats. *Br. J. Pharmacol.*, **94**, 1175-83.

Iwasawa, Y. and Gillis, C. N. (1974). Pharmacological analysis of norepinephrine and 5-hydroxytryptamine removal from the pulmonary circulation: differentiation of uptake sites for each amine. *J. Pharmacol. Exp. Ther.*, **189**, 386-95.

Joiner, P. D., Davis, L. B., Kadowitz, P. J., and Hyman, A. L. (1973). Effects of prostaglandins on canine isolated pulmonary lobar small arteries and veins. *Pharmacologist*, **15**, 208.

Kadowitz, P. J., Nandiwada, P. A., and Hyman, A. L. (1964). Parasympathetic neurohumoral control of pulmonary vascular bed. *Circulation*, **64**, IV-180.

Kadowitz, P. J., Joiner, P. D., and Hyman, A. L. (1974). Effects of sympathetic nerve stimulation on pulmonary vascular resistance in the intact spontaneously breathing dog. *Proc. Soc. Exp. Biol. Med.*, **147**, 68-71.

Kay, J. M. (1983). Comparative morphologic features of the pulmonary vasculature mammals. *Am. Rev. Respirat. Dis.*, **128**, S53-7.

Kilbourne, E. M., Rigau-Perez, J. G., Heath, C. W. J., Zack, M. M., Falk, H., Martin-Marcos, M., *et al.* (1983). Clinical epidemiology of toxic-oil syndrome. Manifestations of a new illness. *N. Engl. J. Med.*, **309**, 1408-14.

Krell, R. D., McCoy, J., and Christian, P. (1978). Accumulation and metabolism of ^{14}C histamine by rat lung *in vivo*. *Biochem. Pharmacol.*, **27**, 820-7.

Lategola, M. T. (1958). Pressure-flow relationships in the dog lung during acute, subtotal pulmonary vascular occlusion. *Am. J. Physiol.*, **192**, 613-19.

Leach, R. M., Twort, C. H., Cameron, I. R., and Ward, J. P. (1992). A comparison of the pharmacological and mechanical properties *in vitro* of large and small pulmonary arteries of the rat. *Clin. Sci.*, **82**, 55-62.

Linder, L., Kiowski, W., Buhler, F. R., and Luscher, T. F. (1990). Indirect evidence for release of endothelium-derived relaxing factor in human forearm circulation *in vivo*. Blunted response in essential hypertension. *Circulation*, **81**, 1762-7.

Lippton, H. L., Pellett, A., Cairo, J., Summer, W. R., Lowe, R. F., Sander, G. E., *et al.* (1989). Endothelin produces systemic vasodilatation independent of the state of consciousness. *Peptides*, **10**, 939-43.

Lippton, H. L., Ohlstein, E. H., Summer, W. R., and Hyman, A. L. (1991). Analysis of responses to endothelins in the rabbit pulmonary and systemic vascular beds. *J. Appl. Physiol.*, **70**, 331-41.

Liu, S. F., Crawley, D. E., Barnes, P. J., and Evans, T. W. (1991). Endothelium-derived relaxing factor inhibits hypoxic pulmonary vasoconstriction in rats. *Am. Rev. Respirat. Dis.*, **143**, 32-7.

Liu, S. F., Crawley, D. E., Evans, T. W., and Barnes, P. J. (1992). Endothelium-dependent nonadrenergic, noncholinergic neural relaxation in guinea pig pulmonary artery. *J. Pharmacol. Exp. Ther.*, **260**, 541-8.

Lloyd, T. C. (1964). Effect of alveolar hypoxia on pulmonary vascular resistance. *J. Appl. Physiol.*, **19**, 1086–94.

Lonigro, A. J., Sprague, R. S., Stephenson, A. H., and Dahms, T. E. (1988). Relationship of leukotriene C4 and D4 to hypoxic pulmonary vasoconstriction in dogs. *J. Appl. Physiol.*, **64**, 2538–43.

Luscher, T. F., Raij, L., and Vanhoutte, P. M. (1987). Endothelium-dependent vascular responses in normotensive and hypertensive Dahl rats. *Hypertension*, **9**, 157–63.

Luscher, T. F., Yang, Z., Tschudi, M., von-Segesser, L., Stulz, P., Boulanger, C., et al. (1990). Interaction between endothelin-1 and endothelium-derived relaxing factor in human arteries and veins. *Circ. Res.*, **66**, 1088–94.

McMahon, T. J., Hood, J. S., Bellan, J. A., and Kadowitz, P. J. (1991). N^W-Nitro-L-arginine methyl ester selectively inhibits pulmonary vasodilator responses to acetylcholine and bradykinin. *J. Appl. Physiol.*, **71**, 2026–31.

McMahon, T. J., Hood, J. S., and Kadowitz, P. J. (1992). Pulmonary vasodilator response to vagal stimulation is blocked by N^W-nitro-L-arginine methyl ester in the cat. *Circ. Res.*, **70**, 364–9.

McMurtry, I. F. (1984). Angiotensin is not required for hypoxic constriction in salt solution-perfused rat lungs. *J. Appl. Physiol.*, **56**, 375–80.

McMurtry, I. F., Hookaway, B., and Roos, S. (1977). Red blood cells play a crucial role in maintaining vascular reactivity to hypoxia in isolated rat lungs. *Chest*, **71 (suppl)**, 253–6.

Madden, J. A., Dawson, C. A., and Harder, D. R. (1985). Hypoxia-induced activation in small isolated pulmonary arteries from the cat. *J. Appl. Physiol.*, **59**, 113–18.

Mann, J., Farrukh, I. S., and Michael, J. R. (1991). Mechanisms by which endothelin 1 induces pulmonary vasoconstriction in the rabbit. *J. Appl. Physiol.*, **71**, 410–16.

Martin, L. F., Tucker, A., Munroe, M. L., and Reeves, J. T. (1978). Lung mast cells and hypoxic pulmonary vasoconstriction in cats. *Respiration*, **35**, 73–7.

Mazmanian, G., Baudet, B., Brink, C., Cerrina, J., Kirkiacharian, S., and Weiss, M. (1989). Methylene blue potentiates vascular reactivity in isolated rat lungs. *J. Appl. Physiol.*, **66**, 1040–5.

Meyrick, B. and Reid, L. (1983). Pulmonary hypertension. Anatomic and physiologic correlates. *Clin. Chest Med.*, **4**, 199–217.

Meyrick, B., Niedermeyer, M. E., Ogletree, M. L., and Brigham, K. L. (1985). Pulmonary hypertension and increased vasoreactivity caused by repeated indomethacin in sheep. *J. Appl. Physiol.*, **59**, 443–52.

Michel, T., Li, G. K., and Busconi, L. (1993). Phosphorylation and subcellular translocation of endothelial nitric oxide synthase. *Proc. Natl. Acad. Sci. USA*, **90**, 6252–6.

Milnor, W. R. (1989). Steady flow. In *Hemodynamics*, pp. 47–50. Williams and Wilkin, Baltimore.

Morganroth, M. L., Stenmark, K. R., Zirrolli, J. A., Mauldin, R., Mathias, M., Reeves, J. T. et al. (1984). Leukotriene C4 production during hypoxic pulmonary vasoconstriction in isolated rat lungs. *Prostaglandins*, **28**, 867–75.

Nishiwaki, K., Nyhan, D. P., Rock, P., Desai, P. M., Peterson, W. P., Pribble, C. G., et al. (1992). N^w-Nitro-L-arginine and pulmonary vascular pressure–flow relationship in conscious dogs. *Am. J. Physiol.*, **262**, H1331–7.

Oka, M., Hasunuma, K., Webb, S. A., Stelzner, T. J., Rodman, D. M., and McMurtry, I. F. (1993). EDRF suppresses an unidentified vasoconstrictor mechanism in hypertensive rat lungs. *Am. J. Physiol.*, **264**, L587–97.

Olson, J. W., Hacker, A. D., Altiere, R. J., and Gillespie, M. N. (1984). Polyamines and the development of monocrotaline-induced pulmonary hypertension. *Am. J. Physiol.*, **247**, H682–5.

Orton, E. C., Reeves, J. T., and Stenmark, K. R. (1988). Pulmonary vasodilation with structurally altered pulmonary vessels and pulmonary hypertension. *J. Appl. Physiol.*, **65**, 2459–67.

Palevsky, H. I., Schloo, B. L., Pietra, G. G., Weber, K. T., Janicki, J. S., Rubin, E., *et al.* (1989). Primary pulmonary hypertension. Vascular structure, morphometry and responsiveness to vasodilator agents. *Circulation*, **80**, 1207–21.

Peake, M. D., Harabin, A. L., Brennan, N. J., and Sylvester, J. T. (1981). Steady-state vascular responses to graded hypoxia in isolated lungs of five species. *J. Appl. Physiol.*, **51**, 1214–19.

Pepke-Zaba, J., Higenbottam, T. W., Dinh-Xuan, A. T., Stone, D., and Wallwork, J. (1991). Inhaled nitric oxide as a cause of selective pulmonary vasodilatation in pulmonary hypertension. *Lancet*, **338**, 1173–4.

Perrella, M. A., Hildebrand, F. L., Margulies, K. B., and Burnett, J. C. (1991). Endothelium-derived relaxing factor in regulation of basal cardiopulmonary and renal function. *Am. J. Physiol.*, **261**, R323–8.

Persson, M. G., Gustafsson, L. E., Wiklund, N. P., Moncada, S., and Hedqvist, P. (1990). Endogenous nitric oxide as a probable modulator of pulmonary circulation and hypoxic pressor response *in vivo*. *Acta Physiol. Scand.*, **140**, 449–57.

Pietra, G. G., Edwards, W. D., Kay, J. M., Rich, S., Kernis, J., Schloo, B., *et al.* (1989). Histopathology of primary pulmonary hypertension: a qualitative and quantitative study of pulmonary blood vessels from 58 patients in the National Heart, Lung and Blood Institute, Primary Pulmonary Hypertension Registry. *Circulation*, **80**, 1198–206.

Post, J. M., Hume, J. R., Archer, S. L., and Weir, E. K. (1992). Direct role for potassium channel inhibition in hypoxic pulmonary vasoconstriction. *Am. J. Physiol.*, **262**, C882–90.

Powels, H. M. M., Smeets, J. L. R. M., Cheriex, E. C., and Wouters, E. F. M. (1990). Pulmonary hypertension and fenfluramine. *Eur. Respirat. J.*, **3**, 606.

Quebbeman, E. J. and Dawson, C. A. (1977). Effect of lung inflation and hypoxia on pulmonary arterial blood volume. *J. Appl. Physiol.*, **43**, 8–13.

Rabinovitch, M. (1987). Prostaglandins and structural changes in pulmonary arteries. *Am. Rev. Respirat. Dis.*, **136**, 777–9.

Raffestin, B., Adnot, S., Eddahibi, S., Macquin-Mavier, I., Braquet, P., and Chabrier, P. E. (1991). Pulmonary vascular response to endothelin in rats. *J. Appl. Physiol.*, **70**, 567–74.

Randall, M. D. and Hiley, C. R. (1988). Detergent and methylene blue affect endothelium-dependent vasorelaxation and pressure/flow relations in rat blood perfused mesenteric arterial bed. *Br. J. Pharmacol.*, **95**, 1081–8.

Rapport, M. M., Greene, A. A., and Page, I. H. (1948). Serum vasoconstrictor (serotonin). *J. Biol. Chem.*, **176**, 1243–60.

Rimar, S. and Gillis, C. N. (1993). Selective pulmonary vasodilation by inhaled nitric oxide is due to hemoglobin inactivation. *Circulation*, **88**, 2884–7.

Robard, S. and Kira, S. (1972). Lobar, airway and pulmonary vascular effects of serotonin. *Angiology*, **23**, 188–97.

Robertson, B. E., Paterson, D. J., Peers, C., and Nye, P. C. (1989). Tolbutamide reverses hypoxic pulmonary vasoconstriction in isolated rat lungs. *Q. J. Exp. Physiol.*, **74**, 959–62.

Robin, E. D., Theodore, J., Burke, C. M., Oesterle, S. N., Fowler, M. B., Jamieson, S. W., *et al.* (1987). Hypoxic pulmonary vasoconstriction persists in the human transplanted lung. *Clin. Sci.*, **72**, 283–7.

Rodman, D. M. (1992). Chronic hypoxia selectively augments rat pulmonary artery Ca^{2+} and K^+ channel-mediated relaxation. *Am. J. Physiol.*, **263**, L88–94.

Rodman, D. M., Yamaguchi, T., Hasunuma, K., O'Brien, R. F., and McMurtry, I. F. (1990). Effects of hypoxia on endothelium-dependent relaxation of rat pulmonary artery. *Am. J. Physiol.*, **258**, L207-14.

Rosenberg, H. C. and Rabinovitch, M. (1988). Endothelial injury and vascular reactivity in monocrotaline pulmonary hypertension. *Am. J. Physiol.*, **255**, H1484-91.

Russ, R. D. and Walker, B. R. (1993). Maintained endothelium-dependent pulmonary vasodilation following chronic hypoxia in the rat. *J. Appl. Physiol.*, **74**, 339-44.

Ryan, U. S. (1990). Endothelial processing of biologically active materials. In *The pulmonary circulation* (ed. A. P. Fishman), pp. 69-83. University of Pennyslvania Press, Philadelphia.

Said, S. I. (1983). Vasoactive peptides. State-of-the-art review. *Hypertension*, **5**, 117-26.

Samet, P., Bernstein, W. H., and Widrich, J. (1960). Intracardiac infusion of acetylcholine in primary pulmonary hypertension. *Am. Heart J.*, **60**, 433-9.

Sato, K., Webb, S., Tucker, A., Rabinovitch, M., O'Brien, R. F., McMurtry, I. F., *et al.* (1992). Factors influencing the idiopathic development of pulmonary hypertension in the fawn-hooded rat. *Am. Rev. Respirat. Dis.*, **145**, 793-7.

Shaul, P. W., Kinane, B., Farrar, M. A., Buja, L. M., and Megness, R. R. (1991). Prostacyclin production and mediation of adenylate cyclase activity in the pulmonary artery. Alterations after prolonged hypoxia in the rat. *J. Clin. Invest.*, **88**, 447-55.

Singhal, S., Henderson, R., Horsefield, K., Harding, K., and Cumming, G. (1973). Morphometry of the human pulmonary arterial tree. *Circ. Res.*, **33**, 190-7.

Smith, W. L. (1986). Prostaglandin biosynthesis and its compartmentation in vascular smooth muscle and endothelial cells. *Annu. Rev. Physiol.*, **48**, 251-62.

Sole, M. J., Drobac, M., Schwartz, L., Hussain, M. N., and Vaughan-Nell, E. F. (1979). The extraction of circulating catecholamines by the lungs in normal man and in patients with pulmonary hypertension. *Circulation*, **60**, 166-3.

Stamler, J. S., Loh, E., Roddy, M., Currie, K. E., and Creager, M. A. (1994). Nitric oxide regulates basal systemic and pulmonary vascular resistance in healthy humans. *Circulation*, **89**, 2035-40.

Stelzner, T. J., O'Brien, R. F., Yaganisawa, M., Sakurai, T., Sato, K., Webb, S., *et al.* (1992). Increased lung endothelin-1 production in rats with idiopathic pulmonary hypertension. *Am. J. Physiol.*, **262**, L614.

Strum, J. M. and Junod, A. F. (1972). Radioautographic demonstration of 5-hydroxy tryptamine-H^3 uptake by pulmonary endothelial cells. *J. Cell Biol.*, **54**, 456-62.

Suzuki, M., Ohyama, Y., and Satoh, S. (1984). Conversion of angiotensin I to angiotensin II and inactivation of bradykinin in canine peripheral vascular beds. *J. Cardiovasc. Pharmacol.*, **6**, 244-50.

Tseng, C. M. and Mitzner, W. (1992). Antogonists of EDRF attenuate acetylcholine induced vasodilation in isolated hamster lungs. *J. Appl. Physiol.*, **72**, 2162-7.

Tseng, C. M., Goodman, L. W., Rubin, L. J., and Tod, M. L. (1993). N^G-Monomethyl-L-arginine paradoxically relaxes preconstricted canine intrapulmonary arteries. *J. Appl. Physiol.*, **74**, 549-58.

Vallance, P., Collier, J., and Moncada, S. (1989). Effects of endothelium-derived nitric oxide on peripheral arteriolar tone in man. *Lancet*, **2**, 997-1000.

Voelkel, N. F., Gerber, J. G., McMurtry, I. F., Nies, A. S., and Reeves, J. T. (1981). Release of vasodilator prostaglandin PGI$_2$ from isolated rat lung during vasoconstriction. *Circ. Res.*, **48**, 207-13.

Von Euler, U. and Liljestrand, G. (1946). Observations on the pulmonary arterial blood pressure in the cat. *Acta Physiol. Scand.*, **12**, 301-20.

Wagenvoort, C. A. and Wagenvoort, N. (1977). *Pathology of pulmonary hypertension*. Wiley, New York.

Weir, E. K. (1978). Does normoxic pulmonary vasodilatation rather than hypoxic vasoconstriction account for the pulmonary pressor response to hypoxia? *Lancet*, **i**, 476-7.

Weir, E. K., McMurtry, I., Tucker, A., Reeves, J., and Grover, R. F. (1976). Prostaglandin synthetase inhibitors do not decrease hypoxic pulmonary vasoconstriction. *J. Appl. Physiol.*, **41**, 714-18.

Wilkinson, M., Langhorne, C. A., Heath, D., Barer, G. R., and Howard, P. (1988). A pathophysiological study of 10 cases of hypoxic cor pulmonale. *Q. J. Med.*, **66**, 65-85.

Wood, P., Besterman, E. M., Towers, M. K., and McIlroy, M. B. (1957). The effect of acetylcholine on pulmonary vascular resistance and left atrial pressure in mitral stenosis. *Br. Heart J.*, **19**, 279-86.

Yanagisawa, M., Kurihara, H., Kimura, S., Tomobe, Y., Kobayashi, M., Mitsui, H., *et al.* (1988). A novel potent vasoconstrictor peptide produced by vascular endothelial cells. *Nature*, **332**, 911-17.

Yen, R. T. and Sobin, S. S. (1988). Elasticity of arterioles and venules in postmortem human lungs. *J. Appl. Physiol.*, **64**, 611-19.

Yen, R. T., Fung, Y. C., and Bingham, N. (1980). Elasticity of small pulmonary arteries in the cat. *J. Biomech. Eng.*, **102**, 170-7.

Yen, R. T., Tai, D., Rong, Z., and Zhang, B. (1990). Elasticity of pulmonary blood vessels in human lungs. In *Respiratory biomechanics: engineering analysis of structure and function* (ed. L. Farrell Epstein and J. R. Ligas), pp. 109-16. Springer-Verlag, New York.

Yoshibayashi, M., Nishioka, K., Nakao, K., Salto, Y., Matsumura, M., Ueda, T., *et al.* (1991). Plasma endothelin concentrations in patients with pulmonary hypertension associated with congenital heart defects. Evidence for increased production of endothelin in pulmonary circulation. *Circulation*, **84**, 2280-5.

Index

ACE inhibitors 396
acetylcholine 291-9
  in atherosclerosis 333
acute myocardial ischaemia 331-2
adenosine 317
adenosine triphosphate (ATP)
  and α-antagonist resistant e.j.p. 188, 197-8
  and cotransmission 210-18
adenylyl cyclase 174
ADH, see vasopressin
adrenoceptor agonists 284
β-adrenoceptor antagonists 395
adrenoceptors 123-4, 193-4, 301-2
α-adrenoceptors 311, 396
β-adrenoceptors 312
affinity 6-7
agonist affinities 18
agonist effect 6-9
  direct methods to determine 6-7
  graphical methods to determine 6-7
agonist efficacies 18
agonist modulation 150-4
agonist potency 105
agonist relative potencies 18
agonists 1-5, 18-20, 149
agonist-stimulated phosphatidylcholine hydrolysis 164-5
agonist-stimulated phosphoinositide hydrolysis 160-2
alcohol intake 393-4
amino acids 318
anaesthesia 75
angiotensin 125, 314-15, 396
antagonist effects 8-9
  direct model-fitting methods and 9
  graphical methods and 8
antagonisist-receptor interactions 1-5
α-antagonist resistant e.j.p. 197-8
antagonists 3, 14
antidiuretic hormone, see vasopressin
antihypertensive therapy 393-7
applanation tonometry 99
L-arginine analogues 241-4
arterial compliance 99
arterial neuroeffector transmission 184-209
arteriolar neuroeffector transmission 184-209
  large 26-8
  small 26-8
  see also under large coronary arteries and also small coronary arteries; see also specific forms
arterioles 28-9
atherosclerosis 328-56, 391-2
  therapy of 350-1
atherosclerotic damage 329-31
ATP-sensitive K^+ channels 141, 143-4
atrial natriuretic peptide (factor) 118, 316
autonomic blockade 84-6
average radius (vascular bed) 76-80

bacteria, and sepsis 369-86
bacterial toxins 114
baroreceptor reflex 86-8
binding, drug 1-2
blood-brain barrier 255, 358-63
  functions of 358
  in ischaemia 361-3
  regulation of 359-61
blood flow 75
blood flow measurements 96
blood pressure 75
blood vessel diameter measurement 92
blood vessel geometry 9
blood vessels 76-80
  neuromuscular junctions 193
  in vitro studies of 25
  viable smooth muscle cells from 43
bolus injection 72
bradykinin 315-16

caged compounds 58-61
  properties of 59-61
  in vascular smooth muscle studies 61-2
calcitonin gene-related peptide 219-20
calcium-activated K^+ channels 139-40, 142
calcium antagonists 395-6
calcium ion channels 120-2, 145-8
  sympathetic nerves and 200-1
calcium ion concentrations, intracellular 54-8
calcium ions 162-3
calcium sensitive K^+ channels 141, 145
cannulated vessels 34-5
5-carboxamidotryptamine 88-91
carotid artery diameter, in conscious dog 82-4
cell signalling pathways 160-83
cerebral circulation 255-75
cerebral ischaemia 357-68

cerebral microvascular endothelium 357–68
cerebrovascular gabaergic systems 257–9
chemical composition, of receptor 106
cholera toxin 114
cholesterol 342
cholinergic receptors 312
collateral artery function 341–56
collateral reactivity 346–9
collateral vessels 335–6
compliance, arterial 99
conductance 34–5, 76
ω-conotoxin 87–8
constant flow perfusion method 38–9
constant pressure gradient perfusion 37
contraction regulation, and protein kinese C
  isoforms 166–8
  G proteins and 166
  sustained 167
  tyrosine phosphorylation and 169–73
    growth factor receptors 170
    MAP kinase and 170
contractions, of isolated coronary arteries
  276–305
coronary arteries 276–305
coronary risk factors 328–9
coronary vasoactivity, abnormal 328–9
coronary vasoconstriction 336–7
cotransmission 210–32
  definition of 212
  intramural nerve 222–3
  parasympathetic nerve 220–2
  sensory motor nerve 219–20
  sympathetic nerve 212–18
cumulative drug additions 13
cyclic adenosine-3,5-monophosphate (cAMP)
  175
cyclic guanosine-3,5-monophosphate (cGMP)
  175
  -dependent protein kinase 175
cyclic nucleotide phosphodiesterases
  175–6
cyclic nucleotides 173–6
cytokines 369–71, 377
  antibodies against 377
  effects of 371–3
    acute 371–2
    chronic 372–3
  kinins 375
  nitric oxide and 373, 375
  PAF 375
  prostaglandins 375
  vascoconstrictors 376–7

dead space 37–8
delayed rectifier K^+ channels 122
diabetes mellitus 391
diacylglycerol 163–4
diet 393–4

dimethoxy O-nitrophenylethylester, *see* caged
  compounds
direct model-fitting methods 7–8
  for agonists 7–8
  for antagonists 9
diuretics 394–5
dopamine 312–13
Doppler flowmetry 99
Doppler velocimetry 96–8
drug additions 13
  cumulative 13
    paired curve 13
    single curve 13
  single exposure 13
drug binding 1–2
drug delivery 72
drug disposition 10–11
drug-receptor theory 1–9
drug selectivity, *in vivo* 88–91

EDRF, *see* endothelium-dependent relaxant
  factor
efficacy 3–7
eicosanoids 318–19
  see also specific types
electrophysiology, vascular cells 47–54
  patch-clamp 50
    single-channel recording 53–4
    whole-cell recording 50–3
  voltage-clamp 47–50
endothelial cells 47
endothelial hormones 396–7
endothelial vasoactive agents 223–5
endothelins 316–17, 412–13
  see also atherosclerosis
endothelium 9–10
endothelium-dependent hyperpolarization
  (EDH) 244–8, 260–1
endothelium-dependent relaxation
  244–8
endothelium-dependent vasodilatation
  mechanisms 233–51
endothelium-derived relaxing factor (EDRF)
  234–7, 260–3, 299, 300–1, 317–18, 388,
  399
  and the lungs 408
endotoxin 371–3, 377
  acute effects of 371–2
  antibodies against 377
  chronic effects of 372–3
  nitric oxide and 373, 375
  PAF 375
  prostaglandins 375
  vasoconstrictors 376–7
equilibrium dissociation constant 14–17
extracellular metabolism 11
extrapolation technique 75
extravascular drug delivery 73

Index

Fick principle 96
flash photolysis 58-61
full agonist 3

GABA transaminase 257-9
G protein-linked receptors 106-16
G proteins 166
 classification of 113-16
 properties 113
 receptor transduction 116
 α-subunit 113-14
 βγ-subunit 115-16
 and vascular smooth-muscle contraction sensitivity 166
gradient perfusion 37
graphical methods 6-9
 for agonist effects 6-7
 for antagonist effects 8
growth factor receptors 170
guanylyl cyclase 174-5
 receptor 118-20

high-affinity antagonists 105
histamine 313
histaminergic receptors 125
homologous desensitization 106
human studies, *in vivo* 91-9
 arterial compliance 99
 blood flow 96-9
  by Doppler velocimetry 96-7
  by indicator dilution 96
  by laser Doppler flowmetry 99
  by plethysmography 98-9
  by thermodilution 96
 blood-vessel diameter 92-5
  by angiography 92
  by ultrasound 92-4
  by venous reactivity 94-5
5-hydroxytryptamine 124, 263-7, 282-3, 299-301, 313-14, 336-7, 346-9
hypertension 387-401
 abnormalities of vasculature in 387
 adrenoceptors and 395-6
 β-antagonists and 395
 antihypertensive therapy 393-7
 atherosclerosis and 391-2
 and other disease states 390-2
 drug therapy of 394-6
  with ACE inhibitors 396
  with calcium antagonists 395-6
  with diuretics 394-5
 function changes 387
 glucose metabolism 391
  and diabetes mellitus 391
 non-drug therapy 393-4
 structural changes in 390
 see also pulmonary hypertension

hypoxic pulmonary vasoconstriction 404-5

indicator dilution method 96
inositol 1,4,5-trisphosphate-induced intracellular Ca^{2+} 162-3
interleukins 370-1
intra-arterial drug administration 84-6
intra-arterial infusions 72-3
 extravascular (topical) 73
 local 72-3
intracellular Ca^{2+} concentration 54-8, 162-3
intracellular metabolism 11
intramural nerve cotransmission 222-3
intravascular ultrasound 92-3
intravenous drug delivery 72, 84
intrinsic activity 3
intrinsic efficacy 4
in vitro coronary artery studies 283-4
in vitro studies 25-41
in vivo studies 70-102
 cerebral circulation 254-5
 in man 91-9
ischaemia 357-68
isolated tissue techniques 25-41

juxtamedullary nephron 310

kidney, *see* renal circulation
kinins 375

large coronary arteries 277-90
 acetylcholine and 288
 coronary atherosclerosis and 288-90
 adrenoceptor agonists 284
 coronary atherosclerosis 285
 endothelium-dependent vasodilators and 285
 functional antagonism 285
 5-hydroxytryptamine (5HT) and 282
 induced phase activity 279
 nifedipine and 285
 reactivity of 277
 spontaneous activity of 279
 structure of 277
large diameter arteries 80-2
laser Doppler flowmetry 99
Law of Mass Action 2
leukotrienes 319
ligands, indirect action of 11-12
local infusion 72-3
L-type Ca^{2+} channels, *see* calcium ion channels
lungs, *see* pulmonary hypertension

maximum effect 5-6
membrane ion channels 136-59

methylene dioxyamphetamine 266
mitogen-activated protein (MAP) kinase 170, 172
multiple receptors 12
muscarinic receptors 125
muscle tone 103–5
myocardial ischaemia 332–5
  adrenergic mechanisms of 332–3
  cholinergic mechanisms of 333
  sympathoadrenergic mechanisms of 334–5
  see also atherosclerosis

neuroeffector transmission 184–209
neuromodulation 212
neuropeptides 267–8
neuropeptide Y 267–8
nifedipine 285
nitric oxide (NO) 237–41, 260–3, 373–5, 377–9, 396–7
  and the lungs 408–9
nitric oxide synthase 221–3, 237–48, 377–9
N^G-monomethy-L-arginine 239–44
N^G-nitro-L-arginine 239–44, 261–2
non-invasive high-frequency ultrasound 93–4

O-nitrobenzylester, see caged compounds
O-nitrophenylethylester, see caged compounds

parasympathetic nerve cotransmission 220–2
partial agonists 3
patch-clamp technique 50
peptide histidine isoleucine 220
perfusion systems 37–9
  constant flow in 38–9
  dead space in 37–8
perivascular nerve plasticity 223–5
pertussis toxin 114
pharmacology, of receptor principles 1–24
phasic contractile activity 279
phosphatidylcholine hydrolysis 163–5
phosphodiesterases, and muscle relaxation 175–6
phosphoinositide hydrolysis 160–2
phospholipid hydrolysis 160–9
plasticity 233–5
platelet activating factor (PAF) 375
platelet activation 336–7
platelet-derived growth factor (PDGF) 118
platelet products 344–6
platelets 344–6
plethysmography 98–9
potassium channels 122, 137–45, 150–4
  ATP-sensitive 122, 141
  calcium-activated 122, 139–40
  delayed rectifying 122
  extracellular calcium-sensitive 141

inward rectifying 201
sympathetic nerves and 200–1
voltage-gated 140
potency 5–6
prostaglandins 126, 318, 337, 375, 379
prostanoid receptors 126
prostanoids 407–8
  see also prostaglandins
protein kinase C 165–6
  isoforms 166
  in smooth muscle relaxation 169
  sustained contraction 167–9
pulmonary circulation 402–3, 406–12
  neural control of 406–7
  prostaglandins and 407–8
  vasoactive agents 407
pulmonary endothelium 407
pulmonary hypertension 402–30
  endothelium in 414–21
  histopathology of 413–14
  vasoconstriction in 404–5
pulmonary vasculature 404
pulmonary vasomotor regulation 405
  tone 405
pulmonary vessels, isolated 406–7
purinoceptors 194–7

radiolabelled agonists 105
receptor classification 14–21, 105–6
receptor concentration 4
receptor-gated channels 149–50
receptor interaction 1–5
receptor-linked ion channels 120
receptor-operated Ca^{2+} channels 121
receptor reserve 3
receptor transduction 103–22
regulation, of smooth muscle contraction, see contraction regulation
relaxation, of smooth muscle, and protein kinase C 169
  cyclic nucleotides in 173–6
    adenylyl cyclase 174–5
    phosphodiesterases 175–6
renal blood flow 306–8
  clearance and 306–8
  direct measurement 308
renal circulation 306–27
  α- and β-adrenoceptors and 311–12
  angiotensin and 314–15
  atrial natriuretic peptide and 316
  bradykinin and 315–16
  cholinergic receptors 312
  dopamine and 312–13
  eicosanoids and 318–19
  endothelins and 316–17
  endothelium-dependent relaxing factor 317–18
  histamine and 313

5-hydroxytryptamine and 313-15
  peptides and 318
  vasopressin and 315
renal microcirculation 308-11
  blood-perfused juxtamedullary nephron 310
  isolated arterioles 309-10
  videomicroscopy, medulla 310-11
renin-angiotensin system 396
resistance 75-6
  see also conductance
resistance arteries, see small arteries

salt, dietary 393-4
Schild plot 8-9, 14-17
second messenger system 106
sensory motor nerve cotransmission 219-20
sepsis 369-86
septic shock 379-81
single cell techniques 42-69
single-channel recording 53-4
single-exposure drug additions 13
small arteries 26-31
small coronary arteries 290-302
  acetylcholine and 291-9
  adrenoceptors and 301-2
  5-hydroxytryptamine 299-301
  vessel isolation 291
  vessel mounting 291
smooth muscle cell membrane receptors 123-6
smooth muscle cells 43-7
smooth muscle responses 103-5
smooth muscle tone 369-86
sodium ion channels 148-54
spontaneous excitatory junction potentials 196
substance P 219-20
α-subunit G proteins 113-14
βγ-subunit G proteins 114-16
sympathetic axons 185-8
sympathetic nerve cotransmission 212-18
sympathetic nerves, trophic effects of 200-1
sympathetic nervous system 255-7
sympathetic neurovascular junctions 189-92
sympatholytic activity 86-8

thermodilution technique 96
thrombosis 336-7
thromboxanes 126, 319, 336-7
tissue preparation 9-10
tissue response stability 12-13
tone, muscle 105

tonic contractile activity 279
tonometry 99
topical drug delivery 73
transduction 1-2, 116
transmembrane domain receptors 106-16
T-type Ca^{2+} channels, see calcium ion channels
tumour necrosis factor 370-1
tyrosine kinase-linked receptors 118-19
tyrosine kinase pathways 170
tyrosine phosphorylation 169-73

ultrasound 92-4

variable affinities 17
variable pharmacodynamics 17
variable properties of tissues 4
vascular cell isolation 43-7
vascular damage 379
vascular dysfunction 329-31
vascular growth regulation 349-51
vascular injury 344-6, 349-51
vascular neuroeffector junction 211-12
vascular reactivity 73-4, 342-4
  in vivo 94-5
vascular response, of smooth muscle 1-24
vascular smooth muscle contraction 160-83
vascular smooth muscle excitation-contraction coupling 136-59
vascular smooth muscle relaxation 160-83
  endothelium-dependent 234-7
vascular smooth muscle tone 103-5
vasoactive intestinal peptide (VIP) 220-2
vasodilatation, endothelium-dependent 233-51
vasodilators, endothelium-dependent 285-8
  nifedipine 285
vasopressin 125-6, 315
venous neuroeffector transmission 184-209
venous occlusion plethysmography 98-9
venous reactivity 94-5
vessel isolation techniques 291
vessel wall injury 341-56
voltage-clamp 47-50
voltage-gated K^+ channels 140, 150-4
voltage-gated Na^+ channels 148-9
voltage-operated Ca^{2+} channels 121

whole-cell recording techniques 50-3
wire-mounted preparations 29-37